The Wisdom of Menopause

ALSO BY CHRISTIANE NORTHRUP, M.D.

Women's Bodies, Women's Wisdom
Creating Physical and Emotional Health and Healing

Mother-Daughter Wisdom
Understanding the Crucial Link Between
Mothers, Daughters, and Health

The Wisdom of Menopause

Creating Physical and Emotional
Health and Healing During the Change

Christiane Northrup, M.D.

BANTAM BOOKS

Many of the stories that appear in this book are composites; individual names and identifying characteristics have been changed. Nevertheless, they reflect authentic situations in the lives of the thousands of perimenopausal women I've seen in my practice over the years. If you think you recognize yourself in these pages, the similarities are strictly coincidental unless I have received your specific written permission to use your story.

THE WISDOM OF MENOPAUSE
A Bantam Book

PUBLISHING HISTORY
Bantam hardcover edition published March 2001
Bantam trade paperback edition published January 2003
Bantam revised edition / November 2006

Some of the material in *The Wisdom of Menopause* was originally published in *Health Wisdom for Women*, Phillips Publishing International.

Published by Bantam Dell
A Division of Random House, Inc.
New York, New York

Author photo by Barbara Peacock
Jacket and cover design by Beverly Leung
Book design by Glen Edelstein

Library of Congress Cataloging-in-Publication Data
Northrup, Christiane.
The wisdom of menopause : creating physical and emotional health and
healing during the change / Christiane Northrup. — Rev. and updated.
p. cm.
Includes bibliographical references and index.
ISBN-13: 978-0-553-80489-8 (hc) 978-0553-38409-3 (tp)
ISBN-10: 0-553-80489-8 (hc) 978-0-553-38409-0 (tp)
1. Menopause. 2. Menopause—Psychological aspects.
3. Menopause—Religious aspects. I. Title.

RG186.N67 2006

618.1'75—dc22

2006021672

Printed in the United States of America
Published simultaneously in Canada

www.bantamdell.com

BVG   20 19 18 17 16 15 14

*This book is dedicated to the pioneering spirit
embodied in the women of the baby boom generation*

Contents

List of Figures

Acknowledgments

I would first like to acknowledge all those whose skills and insights helped me birth the first edition of this book during my own perimenopause back in the early 2000s, especially Mona Lisa Schulz, M.D., Ph.D., and Joel Hargrove, M.D.

For this updated version, I gratefully thank:

Irwyn Applebaum, president of Bantam Books, for years of support and insight.

Toni Burbank and Beth Rashbaum for masterful editing.

Ned Leavitt for being a soul-mate agent.

Barb Burg and Theresa Zorro for veteran publicity skills.

Nancy Etnier and Hope Matthews, my Pilates teachers, for helping me transform my midlife body.

Dixie Mills, M.D., for contributing your compassion and medical expertise concerning breast health.

Erika Schwartz, M.D., for your truth telling, friendship, and integrity-filled approach to menopause and hormone replacement.

Ray Strand, M.D., for having the courage and insight to put your clinical observations into such a useful format for helping people heal and reverse the effects of glycemic stress.

Fern Tsao and her daughter Maureen Manetti for your skill

with Traditional Chinese Medicine and for keeping my *chi* flowing freely.

My team at Hay House, Louise Hay, Reid Tracy, Ron Tillinghast, Margarete Nielsen, Donna Abate, and Nancy Levin, for helping me pleasurably produce my newsletter and PBS shows—and also orchestrating wonderful speaking engagements.

Judie Harvey for her newsletter and e-letter editing skills, and great sense of humor.

Deena Spear, my vibrational healer friend and colleague who helps keep me and my life finely tuned.

Katy Koontz for living out your scribe archetype with such skill, speed, and panache. You've been a godsend during this revision process.

Sue Abel for helping keep my home clean, restful, and beautiful and for taking such good care of my cats when I'm not here.

Mike Brewer for keeping my home and grounds maintained and lovely.

Abby Shattuck for your gardening skills and feeling for plants and the earth.

Chip Gray and the Gray family of the Harraseeket Inn in Freeport for providing delicious gourmet organic food in a beautiful setting. You have created an invaluable oasis of comfort, warmth, and nourishment that I treasure.

The staff of the Royal River Grillhouse in Yarmouth for uplifting and inspiring business lunches every day.

Paulina Carr for your cheerful willingness to do whatever needs to be done. And also your ability to stick with it until you get an answer.

Janet Lambert for your superior bookkeeping skills and general all-around great attitude.

Diane Grover for being the rock at the center of my business—keeping everything organized, clear, and fun. Much gratitude also for cheering me on in my personal life at all times and being an integral part of my family. You are a first-chakra genius for whom I am enormously grateful every day.

Charlie Grover, Diane's husband, whose good humor and willingness to provide backup are precious.

My sister, Penny Northrup Kirk, and her husband, Phil, for being such good friends and perfect business partners in Team Northrup.

My mother, Edna, for continuing to be an inspiration about what's possible in one's eighties. To my late father, George Wilbur, whose work was the inspiration for my approach to women's health. And to my brothers, John and Bill, and their wives, Annie and Lori. I cherish you all more than I can say.

Finally to my two twenty-something daughters, Annie and Katie. You two give me enormous faith in the future and I love you with all my heart.

Christiane Northrup, M.D.

The Wisdom of
Menopause

INTRODUCTION

The Journey Begins

I
n the year or two before I actually started to skip periods, I began
to experience an increasingly common feeling of irritability whenever my work was interrupted or I had to contend with a coworker or employee who was not as committed to accomplishing the
job as I was. Looking back, I recall that when I was in my thirties and
my children were younger, their interruptions when I was in the middle of writing an article or talking on the phone were only mildly
irritating to me. My love and concern for their welfare usually over-
rode any anger or frustration I might have felt.

But as I approached menopause, I found myself unable to tolerate distractions like my eighteen-year-old asking me, "When is dinner?" when she could clearly see I was busy. Why, I wondered, was it
always my responsibility to turn on the stove and begin to think
about my family's food needs, even when I wasn't hungry and was
deeply engrossed in a project? Why couldn't my husband get the dinner preparations started? Why did my family seem to be almost totally paralyzed when it came to preparing a meal? Why did they all
wait in the kitchen, as though unable to set the table or pour a glass
of water, until I came into the room and my mere presence announced, "Mom's here. Now we get to eat"?

The same thing occurred when it was time to get into the car and

1

take off on vacation. Only when I myself made a definitive move toward the door did my family mobilize. It felt as though my presence caused them to lose their own personal initiative to take charge of a situation, be it dinner or a family trip. Still, during my childbearing years I accepted this, mostly good-naturedly, as part and parcel of my role as wife and mother. And in so doing, I unwittingly perpetuated it, partly because it felt so good to be indispensable.

During perimenopause, I lost patience with this behavior on all levels, whether at home or at work. I could feel a fiery volcano within me, ready to burst, and a voice within me roaring, "Enough! You're all able-bodied, capable individuals. Everyone here knows how to drive a car and boil water. Why is my energy still the organizing principle around here?" My indignation grew as I mumbled to myself, "If I were a man in the prime of life and at the pinnacle of his career, I wouldn't be interrupted like this. Everyone would be wondering how to help me, instead of the other way around!"

Little did I know that these little bursts of irritability over petty family dynamics were the first faint knocks on the door marked Menopausal Wisdom, signaling that I needed to renegotiate some of my habitual relationship patterns. Nor did I know that by the time I began to actually skip periods and experience hot flashes, my life as I had known it for the previous quarter century would be on the threshold of total transformation. As my cyclic nature rewired itself, I put all my significant relationships under a microscope, began to heal the unfinished business from my past, experienced the first pangs of the empty nest, and established an entirely new and exciting relationship with my creativity and vocation.

All of the changes I was about to undergo were spurred, supported, and encouraged by the complex and intricate brain and body changes that are an unheralded—but inevitable and often overwhelming—part of the menopausal transition. There is much, much more to this midlife transformation than "raging hormones." Research into the physiological changes taking place in the perimenopausal woman is revealing that, in addition to the hormonal shift that means an end to childbearing, our bodies—and, specifically, our nervous systems—are being, quite literally, rewired. It's as simple as this: our brains are changing. A woman's thoughts, her ability to focus, and the amount of fuel going to the intuitive centers in the temporal lobes of her brain all are plugged into, and affected by, the circuits being rewired. After working with thousands of women who have gone through this process, as well as experiencing it myself, I can say with great assurance that menopause is an exciting developmental stage—one that, when participated in consciously, holds enormous promise for transforming and healing our bodies, minds, and spirits at the deepest levels.

As a woman in midlife today, I am part of a growing population that is an unprecedented 45.6 million strong in the United States alone. This group is no longer invisible and silent, but a force to be reckoned with—educated, vocal, sophisticated in our knowledge of medical science, and determined to take control of our own health. Think about it: more than 45 million women, all undergoing the same sort of circuitry update at the same time. By virtue of our sheer numbers, as well as our social and economic influence, we are powerful—and potentially dangerous to any institution built upon the status quo. It's a safe bet the world is going to change, willingly or otherwise, right along with us. And it's likely to change for the better.

It's no accident that the current movement of psychospiritual healing is composed largely of women in their thirties, forties, fifties, and early sixties. We are awakening en masse and beginning to deliver a much-needed message of health, hope, and healing to the world.

My personal experience tells me that the perimenopausal lifting of the hormonal veil—the monthly cycle of reproductive hormones that tends to keep us focused on the needs and feelings of others—can be both liberating and unsettling. The midlife rate of marital separation, divorce, and vocational change confirms this. I, for one, had always envisioned myself married to the same man for life, the two of us growing old together. This ideal had always been one of my most cherished dreams. At midlife I, like thousands of others, had to give up my fantasies of how I thought my life would be. I had to face, head-on, the old adage about how hard it is to lose what you never really had. It means giving up all your illusions, and it is very difficult. But for me the issue was larger than where, and with whom, I would grow old. It was a warning, coming from deep within my spirit, that said, "Grow . . . or die." Those were my choices. I chose to grow.

MIDLIFE: REDEFINING CREATIVITY AND HOME

For most women, identity and self-esteem are generated by our associations and relationships. This is true even for women who hold high-powered jobs and for women who have chosen not to marry. Men, by contrast, usually get most of their identity and self-esteem from the outer world—the job, the income, the accomplishments, the accolades. For both genders, this pattern may change at midlife.

Women often begin to direct more of their energies toward the world outside of home and family, which may suddenly appear as a great, inviting, untapped resource for exploration, creative expression, and self-esteem. Meanwhile, men of the same age—who may be undergoing a midlife crisis of their own—are often feeling world-weary; they're ready to retire, curl up, and escape the battles of the workplace. They may feel their priorities shifting inward, toward home, hearth, and family.

It's an ironic transposition: the man is beginning to look to relationships for his "juice"; the woman is feeling biologically primed to explore the outer world. In married couples, this often produces profound role shifts. In the best of all worlds, the man retires or cuts back on work, becoming the chief cook and bottle washer at home, and providing emotional and practical support for his wife's new interests. She, in turn, goes out into the world to start a business, get an education, or do whatever her heart dictates. If their relationship is adaptable and resilient, they adjust to their new roles. If not, he may become jealous of her success and independence, and put pressure on her to continue to care for him as she has always done. He may even get physically sick, often in the form of heart disease and/or clinically dangerous high blood pressure. It's important to note that this is not a willful act; he's simply responding to the promptings of our lopsided culture.

A woman often finds herself in the difficult position, then, of having to choose between returning to the role of caretaker to nurture her husband at the expense of her own needs and pursuing her own creative passions. It's an old story, common to women in many cultures, not just our own. The woman in menopause, who is becoming the queen of herself, finds herself at a crossroads of life, torn between the old way she has always known and a new way she has just begun to dream of. A voice from the old way (in many cases it's her husband's voice) begs her to stay in place—"Grow old with me, the best is yet to be." But from the new path another voice beckons, imploring her to explore aspects of herself that have been dormant during her years of caring for, and focusing on, the needs of others. She's preparing to give birth to herself, and as many women already know, the birth process cannot be halted without consequences.

Caring for others and pursuing unexplored personal passions are not necessarily mutually exclusive choices, but our culture makes them seem so, always supporting the former at the expense of the latter. This is part of what makes the midlife transformation so much of a challenge—as I know only too well.

WHY I'M WRITING A MENOPAUSE BOOK NOW

Though I have worked closely with menopausal women for over twenty years, I vowed that I wouldn't write a book on this subject until I entered the process myself. I knew that I would learn something through the direct experience of this transition that I couldn't possibly learn any other way. My personal approach to pregnancy and birth, for example, was completely transformed and deepened when I had my two daughters. The same has been true for the menopausal transition and its attendant challenges.

For some people, it's surprising to hear a doctor revealing anything of her personal life. But I've always been comfortable with the idea that what I have to offer as a woman, wife, and mother is every bit as valuable as what I have to offer as a trained medical professional—that they are equally valid as teaching tools, and that one can augment the other. In fact, I find the idea of dividing myself into a work persona and a home persona unimaginable. It's dishonest, and it creates a barrier to full communication on both fronts. This is why, throughout my professional career as a clinician, surgeon, and teacher of women's health issues, I've approached my patients and students from the fullness of who I am, in all my roles. And because this sharing has resulted in such an outpouring of warmth and acceptance from my patients and readers, I have once again found the courage to share some of my experiences in this book.

The culture in general, and the medical profession in particular, admonishes doctors to keep our personal stories to ourselves, especially when they involve difficult emotions like fear or anger—allegedly because to appear too human would undermine our authority. Yet I've found over the years that nothing illustrates a point quite as effectively or helpfully as an honest personal story. Telling the truth of my own humanness and vulnerability is also helpful to me. This is, after all, one of the reasons why twelve-step programs work so well to help people recover from the grip of addiction and denial. Honest stories help awaken the healer within us. By sharing both the joy and the pain of my own transition, I hope that I can help to illustrate and also demystify the surges of creative energy that erupt in so many of us at midlife. I also bring many personal stories from my patients and my newsletter subscribers, whose experiences reveal how the emotional shifts that occur at menopause, which may at first feel uncomfortable or even frightening, ultimately help us do the work (and play) that await us on our journey.

The dilemma for me and women everywhere is that we often feel guilty about self-revelation, because by being true to ourselves and our own feelings, we feel that we are betraying others, especially family members. I assure you that I have shared the stories printed here with my family. For all other stories, I have sought the explicit permission of those concerned, except where so much detail has been changed that the subject cannot be identified.

BLAZING A NEW TRAIL

Throughout most of human history, the vast majority of women died before menopause. The average life expectancy for a woman in 1900 was only forty. For those who survived, menopause was experienced as a signpost of an imminent and inevitable physical decline. But today, with a woman's life expectancy at eighty-four years, it is reasonable to expect that she will not only live thirty to forty years beyond menopause, but be vibrant, sharp, and influential as well. The menopause you will experience is not your mother's (or grandmother's) menopause.

Women of the World War II generation, whose female role models tended to be like June Cleaver on *Leave It to Beaver,* had an entirely different social and political environment in which to make their transition. Menopause (like menstruation, for that matter) was not discussed in public. Today this is no longer true. As we break this silence we are also breaking cultural barriers, so that we can enter this new life phase with eyes wide open—in the company of more than 45 million kinswomen, all undergoing the same transformation at the same time. And, as you'll soon discover, the changes taking place in middle-aged women are going to act like the power plant on a high-speed train, whisking the evolution of our entire society along on fast-forward, to places that have yet to be mapped. Whether you climb aboard this fast-moving train or step aside and let it pass will play a major role in how far you go and how you feel along the way.

Ultimately, I've found this journey bracing, exciting, and health-enhancing. And I'm certainly not alone. A 1998 Gallup survey, presented at the annual meeting of the North American Menopause Society, showed that more than half of American women between the ages of fifty and sixty-five felt happiest and most fulfilled at this stage of life. Compared to when they were in their twenties, thirties, and forties, they felt their lives had improved in many ways, including family life, interests, friendships, and their relationship with their spouse or partner. In other words, the conventional view of menopause as a scary transition heralding "the beginning of the end" couldn't be further from the truth. So please join me—and the millions of others who have come before and will come after—as we transform and improve our lives, and ultimately our culture, through understanding, applying, and living the wisdom of menopause.

1

Menopause Puts Your Life
Under a Microscope

It is no secret that relationship crises are a common side effect of menopause. Usually this is attributed to the crazy-making effects of the hormonal shifts occurring in a woman's body at this time of transition. What is rarely acknowledged or understood is that as these hormone-driven changes affect the brain, they give a woman a sharper eye for inequity and injustice, and a voice that insists on speaking up about them. In other words, they give her a kind of wisdom—and the courage to voice it. As the vision-obscuring veil created by the hormones of reproduction begins to lift, a woman's youthful fire and spirit are often rekindled, together with long-sublimated desires and creative drives. Midlife fuels those drives with a volcanic energy that demands an outlet.

If it does not find an outlet—if the woman remains silent for the sake of keeping the peace at home and/or work, or if she holds herself back from pursuing her creative urges and desires—the result is equivalent to plugging the vent on a pressure cooker: something has to give. Very often what gives is the woman's health, and the result will be one or more of the "big three" diseases of postmenopausal women: heart disease, depression, and breast cancer. On the other hand, for those of us who choose to honor the body's wisdom and to express what lies within us, it's a good idea to get ready for some boat rocking, which may put long-established relationships in upheaval. Marriage is not immune to this effect.

"NOT ME, MY MARRIAGE IS FINE"

Every marriage, even a very good one, must undergo change in order to keep up with the hormone-driven rewiring of a woman's brain during the years leading up to and including menopause. Not all marriages are able to survive these changes. Mine wasn't, and nobody was more surprised about that than I. If this makes you want to hide your head in the sand, believe me, I do understand. But for the sake of being true to yourself and protecting your emotional and physical health in the second half of your life—likely a full forty years or more—then I submit to you that forging ahead and taking a good hard look at all aspects of your relationship (including some previously untouchable corners of your marriage) may be the only choice that will work in your best interest in the long run, physically, emotionally, and spiritually.

From the standpoint of physical health, for example, there is plenty of evidence to suggest that the increase in life-threatening illnesses after midlife, which cannot be accounted for by aging alone, is partly rooted in the stresses and unresolved relationship problems that simmered beneath the surface during the childbearing years of a woman's life, then bubbled up and boiled over at perimenopause, only to be damped down in the name of maintaining the status quo. The health of your significant other is also at stake. Remaining in a relationship that was tailor-made for a couple of twenty-somethings without making the necessary adjustments for who you both have become at midlife can be just as big a health risk for him as it is for you.

This is not to say that your only options are divorce or heart attack. Rather, in order to bring your relationship into alignment with your rewired brain, you and your significant other must be willing to take the time, and spend the energy, to resolve old issues and set new ground rules for the years that lie ahead. If you can do this, then your relationship will help you to thrive in the second half of your life. If one or both of you cannot or will not, then both health and happiness may be at risk if you stay together.

Preparing for Transformation

At midlife, more psychic energy becomes available to us than at any time since adolescence. If we strive to work in active partnership with that organic energy, trusting it to help us uncover the unconscious and self-destructive beliefs about ourselves that have held us back from what we could become, then we will find that we have access to everything we need to reinvent ourselves as healthier, more resilient women, ready to move joyfully into the second half of our lives.

This process of transformation can only succeed, however, if we become proactive in two ways. First, we must be willing to take full responsibility for our share of the problems in our lives. It takes great courage to admit our own contributions to the things that have gone wrong for us and to stop seeing ourselves simply as victims of someone or something outside of ourselves. After all, the person in the victim role tends to get all the sympathy and to assume the high road morally, which is appealing; none of us wants to feel like the bad guy. But even though taking the victim role may seem a good choice in the short run, this stance is ultimately devoid of any power to help us change, heal, grow, and move on to a more fulfilling and joyful life.

The second requirement for transformation is more difficult by far: we must be willing to feel the pain of loss and grieve for those parts of our lives that we are leaving behind. And that includes our fantasies of how our lives could have been different *if only*. Facing up to such loss is rarely easy, and that is why so many of us resist change in general and at midlife in particular. A part of us rationalizes, "Why rock the boat? I'm halfway finished with my life. Wouldn't it just be easier to accept what I have rather than risk the unknown?"

The end of any significant relationship, or any major phase of our lives, even one that has made us unhappy or held us back from our full growth and fulfillment, feels like a death—pure and simple. To move past it, we have to feel the sadness of that loss and grieve fully for what might have been and now will never be.

And then we must pick ourselves up and move toward the unknown. All our deepest fears are likely to surface as we find ourselves facing the uncertainty of the future. During my own perimenopausal life changes, I would learn this in spades—much to my surprise.

By the time I was approaching menopause, I had worked with scores of women who had gone through midlife "cleansings"; I had guided and counseled them as their children left home, their parents got sick, their marriages ended, their husbands fell ill or died, they themselves became ill, their jobs ended—in short, as they went through all the storms and crises of midlife. But I never thought I would face a crisis in *my* marriage. I had always felt somewhat smug, secure in my belief that I was married to the man of my dreams, the one with whom I would stay "till death do us part."

Delirious Happiness and Shaking Knees

I will always remember the happiness of meeting and marrying my husband, a decision we made merely three months after we met. He was my surgical intern when I was a medical student at Dartmouth. He looked like a Greek god, and I was deeply flattered by his attention, especially since I wasn't at all sure I had what it took to attract such a handsome man with such an Ivy League, country-club background. Something deep within me was moved by him beyond all reason, beyond anything I'd ever felt before with any other boyfriend. For the first five years of our marriage my knees shook whenever I saw him. There wasn't a force on this planet that could have talked me out of marrying him. I remember wanting to shout my love from the tops of tall buildings—an exuberance of feeling that was very uncharacteristic of the quiet, studious valedictorian of the Ellicottville Central School class of 1967.

He, however, was considerably less eager to display his feelings. I couldn't help but notice during the years we were both immersed in our surgical training that my husband seemed uncomfortable relating to me when we were at work, and often appeared cold and distant when I'd try to show affection in that setting. This puzzled and hurt me, since I was always proud to introduce him to my patients when we happened to see each other outside of the operating room. But I told myself that this was because of the way he had been raised, and that with enough love and attention from me, he would become more responsive, more emotionally available.

THE CHILDBEARING YEARS: BALANCING PERSONAL AND PROFESSIONAL LIVES

My husband's life didn't change much when we had our two daughters. Mine, however, became a struggle—one that millions of women will recognize from their own experience—as I tried to find satisfying and effective ways to mother my children, remain the doctor I wanted to be, and at the same time be a good wife to my husband. Nonetheless, these were happy years, for both of us adored our daughters from the beginning and enjoyed the many activities we shared with them—the weekend walks, the family vacations, the simple daily contact with two beautiful, developing young beings.

I did sometimes resent the disparity between what I contributed to the upkeep of our family life and what my husband did. Once, when the children were still young, I asked him if he'd consider working fewer hours so that I wouldn't have to give up delivering babies, an aspect of my practice that I dearly loved. He replied, "You've never seen a part-time orthopedic surgeon, have you?" I admitted that I hadn't, but suggested that this didn't mean it couldn't happen with a little imagination on his part. It was not to be, however. It was I who, like so many other women, became the master shape-shifter, adjusting my own needs to those of everyone else in the family.

In the early years of our family life, I was also becoming increasingly aware that the inequities that bothered me in my marriage were a reflection of inequities that existed in the culture around us. I saw many people like my husband and me—people who had started their marriages on equal grounds financially and educationally, even people who, like us, did the same work—and always, once the children arrived, it was the wife who made the sacrifices in leisure time, professional accomplishment, and personal fulfillment.

Change Yourself, Change the World

During those often exhausting years, I began to put into action some of the ideas I'd been developing about women's health—while always being careful not to say much about those ideas at home, where I knew they would not be welcomed by my husband. Inspired by my own experiences as well as those of my patients, and buoyed by the conviction that my ideas could make a difference in people's lives, in 1985 I joined three other women in the venture of establishing a health care center we called Women to Women. The idea of a health center run by women for women was virtually unheard of at that time. Our central mission was to help women appreciate the unity of mind, body, and spirit, to enable them to see the connection between their emotional health and their physical well-being. I wanted to empower women, to give them a safe place in which to tell their personal stories so that they could discover new, more health-enhancing ways of living their lives.

I knew that sometimes this would involve challenging the status quo, because the inequities of the culture take a terrible toll on women's bodies as well as their spirits. But as I practiced this new, holistic form of medicine, which was quite revolutionary for its day, I realized that the fact that I had a normal, happy family life, as well as a husband with conventional medical ideas who practiced in the same community, provided a kind of cover for me. It made me appear "safe" at a time when my ideas were considered unproven at best, dangerous at worst.

My three partners in Women to Women and I bought an old Victorian house that we could convert into a center for our new practice. We all agreed that we wanted to keep our husbands out of our new venture, lest their participation undermine our enthusiastic but still tender confidence in ourselves as businesswomen.

Of course, in my case, at least, that didn't necessarily mean that I didn't want my husband's support. I clearly remember a day at the beginning of the building and site renovation. Two bulldozers sat on the lawn, workers were everywhere, and the existing building had been torn apart. At that moment the whole project suddenly became real for me, and I realized that my colleagues and I were now responsible for paying for all of this. This was an overwhelming thought. When I came home that evening, I uncharacteristically reached out to my husband for help in calming my fears. "I'm scared," I told him. "I'm not sure I can do this." He replied, "I hate it when you're disempowered like this." I quickly realized that I'd been foolish to expect anything from him.

His response to my uncharacteristic and risky moment of emotional vulnerability simply reinforced the coping style I'd developed in childhood, a stoicism that was a necessity in a household where emotional neediness was frowned upon and we were told to "keep a stiff upper lip." Another favorite saying in my family was "Don't ask for a lighter pack, ask for a stronger back." So, as usual, I pulled myself up by my own bootstraps, dug into my inner resources, and pretended that I wasn't afraid.

As it turned out, Women to Women became a great success. Our work struck a resonant chord with our patients, and the center grew steadily by word of mouth. As excited as I was about what I was doing, I could never interest my husband in any of the ideas about alternative medicine that were at the core of my new clinical practice. We did, however, have enough other areas of mutual interest that I didn't think his attitude toward my work mattered. In fact, I was rather proud of myself for being able to sustain a loving relationship with a card-carrying member of the American Medical Association.

Marrying My Mother

Looking back, I see that in marrying my husband I had made a secret and mostly unconscious vow that I would do whatever it took to make this marriage work and be the woman I thought he wanted—as long as I could also pursue the work that I loved. (Back then, like most women, I didn't know that the secret to happiness for both ourselves and our loved ones requires that we first and foremost become who we really are—not who we think we should be!) Unbeknownst to me, I was re-creating with my husband many aspects of the unfinished business I had carried over from my relationship with my mother, a fact that would only begin to dawn on me some twenty-two years later, as I entered perimenopause.

Until then, in my marriage I would continue to play the role of the eager-to-please child I had once been, while my husband would fill the role of my remote, emotionally unavailable mother. As the quiet, sensitive child in a family of outgoing, athletic siblings who loved to spend every moment of life charging full speed ahead up mountains and down ski slopes, I had always been the type who tended to disappear, going off by myself into a quiet room where I could listen to music, read fairy tales, sit dreamily by a fire, or gaze out onto the ocean. Much more tuned in to the other members of our large, bustling family, my mother always seemed too busy to notice me. And although my father supported my studious side, he, like most men of his era, left the hands-on parenting to my mother.

Longing for my mother's approval, I tried to win her love by being good. So I worked and studied hard, never got into trouble, and made myself into my mother's little helper, cooking, cleaning, creating centerpieces for holiday dinners—whatever I could think of that would prove my worth. Intuiting that my mother was in some pain—though it would be many years before I understood the nature of that pain—I tried to be a comfort as well as a help to her, just as I would later try in my marriage to heal my husband's childhood wounds, to give him enough love to make it possible to overcome his early fears and hurts.

Meanwhile, I looked to my teachers for the applause I couldn't get at home. My search for acknowledgment made me a classic overachiever at school, a pattern that would continue all the way through medical school and into my marriage.

Eventually, just as I had turned to my schoolteachers for the support and approval I didn't get at home, I would one day turn to people other than my husband to meet my emotional needs. But until I began the process of self-knowledge that culminated in the dismantling of my marriage, I simply accepted the fact that, like my mother, my husband could not really see or appreciate me for who I was. In fact, I never expected him to. I was operating under the assumption that I was fundamentally unworthy of being cherished by such a special person.

Had I felt more worthy of love, I never would have chosen someone like my husband. Several of the boyfriends I was involved with before I met him did admire and value me. But when your working belief about yourself is that you have to earn love—earn it both by overachieving in your own life and by rescuing someone from the pain of their own—then you will attract a person who reflects those beliefs back to you. Inevitably the young men who were supportive of me were not the ones I wanted. I wanted precisely the kind of emotional unavailability that felt most like home to me—and I got it.

In this way my husband was a true soul mate, and I do not blame him for what happened between us. It was only when I was able to change my soul—to change from the inside out, in the most fundamental of ways—that we ceased to be life partners. In retrospect, he was one of the biggest gifts of my life!

After my divorce, I found myself face-to-face with my unfinished business with my mother—a very common theme—and eventually worked through that. (See my book *Mother-Daughter Wisdom* [Bantam Books, 2005] for all the details.)

WHY MARRIAGES MUST CHANGE AT MIDLIFE

When we look at the typical dynamics of intimate family relationships in this culture, it's reasonably safe to say that the vast majority of the nurturing, supportive, subordinate roles fall to the women, as does most of the self-sacrifice. Yes, it has become somewhat more common for women to achieve high-ranking positions in corporate, political, and scientific arenas. But whenever career concessions must be made for the sake of the family, it's still likely to be the woman who steps down or cuts back; that's why we have the term "mommy track."

It's true that a woman's biology tends to encourage her involvement with her family at the expense of other interests during the childbearing phase of her life. But it's also true that the culture's atmosphere of gender inequity exploits this tendency to an extreme. This can lead to an incredible surge of pent-up resentment when the hormonal veil lifts and a woman suddenly sees with clarity what has happened in her life.

The emotional changes that come about in the years leading up to and during menopause can feel earthshaking and even terrifying, particularly for those of us who are accustomed to thinking we're in control. It's one thing to resist change from some external force. It's quite another when the change is coming from within, and everything you cling to that's comfortable in its familiarity, including your very identity, is metamorphosing from the inside out. There are only two ways to avoid this abrupt, jolting level of change: defy social and cultural dictates throughout your childbearing years, so that by the time you approach menopause you will already have put into effect many of the changes that cry out to be made at midlife, *or* defy your body's wisdom at perimenopause and ignore its call for truth, creative expression, and personal fulfillment. The latter course can have disastrous consequences for your own health as well as the health of your significant other, not to mention your relationship, which would then be based on something other than mutual respect and love. And you'd never find the treasure that perimenopause is desperately trying to bring to your attention—a life based on true freedom and joy!

How Your Brain Is Hardwired for Relationships

Nothing in our lives can affect us more profoundly, both physically and emotionally, than our relationships with others. The neural pathways that enable us—that actually compel us—to relate to other human beings are laid down in our brains in early childhood. The experiences we have at this critical stage will influence the circuitry that develops and stays with us for life. If, for example, our needs as infants are met by a loving caretaker who responds to our cries by feeding or changing or stroking or rocking us when we are hungry or cold or wet or scared, then we will feel good about ourselves, and trusting of the outside world. Our needs have been validated, our emotional cravings met, with our relationship with another human being serving as confirmation of our worthiness. And certainly the biochemistry of motherhood supports this outcome. The hormones associated with birth and nursing in a happy, healthy, well-supported mother predispose her to fall in love with her baby and to fill the child with a sense of being loved and accepted unconditionally.

Sometimes, however, our parents did not themselves experience this kind of unconditional love and may therefore be unable to give it to us. Then our cries may go unheeded or, worse, meet with active disapproval or resentment, and we will feel that the universe is not a safe place. Our relationships with others will seem undependable, even threatening.

The feelings we develop about ourselves and others as children become etched into the circuitry of our brains and bodies, where they will continue, albeit subconsciously, to affect our relationship choices and responses throughout life. They are part of our basic emotional portfolio, easily accessible and freely expressible, sometimes excessively so. On the other hand, those feelings that were not reinforced by early experience tend to wither away, to become unavailable to us until we make a conscious effort to access our innate power to change our circuitry!

Your ability to live successfully, however you might define success, depends to a great degree on how you relate to other people. If that part of your life is unsatisfactory, the only way you can revise the old relational circuits that determine your current relationships is to expose them and update them. Once you have a better understanding of the environment in which you were born and raised, it becomes possible—though never easy—to change some of the choices you usually make automatically, as a consequence of that old wiring.

But change can occur only when you understand how important it is to change. You must ask yourself why you feel the emotions you feel, choose the mates you choose, act the way you act. The answer is in those early life experiences that served as the architects of your neural circuits and live on today in your very cells.

During and after adolescence we almost invariably find ourselves attracted to mates who enable us to revisit and perhaps heal the unfinished emotional business of childhood. In our culture, romantic love is where we express our deepest longings. Thus each romantic relationship we enter into can serve as a microscope into our emotional circuitry. More than any other aspect of our lives, our intimate relationships bring to light the old wounds still begging for closure. And most women have been taught to put their needs last in relationships because we feel unworthy. Therefore we don't even know what we want until we give ourselves permission to remember!

In retrospect, I can see that this was true of my feelings toward the man who became my husband. I was acting out with him a family drama that was still ongoing for me. And although I can't speak on his behalf, in all likelihood I served a similar purpose for him. It took the hormonal and developmental changes of the climacteric to help me see that the role I played in my marriage was based on old beliefs about myself and my worth, beliefs that no longer served me well and were no longer valid.

Menopause to the Rescue

It may not feel like a rescue at the time, but the clarity of vision and increasing intolerance for injustice, inequity, and lack of fulfillment that accompany the perimenopausal changes are a gift. Our hormones are giving us an opportunity to see, once and for all, what we need to change in order to live honestly, fully, joyfully, and healthfully in the second half of our lives. This is the time when many women stop doing what I call "stuffing"—stifling their own needs in order to tend to everybody else's. Our culture expects women to put others first, and all during the childbearing years most of us do, no matter the cost to ourselves. But at midlife we get the chance to make changes, to create lives that fit who *we* are—or, more accurately, who we have become.

If, however, a woman cannot face the changes she needs to make in her life, her body may find a way to point them out to her, lit up in neon and impossible to ignore. It is at this stage that many women reach a crisis in the form of some kind of physical problem, a life-altering or even sometimes life-threatening illness.

One very common physical problem in the years leading up to menopause, for example, is fibroid tumors in the uterus. Forty percent of all perimenopausal women in our culture are diagnosed with one or more fibroid tumors, and many of them will undergo midlife hysterectomies to deal with the problem. In conventional medicine, we doctors are content to explain that the reason fibroids occur so frequently in women in their forties is because of changing hormone levels, with too much estrogen being produced compared to progesterone.

Though this is true as far as it goes, it is not the whole truth. I know this both personally and professionally, through the experience I had with a fibroid tumor that was first diagnosed when I was forty-one. Bodily symptoms are not just physical in nature; often they contain a message for us about our lives—if only we can learn to decipher it. Sometimes, as happened with me, the message becomes clear only in stages, with its full meaning available only in retrospect. But what I learned firsthand over the course of the eight years during which I was processing the experience of my fibroid is that we attract precisely the illness or problem that best facilitates our access to our inner wisdom—a phenomenon that is both awe-inspiring and sometimes terrifying. Though this is true throughout our lives, it hits us harder and more directly during perimenopause and menopause, as though nature is trying to awaken us one last time before we leave our reproductive years, the era when our inner wisdom, mediated in part by our hormones, is loudest and most intense.

I had a fibroid as my wake-up call. Another woman might have had a flare-up of migraine headaches, or PMS, or breast symptoms, or any of the several other conditions so common at perimenopause. Your body's message to you will be in the language that best breaks through your particular barriers and speaks most specifically to the issues you need to change in your life. The wisdom of this system is very precise.

MY PERSONAL FIBROID STORY:
THE FINAL CHAPTER

My fibroid was initially diagnosed in 1991, several years before my first book, *Women's Bodies, Women's Wisdom*, was published. By then I had been working on the book for over three long years, and for a while there it felt literally like a stuck creation. In my darkest moments I sometimes doubted that the book would ever be published. I assumed at the time that my fibroid was related to my frustration at how long it was taking me to finish the book and get it out into the world. Fibroids can often represent blocked creativity, or creativity that hasn't been birthed yet, usually because it is being funneled into dead-end relationships, jobs, or projects. (Blocked creative energy can also express itself in other locations, such as the ovaries, fallopian tubes, lower intestines, lower back, bladder, and hips, as well as the uterus—all of which are part of the second female energy center, or what Eastern medical practitioners call the second-chakra area.)

When *Women's Bodies, Women's Wisdom* was finally published, it was well received, much to my surprise. I had secretly feared that I'd be vilified by my beloved profession for writing the truth as I saw it about the profound connection between women's lives and their health. Though the book wasn't exactly embraced with open arms by my fellow OB/GYNs, it wasn't rejected, either. And the women for whom I had written it received it with great enthusiasm.

I was happy and relieved about the response I got, and my fibroid remained quiescent. It didn't go away, but it didn't get much larger, either. It remained as a kind of semidormant whisper from my inner wisdom. I knew the fact that it was there was not a fluke. It meant something. So I vowed to remain open to its message.

Over the next few years I continued to heed my inner voice—as far as I was able to understand it. I tried to change relationships that weren't working for me, I found new ones that were more reciprocal, more of a partnership, and I tried to follow my creative instincts wherever they led me. Thus, after more than a decade of what had been deeply fulfilling work with my colleagues at Women to Women, I found that my heart was increasingly drawn to writing and teaching. Because I was eager for my message to reach a larger audience than ever before, I began to reduce my involvement in the center.

I gave up my surgical practice and gradually, ever so gradually, cut back on direct patient care, too. Though I was very excited by the new direction my life was taking, I was conflicted about losing this close connection with my patients. I loved having a regular practice in which I saw the same women year after year, helping them in times of illness, celebrating with them as they learned the skills of creating health. But the pile of charts requiring my attention at the end of each day was increasingly giving me a knot in my stomach.

Meanwhile, the monthly newsletter that I had started in 1994 was doing well, and I was spending a great deal of time researching and writing it each month. I also began traveling around the country teaching and lecturing. All during this time of change I was trying to understand what my fibroid was trying to teach me—especially when, after having been stable for almost four years, it began to grow larger, until finally it was the size of a soccer ball. Although I didn't feel that my life was acutely out of balance in any way, I was aware that the various changes I was making were accompanied by a lot of guilt, and that guilt about doing something we love is always a clue that points to blocked energy. But since I was feeling so fulfilled in my work life (despite feeling guilty that I was having too much fun), I did not understand what the blockage could be.

On Thanksgiving Day of 1996, while trying to find something to wear for dinner that would conceal the now visible swelling in my belly, I finally realized that I was tired of trying to dress around my fibroid, tired of the discomfort it caused me whenever I lay down on my abdomen. I decided that it was time to give up my attempts to shrink it through visualization, homeopathy, diet, and acupuncture. I was ready to ask for help and have my fibroid surgically removed.

After scheduling the surgery, I started to take a GnRH agonist, a medication that decreases estrogen levels and therefore shrinks fibroids. This creates an artificial menopause, with many of the same side effects experienced by women in real menopause, such as memory change, hot flashes, and bone loss. Nonetheless, I decided that the benefits I would get from shrinking the tumor—the smaller the tumor, the smaller the incision, and the lower the risk of excessive blood loss—were worth the inconvenience, especially since I was only going to be taking the drug for two months.

Little did I know that the benefits would extend far beyond the shrinking of the tumor. Looking back on this period now, I see that the two months of artificial menopause brought on by the drug jump-started the changes in my brain—and my life—that set the stage for a complete cleansing and reorganization of some of my closest relationships, including, ultimately, my marriage.

Fired Up and Having My Say

One evening, a couple of weeks after I started taking the GnRH agonist, all of the family, including our household manager and former nanny, whom I shall refer to as Lida, was gathered before the television set watching an episode of *ER*. At the end, one of the nurses was telling a visitor that he should come in and talk to his friend, a man who had been so badly burned that he was near death. Observing that the nurse was not telling the visitor the truth about how serious his friend's condition was, Lida said to me, "Do they teach you to be like that in your medical training?" "Be like what?" I asked her. "Do they teach you to withhold the whole truth when the situation is very dire?" she clarified. After thinking about her question for a minute, I replied that there was indeed an unspoken belief among our teachers in medical school that patients (and family and friends) were not really able to handle the truth, and that this belief resulted in many things being left unsaid—a fact that was beautifully illustrated in what we had seen on television.

My husband stood just then, drawing himself up to his full, quite impressive height, and proclaimed, "Of course they don't teach you that. I don't know what you're talking about!" Something within me snapped. After years and years of down-regulating my personal truth to make myself acceptable to my husband and to every authority figure like him in medical school, I simply couldn't keep still another moment. I told him that I felt that I—and everybody else—had been socialized in a thousand nonverbal ways to talk with my patients in a certain way, and that this way left out a lot of the truth of their experience and mine. Of course there was no Don't Talk to Patients 101 course, I said, but I'd learned by example that a hand on the doorknob, the sight of a doctor racing from bed to bed on rounds, conveyed a world of information to patients about what they could and couldn't expect in the way of communication and contact with their physician.

As the conversation heated up, my husband and I retired to the bedroom to spare the others our anger. And for the next forty minutes I felt myself grow taller and taller with my own truth. I told my husband what I believed—about medical practice, about our relationship, about the inequity in the way we'd been living all these years—and I offered no excuses for what I said, nor any attempt to make it easier to hear. This was one of those amazing volcanic eruptions that occur from time to time when the lid finally blows on the container overstuffed with things we know but can't talk about because we are female and have been taught that in order to survive, we must keep quiet so that authorities (mostly men) will like us. Everything we've tried to ignore and struggled to keep beneath the surface bursts forth in all its unedited glory. At the end, my husband did not look as tall as he had at the beginning, and he was speaking softly and apologizing to me. That was the turning point in our marriage. There was no going back.

What had happened in that moment when I suddenly opted to speak out instead of remaining silent was a direct result of my artificial menopause. Usually menopause comes on gradually, of course. But when it happens more or less instantly because of medication, as it did for me, or because of surgery or radiation, as it does for other women, the sudden hormonal changes can result in insights about our lives that are as dramatic and unexpected as the hot flashes that often plague us at this time. Though my own premature menopause was not permanent and the hot flashes ended as soon as I stopped taking the medication that caused them, the inner change brought about by that brief menopausal interlude *was* permanent. It brought to the surface all the hidden conflicts in myself and my marriage.

FEELING THE JOY OF CO-CREATIVE PARTNERSHIP

Although until that time I had been in a marriage that had silenced my voice at home, it had not stopped me from becoming increasingly vocal in my work, and I was now being heard by people far beyond my immediate circle. My career star was definitely on the rise. I had co-founded a very well-known women's center, become president of the American Holistic Medical Association, and written a book that had brought me enormous validation for my work and my ideas. My faith in my own work—work that I absolutely adored—was growing all the time.

I was also proud of the fact that I was contributing more and more to the family finances, and as usual had looked to my husband for approval—but that was not to be.

As happens for so many women at midlife, around this time I found a new model for partnership. I first met Dr. Mona Lisa Schulz when I was finishing up *Women's Bodies, Women's Wisdom.* Both an M.D. and Ph.D. in neuroscience, Mona Lisa eventually became my research partner as well as one of my closest friends. She appraised my work from the viewpoint of pure science and found scientific validation for it. Up until then, my training had led me to believe that hands-on clinicians weren't really scientists. Scientists were people who didn't dirty their hands with the messy details of patients' actual lives, preferring instead to gather data under perfectly controlled conditions. The kind of medicine I was practicing was anything but controlled, given that I was helping women choose individual solutions to their health care problems based on a partnership between doctor and patient, and between the patient and her own inner wisdom. This, surely, was not science.

But Mona Lisa helped me see myself and my contribution more clearly. Until I met her, I had found precious few local physicians who took the same approach to medicine that I did, and fewer still who were willing to talk about it publicly. That was a time when it still wasn't safe to call yourself "holistic," so there weren't too many other volunteers for possible professional martyrdom. But Mona Lisa was one of them. She shared my vision as well as my willingness to take risks, to speak out.

Mona Lisa's approach to science wasn't limited to the conventionally acceptable. In addition to being a neuroscientist, she was a practicing medical intuitive. She was able to ascertain the emotional and mental patterns associated with a person's illness, knowing only their name and age, and without ever having seen them. Her scientific validation of intuition—defined as the capacity to know something directly without sufficient objective data—contributed to my growing faith in my own inner guidance. I could share with her my life-long interest in mysticism, astrology, and angels. She also taught me how to use tarot cards as a tool to focus my intuition. I, in turn, provided her with a role model of a physician who had successfully combined right-brain intuitive wisdom with left-brain diagnostic and surgical skills.

Our work together was a working model for a partnership between two people who were both peers and friends. Besides ideas and values, we shared many of the same attitudes toward life. We had the same sense of humor, loved going to movies together, enjoyed putting on parties for my daughters, giggled while we helped each other choose "speaking costumes" for the public appearances both of us were making ever more frequently in those days. This experience of working with someone who was fun, happy, fulfilled, and ambitious set a whole new standard for the kind of person I wanted to spend time with.

More Validation: My Message Goes to Television

Early in 1997, I began working on my first two public television specials. Soon after GnRH had jump-started my brain, I met Jack Wilson and Bill Heitz, two producers from Chicago whose wives had suggested they track me down and put my work on television. Co-creating what eventually turned out to be four successful public television specials with Jack and Bill also boosted my self-confidence. Now I had the experience of being truly seen and highly valued not only by a rigorous scientist, but by two people who had believed in me even when I was a complete novice as a television personality.

This was an enormously exciting time for me. However, by this point I was out of the office more often than I was in it. My dream of teaching and writing, of bringing my message to an ever wider audience, had become a full-time reality—and then some. Reluctantly I cut the cord with Women to Women completely, selling my share of both the business and the building to my partners. The work I was doing no longer fit the model that we had started together. I knew it was time to go out on my own.

THE FORCES THAT CHANGE THE GOOSE
ALSO CHANGE THE GANDER

As I was making and experiencing all these changes in my life, my husband was going through changes of his own. His midlife reevaluation started with questioning his career goals. The era of managed care was forcing him to change the way he practiced, and he found himself increasingly unhappy in his work. He was also becoming very anxious about money, a fear that my own success seemed only to intensify, rather than to soothe. I couldn't understand why he worried so much about our finances. After all, I reasoned, I was making good money, and we were in this together.

One reason for his anxiety was that he was thinking about retiring when our younger daughter graduated from high school—which was just two short years away. In contrast, I felt as though I was just hitting my stride, and I had no intention of retiring, then or ever. During the retirement planning sessions my husband scheduled with our accountant, I felt as though we were in two different worlds. There didn't appear to be any computer programs designed to take into account two sets of goals as different as the ones my husband and I described in these meetings.

Like many other men at midlife, my husband seemed to deal with his anxiety about change by trying to exert more and more control over our financial resources—resources that were increasingly from my earnings. Or perhaps he had always exerted that kind of control and I was just now waking up to it. For, like many women, I had always been convinced that my husband was better at money management than I was, so I had turned it over to him. He did all the planning and paid all the bills, spending hours at his computer each week doing so. As he went through his midlife crisis, this task seemed to fill him with ever more dread and worry every time he did it, with the result that he tried to micromanage my own expenditures. A part of me was convinced that we were indeed overspending, and I was always on the verge of succumbing to the same fears that plagued him.

But no matter how hard I tried, I could never live within the budget he considered appropriate to our circumstances. I found myself hiding purchases from him, lest he blow up at me. Of course, the conflict between the ideals I had been promoting all these years to my patients and the reality I was living was not lost on me. But my fear of my husband's anger was very real. I let myself be controlled by it, and silenced by it, for years. Even then I was still in some ways the person who wanted more than anything to please, to appease.

REAL MENOPAUSE HITS

Two weeks after leaving the center I had cofounded nearly fifteen years before, my "official" hot flashes began. They were much less intense than the drug-induced hot flashes I had experienced earlier—flashes so extreme that I routinely removed my winter coat and stripped down to a tank top in the middle of a Maine winter! Nonetheless, they were eloquent enough to make me realize that I was finally entering menopause for real.

It was December 18, 1998—the end of a year and, as it turned out, the end of an era. The separation I had just negotiated from Women to Women was only a warm-up for what was about to happen on the home front—though on the surface things looked fine, even festive. The day my hot flashes started was also the day I, my husband, and our daughters embarked on a long-awaited family ski trip to Austria, where we would spend Christmas with my mother and my siblings. This was something I had dreamed for years about doing.

The trip was wonderful in many ways, and I was very happy to be with my extended family in such a magical place, but I felt the strain in my marriage as never before. When I looked at other couples around us, men and women who were clearly engaged with and enjoying each other, I felt very alone. I found that I was avoiding my husband on that trip, skiing mostly with my daughters, my sister, and my mother. I simply didn't want to use my energy to try to soothe my husband and keep him comfortable, as I had always done before. The coming of my hot flashes had signaled another stage in my own midlife reevaluation—a commitment to setting healthier boundaries, to taking better care of myself, to speaking the truth.

In case I had any doubts, my body reinforced my decision to honor my own needs. I broke out in adult acne, a sign that something had "gotten under the skin" and was now about to erupt. When I turned to the Motherpeace tarot cards I had used to help me access my intuition, I kept drawing the Shaman of Swords card, whose message is about saying what you know to be true. The universe was speaking to me in many guises. I was now ready to hear.

MY MARRIAGE GOES BANKRUPT

Soon after the New Year, at the beginning of 1999, a series of overdraft notices that arrived from our bank seemed to me to symbolize the degree to which my husband and I had failed to create a viable partnership. Our household account had insufficient funds. So did our marriage. When I suggested that I needed my own space for a while and wanted us to consider separate bedrooms during this period, my husband left in a fit of rage. He did not return.

Almost overnight I was handed the opportunity—and the responsibility—to assume complete financial dominion over both my business and my household.

Up until the moment my husband left, it had never occurred to me in all my years of marriage that I would ever end up divorced. My fantasy was always that my husband would change or that I would change or that something would change so that the two of us could become the team I thought we were capable of being. For years psychics and astrologers had been telling me we were meant to be together. This couldn't be happening.

And yet despite what seemed to be in the stars, and despite our three years of couples therapy, I had reached the end of the road. I could no longer allow myself to be in what I perceived was an unbalanced relationship. I needed to come into my own. I was no longer willing to be controlled by another person, emotionally, financially, or physically. I had come too far.

Finally I was ready to do the last part of the self-healing that I'd spent half a century preparing for. Menopause had spurred me to make the ideals I'd been promoting in my work a reality. I knew I now had two choices: to mute my voice so that I could stay in my marriage, or to find the courage I needed to take steps toward divorce. But what a hard choice it was.

Perhaps one reason it was so hard was that the 1950s was the period in which my brain had been wired for relationships. If my marriage had broken up in that era, it would have been widely agreed that I had wrecked our relationship with my ambition. Why couldn't I have just put my husband's needs before my own? Why did I insist on being fully supported and fully met in my marriage relationship? Why did I insist on pushing my husband past where he felt comfortable going? I did it because I had no other choice. Something within me, some voice from my very soul, was urging me on, and I had to trust it.

Nonetheless, I was frightened of what it would be like to live without my longtime mate. And then one day I remembered something one of my daughters had said to me several months before: that things were so unpleasant in our house, she doubted she would come home for vacations once she had left for college. That gave me courage to move forward.

Healing Through Pain

Even though I could see, in retrospect, that I had started the process of letting go of my marriage several years before, I was still not prepared for the deep sense of loss I felt when it ended. Initially I felt as though one of my limbs were missing. For weeks I awoke before dawn, feeling an acute ache in my throat and in my heart as soon as the realization hit me, once again, that my husband was not next to me in bed.

Once out of the house, I found I could sometimes get along okay for days at a time. Then I'd go somewhere and have to fill out one of those forms that are ubiquitous in our lives, and I'd think about how the day was going to come when I would have to check the box that said "divorced." I dreaded that day.

I remembered how hard it was for my mother after her marriage ended. But hers was a happy marriage, cut short when my father died suddenly on the tennis court at the age of sixty-eight. That had been a terrible blow for her. Still, in the early months of my separation, I remember thinking that my own pain was in some ways even worse, because it made me question the most central fact of my life for the past twenty-four years. Even though I knew that 50 percent of all marriages ended in divorce, I felt like an incredible failure. I was afraid I was becoming the kind of woman I'd always heard no one wants to invite anywhere lest she steal another woman's husband: a woman alone at midlife, unclaimed, unwanted, and dangerous to the status quo.

Loss is a recurrent theme at midlife. Even women who don't go through divorce at this time often face other losses—the death of parents or spouse, estrangement from a child, being let go from a job, changes in physical appearance, or the realization that the reproductive years are over. For a woman who has never borne a child and had always hoped that that was in her future, the end of her fertility can be a terrible loss. But no matter what the circumstances, nearly every woman has to give up *some* dream about what she thought her life would be like.

And when that realization hits, it is very painful. Gradually I allowed myself to feel all my grief and pain, secure in the knowledge that it would not destroy me. I knew that only then could I move forward with my life.

Healing Through Anger

I would be lying to you, and perpetuating a grave disservice to midlife women, if I allowed you to believe that my feelings at this time were solely about grief and loss. There was also another feeling brimming up from my depths, and this emotion saved me from the paralysis that I might otherwise have felt.

It was the emotion of anger that gave me the energy to proceed with the onerous task of dismantling twenty-four years of married life—and building another kind of life. I used the volcanic energy of my anger to guide me toward identifying my needs and then getting them met. Having experienced my husband's departure as an abandonment of me and our daughters, I was determined to do whatever I had to in order to make our lives whole again.

At first I wasn't sure I could do it. My anger was tempered by a liberal dose of fear. But every time I teetered on the brink of despair or terror, some piece of evidence would arrive in the mail that compelled me to see the truth: overdraft notices from the bank, credit card bills, and lawyers' letters were showing up with great regularity. Like it or not, I was on my own, financially and in every other way. I was going to have to give up my sentimental fantasies that our marriage could still be saved. My focus would have to be on ensuring my own and my daughters' well-being.

I also had another source of energy during this hard time. My brother had gone through a divorce himself some years before. He seemed to know instinctively when to call me and what to say to give me encouragement. His clear-sightedness proved to be invaluable to me.

Healing Through Acceptance

I began a daily prayer practice to give me the courage to continue the process of letting go of my marriage and my identity as a married woman. This involved taking a walk every morning and stopping halfway through to look out over the harbor. There I would think about all that I had to be grateful for in my life—which was a lot.

Then I would say a prayer of thanks out loud, sending the words down the river to its source. Each day as I stood there I watched the ice on the river receding, the tides changing. Spring would come soon, I knew, and with it the healing energy of rebirth and renewal. I was grateful for winter and the time it gave me to grieve, grateful for having spring to look forward to.

On the weekend just before our twenty-fourth wedding anniversary, about three months after our separation, I felt especially bereft, my feelings of loss temporarily obliterating all my intellectual and emotional reasons for proceeding with divorce. A friend of mine had called that morning and told me how sad she felt about our split, since she could feel that there was still so much love between my husband and me. She told me she would spend part of the weekend burning prayer sticks for us in the ashram where she worships.

Monday, the day of our anniversary, I felt filled with longing. I spent the whole day wanting to call my husband. Then, as I was sitting down to dinner with the girls, the doorbell rang. It was the florist, delivering a dozen white roses accompanied by a card that read, "Thanks for almost twenty-four years together. And our two daughters." I wept and said to the girls, "Never doubt that your father and I have always loved each other."

ARMADILLO MEDICINE: THE POWER OF VULNERABILITY

During the weeks just after my separation, a newspaper reporter interviewed me for a story she was doing about my work. "I have only one more question," she said at the end. "Has Chris Northrup ever really suffered?"

I was shocked. At that very moment I was feeling the loss of the most significant relationship of my life, and feeling it in every cell of my body. How could she assume my life was easy? But I said nothing. It was too soon to discuss my situation publicly. The wounds were too new, too raw.

Earlier that same month Mona Lisa had said to me, "You're not vulnerable enough, so no one feels drawn to take care of you. I, on the other hand, have had so many health problems that everyone feels drawn to take care of me. I attract 'mothers' wherever I go."

This made me furious. It hadn't felt safe to allow myself to be vulnerable with my husband, or before that with my mother. Somewhere along the line I had lost the ability. Besides, it hadn't been an ability I admired. I'd watched far too many women milk the victim role, playing on the sympathy of others to get their needs met. I had never wanted to be such a woman. But I knew that our culture identified so deeply with victims that it doubted the humanity of those who didn't assume that role. That was really what the newspaper reporter had been saying to me with her question.

For two nights in a row after my conversation with Mona Lisa, I sought guidance in a set of animal "medicine cards" that worked something like a tarot pack. Each time I drew I picked the card known as Armadillo (in the reversed position), whose message is this:

> You may think the only way to win in your present situation is to hide or to pretend that you are armor-coated and invincible, but this is not the way to grow. It is better to open up and find the value and strength of your vulnerability. You will experience something wonderful if you do. Vulnerability is the key to enjoying the gifts of physical life. In allowing yourself to feel, a myriad of expressions are made available. For instance, a true compliment is an admiration flow of energy. If you are afraid of being hurt and are hiding from anything, you will never feel the joy of admiration from others.[1]

This message was right on target for me. And once again I was reminded of how well I had learned from my stoic mother to hide my vulnerability. It was now time to change this pattern, as part of letting go of my past.

At midlife, some women seek new satisfactions in the world beyond that of home and family life. They may need to don some armor. But other women need to let the armor down a bit. That was the case for me. And it's also true for many men, who traditionally spend the years leading up to midlife focused on achieving success in the workplace. The point is that at midlife, more than at any other time, the aspects of your personality that kept you alive and functional for the first half of your life may actually put you at risk in the second half. All of us must find the courage to make the changes that will enable us to live our lives in an empowered fashion.

CELEBRATING THE PAST WHILE
CREATING A NEW FUTURE

Our household became much more relaxed once my husband left. The tension was gone. I adopted a couple of kittens from our local animal shelter and found that they brought me and my daughters a great deal of comfort and enjoyment. We had never had pets before, because a dog had always seemed like too much trouble, and my husband was allergic to cats.

Surprisingly, I also found that I was sleeping better than I had in years, waking up easily every morning without the alarm clock. This had never happened before. Looking back now, I can finally appreciate how much energy I had been using in the effort to keep my marriage going.

As the weeks went by, I began the slow process of feeling what it was like to have myself to myself. And on some very deep level I began to feel, ever so gradually, that I was recharging my inner batteries from a source deep within me. As with all grieving and letting go, there were ups and downs to this process. One week, for example, I found myself crying while watching the Thursday night TV shows I used to watch with my husband and daughters as a weekly ritual. But then one week later I was able to spend the evening alone, away from the TV, reveling in the beautiful light on the river outside my home. I was alone, but I was not lonely. I knew I was going to make it. I was happy.

The kind of marriage I had worked well for me for many years, and I am very grateful for having been able to experience all the joys and pleasures of family life with my husband and our two children. Those joys were very real, as I was reminded the day my husband came to claim his share of the paintings that were hanging on our walls. After he removed them, I was left with that awful feeling of loss that newly bare walls give you at such times. To get me past this latest milestone in grief, two friends and I spent an afternoon creating an entire wall of family photos in the dining room—providing concrete and comforting evidence of the good times in my past. A year later I replaced the photos of my husband with those of my daughters and me. Later still, when I remodeled that room, I changed the space yet again. I have learned that letting go is a process, not an event.

I have also learned that part of the process is acknowledging the past value of the relationship you are leaving behind, and doing this not just silently, to yourself, but, when appropriate, to the person who was part of that relationship.

I did this myself five months after our separation, when my husband and I were nearing a settlement. As we were leaving one of our mediation sessions, I asked him to meet with me privately, and then I poured out everything that was in my heart. I apologized for trying to change him. I said how glad I was that neither of us had used an affair to get out of the marriage. I thanked him for the safe haven of the family we had created together, and for the wonderful children who would not have existed without our love for each other. I told him I was grateful for the support and structure he provided for me when I was out blazing new trails in women's health. I also told him that I loved him.

My feelings were so poignant during that outpouring of gratitude that I could easily see why estranged couples might want to keep their anger and resentment alive. That way they wouldn't have to feel all the pain of what they are losing. But I could also see how damaging this could be to their children, themselves, and everyone else involved, and I was glad I had found the courage to express what was in my heart.

I let go of so much that year, including my feelings of failure. Margaret Mead, the renowned anthropologist, once pointed out that in the past, most marriages continued "till death do us part" because after twenty-five years of marriage, one or both members of the couple had died! In other words, at the same age that most of us are going through the changes of menopause, our ancestors were falling ill and dying—or were already dead. "Till death do us part" was much easier to accomplish when lives were shorter. Mead's observation helped me feel less of a failure for being unable to preserve my marriage.

My health remained good throughout the difficult and painful year of my divorce. I allowed my tears to flow freely, my anger to erupt and dissipate. I also called on spiritual guidance unceasingly, and this, together with my new emotional openness, helped me negotiate a period characterized by significant hormonal change with minimal symptoms. I also used a variety of natural approaches to hormonal balance, as I will discuss in chapter 6.

Now it is time for me, as for so many other women of the baby boom generation, to be pioneers in re-creating the second half of our lives on our own terms. As we do so, we must keep in mind that physical and emotional health is our natural state, even during this time of transition. And although the life ahead of many is uncharted territory, fraught with all the uncertainty that accompanies change, I have now gotten to the other side. I can guarantee you that this second stage of life is set up to be the most liberating and fulfilling time of your life if you heed your inner wisdom and follow its dictates.

Have no regrets, whatever you decide. Take advantage of the clarity of vision that is the gift of menopause, and use that gift to let the second half of your life be truly your own.

2

The Brain Catches Fire
at Menopause

A woman once told me that when her mother was approaching the age of menopause, her father sat the whole family down and said, "Kids, your mother may be going through some changes now, and I want you to be prepared. Your uncle Ralph told me that when your aunt Carol went through the change, she threw a leg of lamb right out the window!" Although this story fits beautifully into the stereotype of the "crazy" menopausal woman, it should not be overlooked that throwing the leg of lamb out the window may have been Aunt Carol's outward expression of the process going on within her soul: the reclaiming of self. Perhaps it was her way of saying how tired she was of waiting on her family, of signaling to them that she was past the cook/chauffeur/dishwasher stage of life. For many women, if not most, part of this reclamation process includes getting in touch with anger and, perhaps, blowing up at loved ones for the first time. The events that evoke anger are never new. What is new, however, is our willingness and energy to let that anger be acknowledged and expressed, both to ourselves and to others. This can be the first step toward much-needed change in our lives ... change that is often long overdue.

OUR CULTURAL INHERITANCE

Regardless of where you currently stand in your menstrual or perimenopausal transition, chances are you've inherited a few beliefs about your cycle that boil down to a variation of the following: "The issues that arise premenstrually have nothing to do with my actual life. They are strictly hormonal. My hormones exist in a universe that is completely separate from the rest of my life." I found a superb example of this culturally sanctioned unconsciousness about premenstrual syndrome (PMS) in a popular women's magazine:

> I love PMS! It gives me so much perspective! It makes me cry in the supermarket aisle because they're out of Calamata olives—a deliberate plot by the Stop & Shop stock boy to sabotage the new recipe I'm dying to try on my one day off! It makes me pick fights with my husband over incredibly important stuff—like the fact that he's forgotten to put out my morning coffee cup alongside his, which is incredibly symbolic of something deeper, don't you think? . . . And then, POOF! My period arrives and I wake up to a world that looks rosy. Gone is the pressure to get a divorce, send my kids to reform school, and move to another country. In fact, compared to how I felt the previous week, I feel pretty good indeed.[1]

The writer goes on to explain that her PMS has only intensified as she has gotten older and that her OB/GYN has suggested that she go back on the pill, or try Prozac before her period. In other words, she needs to get "fixed." But she's ignoring potentially important messages from her body. PMS and the escalation of symptoms that is so common during perimenopause are really our inner guidance system trying to get us to pay attention to the adjustments we need to make in our lives, adjustments that become particularly urgent during perimenopause.

If we don't pay attention to the issues that come up for us every month during the years when our periods are regular, our symptoms will escalate as we get older. Every premenstrual issue that this writer blames on PMS is potentially related to a larger and deeper need that is not being met. The issues she raises may appear superficial or even silly at first glance. But if she were to be completely honest with herself, she would realize that the lack of olives at the grocery store and the fact that her husband doesn't put out her coffee cup in the morning may be doorways to deeper needs that she has been ignoring: the need for more time off, a longing for the sensual satisfaction of cooking, a longing to be cherished daily by her husband. When these needs aren't acknowledged, the body ends up screaming louder and louder to get our attention.

By reducing her body's signals to physical symptoms, the writer has bought into the dualistic belief system that pervades Western medicine. Her attitude—one that is all too common—is that troublesome hormones are a woman's cross to bear, but with a variety of remedies and a sense of humor, they can be kept to a low roar, so they're at least tolerable. Instead of seeing an opportunity for insight here, she has diminished and dismissed her inner guidance.

OUR BRAINS CATCH FIRE AT MENOPAUSE

Our brains actually begin to change at perimenopause. Like the rising heat in our bodies, our brains also become fired up! Sparked by the hormonal changes that are typical during the menopausal transition, a switch goes on that signals changes in our temporal lobes, the brain region associated with enhanced intuition. How this ultimately affects us depends to a large degree on how willing we are to make the changes in our lives that our hormones are urging us to make over the ten years or so of perimenopause.

There is ample scientific evidence of the brain changes that begin to take place at perimenopause. Differences in relative levels of estrogen and progesterone affect the temporal lobe and limbic areas of our brains, and we may find ourselves becoming irritable, anxious, emotionally volatile. Though our culture leads us to believe that our mood swings are simply the result of raging hormones and do not have anything to do with our lives, there is solid evidence that repeated episodes of stress (due to relationship, children, and job situations you feel angry about or powerless over, for example) are actually behind many of the hormonal changes in the brain and body. This means that if your life situation—whether at work or with children, your husband, your parents, or whatever—doesn't change, then unresolved emotional stress can exacerbate a perimenopausal hormone imbalance. In a normal premenopausal hormonal state it's much easier to overlook those aspects of your life that don't really work, just as you can overlook them more easily in the first half of your menstrual cycle—the time when you're more apt to feel upbeat and happy and able to shove difficult material under the rug. But that doesn't mean the problems aren't there.

LEARNING TO RECOGNIZE AND HEED OUR WAKE-UP CALLS

Whether you are in early perimenopause at thirty-five or standing at the threshold of menopause, your body's inner wisdom will attempt to catch your attention through four kinds of escalating physical and emotional wake-up calls.

Our First Wake-Up Call: PMS

What happens if, during our childbearing years, we ignore our cyclic nature, disconnect from the body's wisdom, and attempt to

FIGURE 1: THE FIRST TWO WAKE-UP CALLS: PMS AND SAD

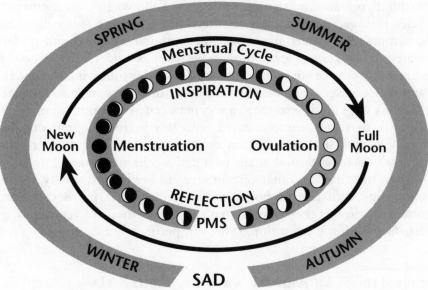

PMS is to the monthly cycle as SAD is to the annual cycle. Both conditions respond to the same treatment while asking us to deepen our connection to our cyclic wisdom.

function as though we were linear beings, with the same drives, the same focus, and the same aptitudes day after day? Very often PMS happens. With its physical and emotional discomfort, PMS is one way a woman's body elbows her every month to remind her of the growing backlog of unresolved issues accumulating within her. Everything from unbalanced nutrition to unresolved relationships can disrupt the normal hormonal milieu, wreaking physical and emotional havoc during the childbearing years. Ignoring these early, relatively gentle nudges month after month sets her up for sharper and more urgent messages. Inconvenient as they are, these pains are our allies, begging us to look up and see what's not working in our lives. Often we don't, however. Most of us are too busy, and the discomfort isn't that bad, after all. It's easier to just ignore it. But the body is insistent!

A Poignant Wake-Up Call: Postpartum Depression

It is well documented that women who have significant PMS are also more apt to suffer from postpartum depression in the first days or weeks after giving birth. Or sometimes those who suffer from postpartum depression will go on to develop PMS when their menstrual cycles resume. Because new mothers often feel far too vulnerable to complain, postpartum depression is underdiagnosed and undertreated in our culture, even though between 10 and 15 percent of all women experience some form of mood disorder following childbirth, ranging from major depression to anxiety disorders such as panic attacks. As with all illness, there are genetic, environmental, and nutritional factors that are associated with postpartum depression. But it is also true that postpartum depression is often a sign from a mother's inner wisdom that she isn't getting the support and help she needs at this time, and that certain areas of her life, especially her relationships with one or both parents or with her partner, require some attention. If these issues aren't resolved, they are very likely to resurface during the hormonal shifts of perimenopause.

An Annual Wake-Up Call: SAD

If the monthly messages go unheeded, a woman's body may send a louder wake-up call on a yearly basis, in the form of seasonal affective disorder, or SAD. It begins with an intensification of the symptoms of PMS during the autumn and winter of the year, when the days are shortest and darkness dominates. Eventually it can evolve into full-blown depression and despair during the time of year when daylight is abbreviated. It is well known that providing two hours of full-spectrum artificial light in the evening, to trick the body into thinking the days are longer, can reverse the weight gain, depression, carbohydrate craving, social withdrawal, fatigue, and irritability of SAD. (Studies have also shown that light therapy helps depression in pregnancy.)[2] But without continued use of the artificial lights, the symptoms return the following autumn... unless the wake-up call is heeded. The link between PMS and SAD is a profound example of how women's wisdom is simultaneously encoded into both our monthly cycles and the annual cycle of the seasons.

Perimenopause: The Mother of All Wake-Up Calls

For many women perimenopause can be, as one of my patients described it, "PMS times ten"—and this is particularly the case for those who, for one reason or another, hit the snooze button instead of heeding their monthly and seasonal wake-up calls. This is not to discount the direct physical effects of changing hormone levels. However, it is a safe bet that any uncomfortable symptoms that reveal themselves during times of hormonal shift will be magnified and prolonged if a woman is carrying a heavy load of emotional baggage. These symptoms are the body's wisdom, pleading yet again that unresolved life issues be attended to. Throughout a woman's childbearing years, a kind of "debt account" is established where existing and future issues accumulate, compounding interest with each passing month that the debt goes unpaid.

Thus the average woman, blessed with approximately 480 menstrual periods and 40 seasonal cycles to bring her to the threshold of her menopause, gets about 500 progress reports. How is her physical health and nutrition? How are her emotions? What's happening in her relationships and her career? Is she scheduling pleasure into her daily life on purpose or putting herself last? There have been approximately 500 opportunities to resolve those issues... or sweep them under the rug. At perimenopause the process escalates. The earnest, straightforward inner self, which has tried for years to get our attention, makes one final hormonally mediated attempt to get us to deal with our accumulated needs, wants, and desires. This is likely to turn into a period of great emotional turmoil, as each woman struggles to make a new life, one that can accommodate her emerging self. Externally and internally, this period is a mirror image of adolescence, a time when our bodies and brains were also going through major hormonal shifts that gave us the energy to attempt to individuate from our families and become the person we were meant to be. At menopause we pick up where we left off in adolescence. It is now time to finish the job.

It should be no surprise, then, that research has documented that those women who experience uncomfortable—even severe—symptoms of PMS are often the same women who have a tumultuous perimenopause, with physical and emotional symptoms that become increasingly impossible to ignore.[3]

As a woman makes the transition to the second half of her life, she finds herself in a struggle not only with her own aversion to conflict and confrontation, but also with the culture's view of how women "should" be. The body's inner wisdom gets its last, best chance of breaking through culturally erected barriers, while shining a light on aspects of a woman's life that need work. To resolve the situation, then, it is up to the individual woman to meet her body's wisdom halfway.

IS IT ME OR IS IT MY HORMONES? DEBUNKING THE MYTH OF RAGING HORMONES

The fluctuating hormone levels that most women experience during perimenopause and during menopause do not, in and of themselves, cause the distressing emotional and psychological symptoms (such as anger and depression) that so many women suffer with PMS and at midlife. But if there is an underlying susceptibility to distress in the first place, there is no doubt that hormonal swings will help bring that distress to the surface.

Though hormone levels and mood do tend to fluctuate widely during our reproductive years, and even more widely still during our perimenopausal years, research has failed to show any appreciable differences between the hormone levels of those women who suffer from PMS-like symptoms and those who don't. What has been well documented, however, is that the *brains* of women who suffer the most from PMS-like symptoms are more susceptible to the effects of fluctuating hormone levels.[4] In other words, it is not the hormone levels per se that are the problem. Rather, it is the particular combination of a woman's hormone levels and her preexisting brain chemistry along with her life situation that results in her symptoms. It is estimated that 27 percent of all women who experience agitation and depression during their periods, and 36 percent of all women who become depressed premenstrually, will be very sensitive to the hormonal changes that occur at menopause.[5]

Though we tend to blame perimenopausal symptoms on hormonal shifts in the body, their origins are far more complex. Several women in my practice, for example, have experienced symptoms such as hot flashes and mood swings in their later forties—despite having been on full hormone replacement for over twenty years as a result of having undergone hysterectomies and removal of their ovaries while still in their twenties. Clearly, changes in reproductive hormones alone do not account for these symptoms. They are signals from our mind and body that we have reached a new developmental stage—an opportunity for healing and growth.

ANATOMY OF MENOPAUSAL WISDOM

Menopause combines the wisdom of the prior stages and brings it to a new level.

Body Process	Encoded Wisdom
MENSTRUAL CYCLE	Cyclic intuitive wisdom and emotional recycling and processing
PREGNANCY/FERTILITY	Capacity to conceive an idea or a life with another, hold it, nurture it, and allow it to be born
MENOPAUSE	Passage into the wisdom years
	Capacity to be open to constant intuitive knowing
	Reseeding the community

Moving Inward

Until midlife, it is characteristic for a woman's energies to be focused on caring for others. She is encouraged to do so, in part, by the hormones that drive her menstrual cycles—the hormones that foster her instincts for nurturing, her devotion to cohesion, and harmony within her world. But for two or three days each month, just before or during our periods, there is a hormonal interlude when the veil between our conscious and unconscious selves is thinner and the voice of our souls beckons to us, subtly reminding us of our own passions, our own needs, which cannot and should not always be subsumed to the needs of those we love.

This fluctuation between inner and outer worlds and the way it is influenced by our hormones was revealed in a fascinating study done in the 1930s by a psychoanalyst and a physician. Dr. Therese Benedek studied the psychotherapy records of patients, while Dr. Boris Rubenstein studied the ovarian hormonal cycles of the same women. By looking only at a woman's emotional state, Dr. Benedek was able to identify where she was in her menstrual cycle with incredible accuracy. The two doctors found that just before ovulation, when estrogen levels were at their highest, women's emotions and behavior were directed toward the outer world. At ovulation, women were more relaxed and content and quite receptive to being cared for and loved by others. During the postovulatory and premenstrual phase, when progesterone is at its highest (and PMS symptoms are also at their peak), women were more likely to be focused on themselves and more involved in inward-directed activity.[6]

I like to think of the first half of our cycles as the time when we are both biologically and psychologically preparing to give birth to someone or something outside of ourselves. In the second half of our cycles, we prepare to give birth to nothing less than ourselves. It is at this time that the more intuitive parts of our brain become activated, giving us feedback and guidance about the state of our inner lives. One of my newsletter subscribers, Lucinda, describes the process eloquently.

LUCINDA: *Healing PMS*

PMS has been an issue for me that has severely limited my life, distorted my children's experience of their mother, and made my husband's life with me very scary. He insisted for years that an alien must take over my body when my hormones fluctuated in preparation for my menstrual cycle! Migraines were part of this pattern, too. I insisted that it was the "true ugly me" that surfaced at a weakened time! One minute I would be rational and peacefully attending to my life tasks, the next I would be argumentative until war broke out!

Then I would cry and feel like the worst person on the planet.

This didn't happen every month, but when it did it was on schedule, around the seventeenth day of my cycle. The consequence of this pattern was that I feared I was crazy, and I could not count on myself for normal planning of life events, making me an unreliable family member. While I longed for intimacy, I was too scary a person to approach. I was caught in the busy schedule of a working wife and mother and couldn't figure out this problem in my life. I limped along, trying to appear normal to the outside world but becoming more and more exhausted.

As the years passed I was introduced to new theories about the mind/body connection and information about the benefits of physically releasing emotional distress, past as well as present, through crying, yawning, sweating, shaking, and so on. These things remained a concept for a long time. I knew the information in my head, but I had not assimilated it into my being for use. I was still fighting the monthly disability of PMS and internally asking why—why did I, who was creative, intelligent, and loving, have this condition that was ruining my life?

Insight came one day as I was getting a migraine and knew what would follow. I consciously asked myself what would happen if, instead of fighting the feeling and judging myself as a defective person, I instead allowed myself to fully feel what was happening in my body. I surrendered my control and focused on just being present with my body for the first time ever.

I felt vulnerable. The shift in my hormones left me feeling vulnerable. That was not a state of being I could tolerate. I was a warrior, not a maiden. I cried, acknowledging my defenselessness. I experienced my feminine side for the first time. In fear, I had raged against it in the past. No wonder I felt like a victim. I was battering my own feminine side—my internal goddess.

I stayed with the feeling. I didn't die. I needed her softness and wisdom. The migraine faded. I eased up on my self-judgment and embraced that part of myself long hidden—even from my own view.

The physical symptoms that had accompanied my PMS lessened. I use the increased energy to do some other things for myself. I have a holistic nutritionist and slowly am improving my diet. I use a good massage therapist. I continue to discharge my past and present feelings. I have fun at whatever I am doing because I see it as important, as my own creative expression. I talk before crisis occurs.

I have continued to be challenged by my body's response to my poor choices. I am grateful for its ability to do so, and now when I wonder, it is more a question of what than of why: what am I doing that denies my feminine inner wisdom and goes against my true spiritual identity?

As I sit present with that question, the answer bubbles up from within. We do come with an instruction kit, if we will just quiet ourselves to receive the information and learn some new skills.

Moving from an Alternating to a Direct Current of Wisdom

At midlife, the hormonal milieu that was present for only a few days each month during most of your reproductive years, the milieu that was designed to spur you on to reexamine your life just a little at a time, now gets stuck in the on position for weeks or months at a time. We go from an alternating current of inner wisdom to a direct current that remains on all the time after menopause is complete. During perimenopause, our brains make the change from one way of being to the other.

Biologically, at this stage of life you are programmed to withdraw from the outside world for a period of time and revisit your past. You need to be free of the distractions that come when you are focusing your mothering efforts solely on others. Perimenopause is a time when you are meant to mother yourself.

It may be no accident that the word *menopause* invites the association "pause from men." We don't really need to withdraw from men per se. We need, instead, to put our focus on ourselves instead of spending so much time and effort pleasing them! In truth, you are being urged, biologically, to pause from everyone—from mankind in general—in order to do important work on yourself. Perhaps as a result of this, one of the most common threads running through women's descriptions of how they feel during the menopausal transition is the longing for time alone, for a refuge that provides peace, quiet, and freedom from distractions and demands.

It's a wistful dream, seemingly out of reach in this busy age of multidirectional tugs-of-war. But those who have the yearning often believe nonetheless that their uncomfortable menopausal symptoms would simply dissolve if only they had the luxury of shutting out the world so they could tune in to the growth process occurring within themselves. This wistful dream is real. It comes from your soul. I've come to realize that you can trust it and believe in it—and that you must do its bidding.

Even if this dream seems out of reach, the simple truth is that

FIGURE 2: CURRENTS OF WISDOM

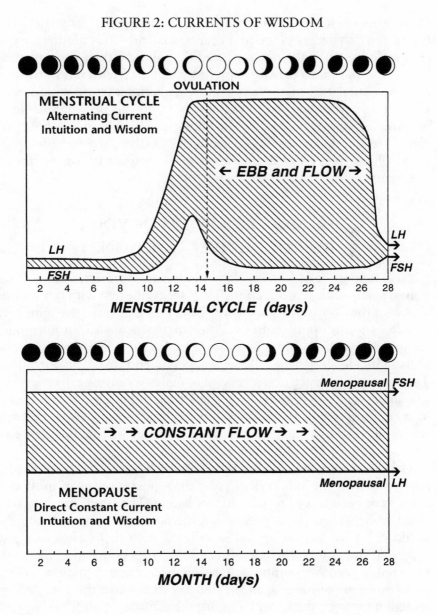

FSH and LH stimulate ovulation and are released cyclically each month up until the years before menopause. They then undergo a change during which ovulation gradually ceases and FSH and LH levels gradually increase. I believe that these high levels have to do with moving from "AC current" to "DC current." The intuitive wisdom that was once available most clearly during only certain parts of the menstrual cycle is now potentially available all the time.

every woman *can* find refuge within her existing environment. Even if you can't charter a plane to a deserted island, odds are that if you acknowledge and validate your need for solitude, then you can clear some time and find a private corner to which to retreat daily. You can insulate yourself from noise, telephones, and interaction with others. I encourage every woman to find a way to do this on whatever level is possible. When we commit to taking this first step, we have the chance to develop a newfound sense of ourselves and our life's purpose, which gives us an exhilarating sense of what is possible for us during the second half of our lives.

THE MULTIPLE ROLES OF YOUR "REPRODUCTIVE" HORMONES

It has long been known that our female hormones are not involved solely with reproduction. They are connected with our moods and with the way our brains work. Boys and girls have the same rate of depression up until puberty. After that, when ovarian hormones surge and cycling begins, depression increases in females, with the highest incidence reached between ages twenty-two and forty-five. The lifetime incidence of depression in males is only one in ten, while in females it is one in four. After menopause, the rates of depression in men and women reach gender parity once again. Cross-cultural studies have shown that women have a higher lifetime incidence of depression in other cultures as well.

I believe that this gender-wide susceptibility to depression is in part related to the subservient roles that most women in most cultures have been forced to play for millennia. That said, it is also true that the menstrual cycle, pregnancy, the postpartum period, and the perimenopausal period are all associated with depression in many women. And those who are susceptible to PMS are also the most susceptible to postpartum depression and perimenopausal mood problems. Part of the reason for this has to do with the complex interaction between the hypothalamus, the pituitary gland, the ovaries, and the multiple hormones that are produced in and interact within these key areas. These key hormones are:

~ *GnRH* (gonadotropin-releasing hormone), which is produced in the hypothalamus

~ *FSH* (follicle-stimulating hormone) and *LH* (luteinizing hormone), which are produced in the pituitary and stimulate, in turn, the rise of estrogen and progesterone during the monthly menstrual cycle

~ **Estrogen,** produced in the ovaries, body fat, and other areas

~ **Progesterone,** produced primarily in the ovaries—which, together with estrogen, prepares the lining of the uterus for implantation and growth of an embryo

The hypothalamus regulates the production of all of these hormones and is in turn regulated by them—and by many others. It has receptors on it not only for progesterone, estrogen, and androgens (e.g., DHEA, testosterone), but also for norepinephrine, dopamine, and serotonin, neurotransmitters that regulate mood and that are affected in turn by our thoughts, beliefs, diet, and environment.

If estrogen, progesterone, and androgen had no other role in the body besides driving reproduction, your levels of these hormones would drop to zero after menopause. But they don't. Similarly, if GnRH, FSH, and LH suddenly were without purpose after menopause, one might expect that there would cease to be any of these hormones circulating in your system after that time. In fact, quite the contrary is true.

During perimenopause, GnRH levels begin to rise in the brain, causing FSH and LH to surge to their highest levels ever. A popular explanation is that this is the body's attempt to "kick-start" the ovaries into resuming their original function, which might make sense if it weren't for one eloquent fact: those elevated FSH and LH levels *stay* elevated, permanently, well after it is physiologically obvious that the ovaries (which are, essentially, out of eggs) have no intention of jumping back onto the reproductive bandwagon. It would seem that your body, in its wisdom, has ulterior motives for continuing to produce the so-called reproductive hormones, and reproduction no longer is the point. In fact, evidence is mounting that at least one of the roles for this off-the-charts production of FSH and LH, and of the GnRH that precipitates this rise, is to drive the changes taking place in the midlife woman's brain.

For biological reasons, females of the human species are often easier to control—intellectually, psychologically, and socially—during their childbearing years than they are before puberty (from birth to age eleven) or after menopause. When we are creating a home and building a family, our primary concern is to maintain balance and peace. We seem to know instinctively that when we're raising a family, it's better for all if we compromise and maintain whatever

FIGURE 3: THE HYPOTHALAMUS-PITUITARY-OVARY CONNECTION

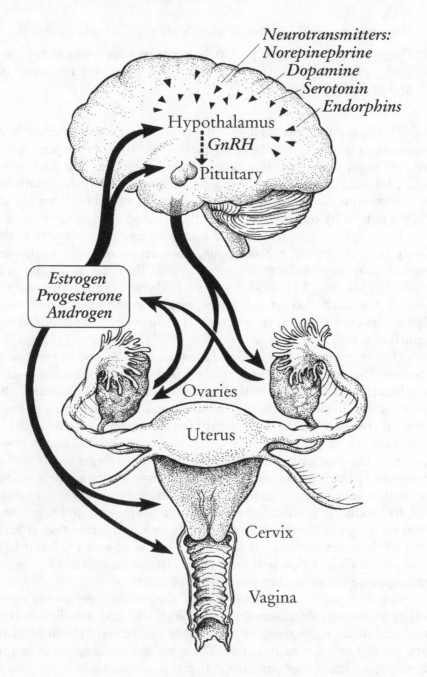

The brain and the reproductive organs are intimately connected by a complex series of feedback loops.

support we have, even if it's less than ideal, rather than risk going it alone. Though this may mean we lose sight of our individual goals, our ability to "go with the program" is in fact protective. A recent medical study done in Sweden, for example, demonstrated that single mothers had an almost 70 percent higher risk of premature death than did mothers with partners. And, surprisingly, this increase in the rate of premature death was the same regardless of socioeconomic or health factors. In other words, even single mothers with adequate economic resources who were physically and psychologically healthy were at greater risk.[7]

This process of sublimating our truest selves begins early, in adolescence. The "activist" mindset of the prepubescent girl, her childlike forthrightness and honesty, and her tendency to jump in when there is conflict all become hormonally sublimated. Though an adolescent girl may be concerned with social injustice, she is likely to be even more preoccupied with her body image and attractiveness to potential mates. Put another way, while a woman is being biologically primed for childbearing, child rearing, and nurturing of others—all vital and species-enhancing roles—the conflicts in the world at large become somewhat blurred to her. Her concern with personal injustices and childhood traumas may also fade or be suppressed. She is likely to give minor offenses no more than cursory attention, for to lick her own wounds, analyze old hurts, or confront long-standing abuses would demand precious energy. She needs to fulfill her primary role, which, biologically speaking, is to reproduce and nurture.

She is rewarded handsomely for complying with this biological agenda. Reproductive hormones are directly responsible for stimulating opioid centers in the brain. These areas actually produce narcotic-like chemicals that swirl into the bloodstream and provide a feel-good sensation, a natural high. Estrogen, for example, is richly provided during the high-fertility phase of the menstrual cycle, when a woman is most "electric" to men and most receptive to their advances. Hormones such as prolactin also flood the system while she is in mothering mode, breast-feeding her baby or nurturing her loved ones. Those strong feelings of attraction, that deep sense of satisfaction, that mantle of loving warmth and purpose that a woman feels when nurturing—all are due in part to natural, narcotic-like chemicals produced by the brain in response to reproductive hormones. Since it feels wonderful, she is encouraged to continue. This is one of the reasons why women are extraordinary caretakers.

Women who are lesbians and/or who choose not to marry or bear children are not exempted from this built-in incentive system, because

FIGURE 4: REWARD ACROSS THE LIFE CYCLE

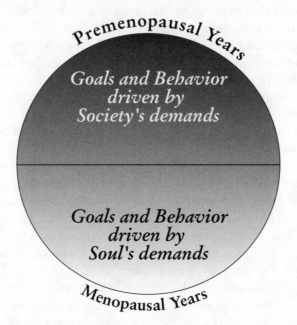

it is stamped into their circuits within the first few days of life as a female embryo. Whether the nurturing behavior is related to pregnancy and child rearing or to other forms of caregiving, the biological feedback is unavoidable, powerful, and very, very positive. Research has clearly shown that when women are under stress, we produce the bonding hormone oxytocin, which promotes supporting others. UCLA professor of psychology Shelley Taylor, Ph.D., author of *The Tending Instinct,* calls this the "tend and befriend" response to stress versus the more male "fight or flight" response.[8]

How Menopausal Hormonal Changes Facilitate Your Brain Rewiring

As a woman enters menopause, she steps out of the primarily childbearing, caretaking role that was hormonally scripted for her. This is not to say that the postmenopausal woman is no longer an effective nurturer. Rather, she becomes freer to choose where she will direct her creative energies, freer to "color outside the lines." Many of the issues that had become blurry to her when the hormones of puberty kicked in may suddenly resurface with vivid clarity as those hormones recede. This is why so many midlife women recall, and decide to confront, past abuses. The concern with social injustices, the political interests, and the personal passions that were sublimated in the childbearing years now surface in sharp focus, ready to be examined and acted upon. Some women funnel this heightened energy into new businesses and new careers. Some discover and cultivate artistic talents they never knew they had. Some women note a surge in their sexual desire, to heights never before experienced in their lives. Some report changes in sexual preference. However they channel it, there's a wonderful sense of living from the inside out!

EMBRACING THE MESSAGE BEHIND OUR MENOPAUSAL ANGER

The GnRH pulses associated with menopause prime the brain for new perceptions—and, subsequently, for new behavior. It is very common for women to become more irritable, even downright angry, about things that were more easily overlooked before. Long before we begin to feel hot flashes from changing hormonal levels, our brains undergo changes in the hypothalamus, the place where GnRH is produced. This same brain region is key for experiencing, and ultimately expressing, emotions such as anger.[9] It is well known that hormones modulate both aggression and anger. Our midlife bodies and brains fully support our ability to experience and express anger with a clarity not possible prior to midlife.

GnRH is just one of several hormones that support the changes occurring in the brain. Estrogen and progesterone molecules bind themselves to areas such as the amygdala and hippocampus, which are important for memory, hunger, sexual desire, and anger. Changing levels of these and other hormones may well help to bring up old memories, accompanied by strong emotions, especially anger. This is not to say that anger is caused by hormonal change. Rather, it means that the hormonal changes simply facilitate remembering and clearing up unfinished business.

Many women are disturbed or frightened when they feel this anger arising. Maybe you don't feel angry. Maybe you're "just" irritable, grouchy, aggravated, envious, overwhelmed, or depressed, or you "just" have high cholesterol or high blood pressure. Believe me, all these emotions and physical conditions are associated with the same thing: anger. Anger in women has a bad rap in general unless that anger arises in the service of others. This probably accounts for the fact that although anger has been studied exhaustively in men, the gender in which it is acceptable, the only kind of female anger that has received a great deal of study is maternal anger, the function of which is to protect a child who is threatened. It is also culturally acceptable for women to express their personal anger by fighting for social justice, which too often becomes a platform for releasing personal anger. Though we're socialized to believe that our anger arises from observing the injustice done to others, the political is always personal: our anger is ultimately about ourselves, and its energy is always urging us toward self-actualization.

That doesn't mean we should abandon social protest, reform, and a quest for justice if we feel passionately about these areas. It simply means that we must be mindful of our personal motivation for participating in these arenas, not allowing them to distract us from self-transformation and self-healing—processes that always render us even more effective as agents for social change.

We need to claim our anger. Especially during midlife, it can play an important role in improving the quality of our lives and our health. It is a powerful signal from our inner wisdom—one we should learn to listen to and act on. It often arises from:

~ Being unable to count on promises or commitments made to us

~ Losing power, status, or respect

~ Being insulted, undermined, or diminished

~ Being threatened with physical or emotional pain

~ Having an important or pleasurable event postponed or canceled to suit someone else's convenience

~ Not obtaining something we feel should legitimately be ours[10]

If, before menopause, a woman hasn't learned to identify her anger and what it is telling her (and this describes many women), perimenopause is her best remaining opportunity to do so. At perimenopause, the rewiring of her brain makes her vision clearer and her motivations easier to identify. Using anger as a catalyst for positive change and growth is always liberating.

In the early stages of perimenopause, the irritability you feel may be subtle. Irritability is a low-voltage form of anger that doesn't usually lead to lasting change—or any change. Irritability is like keeping a pot on simmer but always adding more water or turning down the heat just before it boils. If we do not attend to the things in our lives that irritate us, nature will turn up the flame on the burner in an attempt to mobilize us.

GLADYS: *Never Bringing the Pot to a Boil*

Gladys was a poster child for menopausal irritability. In my office she complained often about her husband, her children, and her job. She had chronic sinusitis, a condition often linked to emotional irritability and anger simmering beneath the surface. Whenever I asked Gladys when she was going to take steps to actually change the aspects of her life that so constantly irritated her, she'd always recover herself immediately, give me a big smile, and say, "But, dear, my husband is really a wonderful man. And my children are really very loving. I really can't complain about any parts of my life." Gladys went to her internist and was put on Prozac, but she never felt as though it, or anything else, ever really helped her. Over the years I cared for her, Gladys's health never improved.

Killing the Messenger: Medicating Our Anger and Irritability to Maintain the Status Quo

In our culture, unfortunately, the usual approach to perimenopausal symptoms such as mood changes and irritability is to prescribe something to soothe us and make us feel better. We seldom ask ourselves—and certainly our doctors rarely ask—"What is out of balance that needs to be changed?" If we look to hormone replacement therapy for relief without addressing the underlying issues, then even appropriate doses of hormones may not help much.

The women who are most vulnerable to the effects of hormonal swings and have the most difficulty finding relief from hormone replacement regimens and other medication are those who have had problems with mood during menarche, postpartum, and during perimenopause.[11] If the emotional issues in their lives are not attended to, if their midlife losses are not fully grieved and released (if, in other words, they don't listen to their anger and take action), they may end up with full-blown depression—which is sometimes described as anger turned inward. Depression, in turn, is a very well documented independent risk factor for heart disease, cancer, and osteoporosis.

Emotional turmoil affects the brain and all its functions. Continuing in the same upsetting situation virtually guarantees that a woman's hormones will stay unbalanced. The longer she allows negative situations to persist, the more out of whack her hormones will become, and the more physically uncomfortable she will feel. A prescription for estrogen may stop this cycle temporarily, but the body will eventually demand that its message be heard.

DORIS: *Bypassing Anger*

Many women downplay their pain by comparing themselves to someone else who is much worse off. If unresolved, this pattern can be a setup for health problems, especially at midlife. Here's an example from my practice.

Doris was suffering from high blood pressure and slightly elevated cholesterol, both of which were getting worse as she approached the end of her menopausal transition at age fifty-two. Doris told me that her socialite mother had devoted herself to her husband and his career in an unbalanced way that led to rather significant emotional neglect of her children, who were cared for by nannies and household help. Doris had unwittingly created the same pattern with her husband, who was so caught up in his work that he simply wasn't available to her emotionally. But she would not permit herself to state her needs for emotional support to either her husband or her mother. Doris, like so many women whose lives appear relatively privileged, said to me, "I feel so selfish and foolish for feeling sorry for myself. I really have nothing to complain about. After all, there are all these women who've been raped or been victimized by incest, or whose husbands have left them penniless at midlife. I have so much to be grateful for."

I call Doris's approach the intellectual bypass—intellectual because the logical part of our brains can always come up with good reasons why we have nothing to complain about. And on the surface this may well be true. However, there's a deeper problem. Comparing our pain to that of someone else invariably takes us away from our own emotions and what we need to do about them. This is because the part of the brain that allows us to feel emotions has far richer and more complex connections with our internal organs, such as the heart and cardiovascular system, than does the area associated with logical, rational thought.[12] Comparisons keep us stuck in our intellect. It's not enough to simply think about our feelings or talk about them. Remember, the word *emotion* contains the word *motion* within it! Our feelings are meant to move us.

Healing doesn't take place until we surrender to our feelings and allow them to wash over us. Doris won't be able to create full cardiovascular health until she allows herself to feel how painful it is to have a husband who is emotionally unavailable to her, a situation that mirrors so many aspects of her childhood. When she finally surrenders to the grief and rage that have been bottled up for years, first during her childhood and again during her marriage, she will be on her way to creating not only cardiovascular health, but the gift of a healed life as well. She will find that hiding behind her grief and rage are desires and dreams that have been patiently waiting for years to find expression.

EMOTIONS, HORMONES, AND YOUR HEALTH

Your emotions, desires, and dreams are your inner guidance system. They alone will let you know whether you are living in an environment of biochemical health or in an environment of biochemical distress. Understanding how your thoughts and your emotions affect every single hormone and cell in your body, and knowing how to change them in a way that is health-enhancing, gives you access to the most powerful and empowering health-creating secret on earth.

Natural foods, supplements, herbs, meditation, acupuncture, and so on are all powerful tools for building and protecting your health. But regardless of what supplements you take and what kind of exercise you do, when all is said and done it is your attitude, your beliefs, and your daily thought patterns that have the most profound effect on your health. How many times have you heard someone say, "I don't understand it—she always ate right and exercised. How come she, of all people, got sick?" On the other end of the spectrum is the person who smokes cigarettes and drinks too much alcohol, yet lives without any apparent illness well into healthy old age. The answer lies at least in part in the individual's attitudes and emotions. Attitudes and beliefs also influence how well your food is digested and how effective your exercise is. You have, within you, the power to create a life of joy, abundance, and health, or you have the same ability to create a life filled with stress, fatigue, and disease. With very few exceptions, the choice is yours.

Specific Emotional Patterns Are Associated with Specific Illnesses in Specific Parts of the Body

It has now been scientifically documented that specific patterns of emotional vulnerability affect specific organs or systems of the body.

There are dozens of medical studies on breast cancer alone showing that feelings of powerlessness in important relationships and an inability to express the full range of emotions raise the risk of developing breast cancer and lower survival rates from it. Similarly, dozens of studies have suggested that difficulties in handling negative emotions, especially hostility, are linked to sudden death from heart attack.[13] Beyond these are literally hundreds of studies showing that lack of social support, loss of or separation from one's family, or difficulties balancing a feeling of belonging with a sense of independence can affect the immune system and increase susceptibility to infection and autoimmune diseases.

Clinical practitioners have known for hundreds of years that the connection between emotions and states of health is direct and powerful. Amazingly, our outward-focused, cause-and-effect, data-driven culture simply ignored the evidence. Even as late as the 1970s, the pioneering work of scientists such as Walter B. Cannon and Hans Selye, who did groundbreaking research on stress and the mind/body connection, was not accepted in the mainstream. It was scientifically accurate and compelling, but our culture simply wasn't ready for it.

We midlife women *are* ready, and we have the perfect opportunity right now to live this knowledge for ourselves, while also sparking the fire of change in the culture at large.

Our state of health and happiness depends more upon our perception of life events around us than upon the events themselves. This is a truth that our culture does not teach. Instead, we are taught from an early age that our health is largely the result of our genetic heritage, whether or not we've been immunized, how many supplements we take, and how much exercise we get. There is no doubt that these factors can contribute to our state of health. But their influence pales in comparison to the power of our beliefs and attitudes.

How Your Thoughts and Perceptions Become Biochemical Realities in Your Body

Your autonomic nervous system is the system that helps transform your thoughts and emotions into the physical environment that,

over time, becomes your actual physical body. This part of the nervous system, which also governs the day-to-day activity of all your
internal organs, is divided into two parts: the *parasympathetic* nervous system and the *sympathetic* nervous system. These two systems
innervate every organ of your body, including your eyes, tear ducts,
salivary glands, blood vessels, sweat glands, heart, larynx, trachea,
bronchi, lungs, stomach, adrenals, kidneys, pancreas, intestines, bladder, and external genitalia.

In general terms, the parasympathetic nervous system (PNS) is
the brake in your body. It promotes functions associated with growth
and restoration, rest and relaxation, and deals primarily with conservation of bodily energy by causing your vital organs to "rest" when
they are not "on duty."

In contrast to the PNS, the sympathetic nervous system (SNS) is
the gas. It revs up your metabolism to deal with challenges from outside the body. Stimulation of the SNS quickly mobilizes your body's
reserves so that you can protect and defend yourself. This is where
the fabled fight-or-flight mechanism kicks in: Your eyes dilate, the
rate and force of your heart's contractions increase, and your blood
vessels constrict, so your blood pressure rises. Blood is borrowed
from the intestinal reservoir and shunted to your major muscles,
lungs, heart, and brain, preparing you for battle. Bowel and bladder
function shut down temporarily, conserving energy needed to power
your muscles, whether you choose to stay and fight or run away.
(This is the exact opposite of the PNS's function, which is to constrict
the pupils, slow the heart, make the bowels move, and relax the bladder and rectal sphincters.)

Since the parasympathetic nervous system deals primarily with
restoration and conservation of bodily energy and the resting of vital
organs, any activity or thought pattern that engages the PNS puts deposits into your health bank. Conversely, SNS action makes withdrawals from that bank.

It is at this point that perception becomes so important. What is
experienced in the body as a challenge from outside—a stressor—will
vary from person to person, influenced by each individual's past history, childhood, family background, diet, job, and activities at the
moment. Many midlife women live in a state of constant anxiety
overload, much of which is a side effect of the culture around us. We
want to be good women. We want to do what is right. But the culture
around us is changing so fast, and the information overload that it
generates is so huge that we easily become overwhelmed and confused, dancing faster and faster just to keep up. Not knowing what to

choose, and what to avoid, we give our bodies mixed signals. We may step on the gas and the brake at the same time. Or we may let the gas get stuck in the on position, living in a constant state of fight-or-flight—and making far too many withdrawals from the health bank.

Biologically speaking, we may be undergoing an evolutionary process that will enable our species to handle all this stress more gracefully and healthfully. Frankly, I believe that the multimodal brain of the midlife woman is leading the way. We've always had to be able to do at least three tasks at once. And now, at midlife, when the dictates of our souls make themselves known more fully than ever, we wake up to discover that our brains and bodies are being re-tooled to facilitate this beautifully.

Stress and Your Temperament

Scientific studies have found a link between temperament, personality, and the ability to deal with stressors. Have you noticed that some people, regardless of what happens to them in their lives, seem to be happy, while some are down even when life seems to be on the upswing? Or that others are anxious or fearful even when they're safe and secure? To a degree, we are born with one of these temperaments, and there is evidence of measurable *biological* differences that go along with each temperament. For example, Stephen Porges, M.D., has found that each individual has—from birth—his/her own characteristic balance between the PNS and SNS, resulting in what is known as "vagal tone."[14] Your individual balance is visible on a type of EKG (electrocardiogram) and illustrates how your heart rate coordinates with your breathing rate, yielding valuable information about your metabolic balance and inherent resilience to stress. Porges has found that, even in premature babies, those who have higher vagal tone, meaning that their parasympathetic nervous system is more activated, are less stressed by external events in the nursery (such as being handled and having IVs started) than are babies with low vagal tone. He has also observed that the personality characteristics that go along with high vagal tone are happy, resilient, and trusting *vs.* low tone, which are melancholy, anxious, fearful, and down, tendencies that follow each individual throughout life. These differences are also reflected in genetic differences in the body's ability to metabolize adrenaline!

This explains much about our individual responses to life situations. For instance, it has been clearly shown that one patient may feel great stress while undergoing a relatively simple medical procedure, while a much more difficult procedure might cause little stress in another patient. However, it is also true that the same person may respond minimally to an experience at one time, and then have a massive physiological response to the same experience at another time. This is why attempts to rate stressors are not very useful. A study by Charles B. Nemeroff, M.D., Ph.D., at Emory University School of Medicine found that women who were sexually or physically abused in childhood, compared to those without this history, show very exaggerated physiological responses in later life to stresses like giving a speech or solving arithmetic problems in front of others. They are also at greater risk for depression, anxiety disorders, and other emotional illnesses later in life.[15] Given the large number of women with a history of abuse of some kind, it is not surprising that so many women have mood and other problems during perimenopause.

One of the worst things people can do to themselves is beat themselves up for their inherent temperament or pattern of response to stress. That's why I don't want to suggest that there is some gold standard of emotions that is ideal. This would be no different from telling women they should strive for an ideal weight, height, dress size, and so on. Besides, each temperament appears to predispose people to certain types of genius. If you spent your life wishing you had a "healthier" kind of temperament, for example, you would not be embracing your full genius or taking full advantage of your natural gifts.

How Menopausal Emotions Affect Our Health

Imbalances between the sympathetic and parasympathetic nervous systems, combined with the changing hormonal milieu of menopause, can increase our body's susceptibility to symptoms or disease. The thymus (which creates your immune system's T cells), the lymph nodes (which create your immune system's B cells), and the bone marrow (which creates your red and white blood cells) are all innervated by the autonomic nervous system. Therefore, each area that creates immune system cells has both a gas pedal (sympathetic tone) and a brake pedal (parasympathetic tone).

Why is this important? Because it is via this system that your body records and processes your emotions and the hormones and neurochemicals they promote. As I've noted, if you have a backlog of unprocessed emotions, they are going to surface around the time of menopause. As a result, your susceptibility to illness may increase. Over time, if the fear-driven fight-or-flight response is triggered again and again, you can fall victim to diabetes, hypertension, or possibly even an autoimmune disease such as lupus or rheumatoid arthritis. Where you are affected will be determined by the weakest link in your body, the place where your genetic structure plus your child-hood programming and beliefs have made you most vulnerable.

The bottom line is that whatever goes on in your mind has well-documented effects on every cell in your body via either parasympathetic or sympathetic nervous system activity.[16] Every thought and every perception you have changes the homeostasis of your body. Will it be the brakes or the accelerator, a health account deposit or a health account withdrawal? This, in a nutshell, is how your autonomic nervous system translates how you view your world into the state of your health.

How Thoughts Affect Hormone Levels at Menopause

The "language" spoken by your autonomic nervous system is translated to the rest of your body by hormones. The primary messengers of the sympathetic nervous system are hormones called norepinephrine and epinephrine, which are often referred to together as adrenaline. They are produced in the brain and in the adrenal glands. Every time adrenaline levels go up, levels of another adrenal hormone, cortisol, also go up.

While cortisol provides a much-needed boost in the short run, helping you get through an occasional crisis, it has its dark side. If you live in the SNS's "fast lane" for a long time, prolonged elevation of cortisol can cause a number of problems. Initially cortisol sparks up your immune system, but if stress keeps the body in a constant state of fight-or-flight readiness, cortisol's effects on the immune system quickly become a liability. White blood cells get dumped into the bloodstream, flooding the system with germ-fighting warriors. Over time, the immune system and the bone marrow become depleted. Long-term overexposure to cortisol causes your skin to become thin, your bones to become weaker, your muscles and connective tissue to break down, your body to develop abnormal insulin metabolism, your tissues to retain fluids, your arms and legs to bruise more easily, and your moods to tend toward depression.

If you persist in the perception that events and demands in your life are stressful and uncontrollable, you are adopting the mindset that continually whips your adrenals into producing more and more cortisol. Over time, your adrenals may become exhausted, losing their ability to keep up with the demand for increasing amounts of this hormone. This is often coupled with suboptimal nutrition, impaired digestion, and poor assimilation of nutrients, all of which go hand in hand with a stressful life. The resulting immune system incompetence increases susceptibility not only to infectious diseases, but also to autoimmune disorders and all cancers.

The overstimulated sympathetic nervous system also causes an imbalance in a group of hormones known as eicosanoids, resulting in impairment of the cells' ability to metabolize fatty acids. This is associated with weight gain, as the body tends to break down muscle and replace it with stored fat and excess fluid. Imbalanced eicosanoids are also associated with tissue inflammation, which increases the discomfort felt in a host of chronic diseases such as lupus and rheumatoid arthritis. They have also been shown to increase the speed of tumor growth in individuals already harboring cancer.

In a healthy, normal body, cortisol levels are highest upon awakening in the morning. During the night, the parasympathetic nervous system has done its job of providing rest and renewal to your organs. In other words, a deposit has been made into the "health bank." The morning's increased cortisol levels help you get out of bed and get ready for the day ahead. As you wind down in the evening, cortisol levels normally decrease, reaching their lowest at about midnight, easing you into a rejuvenative, restful night. For many stressed-out women, however, the rise-and-fall pattern of cortisol secretion begins to invert itself. Levels are lower in the morning, affording little or no "gas in the tank" to start the day, and they're higher at midnight, making it virtually impossible to wind down and rest.

It does not end there. In addition to causing deranged output of cortisol, overstimulation of the sympathetic nervous system also causes decreased production of progesterone, one of your body's natural calming agents. The result is that women who are chronically stressed also tend toward hormonal imbalance between estrogen, progesterone, and testosterone (which is important in women as well as in men).

Soothing Your Emotions Before They Become Disease

First of all, there is nothing to be gained by categorizing emotions as "good" or "bad." Instead, think of them as guidance. The emotions that feel good are guiding you toward health, while the ones that feel bad are trying to get your attention so that you can change either your perception or your behavior. It truly is as simple as that.

Emotions can also become toxic if they are allowed to persist unresolved, rather than being worked through fully and released. Consider, for example, the woman who lost a child and fifteen years later, now well into menopause, still hasn't moved anything in that child's room, keeping it exactly as it was the day the child died. The emotions that drive her to enshrine that room—the unresolved grief, the refusal to move forward in life, the denial—are toxic. They have not only robbed her of fifteen years of life, but also are setting her up for physical illness, especially given the intensity with which our unresolved baggage from the past arises at menopause.

The ill health and pain you may experience at midlife are not caused by difficult emotions per se, but rather by a willingness to let those emotions persist unresolved—or by a misperception of what they mean in your life. Unresolved, "stuck" emotions keep setting up the same body biochemistry over and over again. The effect of emotions on our bodies can be likened to water in a river. Our bodies stay clean and fresh as long as our emotions keep flowing, triggering changes in our perception and behavior. The minute that water stagnates, all manner of decay and germs start to flourish.

One of my menopausal patients arrived at a wonderful insight. She began to realize that whenever she feels happy, she also begins to feel nervous, because it is her perception that whenever good things happen in her life, she has to leave behind past aspects of her life that have supported her. Getting a promotion at work, for example, had always been tainted with pangs of regret, because she knew that moving up changed the dynamics of her old relationships. The people she had been friends with before didn't accept her in the same way anymore. I have certainly had the same experience in my own life. The silver lining in that cloud, however, is that by allowing yourself to continually move toward ever-increasing success and joy, you attract new friends and circumstances that support you fully for who you are becoming. The key for this woman is to focus on all the good that has come from allowing herself to become happier and more successful.

Focusing on the positive side of a situation can have a powerful effect on our health. Dr. Bernie Siegel tells a story about a patient who overheard doctors say that he had a "gallop rhythm" in his heart. A gallop rhythm is a dangerous condition, but this patient thought it meant that his heart was as strong as a horse. Because of that perception, the patient's overall status improved dramatically, and he got out of the coronary intensive care unit in record time.

Again, however, beware the oversimplification that "happiness" is good and "sadness" is bad. Both emotions are necessary to function as a normal human being. Without sadness, the experience of happiness would lose its sweetness. The healthy way is to strive for a balance of emotional chemicals in your body that support health, and to have those emotions wash in and out like the tides of the sea. Just as the tides are essential for cleansing the ocean, our emotions cleanse our mind and body. At midlife, sadness and regrets from our past may take on a heightened role for a time, helping us to truly clean out the silted-up river bottoms of our emotional lives, thus setting the stage for more fulfillment and joy to come in.

Are We Responsible for Our Health?

Critics of the mind/body connection say that focusing on the emotional dimension of illness makes people feel worse when they are already vulnerable, as though they are guilty of causing their own disease. I agree that there is the potential to carry this philosophy too far and blame ourselves for ill health. However, the value of the mind/body connection is too great to discard. The simple truth is that the people who heal fastest and remain healthiest the longest are those who feel that their lives are fulfilling and joyful. Even when they're sick, they feel that their life has meaning and that they have some locus of control. Those who think, "The world is doing it to me.... There's nothing I can do about it.... I can't get a break.... The world is out to get me.... This is just the way the world is," et cetera, are disempowered by their thoughts and perceptions. This directly contributes to an imbalance in the autonomic nervous system and associated hormonal systems. Twenty years of medical practice have shown me so clearly that emotions are the primary energy at work, tipping the scales one way or the other, toward illness or toward health, and that the victim mentality from adverse childhood programming is at the root of many illnesses. Cellular biologist Bruce Lipton, Ph.D., has documented the most recent and groundbreaking research on the profound impact of our beliefs on our states of health in his book, *The Biology of Belief* (Mountain of Love/Elite Books, 2005). In almost every case, beliefs are more powerful than genes. In fact, belief and perception control how genes are expressed!

Despite what we learn daily about healthy exercise practices, healthy diets, and good medical care, the bottom line is that the most significant way of contributing to our own good health is through the quality of our thought processes. This power is a valuable gift, in light of the absolute lack of control we have over other aspects of life. Think about being on a turbulent flight in bad weather. You have no control over the winds, or the skills or the mental state of the pilot flying the plane. But you do have the power to minimize your discomfort. You can decide to read a book, strike up a conversation with the person next to you, take your antioxidants, wrap up in a warm blanket, sleep, listen to music, or watch the movie. Alternatively, you can listen to every engine noise and allow yourself to be debilitated by worry the entire flight. It's your choice.

Ultimately, you are the only one who can make significant deposits into your health bank account. This is not the job of your doctor, your nutritionist, your lover, or your parents. There is no supplement, no health care provider, and no exotic herb that can possibly do for you what you can do for yourself.

The key is compassion for yourself. The well-known therapist Gay Hendricks has noted that any area of pain, blame, or shame in our lives is there because we have not loved that part of ourselves enough. No matter what you're feeling, the only way to get a difficult feeling to go away is simply to love yourself for it. If you think you're stupid, then love yourself for feeling that way. It's a paradox, but it works. To heal, you must be the first one to shine the light of compassion on any areas within you that you feel are unacceptable (and we've all got them). The hormonal shifts you experience around the time of menopause can facilitate this.

HOW OUR MIDLIFE BRAINS AND BODIES
ARE SET UP TO HEAL OUR PAST

Though memories are distributed throughout the body and the brain, certain areas of the brain, notably the amygdala and hippocampus, are especially important for the encoding and retrieving of memories. Interestingly, these areas of the brain are particularly rich in receptors for estrogen, progesterone, and GnRH, the hormones that fluctuate the most during the perimenopausal years. Given the

FIGURE 5: WHY TRAUMATIC MEMORIES MAY BE
RELIVED AT MIDLIFE

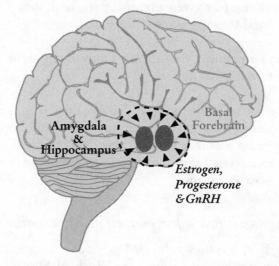

The brain's memory centers are rich in receptors for the hormones that fluctuate in perimenopause.

heightened activity of these hormones in these areas, it makes sense that memory activation and retrieval would be enhanced during the years immediately surrounding menopause.[17] Hurts and losses we've managed to forget or minimize for many years, even decades, may suddenly become overwhelming—even if we think we should be "over" all that pain from the past.

CHRISTINE: *Midlife Brings Self-Healing*

On the tenth anniversary of the day she was raped, Christine wrote, she awoke with a greater rush of energy than ever before. These torrents of feeling had become increasingly powerful as she advanced through perimenopause, like exaggerations of the hormonal crests and troughs of the monthly cycles she described as "like PMS times ten." Uncomfortable physical symptoms increasingly accompanied these waves, as her body begged for attention to the wounds left by her sexual assault.

Headaches, body aches, queasiness, insomnia, anxiety attacks, diarrhea, toothaches, and many other symptoms manifested themselves along the way to my recovery again and again. Over time, I learned to quiet myself and fully experience what I was feeling as each of these "illnesses" struck me. Each time, strong emotions came up and were eventually released, sometimes within minutes—and the symptoms disappeared.

Christine's openness to the messages being sent by her body helped facilitate her healing.

The most incredible insight that became clear to me during the process of discharge, release, and healing that occurred time and time again was that I am my own healer. It was amazing to me how interrelated my emotions were with the various symptoms I was experiencing.

SUSAN: *Standing Up for Herself at Menopause*

At forty-five, Susan wrote, "Menopause for me is the courage and push I've needed all of my life." Both of Susan's parents were weekend alcoholics, and while they "partied," she and her brother took care of their younger sisters. She left home at eighteen to marry.

Naturally I married an alcoholic, but I didn't know it until years later. The relationship was very controlling and abusive—mentally, emotionally, and physically. He controlled my every decision, from when I could see my family to where I worked, what furniture to buy, what cars I drove, and the decision to not have children. I convinced myself that we had a wonderful, close relationship. We became my parents, partying and drinking on weekends just like they did—I drank to keep my husband company and to be "part of" something. I also started smoking up to two packs a day. When I became pregnant at age thirty, he convinced me to get an abortion, saying he was under too much pressure, promising we'd try again the following year. Instead, he had an affair. I hung in there, and eventually he ended it and came back to me. I took this to be proof positive that he truly loved me.

Four years later Susan sought couples therapy, but at the last minute her husband refused to go. Rather than cancel, she went alone. Through her counselor, she started attending meetings of Adult Children of Alcoholics and Al-Anon, where she learned that she was not alone. This marked the beginning of a new life for her. For Susan, the first major milestone was talking about her abortion. Next she quit smoking. "That opened up a whole new world for me. I no longer had to stuff my feelings and light up a cigarette. I had a mouthpiece. I had something to say, and oh, I said a *lot*—I had diarrhea of the mouth. And such honesty!" Then she quit drinking. "My husband didn't like this new me at all. I no longer was a party girl, at his beck and call."

As Susan changed, she felt herself being torn in two, because the life around her, the life her husband had laid out for her, was not changing at all. "I became a married woman living a single life. We no longer went anywhere or did anything with each other." There were a series of attempts at marriage counseling, separation, reconciliation, and alcoholism therapy for him, all to no avail. Then came the ultimate boost—menopause! Susan wrote: "I became perimenopausal at forty-two. I really feel this gave me the courage and the push and the honesty to look at my life with an eye for what I wanted and needed." She started doing "so many things I've been wanting to do and never did." Eventually she filed for divorce and started the life she'd always wanted to have, three thousand miles away from her native New York. "I had such an easy transition," she marveled. "I walked away from my whole life there—husband, job, friends, and all but the few things I packed when I left—but I guess I did my grieving while I lived in the marriage. My life is so full today."

The primary defense against unpleasant memories and emotions is avoidance. This subterfuge often works reasonably well until the perimenopausal transition, when the hormonal shift of focus and accompanying changes in brain activity conspire to call buried traumas and unresolved issues into the light, expressing them through physical symptoms that cannot be ignored. Whatever causes a woman's lingering wounds, perimenopause can be seen as a built-in support system that sets her up to do deep healing and reclaiming of the treasure within. Although it may not be seen this way at first, it is a gift.

In addition to providing the clarity and courage to face past abuses or pain, menopause can help a woman step back, acknowledge the necessity to change, and do whatever is necessary to separate herself from long-term destructive life patterns. Even the most deeply ingrained patterns can be changed with the support of menopause-induced shifts in the brain, energy, and focus. Sometimes the most effective way to make these changes is to begin adding pleasurable activities that you've always wanted to do, e.g., manicures, pedicures, dancing lessons, etc.

Caution: Reinforcing Past Trauma

The disturbing memories and the depression that so often arise at menopause are much less scary and disabling if we see them for what they are. They are evidence that we are now strong enough, deep within, to allow the pain and secrets of the past to rise to the surface and be cleared out once and for all. The midlife investigation and release of the painful patterns from the past is necessary if you are to truly heal. Trust your brain and body to give you the information you need to handle when you're prepared to handle it. You don't need to dwell on it. Think of it as an emotional "catch and release" program.

It is valuable to have someone else witness and validate your pain. Many people have found that it was not just the painful experience itself that was so wounding to them as children, but also the fact that there was no one to whom they could safely turn, no one who could understand or validate their reality at the time.

You may choose to work with a therapist, and you may also consider a course of medication to deal with the sleep problems, anxiety, or panic that may arise. However, note that many antianxiety drugs are highly addictive. Far too many women have been put on drugs such as Xanax or Valium during their menopausal transition, only to find themselves dependent on them for the rest of their lives. If you're willing to work in therapy and make the requisite changes in your life, you probably won't need to remain on medication for more than six months to two years. (See chapter 10, "Nurturing Your Brain," for more information on prescription medications and over-the-counter alternatives.)

While I cannot outline the course of recovery in detail here, I do want to caution you about one pitfall: some forms of therapy actually reinforce negative patterns both in your brain and your body. These include "reliving" the trauma repeatedly and digging for buried memories. Here's why: Significant stress of any kind, including the reexperiencing of past painful memories, is associated with high levels of cortisol. This is the very hormonal milieu that increases the likelihood of laying down memories of all kinds, especially traumatic ones, which are mediated through an area of the brain known as the amygdala.[18]

If you are a highly sensitive or suggestible individual, receptive to mental imagery, and you have a lot of cortisol in your bloodstream (as when you're stressed), it is very possible for you to incorporate new traumatic "memories" into your brain and body that have no basis in your past experiences. Instead, they may be the product of your current environment, combined with the suggestions and imagery you picked up from a well-meaning therapist. For example, if a therapist asks you, "Did your father rape you when you were three?" and you are in a susceptible biological state, your brain may simply incorporate the question as fact—"My father raped me when I was three"—whether or not that actually happened. This scenario may then be encoded as a new trauma memory—one that you'll have to cope with on top of the original memories that have arisen on their own.

Ultimately, make it your goal to move on to forgiveness of yourself and those involved in causing you pain in the past. Forgiveness doesn't mean that what happened to you was acceptable. It simply means that you are no longer willing to allow a past injury to keep you from living fully and healthfully in the present.

FINDING A LARGER MEANING

In some cultures, such as that of Hindu India, midlife is a time associated with the serious pursuit of the spiritual dimensions of life. I see something comparable occurring in this country, where the vast majority of attendees at conferences on the connection between the body and soul are midlife women. With our child-rearing years behind us, our creative energies are freed. Our search for life's meaning begins to take on new urgency, and we begin to experience ourselves as potential vessels for Spirit. I've long believed that each of our lives is directed by a force that I think of as God. This force is much bigger than our own intellects, and it always moves us toward our highest possible purpose, working directly through the unique expression that each of us represents. My lifelong interest in metaphysics and astrology has provided me with very clear evidence for this truth.

Barbara Hand Clow, an author who specializes in using astrology to give us more access to our power, explains that all of us must go through several key life passages in order to reach our full wisdom. Each passage is associated with very specific and predictable shifts that, if negotiated consciously, open us to our full potential. In her 1996 book, *Liquid Light of Sex: Kundalini Rising at Mid-Life Crisis,* Clow writes, "We *form* at age 30, we *transform* at age 40, and we *transmute* at age 50."[19]

Around age forty, the universal energy known as kundalini (which is depicted as a snake in many ancient healing traditions) begins to rise naturally and gradually from the base of our spines, activating

THE SEVEN EMOTIONAL-ENERGY CENTERS
The Physical Effect of Mental
and Emotional Patterns

Emotional Center	Organs	Mental, Emotional Issues
7	Can involve any system	Ability to sense or trust in life's purpose Connection to God or universal source of energy Ability to balance responsibility for life events with acceptance of things we cannot control
6	Brain Eyes Ears Nose Pineal gland	Perception: clarity vs. ambiguity Thought: left brain vs. right brain; rational vs. nonrational Morality: conservative vs. liberal; social rules vs. individual conscience Repression vs. lack of inhibition
5	Thyroid Trachea Neck vertebrae Throat, mouth, teeth, and gums	Communication: expression vs. comprehension (speaking vs. listening) Timing: pushing forward vs. waiting Will: willful vs. compliant
4	Heart, lungs Blood vessels Shoulders Ribs, breasts Diaphragm Upper esophagus	Emotional expression: capacity to feel fully, express joy and love, resolve anger, hostility, and grief; experience forgiveness Relationships: capacity to form mutual reciprocal partnerships with balance of nurturing of self vs.

Emotional Center	Organs	Mental, Emotional Issues
		nurturing of others; intimacy with others vs. capacity to be alone
3	Abdomen Upper intestines Liver, gallbladder Lower esophagus Stomach Kidney, pancreas Adrenal gland Spleen Middle spine	Self-esteem, self-confidence, and self-acceptance Personal power; competence and skills in the outer world Overresponsibility vs. irresponsibility Addictions to sugar, alcohol, drugs, and tobacco Aggression vs. defensiveness Competitiveness vs. noncompetitiveness; winning vs. losing
2	Uterus, ovaries Vagina, cervix Large intestine Lower vertebrae Pelvis Appendix Bladder	Personal power: sex, money, and relationships Fertility and generativity: individual creativity; co-creation with others Boundaries in relationships: dependency vs. independence; giving vs. taking; assertiveness vs. passivity
1	Muscles, bones Spine Blood Immune system	Safety/security in the world; knowing when to trust or mistrust Knowing when to feel fear and when not to Balance between independence and dependence

Sources: C. N. Shealy and C. M. Myss, *The Creation of Health: Merging Traditional Medicine with Intuitive Diagnosis* (Walpole, NH: Stillpoint Publications, 1988). Scientific documentation of the human energy system and updated information from Mona Lisa Schulz, M.D., Ph.D., *Awakening Intuition: Using Your Mind-Body Network for Insight and Healing* (New York: Harmony Books, 1998).

FIGURE 6: EMOTIONAL ANATOMY

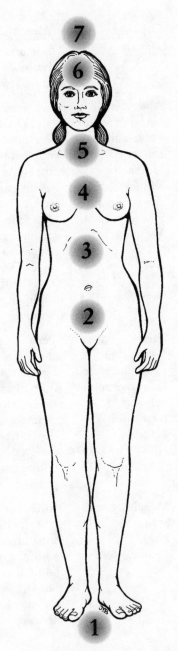

The connection between emotions and physical anatomy comes together in the seven emotional centers. These correspond roughly to traditional energy maps of the body that delineate seven energetic centers or chakras.

each energy center (or chakra) of our bodies as it does so. Sometimes the resulting sexual energy that is released at this time can be quite intense, driving some women to have affairs or to channel this energy into painting, building a new home, or some other creative pursuit.

This energy activation may also manifest in bodily symptoms. The degree of unfinished business we have in each of these energy centers will determine the type and severity of symptoms we will experience in that area. For example, I personally experienced several bouts of rather severe chest pain in the year when I started to skip periods and have hot flashes, an indication of grief and despair, emotions of which I hadn't been fully conscious. Many other women find themselves feeling heart palpitations, anxiety, pelvic pain, or indigestion at midlife.

When we reframe our symptoms and see them as our inner guidance knocking on the door of each emotional center, asking us to allow more light and wisdom into that particular area, then we don't feel victimized by our bodies and we have the opportunity to feel empowered by the life energy that is coursing through us at midlife.

For example, my divorce culminated during what is astrologically known as my Chiron return, the peak time for me to transmute and connect more powerfully than ever with my spirit and my life purpose. Simultaneously I had been under the influence of an astrological configuration known as a yod, which means "the finger of God." The purpose of this was to move me out of my old life so that I had the time and motivation to create new, healthier relationships— which I eventually formed. Though this knowledge did not entirely free me from the suffering I went through, I took great comfort in knowing that there was a larger purpose and meaning in the events that coincided with perimenopause—that my experience amounted to something more than a painful divorce and the onset of hot flashes.

3

Coming Home to Yourself: From Dependence to Healthy Autonomy

The need and desire to assume more dominion over our lives becomes a burning issue at menopause. Suddenly we find ourselves questioning the meaning and value of many of the relationships that we'd never dared to look at too closely before. Although we all want to maintain the relationships that support us at the deepest levels, we often discover that our old ways of feeling or behaving with those closest to us—whether parents, children, spouses, friends, or bosses—need updating. And anytime we update our lives, we have to grieve for the old life that has been lost. Having the courage both to embrace the necessary changes of midlife and to feel the loss that is associated with those changes is a crucial part of creating a firm foundation for health in the second half of our lives.

THE EMPTY-NEST SYNDROME

You don't have to be a mother to experience the empty nest, that aching sense of personal loss, loneliness, and limbo that so often results when your life undergoes significant change. No matter how secure and settled a woman may feel prior to midlife, the transformative passage into the second half of life almost invariably involves an exodus of some kind. Whether it's the final breakup with a husband from whom you have long been estranged, career changes or reversals, the departure of children who have come of age and left home to start lives of their own—lives that no longer include you as an everyday presence or necessity—or all of the above, when your once-bustling home becomes quiet and/or your daily routine suddenly changes and leaves you feeling at loose ends, the experience is not unlike the unexpected death of a loved one. And even if you saw it coming and thought you were prepared for it—even if, in fact, you are the one doing the leaving—it's painful. This is because it's impossible to fully prepare for the kind of upheaval that is so profound, it holds the potential to completely transform you from the inside out.

One of my friends, a woman who has managed to maintain a high-powered corporate career while also raising two children, recently told me, "When my youngest left for college this fall, I was very busy consulting with a wealthy, creative upscale company, which sent me on frequent trips overseas. Though my days were full of excitement, newness, and adventure, I nevertheless found myself bursting into tears at stoplights while driving. I sometimes feel as though a part of my heart has been ripped out of my chest. After all those years of purposeful and fierce mothering, always managing to put my children first in spite of my career, I have been surprised at how very physical and painful this loss feels. And there was no way I saw it coming."

I can relate completely. As a sneak preview into my own empty-nest scenario, my younger child left home the summer before her senior year of high school for a month at camp, just two weeks after my firstborn left for another summer program in preparation for starting college in the fall. With my husband gone and the divorce nearly complete, this marked the first time in my life since college and medical school that I had been truly alone in my house. For a while it felt okay. My house was cleaner than it had been in years (not that this was ever a goal of mine), and the freedom from other people's chaos was a pleasant side effect as I began the process of re-creating the house on my terms. I ate whatever and whenever I wanted, worked whenever I felt like it, lit candles, and watched movies late into the night. I slowly began to enjoy the opportunity to be still and contemplate my life without interruption. After all, I told myself, I wasn't really alone. My daughters would be home soon enough.

But I had a head-on collision with grief and loneliness a month later. I'd picked up my younger daughter at camp, and together we had driven to Dartmouth for a tour, since she was beginning to contemplate her college options. As my medical school alma mater, not to mention the place where I first met my husband, Dartmouth held many fond memories for me. I remembered vividly the exhilaration I'd felt on arriving twenty-eight years before, when I was completely smitten by the place. Now I was standing on that same campus, a fifty-year-old, newly divorced mom watching the second of her two children make plans for her own life. I was facing not only the loss of my husband and my daughters, but also of all the dreams I'd had for my future. During the three-hour drive home, my daughter slept the whole way, and I realized with surprise that I felt even more lonely than I had when she was gone.

Back at home the next morning, I awoke feeling acutely grief-stricken, and I said to myself, "Ah, this is the empty-nest feeling I've heard about, the feeling that says, 'You're not at home in your new world, and your old world no longer fits you.'" I was in limbo, aching for what was and for what might have been. Intellectually I knew this was a growth phase, a kind of labor pain that would yield wonderful things if I could just allow myself to go through it. (It helped to know that I didn't really have a choice.) Rather than smooth it over and find mind-numbing ways to spare myself the anguish, I let myself feel it. I was lonely, disappointed, heartbroken, and scared, and I sat on my bed and cried for everything about my life that was dying.

But there is good news, too. Anyone who has undergone the emotional upheaval of midlife changes can tell you that though the painful feelings associated with the empty nest arise again and again, over time they come less often, their stay is briefer, and their pain penetrates less deeply with each revisit. So our job is simply to be present with them. My own experience, and that of all the women who have shared their empty-nest experiences with me, indicates that the ultimate reward for fully participating in the emotions that wash over us at this time is that the struggle is over sooner than it would be if we tried to resist or deny them. Whether or not a woman realizes it going in, that hollow, unsettling, empty-nest experience is a blessing in disguise. Think of it as a kind of labor pain. What you are trying to give birth to is your new life, which your hormones, your brain, and your body have already welcomed and embraced, even though you may not yet be consciously aware of it. To create a renewed life, it is necessary to go into the abyss, into the emptiness you may have spent a lifetime using relationships and busyness to avoid. Having looked into the abyss myself, I can understand why a woman entering it might find the prospect of a positive outcome very difficult to believe in. But now that I have come out on the other side, I know the journey was worth the pain.

PATRICIA: *Delaying the Inevitable*

Many women do everything in their power to try to resist change and transformation, often retreating into the kind of nurturing and caretaking they've participated in for their whole lives. They spend precious energy trying to keep vital life changes at bay, in essence paddling upstream rather than letting the current carry them into new, uncharted waters. Often their fear of going forward is so great that it leads to a step backward instead.

After raising five children, Patricia came to a crossroads that took her completely by surprise.

My husband always ruled the roost, made all the decisions— what groceries to buy, which children helped with which chores, what color to paint my kitchen—and over the years I learned to deal with it by clamming up and withdrawing into the world I'd created with my kids. When our youngest left home, it hit me like a ton of bricks: it was just me and him. I'd frankly never even thought about that before. We got along okay, but mainly because he did his thing and I did mine. Whenever our purposes crossed, I was submissive and compliant—it had become my habit, and it was easier. Now that the kids were all out of the house, I suddenly realized that this could be my time for *me*. But my husband had never allowed it before; I knew he wouldn't allow it now.

Marriage counseling and divorce were taboo subjects in her husband's family, and Patricia realized that she was unwilling to make further concessions in order to "color within the lines" of the way he'd sketched their lives. Instead she decided to avoid the unacceptable future by trying to re-create the past. At the age of forty-seven, she talked him into adopting a baby girl.

I didn't realize it consciously at the time, but looking back, I guess I knew the baby would spare me from having to put our marriage under lights. I wanted to set the clock back. Going forward was too scary. In some ways it did the trick—it kept me occupied. But even though raising children was my joy in my younger years, I realized—too late—that I'd changed. Devoting my life to children was my past life. Now, in my mid-fifties, I know it's not at all what I want to do at this stage in my life. I'm so tired all the time that I feel sedated, and it's not that it's such hard work physically—it's that my heart isn't in it. I feel tugged, like some force is trying to pull me away from here. I feel like I age ten years for every two. But I'm committed to this little girl now, who deserves all I can give her. I hope I can last until she's grown.

BOOMERANG BABIES

Variations on Patricia's theme are becoming more and more common, thanks to the higher-than-ever numbers of adult children who, for one reason or another, boomerang back home—often with kids of their own for Grandma to raise while they try to get their feet under them. If a woman is to claim the second half of her life for herself, to explore her own creative potential and choose the endeavors onto which she focuses her life energy, then she must find a way to stand firm against forces that could induce her to shoulder someone else's long-term responsibilities—forces such as guilt and the compulsion to shield her children from the consequences of their own choices. When decisions and outside circumstances conspire to keep the nest full, there is the strong potential for a woman's new life to become a tired rerun of the old one.

ANITA: *Finally Cutting the Cord*

When Anita and Ralph's newlywed (and pregnant) daughter and her husband rented an apartment in their complex, Anita was thrilled. But over the ensuing months something began to feel wrong.

At first I thought I was in heaven. Jenny was over here all the time, sometimes to do laundry (claiming she was perpetually having trouble with her machine and Jim didn't have time to fix it), sometimes to bum a cup of sugar, sometimes just to "hang." I thought it was great—it was as if I'd never lost my daughter. Instead of an empty nest, I had the promise of keeping her and having a new little baby around, too. But then, gradually, I started peeling back the layers of what was bothering me. I thought back to when I was a newlywed, and although I adored my folks, I didn't spend nearly as much time with them as Jenny was spending with me. I began to watch for signs of trouble in her marriage, not realizing that I already had recognized a big one—Jenny hadn't really left home yet.

A month later Jim got a promotion, which meant a transfer to the West Coast. I felt as though I'd been kicked in the stomach. Jenny is our only child, and she had been my whole life. It was to be a quick move—they had six weeks to tie up loose ends and get settled in California—but I noticed that in the midst of all the preparations for moving, Jenny started spending even more time with me.

Two weeks later there was a big fight, and the next thing I knew there she was on our doorstep, ready to move "back home," with a look on her face that was both anguished and maybe a little triumphant at the same time. She told me later that she thought I'd be pleased—she knew how much I was going to miss her. That's partly why my response really surprised her.

It was heart-wrenching for me. I hated to see my daughter hurting, her face blotched from crying and her belly beginning to show evidence of her pregnancy. But somehow, fortunately, I woke up, and none too soon. I told her that moving back was not an option. I told her it was time to move forward, not back. I realized that I needed to cut the cord and start exploring my own life, and she needed to do the same—otherwise we'd both be stuck in a phase of life that we'd outgrown.

As a woman faces the prospect of an empty nest, daunting though it may be, the bottom line is this: Separation is a necessary and, ultimately, blessed thing, clearing the way for her next developmental phase. To block that process can be akin to leaving a pot-bound plant, restricted and stunted, in a too-small container. A woman can choose to facilitate her growth, which may be initially painful, or she can choose to block that growth, a path that results in accelerated aging and loss of vitality—just as it would for that pot-bound plant. Staying in place, in other words, is not a viable option. Grow—or die.

POWERFUL FEELINGS, POWERFUL HEALING

In order to take a new path, you must leave the old path behind. This can be one of the most terrifying aspects of the midlife transformation—leaving behind what is familiar and embracing what is unknown. During the first summer after my divorce, for example, I watched my daughter and former husband pull out of the driveway one perfect summer day to go sailing together, a family activity that we had enjoyed for years. I felt left behind, wondering what had happened to my life. In fact, I felt as though, other than my work, I no longer had a real life. When we are standing at a crossroads in our lives, doubts inevitably arise. "Am I capable of pulling this off? Do I have the talent? The strength? Can I make it out there?" Or, as in my case, "What's the use of having made it out there if I have no one to come home to?" Plucked from the milieu in which she has already proven herself, and cast adrift in unfamiliar surroundings, a woman would have to be extraordinary not to be afraid. Her self-doubt may be magnified by the fact that as she faces loss, very often the path that will lead to her new life is not clear.

It is vital to a woman's comfort level to understand that the direction of her new path, and her willingness to try it, will come...in time. Those directions are, after all, already inside her. The steps that separate her old life from the new one were not meant to be easy, any more than the birth process is meant to be easy. As difficult as it is to accept, especially in our quick-fix culture, the struggle that accompanies a woman's midlife transformation appears to be an integral part of the learning process, without which she would not have the incentive to set one foot in front of the other. Your empty nest, your altered living space, your disrupted life focus, that directionless feeling—all must first be acknowledged and experienced, with the attendant emotions, in order for the healing process to begin. In the interim, while we experience the upheaval and wait for the new path to become clear, we have to hang out in the "underworld" for a while, allowing our fears and grief and confusion to be fully experienced. Then, and only then, will the fog begin to lift, revealing hints of new doors, new directions, and a new focus for that shining new life.

Well and good, you might say. But how does one go about fully experiencing powerful emotions without dwelling on them excessively or becoming engulfed in self-pity?

Identifying Your Emotions in Your Writing

There is a writing technique that has been proven effective in helping a woman acknowledge, identify, and express those feelings with focused attention, then release them proactively, on a moment-to-moment basis as they come up, unbidden. It is a skill that requires practice, but the rewards are immediate—and they only get better as your skill level grows. Here's what's involved.

Make a commitment to honor and respect your body by being willing to learn from the emotions that affect it, even if that simply means bringing your loving awareness to it. In other words, be willing to be there for your body and your emotions, just as you would for a child or anyone else you love. If you feel suddenly overwhelmed with sadness or anger, for example, choose to stop and identify that feeling, rather than simply react to it. Acknowledge it. Say to yourself, "I feel sad" or "I feel angry."

Gaze upon your sadness without trying to fix it. The essence of being a good listener—to yourself or to a dear friend—is simply allowing emotion to be expressed freely and honestly. Over time, your caring focus can change pain to compassion. Make the effort to notice your emotions and be with them rather than try to change them, shrug them off, or stuff them into a private corner. Then, once you've focused on them, take the time to write them down.

When I feel strong emotions that stop me in my tracks, I'm almost always helped by writing about the experience as soon as I can find a moment.[1] I sit down, light a candle, put on a tape of some adagio baroque music, take three breaths, and come up writing, recording my thoughts like a good secretary. When a particular thought has a certain buzz or energy associated with it, I urge myself to go deeper, asking what I mean by "sad," "angry," "irritated," or whatever. Within ten to fifteen minutes, I've generally figured out exactly what the emotion was trying to teach me as well as what old, outmoded beliefs and thoughts the emotion was based on. And, more than that, I find that the writing moves my energy to a whole new place. Then I'm in a position to shift my focus to something more pleasurable.

Identifying Your Emotions in Your Body

A related form of awareness involves tuning in to bodily sensations. When you feel the muscles in your temple tighten, for example, simply observe them, and notice how they relax because of your focused attention. Step back and try to recognize the many ways in which each emotion manifests in your body—the slump of your shoulders, the lump in your throat, the tension in your jaw muscles, the trembling weakness in your legs, the hollowness in the pit of your stomach, the congestion in your nasal passages as tears flow. Apply the healing power of your awareness to all of these sensations, the emotional and the physical. Your mindfulness first validates the emotions, then eventually clears away any blockage to your ability to be healthy and fully present in your life. The grace and beauty of this approach is that it allows your suffering to have its time, so it can then flow through and out of you, which it will do. In so doing, you are setting the stage for your own healing... and for your own ability to move on. You can also move difficult emotions through more efficiently by crying, moving, and breathing fully.

CARING FOR OURSELVES, CARING FOR OTHERS: FINDING THE BALANCE

We are all knit together by continuity of care, which is one of the feminine values that the world needs more of, not less. Yet it is also true that women's lives are sometimes unnecessarily sacrificed to this virtue.

Women of my age are often referred to as the "sandwich" generation because so many are caught between caring for their still-dependent children while increasingly being called upon to take care of elderly parents or other relatives. This is a time when our programming and our desire to be good daughters, good mothers, and good wives—roles that bring us the love and approval of others—runs headlong into the increasingly urgent need to care for ourselves and the needs of our souls. The resulting competition between those two strong but apparently conflicting desires can wreak havoc with our health if we don't examine these desires carefully and set priorities.

I've watched hundreds of women run themselves ragged at midlife trying to care for a parent with Alzheimer's, hold down a full-time job, and also run a home and family. This three-ring-circus approach to life too often contributes to health problems such as increased blood pressure and cholesterol, anxiety attacks, heart palpitations, severe hot flashes, and insomnia. In fact, research has documented that people who care for parents with chronic disease have more medical conditions requiring treatment than those who don't have this responsibility.[2]

SHARON: *Too Good for Her Own Good*

Sharon first came to see me when she was fifty-one years old, complaining of hot flashes and inability to fall asleep. When I asked her what her exercise and eating habits were like, she shrugged and said, "Who has time to exercise or eat well?" Though Sharon was about thirty pounds overweight and said she wanted to lose weight, she simply couldn't see how she was going to make the time to improve her lifestyle in any way. As I discovered, Sharon was the eldest of five siblings and the only daughter. When her mother died, she was left to care for her father, a man who, at age seventy-two, had been somewhat abusive and distant to his children for most of Sharon's life. His health had mildly deteriorated after Sharon's mother died. Though Sharon's father didn't require skilled nursing care, he did need someone to come in and cook his meals, do the laundry, and keep the house clean—tasks that had always been done by his wife.

Sharon automatically added these tasks to her own day even though her father lived about thirty minutes away from her and even though she was holding down a full-time job as a nurse, was married, and had two teenage sons still living at home. The first thing I asked Sharon was, "Where are your brothers?" She told me that two were living out of state, but two lived in the same town as their father. The obvious next question was, "Are your brothers pitching in with your father's care?" Sharon said that she couldn't really rely on them to help out. After all, they had jobs, wives, and children of their own. "Besides," she added, "they aren't very good at cooking and cleaning. Also, my father really wants me to be the one to come into his house to help out."

I pointed out to Sharon that if she didn't get some help with her caregiving and also add some pleasure to her life, chances were she was going to end up with a health problem herself. Then she wouldn't be able to help her dad at all! I've seen this many times in my practice and in my life. I also validated her fear that her brothers might be quite resistant to her need for their help and that they would be likely to resent her for a while. Her willingness to take on the whole job herself had made it quite comfortable for her brothers, a perk they weren't likely to give up easily. And her willingness to sacrifice herself for their approval brought her love, gratitude, and a sense of purpose.

Though Sharon felt victimized by her situation, it had never occurred to her to ask her brothers for help. Nor did she like hearing that suggestion from me. But when I raised the possibility that her weight problem and increased blood pressure were related to her current workload, she could see that something had to give. The first thing I advised was that Sharon take a long, hard look at her beliefs about caregiving.

Sharon, like her mother before her, truly believed that "if I don't do it, it won't get done." She had grown up in a household full of boys, none of whom cooked, cleaned, or washed dishes. She and her mother, a woman whom the family described as "a saint," did all the household work. Not surprisingly, Sharon married a man who didn't share in the household tasks, either. And her brothers all married women who were happy to stay home, like their mother, and care for their homes and children.

Unfortunately, this sort of martyrdom had already claimed Sharon's mother, who was only sixty-eight when she died of a heart attack. If Sharon wanted to escape the same fate as her mother, she was going to have to revise her beliefs and behaviors about sacrifice and caregiving.

Changing this kind of pattern is rarely easy, however, because when a caregiver like Sharon finally takes a stand, a kind of emotional domino effect gets put into action. When I saw Sharon several months later, she had spoken with her brothers about chipping in toward their father's care. One was so angry with her, he didn't speak to her for a month. But another was a bit more understanding. As of this writing, Sharon tells me that there has been a split in the family over the stand she has taken. Her brothers have assumed about 40 percent of their father's care. Their father is learning to do more for himself, and Sharon has lost some weight as well as lowered her blood pressure. Though she feels bad about the rift she "caused" in her family, she also feels encouraged by the positive changes that have taken place in her health. She knows she is on the right track.

Breaking the Chain of Self-Sacrifice

Every one of us makes choices every day. For every choice we make, there will be consequences. The more honest we are with ourselves about the motivation that drives our choices, the healthier we will be. This is as true for caregiving as it is for any other area of our lives, perhaps even more so. The following steps are designed to help you consciously care for yourself while caring for others if and when the need arises.

STEP ONE: Acknowledge that women have inherited a cultural and personal legacy of self-sacrifice that has been passed down to us for generations. If you routinely sacrifice yourself for others, relax. You're normal. We've been socialized to value our contribution to our family or social group—our social worth—more than we value ourselves and our relationship with our soul. For at least the past five thousand years, a woman's worth has been largely determined by how well and how much she serves those who have more power and clout than she has. If you doubt this, remember that American women won the right to vote only in 1920, a mere eighty-six years ago. Before that, women's opinions and lives didn't even receive official recognition in the government. We haven't had much time in which to shed the automatic caretaking roles that have won us so much praise for millennia, let alone replace them with new beliefs and behaviors associated with taking our lives as seriously as we take those of others, particularly men. Despite this legacy, thousands of women all over the world are now taking themselves and their own fulfillment seriously. We are in the midst of a very fast-forward—and often delightful—evolution in this area!

STEP TWO: Learn the difference between care and overcare. True care of others, from a place of unconditional love, enhances our health, in part because it's associated with oxytocin, the bonding hormone. That's one reason why volunteering and community service feel good and are associated with improved health. Overcare and burnout result from not including ourselves on the list of people who require care. Burnout destroys our health and run our batteries down. Overcare is often motivated by guilt and unfinished business, for which we hope to somehow compensate through the caregiving role. The way to tell the difference between the two is to be aware of how caring for another makes you feel. You must also be 100 percent honest about what you're getting out of excessive caregiving.

One of my friends told me, "When I do things to make my family happy, I feel good and loved. The more I do, like baking, cooking, and keeping the house picked up, the more compliments I get. Though this can be exhausting, and though I keep saying that I need to get a life for myself other than work and cleaning up after everyone, I'm secretly afraid that if I take a stand and delegate responsibility to other family members for some of the caregiving work, they will resent me and not love me as much. So the payoff of doing it all myself is that I get my parents' love and my husband's love." When I hear something like this, I have to wonder whether it really is pleasure that motivates the caregiving, as she believes, or fear. (This year, I seriously contemplated not putting up a Christmas tree—then relented at the last minute. I didn't really want one, but I thought my daughters would enjoy it when they were home. Turns out, they didn't care one way or another. This was another lesson for me in examining my care versus overcare behavior.)

Each of us needs to examine what we get from martyring ourselves. One of my patients, a woman whose mother was physically and verbally abusive, learned early on that the only way to avoid being hit was to make all the meals, scrub the floors, and clean the rest of the house. To this day whenever she meets new people, she feels compelled to cook, clean, and bring them gifts to earn their love. She recently told me that she'd had the following insight: "If you act like a saint, no one ever confronts you—no one beats up on you. You become a valued part of every group you're in."

Sainthood of this kind seems mainly an avoidance strategy. On the other hand, the desire to nurture others, including plants and animals, is a positive emotion that is built right in to the biological programming of most women (and many men as well). Studies have shown, for instance, that when volunteers in nursing homes are taught how to give massages to the residents, the health of the volunteers is enhanced as well as that of the recipients. Who hasn't enjoyed the satisfaction gained from making a special school lunch that surprises and delights a child, or helping out a sick friend who needs a meal or someone to watch her children?

It feels good deep inside me to bring comfort to those who are suffering. In fact, my entire career is based on helping others feel better. Oftentimes, as I give health assistance to someone, I feel as though I'm in touch with a power that is greater than me but moves through me, helping me as it helps the other person. But many women, including myself, have learned over the years, sometimes through the wisdom of personal illness, that we cannot be available to another in a healthy way unless we're also getting our own needs met. And those needs must include time for pleasurable activities such as eating well and getting enough sleep.

STEP THREE: Learn the health benefits of benign self-interest. Here's a basic scientific truth: our health is best served by participating in those activities that are in our own highest and best interests and that bring us the most pleasure. This is not selfish. It is the very basis for a healthy life. There is not a single cell in our bodies that flourishes through sacrificing its own health for the health of the surrounding cells. It simply doesn't make sense. Instead, cells communicate with one another constantly. The health of one affects the health of them all. The more fully you are participating in the work and activities that brings you the most joy, the healthier you and your entire group become.

STEP FOUR: Understand that caring for parents or aging relatives can be an attempt to heal unfinished business from our family past. Claris, one of my menopausal patients whose diabetes was particularly difficult to bring under control while she was caring for her dying father, told me that the very thought of not caring for her father, who was dying of cancer, caused her to feel overcome with guilt. She said, "Daddy didn't want any strangers in the house, so I didn't feel as though I could hire a nurse or home health aide even though the money was available. To tell you the truth, his insistence that I be the only one to help him made me feel special." When Claris entered therapy after her father's death, she realized that she had never felt her father valued her as much as her brothers, so she tried to prove her worth through caregiving, something she did better than her brothers. She came to see that being constantly available for her father, even though other choices were available, was a way of trying to win the love and approval she had never felt from him in childhood.

STEP FIVE: Learn to delegate and ask for help. Caregiving at midlife is yet another opportunity to learn how to have healthy boundaries, set limits, and get clear about the ways that other family members assume some of the burden or pay for your help. If your husband isn't working or is working fewer hours than you are, for example, there's no reason why he can't pitch in. (You will have to learn the skill of asking for it without anger and resentment in order to get what you want. And in order to do that, you first have to believe that you deserve and are worthy of help. You are!)

I'm well aware that many women are not in a financial position to hire outside help to provide care for family members. But in almost every case there is a caregiving solution that needn't fall squarely on only one woman's shoulders. It's time that all men learned the basics of cooking and cleaning. Or, if no one else in the family can or will pitch in, another tactic would be to figure out what your caretaking time is worth, by finding out what it would cost to hire someone to come in and do the work you are doing. Then you could ask your brothers or other family members to pay you directly so that you can cut back on the hours you work elsewhere. That way you would have more time to replenish yourself each day, including time to exercise and eat well.

Like Sharon, you may have to recover from the family programming that leads you to believe your role as a woman must include self-sacrifice. Sharon had to let her father know that he needed to learn how to receive care from someone other than her. And her father also needed to undo a lifetime of conditioning telling him that all his household tasks would automatically be taken care of. It is well documented that older people, including men, can learn and grow until the end of their lives. There's no reason a man can't learn how to boil an egg, broil a piece of chicken, or stick a load of clothes in a washing machine! Parents who truly love us want what is best for us, even if that means making some adjustments in their behavior and expectations.

STEP SIX: Plan ahead. Don't wait until a parent or relative is in need of care before discussing a potential plan with your siblings. That way you can avoid the emergency caregiving that seemingly "just happens" to us but in reality was set in motion by our beliefs and choices years before. One of my friends, an eldest daughter who has just turned forty, has already made it clear to her younger sister, who lives in the same town as their mother, that she has no intention of allowing the mother, a very dependent woman, to come live with her should something happen to their father. My friend is not being selfish. She's being realistic. She loves her mother but does not intend to sacrifice her life and career for her. Her unblinking approach concerning her mother's possible future care alerts other family members that they can't automatically rely on her to house her mother in the future should the need arise. This breaks the chain of eldest-daughter sacrifice before it even gets welded in the first place.

HITTING PAY DIRT: GETTING CLEAR ABOUT MONEY AT MIDLIFE

Whatever the changes that precipitate a woman's empty-nest experience, the only path that will allow the full expression of her creative potential in the second half of her life is the path that establishes her true independence, both financially and emotionally. Even if she currently has a husband who supports her or money coming in from her family, it's important for her to know that if the need arose, she could manage alone. Inability to support themselves financially is the number-one reason why women stay in less-than-ideal relationships in which they are not treated as autonomous individuals with equal decision-making power. Being able to care for ourselves financially opens up a whole new world of pleasurable possibilities.

Though I do not claim to be a financial expert, I do know this: how, what, where, when, and on whom a woman spends money, and where she gets that money, tells you more about her true values, beliefs, and priorities than any other aspect of her life. Our behavior around making, spending, and saving money lays bare our core beliefs about ourselves and our worth in the world, pure and simple.

The dynamics of money also holds up a mirror to our relationships, telling us how each partner's contribution is valued and whether we are in a truly co-creative partnership. That's why discussing who pays for what and who does what tasks in a relationship is such a loaded and often unpleasant topic.

Cultural Ambivalence About Women and Money

Even though many women now make more money than their mates, the data suggest that we are still not comfortable, as individuals or as a culture, with that pattern. Consider the following research: Although a study from the University of Missouri–St. Louis showed that women now outearn their husbands in one out of five marriages, only 56 percent of men surveyed in the Virginia Slims Opinion Poll 2000 said that it would be acceptable for their spouses to be the primary wage earners. Many women agree with this. In the same poll, only 61 percent of women felt that it would be acceptable for them to be the primary wage earners.

When a woman does earn more than her husband, it doesn't wipe out the power differential. If anything, it seems to exacerbate it, due to the ambivalence couples feel about their status reversal. Julie Brines, a sociologist at the University of Washington who studies status-reversal couples, found, for example, that the more women contribute to the family account, the *less* likely their husbands are to contribute to the housework. In fact, when women made all the money while their husbands stayed home, these men actually did less housework per week than men who worked outside the home![3] Brines also found that in status-reversal marriages, women cede much of the decision-making power to their spouses. This is the opposite of what happens in traditional marriages, where the husband, who brings home the bacon, tends to call the shots. In other words, when women are the major wage earners, there's not a straightfor-ward relationship between income and power. Instead, there's an effort to achieve balance, even though this so-called balance is any-thing but.

The implications of this research are clear: no matter how much of the financial burden we shoulder, we still feel responsible for keeping our husbands happy, for making them feel good about themselves—especially if they're not making as much money as we are.

The sad truth is that many of us are still unsure of our worth as women in relationship to men—which is perfectly understandable given our history. So we do even more than our share to keep the men in our lives happy, lest they leave us for someone who appreciates them more than we do. Secretly we're afraid that if we demand too much, we'll be left alone. We don't realize how much inner power we have to create the life of our dreams because we've been talked out of it!

And then there's that other deeply feminine desire: We want to be cherished and taken care of. We keep hoping (sometimes despite am-ple evidence to the contrary) that to have a husband means that we will be taken care of. I grew up loving Tarzan movies. Recently I watched the classic *Tarzan and His Mate,* which I hadn't seen in years. This time I saw it through a new lens. The programming about gender roles was very clear: Jane provided the playfulness and the sex, while Tarzan protected Jane by fighting off wild things and do-ing a lot of heavy lifting to make sure she had a secure, comfortable home. Very compelling. Very appealing. And like most women, I want to get in on the good parts of this but without having to sacri-fice myself to do so. I finally figured out how to do this, but I first had to reprogram my subconscious beliefs and behaviors around rela-tionships. This took several years, and I'm still learning daily.

In my own family, as soon as my brothers turned eighteen my fa-ther sat them down and told them that they had to start supporting themselves. But he paid for my college tuition without question. I did put myself through medical school with student loans and scholar-ships, but when I got married, during my last month of med school, I gladly let my husband take care of all the details of buying our first home—a process that mystified and terrified me at the time. He used the last of his educational trust fund as a down payment, and I felt unbelievably lucky to be living this fairy-tale life! We paid off my medical school loans without difficulty.

My husband also made all the decisions about charitable donations and investments, though our incomes were basically equal. Donations went to the educational institutions and charities he favored. I never questioned this. I found the topic of money burdensome until I was forced to wake up at midlife. I'm not alone; many women find themselves in the same situation. Though we went through women's liberation in college, in the interest of creating a happy home and family life we were always willing to do "a little more" housework and child care than our husbands. Now our generation is taking the next step and waking up financially.

When I first went through my divorce, I secretly hoped that my life would be miraculously fixed by meeting a financially savvy and successful new man to marry so that I could get squared away again. Yep, I admit it. I was hoping that Prince Charming would ride up on his white horse and save me. (I saw how thoroughly this old programming lived in me, despite my career success.) As time went on, however, and no Prince Charming rode up to my door, I was forced to learn how to save myself. I learned that saving myself was not only fun, it was exhilarating. As the scales fell from my eyes and I learned to trust and value myself, my desires, and my financial savvy more and more, I was finally able to withdraw my projections from men, too. They were human and flawed, just like me. No better. No worse. Through my dealings with bankers, brokers, insurance agents, and accountants, I learned that men didn't have any more financial or other "magic" than I had! In fact, the more I saw myself as the source of my own magic, the better my life became. And from this new perspective, flush with pleasure and delight at my new, more prosperous way of being in the world, I began to appreciate men more than ever! And I found out that when you're clear with them about what you want and ask nicely—without any anger or neediness—they're often more than happy to provide it for you! This past Christmas, for example, I told my oldest brother that I wanted a bonfire outside on the Solstice. When I arrived at his house, he and my younger brother had prepared a pile of wooden pallets so substantial that I was sure my Solstice bonfire could be seen from space! I was completely moved and gratified by this gesture of support! This past spring, a male friend came over to the house and replaced my car battery when the car wouldn't start. I realized that all I had to do was ask instead of being determined to figure it out myself. My old stoic, "I don't need anybody" attitude began melting away in my warm glow of self-acceptance, compassion, and vulnerability. But this magic all started only when I no longer looked to a man to "complete" me or make me happy. When I discovered that I had what it took to make myself happy, and I gave up the futility of self-sacrifice as a way to get my needs met indirectly, my whole world changed. And so can yours.

MARY: *It's Never Enough*

Forty-six-year-old Mary had long been convinced her husband was better at finances than she was. He paid all the bills and did the taxes every year. But these activities always upset him. His mantra seemed to be "There's never enough. There's never enough." Increasingly Mary felt as though she couldn't ask her husband for money for anything but the barest of essentials, and it seemed the only way she could help the situation was to spend less. Finally, after much soul-searching, Mary decided to get recertified as a nurse, the profession she'd had when she had met and married her husband. Given the nursing shortage and the fact that they lived in a city with several large hospitals, Mary had no difficulty getting a job with a good salary and decent benefits. Within a year or so she began to make substantial contributions to the family income. This made her feel good, even though she hated the on-call part of her job. Despite her contribution, however, her husband continued to exercise iron control over all their financial decisions.

Mary suspected that one reason her husband was reluctant to share the financial decision making, as unhappy as it seemed to make him, was that he was going through his own midlife crisis at work. He seemed depressed about his career and the fact that he hadn't reached the success he thought he should have during his forties—a time he referred to as his "power years." He had started talking about retiring early, selling the house, and traveling around the country in an RV. Mary hoped that her husband was just going through a phase and would recover soon. She suggested that he get some individual counseling, but he became angry with her and said absolutely nothing was wrong with him and that he was not depressed.

Meanwhile, bringing home a paycheck had allowed Mary to become much more empowered in the world, if not at home. Nevertheless, she began to suffer from a host of health problems, including palpitations, severe hot flashes, and lower back pain. Her periods also became very irregular and very heavy. It was at this point that Mary came to see me, and I asked her what was going on in her life. When she told me, I gave her a series of recommendations to help her physical symptoms. (I will discuss these in later chapters.) I also suggested that she begin to assume a more proactive role in managing the family finances, which she agreed to do.

When she came back three months later, many of her menopausal symptoms were better. She reported that at first her husband had been resistant to her desire to know about their finances and help with spending decisions. However, soon after she initially raised the issue, he started to experience chest pain, which was diagnosed as angina. He realized that if his life continued in the way it had been going, he could die of a heart attack. This was his own midlife wake-up call, and it made him realize that he, too, needed to revamp some of his outmoded beliefs and behaviors.

In the meantime, Mary took steps on her own to increase her financial knowledge. Her new confidence forced changes in her marriage, of course. She told me that she and her husband had to completely rework their agreements about money and household chores. It wasn't easy. But in time, Mary's husband realized that it was in both his and Mary's best interest if both of them knew everything about their mutual finances and agreed upon their spending habits.

Changing Your Cultural Legacy

Middle-class women of my mother's generation were brought up to believe that they would be taken care of by their husbands. With the help of life insurance policies and the unprecedented economic growth that followed World War II, many of them were. The majority of my mother's friends, women now in their sixties, seventies, and eighties, never worked after marriage and never had to return to work after they became widows. The women's movement brought to our collective consciousness the price that our mothers paid for being taken care of in this way, and my generation vowed that we wouldn't become our mothers. (My mother tells me that she is routinely dismayed at the dismissive and abusive ways in which many of her friends' husbands treat their wives.) Though we've come a very long way when it comes to earning and handling money, the truth is that far too many women still lack basic money skills and are overly dependent upon husbands, employers, or family members to do their financial planning for them. It boils down to this: Many women were raised to think that someone else will take care of us financially if we do all the other kinds of caretaking. We invest in the people (usually husbands, but not always) who we believe will provide for us and love us. We women are actually really good at handling and managing money once we realize that money is simply the manifestation of life energy and not something that is beyond our grasp. The best way to become financially literate is to realize that we have the innate ability to deal effectively with money—with a little education. If our bodies have the skill and know-how to turn our life energy into an entirely new human being from our own flesh and blood, it ought to be a piece of cake to manage the life energy that money is simply a symbol of!

The news is good. Women, particularly midlife women, have now been identified as a lucrative new market for the financial industry. And it turns out that we're good at managing our money. Studies have shown, for example, that women's investment groups do better over the long haul than men's. Women tend to focus more on long-term financial goals rather than short-term performance, perhaps because we live longer and know that we are more likely to be supporting children or aging parents.

The Value of Becoming Financially Savvy

Regardless of your current circumstances, it is crucial that you get very clear about your beliefs about money so that you can begin to assume dominion over your money in the same way you are daily assuming dominion over your health. Money is a very concrete form of energy—it is power in our society, allowing you to go where you want to go and stay where you want to stay. Having control over your money gives you a sense of freedom and safety. In study after study, higher socioeconomic status is consistently associated with better health. But I believe it is the sense of empowerment and control, not the absolute number of dollars involved, that makes the real difference.

Many women report that in the early stages of taking financial control, they feel fueled by both anger and fear. I was no exception. In those first few months after my separation, I found myself possessed by a new sense of purpose, driven by the need to get my life free, clear, and settled. I had to get myself out of debt, pay off the overdrafts, and get the household accounts reorganized. It seemed scary and burdensome at first, but it quickly became exhilarating as I came to the realization that I *could* do it all by myself. The truth is, I had never actually acknowledged the fact that I had doubted that ability before. I learned I could manage my household finances just as effectively as I had for many years managed my professional and business finances—all without my husband's income, advice, or support. This is not to minimize or disparage his contribution during all the years of our marriage. Rather, it is to acknowledge the personal empowerment that comes from becoming financially independent.

From Poverty Consciousness to Prosperity Consciousness

The rubber really hit the road for me when I came to the realization that I was the one who was responsible for paying the mortgage and the vast majority of two private college tuitions. I had dabbled in reading about the universal laws of prosperity, but had never really been "up against it" enough to apply them in my life. Not so anymore. Every day, as I ran on my treadmill, I read *Think and Grow Rich* (Briggs Publications, revised edition, 2003) by Napoleon Hill— about how desire and consciousness create the mindset that attracts prosperity, Suze Orman's *The Courage to Be Rich* (Riverhead Books, 1999), and also everything by Robert Kiyosaki, author of *Rich Dad, Poor Dad* (Doubleday, 1999). I played his brilliant game, Cash Flow 101, over and over until I could easily get out of the "rat race" (living from paycheck to paycheck) and into the "fast track"—having residual income from businesses and investments that come in regularly whether you work or not. For the very first time in my life, I began to see myself as a business that was producing a product. I saw that my books, CDs, and newsletter were all "products" and all marketable.

I also saw how clearly my beliefs about money and prosperity were reflected in my bank accounts. At around this time, I met Suze Orman in the green room at the *Today* show. She told me that you can see people's ill health in their money and cash flow first because money has nowhere to hide an energy imbalance. You either have positive cash flow or you have debt. Simple. Sooner or later, if the behavior patterns and beliefs that create money problems are not addressed, they will manifest as health problems in the body. At the time, I was complaining to her about having to shoulder all the financial responsibility for my daughters. She said, "The only thing holding money back from you is anger and fear." I realized that she was right on the mark. My anger at my ex-husband, who by this time was remarried with a baby on the way, had left me full of resentment. And it was time to let it go instead of staying stuck in the prison I'd created for myself. Suze's remark was a wake-up call. Instead of seeing myself as a victim, I decided to be grateful for the opportunity to really learn how to support myself. I decided then and there to manifest more prosperity than I ever dreamed possible. I realized that what my ex-husband did or didn't do with his life or his money didn't have to affect me adversely at all—if I didn't allow it to. I realized that I could manifest the money I needed—and support myself and my kids even better than before. I read Catherine Ponder's *The Dynamic Laws of Prosperity* (De Vorss & Company, revised edition, 1985) and began to do affirmations about prosperity regularly. I still do them every day to ward off the ill effects of the poverty conscious- ness that pervades most people's way of thinking—and attracts its equivalent. Read the following and see how it makes you feel.

> I am now experiencing perfect health, abundant prosperity, and complete and utter happiness. This is true because the world is full of charming people who now lovingly help me in every way. I am now come into an innumerable company of angels. I am now living a delightful, interesting, and satisfying life of the most widely useful kind. Because of my own increased wealth, health, and happiness, I am now able to help others live a de- lightful, interesting, and satisfying life of the most widely useful kind. My good—our good—is universal.

Now imagine thinking thoughts like this day in and day out. It changes your life. As a result of my efforts in this area, my financial status is now light-years better than it ever was when I was married. And so are my mental and physical health. In fact, I've been so im- pressed with the result of this approach in my own life, and in the lives of my daughters, family members, and close friends, that I have started to include prosperity consciousness as a crucial part of creat- ing health.

Getting Started

Many women already run their own businesses and also do the family finances. If you're one of them, I urge you to update your prosperity consciousness so that you can do even better than you're doing now. I also recommend the book *Secrets of Six-Figure Women* (HarperBusiness, 2004) by Barbara Stanny and the website www. debtfreedivas.com to learn the self-worth/net-worth connection.

Women who are currently being supported by a husband or other family member can put themselves on the road to financial compe- tence by doing the following exercise for one month: pretend you are divorced, widowed, or suddenly faced with supporting yourself. Continuously ask yourself questions such as these: "Where are the insurance papers? The deed to the house? The mortgage papers? The pension plan? The tax forms from past years? What is the appraised value of the house? What is my net worth? When was the last time I filled out a financial statement?" Having a firm grasp on this type of information can help ensure that you remain in your relationship for all the right reasons—because it fulfills you and makes your life better on many levels—rather than because you believe you would fall apart without it. You simply cannot be available for true partnership and exhilarating co-creation with another until you know how to pull your own weight and have faced your own dependency squarely— and then done something about it.

COMING HOME TO YOURSELF

When I wrote the first edition of this book, I was well into peri-menopause, a time when I should have been in the throes of what many call "hormone hell." Yet I felt better than I had in years. The severe hot flashes I was experiencing in the last few months of my marriage virtually disappeared after my husband left—a phenomenon I've seen repeatedly in other women who've had the courage to leave dead-end relationships. Over and over I've watched perimenopausal symptoms resolve in women who've had the courage to negotiate the rapids of their midlife transitions consciously and in an empowered way in which they finally give their own needs high priority.

But I've also watched something even more profound occurring: the emergence of what can only be described as pure joy, the feeling that arises when a woman is truly coming home to herself. My own experience bears this out. I marveled at the power of my newfound nesting instinct and at how differently I chose to do things once I had set both feet across the threshold of my new life.

One of the most striking things I discovered after my husband left was an almost physical need to reclaim and redecorate my home, especially the family and guest rooms. One day, with catalogs, telephone, and credit card in hand, within less than an hour I bought a couch, a rug, end tables for the guest bedroom, and even curtains, something that at the age of forty-nine I had never done. My work in combination with my mothering had left no time or inclination to contemplate decor, let alone participate in choosing it. But that was my old life. Now, with my inner landscape rapidly changing, I felt a powerful compulsion to make my outer surroundings reflect the rejuvenation that was going on inside me.

I discovered that feng shui, the Chinese art of placement, helped me enormously in this process. I came to see that our homes reflect our lives, and that by consciously changing them according to the principles of feng shui, we can actually create improvements in our lives on all levels. By using a tool known as the *baqua* map, one can determine which areas of a room or an entire home correspond to specific aspects of life—for example, health and family, wealth and prosperity, helpful people and travel, love and marriage. This information allows you to enhance and change your physical space in order to enhance and change that particular area of your life. And as with all things in life, when you do this, things sometimes get worse before they get better—kind of like taking out the garbage as part of the process of spring cleaning. When my friend and colleague Terah Kathryn Collins, the author of the 1999 book *The Western Guide to Feng Shui,* did a consultation with me, we both laughed when we realized that my husband had left within four months of the time I had "enhanced" the love-and-marriage area of our property with a beautiful arbor. She said, "I see this over and over. When you enhance an area of your life that isn't working, you first have to let go of the parts that are standing in the way of getting what you really want." I also put a lighted lamppost in the helpful-people-and-places area of the property. Within two months my life became filled with skillful people who help me on all levels of my life, both at home and at work. (See Resources for feng shui information.)

I wanted my home to be the kind of place where people felt comfortable and welcome. And I wanted to feel at home there, surrounded by colors and textures that drew me in. For the first time in my life, I knew exactly what my personal style was and exactly how I wanted my rooms to look and feel. As the furniture began to come in and the rooms took shape, I felt delighted with the results, going back to look at them over and over again. Slowly it began to dawn on me what I was really doing: I was creating a potential space for all the new energy that was beginning to stream into my life. Whereas before I had been grieving the empty nest, now I was re-creating my old nest into a new place that reflected who I was becoming. It was a nest that would, of course, comfortably accommodate my children, their friends, and the new people who, I felt sure, would be coming into my life. And they have!

PAMELA: A Home of Her Own

While for me the process of coming home to myself meant accepting the breakup of my marriage, Pamela found a different—and very unconventional—path. She wrote:

I am forty-seven years old and have been in a relationship with Don for eight years, married for five. He's twelve years older, and his philosophy of life is pretty much "My way or the highway." Don's unilateral decisions aren't always supportive of me, and last year I decided that I needed to make choices that reflected my beliefs and prepared me for my future. He travels frequently for business and pleasure, and I spent a good deal of time alone in a house that didn't feel like home. I had even created a room of my own, but it wasn't enough.

So I've bought a home of my own. The marriage has had to undergo a transformation now that we are not together on a daily basis, and it could have failed. Don lives where he wants to, and I live where I need to. I cannot describe the joy I feel at living in a place that supports me emotionally and spiritually. I am moved to nurture my home and garden just as it nourishes me. I am delighted by the simplest things. Friends who have visited agree that it is me.

I am grateful that I earn a living and am capable of being financially independent of Don. And perhaps finally succeeding at my career gave me the confidence to create my dream home. After a lifetime of determining my worth through male approval, I am now living from my heart rather than from obligation.

VOCATIONAL AWAKENING AT MIDLIFE

For some women, the home—which had been the central focus before midlife—becomes secondary to a new passion, which reveals itself in the form of a vocational calling. Other women leave their previous work "home" to start their own businesses or change careers. Still others are simply forced by life circumstances into a new path.

The breadth of a woman's interests and contacts outside the home during the childbearing years will have an impact on the ease with which she moves into her new life. Some experimentation may be required before a woman can discover where her passions lie, and it may take longer for some to find their niche than others. Those who continue to define themselves by the roles they no longer have—such as mother or wife—and who have long lived enclosed in those roles may be overwhelmed by fear and lapse into immobility. But the key to finding new passions is getting out and getting moving, even if you don't know where you are going. Sometimes it's simply a matter of stumbling from point A to point B with your eyes wide open to the possibilities.

SYLVIA: *Discovering the Artist*

Sylvia retired from teaching the same year her youngest son married and moved to California. It was difficult for her to simultaneously relinquish her role of mother and mentor to her own children as well as to the third-grade students she'd taught for the past twenty-five years. She kept in contact with me through the grieving process, and she admitted there were times she felt she'd never find herself.

"Everything about who I am is wrapped up in kids," she wrote. "On one hand, the extra free time made it more difficult, because I didn't know what to do with myself. The days were so long and bleak." But in retrospect that time was a luxury, because it allowed her to give focused attention to her feelings and let them out—loud and clear. "My husband continued to go to work, so I was able to cry out loud, wail, even roar in frustration. I made some pretty anguished, animal-like sounds alone in that house—just me and those powerful feelings, bouncing off the walls."

Then, a few weeks later, Sylvia started looking at her house as though it were real estate she was contemplating buying—it had lots of potential but needed adjustments to fit her new life. She knocked down walls and incorporated the kids' rooms into the main living space, creating a great room that could accommodate her monthly meetings with local career women who gathered for the camaraderie and to share new skills, projects, and philosophies. Sylvia did much of the remodeling work herself, despite never having hung wallboard or laid ceramic tile before. When it was Sylvia's turn to demonstrate a new skill to the group, she showed them the tilework she'd done in her bathroom. Sylvia started tiling bathrooms for her friends, using handmade tiles and innovative patterns. What started out as a project spanning several weekends has turned into a second profession: two years later, through word of mouth, she has landed clients as far away as New York, and she's hired and trained two women to help her keep up with the demand. "I love the travel—I've always been a homebody, and I never went anywhere without my husband. Now I traipse off to visit beautiful homes and work my magic to make those homes even more beautiful, while my husband stays here and runs the household. Several clients asked me to sign my name on a prominent tile in their finished bathroom, like an artist signs paintings. I feel exhilarated and free as a bird. I love this new life."

JUDITH: *Finding Her True Vocation*

For many women, the key to finding their niche at midlife is in identifying the passions they've always had but never pursued full time. At fifty-four, after more than thirty years in the corporate world, Judith chose to take early retirement. Having looked back over her many years of doing volunteer work, she realized that caring for the elderly was a dream she wanted to pursue. Rather than make excuses for herself because of her age, she undertook a demanding graduate program to prepare for her new work. She wrote:

> I chose to leave my position as a business analyst and embark on a career change. I left with a mission statement: to dedicate my life work to the self-enlightenment, creative development, and joy of being an elder, and to provide services to elders that enhance their physical, mental, and spiritual growth. I interviewed with day-care directors and program managers while continuing my volunteer efforts by delivering hot meals to elderly shut-ins. This past June I completed the required coursework and internship for a master's degree in gerontological psychology.
>
> I have learned that although it can be extremely painful at times, it is only through the process of transition, with eyes and heart wide open, that an individual can truly succeed in personal growth. Now I feel the excitement and fear of taking my plan to fruition—actually doing what I have been studying and talking about doing! My daughter says, "Mom, who will hire you at your age?" My husband wishes me to succeed. I know I have *inner resources unlimited* and that new birth is emerging as I enter this new phase of my life.

Many midlife women discover that as they find new direction in life, they themselves become new, and so they attract new friends. One patient put it to me this way: "I became more interesting. I had more to offer on a personal level—I had more to talk about than kids and soccer practice and my husband's promotion. This new me is someone I really like!"

A ROAD MAP FOR NAVIGATING UNKNOWN TERRITORY

Taking those first steps on your journey home to yourself may be one of the hardest things you'll ever do. But as you venture onto this new path you will find that it loses its intimidating aspects and becomes instead a voyage of exploration and discovery. Here are a few signposts to help you along.

TAKE HEART. Though painful, your feelings of loneliness, like all feelings, will gradually lessen and change as time goes on, especially as you choose new and healthier ways of thinking and being in the world. Be present for your own experience while it's happening. The depth to which you allow yourself to feel pain is the depth to which you will also feel joy. And you have to trust that joy will come again, even though your life will never be exactly the same again. The news is good. I've been hearing about it for years. And I'm a living example myself.

One of my newsletter subscribers wrote:

I haven't felt this good since the whole nonsense started in my early teens. After a hideous perimenopausal epoch in my forties, I look forward to my fifty-second birthday with a big smile! All those years of chasing relationships to make my identity! I now live blissfully alone (except for Harriet the cat) and have an interesting relationship with an unusual man that does not define me. Even though my body will no longer put up with whatever I want to do to it, the aches and pains are treated with acceptance and equanimity. Life is filled with possibilities and delightful friendships, home and garden, dancing the Argentine tango, travel, lots else to do—but great respect for quiet, restful, self-indulgent times.

EMBRACE THE WISDOM OF ROUTINE AND DISCIPLINE. Either start or continue at least one activity that is scheduled regularly. You cannot imagine how healing a regular routine is. In my case, this routine includes daily exercise and a twice-weekly Pilates class. Pilates is a demanding type of exercise that involves moving from and focusing one's attention on what is known as one's "center" or "powerhouse," the muscles of the deep pelvis, buttocks, and abdomen that form a band around the lower body. No matter what else is going on in my life, I make the time to go to the studio and work on the link between my muscles and my brain. The sameness of it and the discipline involved in this activity are very anchoring for me—a part of my life that hasn't changed or gone away. In fact, on the morning my husband left, I went to my class as usual. Though I had no idea what would happen to our marriage at the time, and though my heart was racing and I was scared, getting on the Pilates equipment and going through my usual routine was very calming and reassuring. Though a significant part of my world was falling apart, I could still concentrate on my breathing, the strength of my muscles—and the fact that the planet was going to keep spinning. Pilates has been a key discipline that has transformed my body—making it stronger and more flexible than ever before.

ENHANCE YOUR DAILY LIFE. In the first few months of my almost-empty nest—my younger daughter was still home but deeply involved in her own activities—I began the practice of lighting a fire every night and keeping the doors of the woodstove open so that I could enjoy watching the flames as I ate dinner. In all our years of marriage, my husband and I had rarely opened the doors of this stove because it lessens the amount of heat that is produced. But now I was much less interested in thermodynamics, and instead simply wanted to bring the comfort of firelight into my home—especially at dinnertime, when the prospect of facing an evening alone loomed large before me. I also lit candles at dinner each night and played my favorite CDs. Six months later, when my second daughter left for her first semester away and I was truly faced with being alone every night, I was determined to use my time to tune in to and deepen my relationship with myself and my spirit. Mostly I wanted to heal the parts of myself that had led to my need to go through a divorce in the first place. And I wanted to get comfortable enough being alone in my home that I didn't need to jump into a new relationship right away just to avoid the pain of my husband's and daughters' absence. I knew that to do so might result in a relationship that simply repeated old, unhealed patterns. I've noticed that the people who allow themselves this time tend to end up with much healthier and happier relationships down the road.

KNOW THAT THE FEAR OF LOSS IS OFTEN WORSE THAN THE ACTUAL LOSS. I found that my dread of the empty nest was much worse than the actual experience. In fact, I was so busy with work that I enjoyed having only myself to take care of. Besides, I learned that I like reading in bed as late as I want, going to as many movies as I feel like, taking a bath at any hour of the day or night, and generally discovering what my own needs and desires actually are. Though I had originally planned to have my mother come visit and go skiing with me during my first empty-nest winter, the time flew by so quickly that we never got around to it. Nevertheless, it felt good to know that she was willing to come and provide support and recreation if I needed it.

REMEMBER THAT WE'RE STRONGER AND MORE RESILIENT THAN WE MAY THINK. On the day that would have been my twenty-fifth wedding anniversary, I awoke and just stayed in bed, allowing myself to experience my emotions for a few minutes. I hadn't made it to the quarter-century mark in my marriage, and I felt bad about that. I thought I might spend the whole day feeling sad. But to my surprise, I didn't. Diane, a woman who has worked with me for over twenty years, gave me a funny card. On the cover there was a ridiculous photo of a muscular man dressed up in a tutu with a snake draped over his shoulder. When you opened the card, the greeting read, "Still looking for Mr. Right!" I laughed out loud and put the card in my journal. Later I went out to dinner to celebrate a friend's birthday. The day came and went and I stayed calm and happy. The previous year my heart was breaking on the day of my anniversary, and I dissolved in tears at dinner that night with my two daughters. One year later I was renewed and at peace.

I won't pretend that going through a divorce and seeing both my daughters leave in the same year was easy. That first empty-nest year was the most difficult time of my life, as I experienced the crumbling of everything I had always thought I could count on. Paradoxically, that year also proved to be one of the most strengthening and exhilarating of my entire life. Looking back, I marvel at how far I've come. By turning my life over to Source energy and being willing to roll up my sleeves and rebuild my life, I've become infused with the energy of hope, joy, and new beginnings. Every day I'm reminded that the energy that supports new life abounds. We just have to believe in it, surrender to it, and ask for help.

4

This Can't Be Menopause, Can It?
The Physical Foundation
of the Change

Many women are caught off guard by the first signs of the climacteric. They don't expect symptoms to occur until they've reached the end point—the absolute cessation of periods. But a woman's last period is usually preceded by a long period of transition, which may include symptoms such as hot flashes, mood swings, difficulty sleeping, and night sweats. In fact, so-called menopausal symptoms are worse during perimenopause and then cease within a year or so after the last period.

Doreen was a vital, youthful-looking woman of forty-six when she had her first hot flash. She'd noticed a certain irritability in the way she related to her husband, who had begun to tease her about being menopausal, but she adamantly denied the possibility. "I'm still having my periods like clockwork," she argued. "My mom was fifty-three when she hit menopause. I'm not old enough to be going through the change!"

It is true that the age at which a woman's mother had her last period is probably the best predictor of when it will happen to her. (Though there are certainly exceptions.) But if she doesn't understand that the first symptoms of the climacteric may reveal themselves well before that time—sometimes ten or more years earlier—she is likely to protest, with Doreen, "This can't be menopause...can it?"

The quick answer is this: if you have reason to ask, then it probably is.

WHAT IS HAPPENING IN YOUR BODY: HORMONAL CHANGES

Menopause is officially defined as that point in time when our periods stop permanently. A woman undergoing natural menopause really has no way of knowing whether any given period is truly her last until a year has passed. As menopause approaches, cycles can become quite erratic, and it's not uncommon for several months to go by between periods. By the age of forty some of the initial hormonal changes associated with perimenopause (peri- means "around" or "near") are well under way. Research has shown, for example, that by age forty many women have already undergone changes in bone density, and by age forty-four many have begun to experience periods that are either lighter and/or shorter in length than usual, or heavier and/or longer. About 80 percent of women begin skipping periods altogether.[1] In fact, only about 10 percent of women cease menstruating altogether with no prolonged period of cycle irregularity beforehand. In an extensive study of more than 2,700 women, most experienced a perimenopausal transition lasting between two and eight years.[2]

Unless you've gone into menopause abruptly because of surgery or medical treatment, perimenopause can be thought of as the other end of a process that began when you first started your periods. That first menstrual period is usually followed by five to seven years of relatively long cycles that are often irregular and frequently anovulatory. Eventually, in the late teens or early twenties, cycle length shortens and becomes more regular as a woman reaches her prime reproductive age, which lasts for the next twenty years or so. In our forties, our cycles begin to lengthen again. Though most of us have been led to believe that twenty-eight days is the normal cycle length, research has shown that only 12.4 percent of women actually have a twenty-eight-day cycle. The vast majority have cycles that last anywhere between twenty-four and thirty-five days, and 20 percent of all women experience irregular cycles.[3]

Two to eight years prior to menopause, most women begin skipping ovulations. During these years, the ovarian follicles, which ripen eggs each month, undergo an accelerated rate of loss, until the supply of follicles is finally depleted. Research suggests that, in this culture at least, the acceleration in follicle loss begins around age thirty-seven or thirty-eight. Inhibin, a substance produced by the ovaries, decreases, which results in rising levels of FSH, the follicle-stimulating hormone produced by the pituitary gland. (This doesn't mean you can't get pregnant. For further information about fertility during this time, see my book, *Women's Bodies, Women's Wisdom*, chapter 11, "Our Fertility.")

Contrary to the standard belief, our estrogen levels often remain relatively stable or even increase during perimenopause. They don't wane until less than a year before the last menstrual period.[4] Until menopause, the primary estrogen a woman's body produces is estradiol. However, during perimenopause the body starts making more of a different kind of estrogen, called estrone, which is produced both in the ovaries and in body fat.

Testosterone levels usually do not fall appreciably during perimenopause. In fact, the postmenopausal ovaries of many women (but not all) secrete more testosterone than the premenopausal ovaries.

On the other hand, progesterone levels do begin to fall in perimenopause, often long before changes in estrogen or testosterone. As I will discuss below, this is the most significant perimenopausal issue for the majority of women.

The prevailing message appears to be this: although reproduction is no longer the goal, there continue to be important roles for these so-called reproductive hormones—vital, health-enhancing roles that have nothing to do with making babies. Evidence for this can be seen in the fact that steroid hormone receptors are found in almost every organ of our bodies. Estrogen and androgens (like testosterone) are important, for example, in maintaining strong and healthy bones as well as resilient vaginal and urethral tissue. And both estrogen and progesterone are important for maintaining a healthy collagen layer in the skin.

PERIMENOPAUSE IS A NORMAL PROCESS, NOT A DISEASE

The main thing to keep in mind about perimenopause is that it's a completely normal process, not a disease to be treated. But in order for her body to continue producing levels of hormones adequate to support health, a woman must be optimally healthy going in—physically, emotionally, spiritually, and situationally. In other words, her future well-being depends not only on the health of her physical body, but also on her nonphysical support system, both of which are a reflection of how she cares for herself today and how she has lived up to this point. Because perimenopause occurs at the mid-point of our lives, it is a very good time to take stock and make sure that we are doing everything possible to restore or build our health.

Despite all the media focus on supplemental hormones—which ones to take, what dose, natural versus synthetic, and so on—it is important to bear in mind this often-forgotten fact: a woman's body begins life fully equipped to produce all the hormones she needs throughout life. All of the so-called sex hormones (estrogen, progesterone, and the androgens) are manufactured from the same ubiquitous precursor molecule—cholesterol. In addition, our bodies also have the ability to convert one type of sex hormone into another. So, for example, estrogen can be converted into testosterone, and progesterone can be converted into estrogen. Whether or not these conversions actually take place depends upon our body's minute-to-minute needs, our emotional state, our nutritional state, and so on.

What all this means is that not all women will need or want hormone supplementation. In many cultures hormone supplements are infrequently prescribed, yet women in those cultures rarely have uncomfortable perimenopausal symptoms. How can this be?

First of all, the ovaries only slow down; they do not shut down. Moreover, a woman's body is designed to produce estrogen, progesterone, and testosterone at other sites besides the ovaries, and it is ready and willing to increase or mediate the output from those auxiliary sites when the need arises at midlife. Research has shown, for example, that estrogen, progesterone, and androgen are produced in body fat, skin, the brain, the adrenal glands, and even peripheral nerves! But whether or not adequate production occurs depends on what else is going on in a woman's life.

If, for example, a woman is under significant stress—if she is overworked, if her diet fails to meet her body's needs, if she is physically ill, if she smokes and/or drinks, if she is avoiding spiritual issues that are beckoning her, or if she is involved in relationships in which the energy outflow is not matched by the energy coming back—then she may find that her ability to keep up with the demands on her endocrine system is diminished. It will remain so unless and until she is able to implement some changes in those areas of her life that need work. The result may be a tumultuous midlife transition, fraught with her own individual combination of symptoms—from headaches, hot

FIGURE 7: HORMONE-PRODUCING BODY SITES

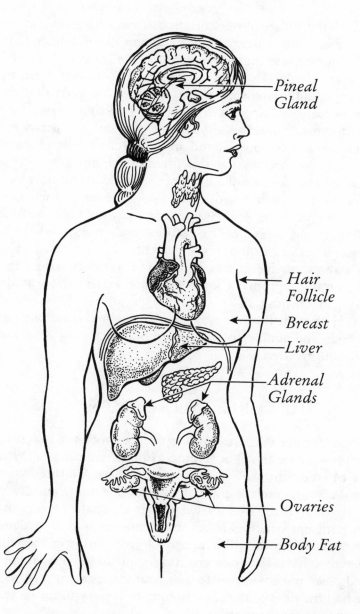

The healthy body is equipped to produce all the hormones a woman needs throughout her life. This natural ability can be supported or thwarted, depending on lifestyle patterns and the state of a woman's health—physically, emotionally, spiritually, and situationally.

flashes, bloating, and fading libido to mood swings and sleep disturbances.

Given the nature of our current culture, with its ever-accelerating
pace of life, about 75 percent of perimenopausal women have symptoms of menopause that are uncomfortable enough to cause them to
seek relief, whether through supplemental hormones, dietary change,
exercise, or alternative therapies. If a woman finds that she needs
supplemental hormones in order to reestablish a physical and emotional comfort zone, this should not be seen as a personal failure.
Rather, it is a wake-up call and an opportunity to implement much-
needed change. A woman in this situation might want to consider accepting what I like to call a dusting of supplemental hormones—just
enough to provide her with the support she needs for comfort and
health, and no more. At the same time she would also be wise to pay
attention to the messages her body is sending. It is asking for more
than just a prescription or a supplement.

The bottom line is this: before you take something to relieve
menopausal symptoms, acknowledge and listen to your body's inner
wisdom in creating those outward symptoms. They are uniquely
yours. How your hormones behave during perimenopause and how
your body and mind respond to hormonal changes is as personalized
as your fingerprints.

THE THREE TYPES OF MENOPAUSE

Imagine that you are standing at the foot of a beautiful mountain. You can see the light shining from behind the peak, and you're
eager to enjoy the view from the top. There are three ways to get
there: You can take the gradually sloping, winding path, which may
require you to climb over a few rocks now and then. You can take the
short path up, which is much more difficult and will require more
equipment and technical support. Or you can skip the climb altogether and have someone else take you up via helicopter—which
sounds easy until you realize that your muscles and organs will not
have had the time or the conditioning to cope with the cold and lack
of oxygen at the summit.

~ NATURAL MENOPAUSE (the sloping, winding path) occurs gradually, usually between ages forty-five and fifty-five, in a woman who
   has at least one of her ovaries. Duration, in most cases, is five to
   ten years, though the entire process sometimes takes up to thirteen

years. During this time, periods may stop for several months and then return, and they may increase or decrease in duration, intensity, and flow. All other things being equal, women who are going through a natural menopause may or may not need any treatment for the sake of physical comfort, because their overall health may be strong enough, and their transition may be occurring gradually enough, for their bodies to keep up with the changing demands. It will depend, in other words, on what else is going on in their bodies and in their lives.

~ PREMATURE MENOPAUSE (the short path) occurs somewhat faster as well as earlier, in women in their thirties or early forties who have at least one ovary. Approximately one in a hundred women completes the menopausal transition by age forty or younger. She may have an illness (such as an autoimmune disease or nutritional deficiency) or some chronic stress (including excessive athletic conditioning) that has adversely affected hormone-related reproductive functions. Duration usually is shorter than natural menopause, one to three years. Because the transition is quicker, and because the early change is often linked to a preexisting physical condition, there is a strong likelihood a woman undergoing premature menopause will need supplemental hormones during the adjustment.[5]

~ ARTIFICIAL MENOPAUSE (the helicopter ride) can occur quite abruptly, induced by surgical removal or disruption of the reproductive tract (including removal of ovaries or surgical disruption of the blood supply to the ovaries), by radiation or chemotherapy, or by administration of certain drugs that induce or mimic menopause for medical reasons (such as to shrink uterine fibroids).

Even tubal ligation has been shown to lower progesterone levels for at least a year following the procedure.[6] (The newest tubal occlusion procedure, Essure, is not likely to have this effect because it doesn't alter ovarian blood supply.) And many women who undergo hysterectomy *with* preservation of their ovaries experience symptoms of hormonal change—in addition, of course, to the loss of their periods.

Current estimates are that approximately one in every four American women will enter an abrupt, artificial menopause. Because there's no opportunity for gradual adjustment to the hormonal drop-off, the symptoms of artificial menopause can be severe and debilitating. Almost invariably, supplemental hormone therapy is elected in order to alleviate physical discomfort.

PATTI: *Artificial Menopause*

Six weeks after vague symptoms (night sweats, weight loss, and a persistent rash in her bikini area) had been misdiagnosed at an urgent-care center as "perimenopause and stress," Patti, a forty-one-year-old single mother and owner of a small business, was diagnosed with Hodgkin's disease, a type of lymphoma. Two six-week courses of chemotherapy left her feeling temporarily exhausted and without her curly blond hair ... but cured. The one side effect that turned out not to be temporary was the loss of her periods.

She wrote, "A couple of weeks after the chemo was over, when I began to get some of my energy back, I started having night sweats again. This scared me, because I thought it was the cancer coming back, and I thought my mood swings were just due to the constant worry." Her internist ran hormone tests and confirmed that Patti had undergone menopause, and she prescribed the appropriate hormone replacement therapy in the form of a skin patch, which gave Patti's body gentle doses of hormone slowly, throughout the day and night. "I felt much better within just a few days, and I think in my condition—after all I'd been through—it really helped me recover quicker, because my body was pretty traumatized and my mind was frazzled."

PERIMENOPAUSE AND HORMONAL LEVELS

The conventional view of what happens at perimenopause is that estrogen levels plummet. This is a gross oversimplification and too often leads to treatment that can make mildly uncomfortable symptoms worse. In natural menopause, the first hormonal change that occurs is a gradual decline in levels of progesterone, while estrogen levels remain within the normal range or even increase. Because progesterone and estrogen are meant to counterbalance each other throughout the menstrual cycle, with one falling while the other rises and vice versa, an overall decline in progesterone allows estrogen levels to go unopposed—that is, without the usual counterbalance. The result is a relative *excess* of estrogen, a condition that is often called estrogen dominance—which is precisely the opposite of the conventional view.

If a woman begins to experience uncomfortable symptoms at this stage, it's because her body can sense—and attempts to adjust to—that relative estrogen excess. Estrogen excess is also exacerbated by high insulin and stress hormones. Unfortunately, however, there's a great deal of overlap in the symptoms of various hormone imbalances, and it's not uncommon for a woman experiencing symptoms of estrogen or stress hormone excess to be given a prescription for more estrogen or even antidepressants. Not surprisingly, her mild symptoms can worsen as a result.

As the transition goes on, progesterone continues to decline, and eventually estrogen levels may begin to swing widely. The estrogen highs occur because the ovaries have begun to allow entire groups of follicles to grow and mature during successive menstrual cycles, instead of only one at a time, as though attempting to hurriedly "spend" those remaining eggs. (This is the reason why the incidence of twin pregnancies increases with age.) The progesterone decline occurs because fewer and fewer of those maturing eggs actually complete the entire ovulation process.

Levels of the hormones FSH and LH, which the pituitary gland in the brain normally releases in precisely metered amounts to stimulate controlled follicular growth and ovulation, become erratic as our ovaries start to skip ovulations. Closer to menopause, hormonal levels start to stabilize. FSH and LH levels smooth out and climb to their new, higher cruising altitude, where they stay for the rest of our lives.

SYMPTOMS OF DECREASED PROGESTERONE AND ESTROGEN DOMINANCE

- Decreased sex drive
- Irregular or otherwise abnormal periods (most often, excessive vaginal bleeding)
- Bloating (water retention)
- Breast swelling and tenderness
- Mood swings (most often irritability and depression)
- Weight gain (particularly around the abdomen and hips)
- Cold hands and feet
- Headaches, especially premenstrually

IS THERE A TEST I CAN TAKE?

For years the diagnosis of menopause was simply based on your age and symptoms. Now it's becoming more mainstream to use laboratory confirmation of your hormone levels. Here's why: First, as illustrated by the story of Patti, there are illnesses that mimic perimenopause rather convincingly. (Hypothyroidism is another example; see page 119.) By having your entrance into the climacteric confirmed, you'll simultaneously be ruling out an unexpected medical problem. Second, by determining your levels of the relevant hormones—estrogen, progesterone, and testosterone, and possibly DHEA and thyroid hormone as well—you and your health care provider can better determine where you stand in the perimenopausal timeline and what approach to take to your symptoms, if any. One caveat about hormone testing: menopausal symptoms do not necessarily correlate well with hormone levels. For example, many women with low testosterone levels have normal libido. And some women with normal testosterone levels have low libido. Bottom line: I think it's useful to get your hormone levels tested. But it's far more useful to tune in to how you're feeling than to focus on a lab test, which gives, after all, just a single snapshot of an ever-changing process.

If you decide to seek laboratory confirmation, it is important that you understand what tests are available, and what they can (and cannot) reveal about your current status.

Hormone Levels: FSH and LH

The testing method employed by many medical practices is to test FSH and/or LH levels either through blood or saliva. This is based on the fact that at menopause and thereafter, a woman's FSH and LH levels rise to their highest ever. But there are problems with this method. First of all, it will tell you nothing about estrogen levels, because FSH is controlled by inhibin, not by estrogen. (This is one of the reasons why estrogen replacement doesn't decrease FSH levels after menopause.)[7] In addition, during the five or ten years of perimenopause—before menstruation ceases for good—FSH and LH levels can fluctuate widely. The ovaries may become inactive for a few days or weeks and then resume production of eggs. It is possible, for example, for a woman's FSH levels to reach postmenopausal levels (greater than 30 IU/1 for blood) while she is still having normal periods. Her LH levels, meanwhile, will remain in the normal pre-menopausal range. For that reason, a single high FSH/LH level can't be used to determine whether or not a woman is in menopause. Until a woman has had no periods for a year and has FSH/LH levels well within the postmenopausal range—FSH greater than 30 IU/1 and LH greater than 40 IU/1—it is even possible for her to get pregnant. This is why it's prudent to use contraception for a year after you think your periods have stopped.

Hormone Levels: Estrogen, Progesterone, and Testosterone

Another common blood test analyzes the total amount of estrogen, progesterone, and testosterone in the bloodstream. The largest drawback to this method is that most of the hormone so measured is inactive. The healthy woman's body produces upward of ten times more of these hormones than she can use, so specialized proteins hook themselves to more than 90 percent of the hormone molecules produced, inactivate them, and lock the "doors" that would otherwise allow them to leave the bloodstream and enter the tissues. The biologically active form of the hormone is the part that is unbound or free. This goes quickly into the tissues instead of hanging around in the bloodstream. Thus the standard blood test, which does not distinguish bound from free hormone, will give an irrelevant result, because it measures primarily inactive, unusable, protein-bound hormone.

Preferred Testing Methods

With the individualized approach to menopause that has become the new standard of care, many clinicians are finding that measuring hormone levels can provide helpful information for balancing hormones either through nutritional means or bioidentical hormone replacement. Though I used to advocate the measurement of salivary hormone levels—and the initial research was promising—there is still insufficient evidence in the published scientific literature to draw any conclusions about the accuracy of this method for the monitoring of menopause and aging.[8]

Most clinicians who work with menopausal women now prefer

serum testing from labs specializing in this area. New and improved FDA-approved assays are now available that measure not only biologically active levels of estrogen, progesterone, and testosterone, but also their breakdown products. A growing body of research is showing that hormone balance can affect bone turnover, lipid metabolism, immune function, as well as hormone-dependent cancers, including breast and uterine. Since blood test results can be modified by changes in lifestyle, including supplementation, diet, exercise, and possible hormone replacement, it is probably worthwhile to have a hormone profile done if you're having a lot of symptoms or are planning on using hormone replacement. It's important to work with a health care practitioner who is familiar with this kind of hormone testing. I recommend the Women's Hormonal Health Assessment from Genova Diagnostics. (See Resources.)

Double Testing: If You Test, Test Again

If you're having symptoms and are actively working with a program to improve hormone balance, I recommend double testing, which acknowledges the fact that hormone levels fluctuate, especially during perimenopause. The best time of day for sample collection is the early morning, and the best time of the month is between days 20 and 23, when progesterone levels are apt to be highest. If your periods are irregular, it is more difficult to accurately assess progesterone levels with just one sample—another reason for double testing. With double testing, the sample is drawn or collected and assayed on at least two different occasions *before* treatment. (If symptoms are really severe, you needn't delay treatment. Just get another set of levels about one month after starting treatment so that adjustments can be made.)

Double testing increases the chance that testing will reveal natural biological variation as well as perimenopausal fluctuations. If the results of the second test are vastly different from those of the first, it may be necessary to run one or more additional tests to determine whether the difference is due to laboratory error or to natural fluctuations. Making this distinction can help avoid getting a hormone prescription that at best fails to meet the body's needs or at worst exacerbates the problem. Because hormone levels so often normalize or improve with lifestyle changes, it's empowering to have this improvement documented through hormone testing.

MENOPAUSE AND THYROID FUNCTION

The ovaries are the organs that we focus on most commonly at menopause, but the physical foundation of a woman's menopausal experience actually rests on the health of all her endocrine (hormone-producing) organs. Thyroid problems are very common during the perimenopausal and postmenopausal years. While many women with these problems are completely asymptomatic, others may have a wide variety of symptoms. Among the most common symptoms are mood disturbances (most often seen in the form of depression and irritability), low energy level, weight gain, mental confusion, and sleep disturbances.

Thyroid problems are intimately intertwined with menopause, and not just because of the epidemiological fact that about 26 percent of women in or near perimenopause are diagnosed with hypothyroidism.[9] According to the late John R. Lee, M.D., a noted clinician and author, there appears to be a cause-and-effect relationship between hypothyroidism, in which there are inadequate levels of thyroid hormone, and estrogen dominance. When estrogen is not properly counterbalanced with progesterone, it can block the action of thyroid hormone, so even when the thyroid is producing normal levels of the hormone, the hormone is rendered ineffective and the symptoms of hypothyroidism appear. In this case, laboratory tests may show normal thyroid hormone levels in a woman's system, because the thyroid gland itself is not malfunctioning.

It is no surprise, then, that this problem is compounded when a woman is prescribed supplemental estrogen, leading to an even greater imbalance. In that circumstance, a prescription for supplemental thyroid hormone will fail to correct the underlying problem: estrogen dominance. Estrogen dominance and also glycemic stress (see chapter 6, "Foods and Supplements to Support the Change") are very often accompanied by high adrenaline levels. And this metabolic situation can exacerbate thyroid problems. Here's what happens. Adrenaline stimulates the sympathetic nervous system, as does glycemic stress. This includes increasing the heart rate and blood pressure, which can lead to palpitations. But it also causes estrogen to be metabolized into substances known as catechol—estrogens that themselves have adrenaline-like effects. The main thyroid hormone, thyroxine, also stimulates the heart and the sympathetic nervous system. To adjust to the already too-high level of adrenaline in the system, the thyroid gland often shuts down a little to lower thyroxine stimulation—which is reflected in slightly high TSH levels.

Hypothyroidism can be confusing because there's a continuum between overt and subclinical hypothyroidism, with a great deal of overlap between the two. Depending upon which expert you talk with and which criteria are used for the diagnosis, as many as 25 percent of perimenopausal women have some kind of thyroid problem. Most of these are cases of subclinical hypothyroidism. Although symptoms may be present, tests of thyroid function are only slightly abnormal (thyroid stimulating hormone, or TSH, of 0.5–5.0, with normal levels of T3—triiodothyronine—and T4—thyroxine). Increasingly, clinicians who specialize in individual hormone solutions are finding that the old "normal" range for TSH in most labs (0.5–5.0) is too broad and that the ideal should be somewhere between only 0.5–2.0. I've found that many women with TSH levels over 2.0 do well with a little thyroid replacement, at least during perimenopause.

Once adrenal stress, glycemic stress, and estrogen dominance are addressed through modalities such as supplementation, adequate rest, and natural light, thyroid levels also recover. In the meantime, it's often helpful to take a small dose of thyroid replacement that is comprised of both types of thyroid hormones (T3 and T4). These are available from formulary pharmacies. (See Resources.)

Even if supplemental thyroid hormone does help alleviate the existing hypothyroidism, in a significant portion of these cases the symptom of depression persists, for a separate and rather surprising reason: depression itself can result in thyroid dysfunction. Treating the hypothyroidism, in other words, may be treating a symptom rather than the underlying cause.

Allow me to explain. In many women thyroid dysfunction develops because of an energy blockage in the throat region, the result of a lifetime of "swallowing" words she is aching to say. In the name of preserving harmony, or because she has learned to live as a relatively helpless member of her family or social group, she has learned to stifle her self-expression. She may in fact have struggled to have her say, only to discover that it doesn't make any difference—because in her closest relationships she has been defined as insignificant. In order for this complex, entangled state of affairs to be resolved, a woman might need to take not only supplemental progesterone and thyroid hormone, but also an unblinking look at what parts of her life and interpersonal relationships need to change.

MENOPAUSE AND ADRENAL FUNCTION

The two thumb-sized adrenal glands secrete three key hormones that help us withstand many of the stresses and burdens of life. However, if a woman has lived for a long time with the perception that her life is inescapably stressful, or if she is chronically ill, then chances are she has asked too much of her adrenal glands and has not given them adequate time to replenish themselves. She may be one of the many today who enter menopause in a state of adrenal exhaustion.

To understand what chronic exhaustion may do to the body and how it affects your menopausal experience, it's important to know what the adrenal glands do for you on a day-to-day basis, through the effects of three distinct but complementary hormones they secrete.

- NOREPINEPHRINE (adrenaline) is the fight-or-flight hormone, produced when something is threatening you (or when you think that something is threatening you). It makes your heart pound, your blood rush to your heart and large muscle groups, your pupils widen, your brain sharpen, and your tolerance for pain increase, so you can be at your best in battle. In modern-day life your battles are likely to consist of daily challenges such as pushing your body to keep going when it's fatigued, dealing with a stressful job, and reacting with quick reflexes to avoid a traffic accident. Think of these adrenaline surges as withdrawals from a bank, to help you get through life's rough spots. If you have gotten into the habit of withdrawing adrenaline from your account too often, you'll eventually be overdrawn. Your adrenal glands will be overwhelmed, and you'll have too little adrenaline when you really need it.

- CORTISOL increases your appetite and energy level while taming the allergic and inflammatory responses of your immune system. It stimulates the liberation and storage of energy in the body, helps the body resist the stressful effects of infections, trauma, and temperature extremes, and helps you maintain stable emotions. Synthetic versions of cortisol—prednisone and cortisone, for example—are prescribed often in human and veterinary medicine to help the patient perk up and feel better so he/she will eat, drink, and move around more and therefore be better able to fight off illness or heal from an injury. Ideally, cortisol is released into the system only on an occasional basis, rather than in response to chronic stress. Undesirable side effects can occur if cortisol levels become too high for too long. These include loss of bone density, muscle wasting, thinning of the skin, decreased ability to build protein, kidney damage, fluid retention, spiking blood sugar levels, weight gain, and increased vulnerability to bacteria, viruses, fungi, yeasts, allergies, parasites, and even cancer. If you've ever seen anyone on high-dose prednisone, you've seen how this drug can adversely affect the body.

~ DEHYDROEPIANDROSTERONE, also known as DHEA, is an androgen that is produced by both the adrenal glands and the ovaries. In both women and men, DHEA helps to neutralize cortisol's immune-suppressant effect, thereby improving resistance to disease. (Cortisol and DHEA are inversely proportional to each other. When one is up, the other goes down.) DHEA also helps to protect and increase bone density, guards cardiovascular health by keeping "bad" cholesterol (LDL) levels under control, provides a general sense of vitality and energy, helps keep the mind sharp, and aids in maintaining normal sleep patterns. Like norepinephrine and cortisol, DHEA also improves your ability to recover from episodes of stress and trauma, overwork, temperature extremes, and so forth. And if a woman is experiencing a decline in libido due to falling testosterone levels, often it is declining DHEA levels that are at the root of the testosterone deficiency, as DHEA is the main ingredient from which the body manufactures testosterone.

There is a price to pay for making too many demands on your adrenal glands. Excessive exposure of the body to adrenaline and cortisol can result in mood disorders, sleep disturbances, reduced resistance to disease, and changes in vital circulation, all of which are common complaints in today's living-on-the-edge lifestyle. And because these side effects are not uncomfortable enough to be intolerable, the self-destructive lifestyle often continues. DHEA, which helps the body recover from this sort of chronic abuse, finds itself on duty full time instead of only episodically. Gradually the adrenal glands become seriously exhausted, with the first and most profound effect being their waning ability to produce DHEA. As levels of this restorative hormone fall, cortisol and adrenaline levels begin to fluctuate as well, as the adrenal glands attempt to fill increasingly impossible orders for more support. One of the cardinal signs of adrenal exhaustion—relentless, debilitating fatigue—becomes a prominent complaint. Though this fatigue is often accompanied by depressed mood, irritability, and loss of interest in life, this doesn't mean that the adrenal problem is necessarily the cause of the mood change, any more than similar problems are always caused by thyroid malfunction. That is why these emotional symptoms do not always go away with treatment—the underlying issues remain unresolved.

A woman in a state of adrenal exhaustion is likely to find herself at a distinct disadvantage when entering perimenopause, because in the simplest terms perimenopause is another form of stress. Furthermore, adrenal exhaustion suggests that there are long-standing life problems in need of resolution. These issues will loom all the larger when seen with the no-nonsense mental clarity of perimenopause, but not only will adrenal exhaustion make the transition needlessly unpleasant, it also can deprive a woman of the resources she needs to address those issues and to take full advantage of the creative promise of the second half of her life.

If a woman is feeling chronically tired or depressed, if she begins her day feeling inadequately rested, or if she finds that ordinary stresses are having an impact that is out of proportion to their importance, she may be suffering from adrenal gland dysfunction.

Adrenal Testing

Salivary or serum DHEA and cortisol levels can be easily tested through accredited laboratories. (Laboratories that can do this with a doctor's prescription include Genova Diagnostics, 800–522–4762; www.gdx.net; and ZRT Laboratory, 503–466–2445, www.salivatest.com.) Conventional blood tests, taken at whatever time your doctor has scheduled your appointment, might indicate that your adrenals are "normal." However, a better diagnostic approach will test your levels at different times of the day, which is much more likely to reveal an out-of-whack pattern of cortisol or DHEA secretion. If you want to be tested for adrenal function, see a health care practitioner who understands the complexities of adrenal testing.

ADRENAL STRESSORS

The following stressors can lead to fatigue and, ultimately, adrenal dysfunction—which may, in turn, make some stressors worse:

- Excessive, unremitting worry, anger, guilt, anxiety, or fear
- Depression
- Excessive exercise
- Chronic exposure to industrial or other toxins
- Chronic or severe allergies
- Overwork, both physical and mental (this applies only if you're doing work that doesn't fulfill you)
- Chronically late hours or insufficient sleep
- Unhealed trauma or injury
- Chronic illness
- Light-cycle disruption: shift work
- Surgery

How to Restore Your Adrenal Function

If, after testing, you find that you are producing inadequate levels of adrenal hormones, there are several available routes for increasing either DHEA, cortisol, or both. One is by taking the hormone directly. The other—which is far better over the long run—is to restore adrenal health and function so that these glands are eventually able to produce the hormones you need without outside supplements. That will require making changes in the lifestyle that caused the adrenal depletion. If you supplement your adrenal hormones in dosages that are too high, or if you take supplements for too long, the result can be permanent depression of adrenal function.

DHEA: DHEA is available as tablets, transdermal creams, or sublingual tinctures. Though DHEA is available over the counter in natural food stores, quality varies widely. It is always best to work with a health care provider who can help you monitor your dosage and your blood or salivary levels. Also I recommend making sure you are taking pharmaceutical-grade DHEA. (See Resources.) Regardless of how you take your DHEA, blood or salivary levels should be retaken regularly until they return to normal. When levels return to the normal range, the dose should be gradually tapered until you're off the hormone completely.

DHEA can also be increased by focusing more on loving thoughts that bring you pleasure (such as thinking about loved ones, favorite pets, a delicious meal, or a sweet memory) and less on thoughts that are stressful. This learning to "think with your heart" may be challenging at first, but because it short-circuits the harm done by the body's physiological reaction to stress, it's a valuable skill. I recommend the training programs and books from The Institute of HeartMath. (For more information on HeartMath, call the institute at 800–450–9111 or visit www.heartmath.com; I also recommend the book *The Amazing Power of Deliberate Intent* [Hay House, 2006] by Esther and Jerry Hicks.) In addition, do more things that bring you pleasure and make you laugh and fewer activities that feel like obligations. Spend more time with people who make you feel good and less with people who are draining. Dwell more on what you like about yourself and less on what you see as your limitations. In short, have more fun! Make pleasure a priority instead of a luxury. This takes courage, and it's worth it.

CORTISOL: Some individuals require very small doses of hydrocortisone, which can be used safely and effectively if prescribed by a health care provider knowledgeable about how and when to use it.[10]

DIET: The food plan outlined in chapter 7 is designed to support and recharge your adrenals, among other benefits. Be sure to get enough protein; every meal or snack should contain some protein. Remember that caffeine whips your adrenals into a frenzy; avoid it altogether. Also avoid fasting or cleansing regimens.

NUTRITIONAL SUPPLEMENTS: Supplement your diet at the higher ranges of the nutrients listed in chapter 7 for at least three months for best results. After that, you can reduce them depending upon how you feel. Be sure you're taking plenty of vitamin C (1,000 to 2,000 mg a day in divided doses), a B complex (25 to 50 mg a day), zinc (15 to 30 mg daily), and magnesium (300 to 800 mg per day in divided doses—in fumarate, citrate, glycinate, or malate form). My colleague Norm Shealy, M.D., Ph.D., has had much success with transdermal magnesium (which you can order from his company, Self-Health Systems; for more information, call 888–272–6109 or visit www.normshealy.com). Dr. Shealy's Youth Formula supplement is specifically designed for raising DHEA.

SLEEP: Sleep is the most effective approach to high adrenaline levels. Sleep restores adrenal function better than almost anything else. (When I'm stressed, I routinely sleep ten hours or more a night! Shoot for at least eight solid hours per night.)

EXERCISE: Regular light-to-moderate exercise, but not so much that you feel depleted afterward.

SUNLIGHT: Exposure to sunlight is not only good for your adrenal glands, but it boosts vitamin D, as well. But do this wisely. Sunbathe only in the early morning or later afternoon, never in midday, and never enough to burn or even redden your skin. Work up to ten to fifteen minutes of exposure three to four times per week. This type of brief exposure will not increase your risk of skin cancer.

HERBAL SUPPORT: Because one of the components of Siberian ginseng is related to a precursor for DHEA and cortisol, taking this herb can be very helpful in restoring proper adrenal function. Try one 100 mg capsule two times a day. It can have a stimulating effect, though, so if it interferes with your sleep, take it before three P.M. Licorice root can also help your adrenals because it contains plant hormones that mimic the effects of cortisol. Take up to one-quarter teaspoon of 5:1 solid licorice root extract three times a day.

WHAT TO EXPECT IN YOUR TRANSITION

Despite the fact that there are stacks of books describing the "normal" symptoms of perimenopause, many women escape most or all of them. Nonetheless, there are a number of symptoms that women in this culture report frequently, and you may want to review the list on the following pages in order to be informed and prepared. It may also decrease your anxiety about a particular symptom to know that it is related to a normal transition.

Bear in mind the following caveat: it is possible for your expectation of your menopausal experience to become your reality simply because it's what you believe will happen. Remember that in some

FIGURE 8: MENOPAUSAL SYMPTOMS TIMELINE

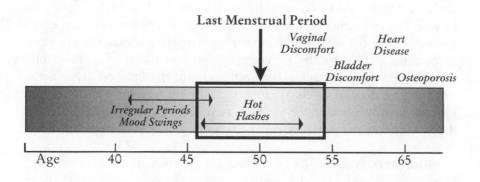

cultures women rarely report any symptoms from perimenopause, and it is not necessarily written into your biological script that you will have any discomfort, either.

Keep in mind also that your mother's menopause experience probably created a powerful unconscious blueprint for you. If your mother's experience was negative, do not assume that you will follow in her footsteps. Focus instead on the ways in which you are different from your mother, and choose a new and improved script for yourself. (See my book *Mother-Daughter Wisdom* [Bantam Books, 2005] for information on how to update the beliefs and behaviors you learned from your mother.)

The quotations that describe the symptoms below come from patients or newsletter subscribers. I have indicated the chapters in which symptoms and solutions are discussed in more detail.

Hot Flashes

"I've had to give up wearing sweaters because I can suddenly get so hot that I feel the need to open all the windows (even in the winter) and peel off as many layers as I can."

Hot flashes are the most common perimenopausal symptom in our culture, occurring in about 70 to 85 percent of all perimenopausal women.[11] They can be very mild or so severe that they result in sleep deprivation and subsequent depression. They begin as a sudden, transient sensation of warmth that can then become intense heat over the face, scalp, and chest area; it may be accompanied by redness and perspiration. They are also sometimes accompanied by an increased heart rate, tingling in the hands, a crawling sensation under the skin, and/or nausea. In some cases the hot flash is followed by a feeling of being chilled. In the majority of women, hot flashes often start just before or during the menstrual periods during perimenopause. Triggered by falling estrogen and rising FSH, they tend to become more frequent as we approach our final period. That is the time when estrogen levels are lowest and FSH levels are highest. Hot flashes usually go away a year or two after actual menopause, although in some (relatively rare) cases they may continue for many years.

Also known as vasomotor flushing, the hot flash occurs when blood vessels in the skin of the head and neck open more widely than usual, allowing more blood to shift into the area, creating heat and redness. Besides hormonal changes, external factors can influence the intensity and duration of a woman's hot flashes. Anxiety and/or tension can magnify them, as can a diet high in simple sugars and refined carbohydrates such as are found in fruit juices, cakes, cookies, candy, white bread, wine and beer, and so on. Coffee—even decaf—also triggers them in some women.

There are many approaches to cooling hot flashes. Estrogen replacement is about 95 percent effective, and it is considered the "gold standard" for hot flash relief. A 2 percent progesterone skin cream also works in many perimenopausal women; as little as ¼ tsp rubbed into the skin once per day may provide relief.[12] (See chapter 5, "Hormone Replacement.") In addition, meditation and relaxation techniques (such as Dr. Herbert Benson's famous Relaxation Response) have been successfully used to cool hot flashes in 90 percent of women, without any hormonal therapy at all.[13] This is because meditation lowers stress hormone levels.

Many women also find relief when they improve their diets. (See chapter 7, "The Menopause Food Plan.") Soy foods (a total of 45–160 mg of soy isoflavones per day) provide relief, as do many herbs, such as black cohosh, dong quai, or chasteberry. Acupuncture can also be very effective. (These approaches are detailed in chapter 6, "Foods and Supplements to Support the Change.")

Night Sweats

"I sweat so much at night, I have to get up to change the sheets."
Night sweats are on a continuum with hot flashes. Traditional
Chinese Medicine tells us, and many of my patients have confirmed,
that three to four A.M. is the most common time for night sweats,
which may wake you up drenched with perspiration. (This often happens postpartum, as well. I like to think of it as the body's way of
detoxing.)

Heart Palpitations

*"It's like all of a sudden I'm aware of my heartbeat, whereas be-
fore my heart just did its job without me noticing it."*
Like hot flashes, palpitations can range from mild to severe. They
are rarely dangerous, though they can sometimes be very frightening.
They are the result of imbalances between the sympathetic and
parasympathetic nervous systems triggered by stress hormones and
are often related to fear and anxiety. If they persist, see your doctor.
(See chapter 14, "Living with Heart, Passion, and Joy.")

LESLIE: *Power Surges at Menopause*

Leslie is an art teacher at a local high school and doubles as an
unofficial counselor for her students, who uniformly respect and love
her for her obvious devotion. "I'm one of those art teachers you can
spot a mile away," she wrote. "I look the part, I guess. I try to do
more than just teach kids how to paint or sculpt—I mean, there's art
all around us in this world, and much of the joy of life is in appreci-
ating it. I try to demonstrate that in the way I live."
Leslie likes the image of hot flashes as "power surges," symboliz-
ing a positive, transformative process, and she did not find her hot
flashes or any of her other symptoms to be troublesome, nor did she
want to mask or muffle them with medication. "My doctor wasn't
surprised when I told her I chose to forgo hormone replacement therapy. She knew I saw this as a way of honoring my body and the natural changes going on within me. At the same time, I did want to
provide my body with support and help it adjust, so my symptoms
wouldn't be severe." Leslie chose to provide that support through
improved nutrition, herbs, and plant-based hormones (phytoestrogens). She takes black cohosh root, which softened her hot flashes

within the first week and kept them mild enough that they were merely "interesting" rather than intrusive. She also drinks a glass of vanilla-flavored soy milk every morning and evening.

Migraine Headaches

"Ever since I turned forty, I've gotten a pounding headache the day or two before my period is due. This has never happened before."

Imbalanced hormone levels contribute to so-called menstrual migraine during perimenopause and menopause. This type of headache usually comes just before your period, when both estrogen and progesterone levels can fall dramatically. Hundreds of women have been able to completely recover from menstrual and menopausal migraines through the use of 2 percent progesterone cream. Apply ¼–½ tsp on your skin daily for the two weeks prior to your period, or three weeks out of every month if you're no longer having periods. (For other headache remedies, see Resources.) Acupuncture and herbs (e.g., feverfew) also often help migraines.

Breast Swelling and Tenderness

"My breasts are sometimes so tender, it hurts to hug my children."

Many women have tender breasts just before their periods. But during perimenopause, you may notice that your breasts feel tender or swollen much more often. This is far more common when a woman is experiencing estrogen dominance. Relief can often be achieved by following a hormone-balancing diet (see chapter 7, "The Menopause Food Plan"), ensuring an adequate intake of B vitamins and omega-3 fats such as EPA and DHA (1,000 to 2,000 mg once or twice daily), stopping caffeine, and/or using 2 percent progesterone cream (¼ tsp twice per day). The addition of whole soy foods to the diet can also be very helpful. (See chapter 13, "Creating Breast Health.")

Heavy Menstrual Periods

"My periods have become so heavy that I soak through a couple of tampons and an overnight maxi pad in fifteen minutes. Sometimes I even soak through my clothing at work."

When estrogen levels are high or even normal but progesterone levels are too low from lack of ovulation, the monthly estrogen-driven buildup of the uterine lining (the endometrium) continues unopposed. When it finally breaks down, the result can be erratic, heavy bleeding that can go on for days at a time.

The problem can become so troublesome that some women resort to hysterectomy as a solution, but because heavy bleeding often resolves as a woman approaches menopause, hysterectomy is rarely necessary. The unopposed estrogen can often be treated with various types of progesterone or birth control pills. Since the problem is often worse in women who have too much body fat (fat produces estrogen), exercise and diet often help. Alternatives such as acupuncture and Traditional Chinese Medicine are also often helpful. In severe cases, the lining of the uterus can be cauterized via laser surgery in a procedure known as endometrial ablation. (See chapter 8, "Creating Pelvic Health and Power.")

Irregular or Erratic Periods

"I never know when I'm going to get a period. Sometimes I have a normal period. Then one week later I'll have some spotting. Then I'll go for three months before I have any bleeding again. I have to carry pads with me all the time, just in case."

When a woman is going through the hormonal changes of perimenopause, just about any kind of uterine bleeding is possible, ranging from periods that become very light and short to periods that space out to every three months or more. And some women have bleeding patterns that are so erratic, they don't seem like periods at all.

If you can live with erratic periods for a while, the problem will go away. It's not really abnormal. But if you also have other symptoms, such as mood swings or headaches, or simply want more regular periods, a very wide variety of treatments are available, ranging from conventional birth control pills to effective alternatives like natural progesterone skin cream or the herb chasteberry (*Vitex agnus-castus*), which helps regulate the hypothalamic-pituitary-ovarian axis to produce more progesterone. (See chapter 8, "Creating Pelvic Health and Power.")

Fibroids

"I was having irregular bleeding, and when I went in for my annual visit with my gynecologist, she told me that I had a growth in my uterus that was a fibroid. An ultrasound confirmed my doctor's diagnosis. My doctor tells me that we can just watch it."

About 40 percent of women develop benign fibroid growths in the uterus during perimenopause. Their growth is stimulated by estrogen, and they can become quite large. Fibroids shrink dramatically after menopause and, like heavy bleeding, do not usually require surgery or other treatment, especially if they don't produce symptoms. Some fibroids, however, can cause heavy bleeding, depending upon their position in the pelvis. Small ones can be removed through laparoscopic surgery or sometimes by surgical removal through the vagina. Uterine artery embolization (UAE) or ultrasonic treatment (such as Exablate) are other nonsurgical treatments. Weight loss, acupuncture, herbs, dietary change, and natural progesterone are all effective alternatives in many cases. (See chapter 8, "Creating Pelvic Health and Power.") Many medical centers, such as The Cleveland Clinic and Johns Hopkins, now have fibroid treatment centers that offer women a wide range of different options.

Loss of Sexual Desire

"There's nothing wrong with my marriage. I love my husband. But quite frankly, I don't even get turned on by Matthew McConaughey anymore, let alone my husband."

The first thing that needs to be checked in a woman with loss of sexual desire is her hormone levels. For reasons that aren't clear, some women experience a drop in their testosterone levels during perimenopause; this can result in lack of sexual desire. Adrenal exhaustion can be another factor. If these levels are low, supplementation with small amounts of testosterone or its precursor, DHEA, will sometimes restore libido to normal levels. For some women, libido problems are related to lack of estrogen or thinning of the vaginal tissue. (See chapter 9, "Sex and Menopause.") Women who've undergone removal of their ovaries surgically, or whose ovarian function has been compromised by illness, chemotherapy, or radiation, have lost a major source of their normal hormone production. A variety of safe alternatives, such as high-dose soy isoflavones, can often help in situations such as these.

Vaginal Dryness and/or Painful Intercourse

"I just don't seem to be able to get lubricated during sex anymore. And when we do have intercourse, it hurts!"

The lining of the outer one-third of the urethra and the lining of the vagina are estrogen-sensitive. Symptoms may arise from a lack of estrogen, as well as from decreases in muscle tone and subsequent blood supply in the urogenital area.

For many women, the first sign of perimenopause is a decrease in normal vaginal discharge. This is a direct result of decreasing estrogen levels. Some may need to use a vaginal lubricant (e.g., K-Y Jelly or Crème de la Femme) during intercourse because arousal and full lubrication take longer. Topical estrogen cream, vitamin E suppositories, systemic estrogen therapy, or increasing intake of phytoestrogens such as soy can be very helpful. Some of my patients have been able to increase vaginal lubrication through creative visualization. (See chapter 9, "Sex and Menopause.")

Urinary Symptoms

"I keep getting symptoms that feel as though I have a urinary tract infection. I feel as though I have to urinate all the time, but my urine tests don't show any evidence of infection."

"I got my first-ever UTI at age forty-five—as it turned out, the first of many."

"Sometimes I lose urine when I cough or sneeze. I'm worried that if this continues, I'm going to end up using adult diapers!"

Recurrent urinary tract infections or urinary stress incontinence (the loss of urine with coughing, sneezing, laughing, etc.) may occur because of the thinning of the estrogen-dependent lining of the outer urethra. Urinary symptoms often resolve through the use of a small dab of estrogen cream applied locally. Kegel exercises can also increase blood flow to the area and help with stress incontinence. (See chapter 8, "Creating Pelvic Health and Power.")

Skin

"Almost overnight it feels as though my skin has become dry and crepey, especially around my eyes."

The collagen layer of our skin becomes thinner as our hormone levels fall. A wide variety of highly effective skin treatments is now available that help build collagen, resurface the skin, and prevent wrinkles. Systemic or topical hormones; foods rich in phytoestrogens, such as soy; and antioxidant supplements such as vitamin C, vitamin E, glutathione, and proanthocyanidins (from grape seeds or pine bark) also help build collagen and rejuvenate the skin. (See chapter 11, "From Rosebud to Rose Hip.")

Bone Loss

"My grandmother gets shorter every year, and more bent over. I don't want that to happen to me."

For many women, bone loss through the insidious process known as osteoporosis begins as early as age thirty—or even earlier. Because of chronic dieting, undereating, overexercising, lack of nutrients, or anorexia, many women do not reach the peak bone density they should when they are in their teens, twenties, and thirties. (Ideally, osteoporosis prevention should begin in childhood!) So when a woman turns forty and her hormonal levels begin to shift, her bone density may already be compromised. When estrogen, progesterone, and androgen levels start to shift, the collagen matrix that forms the foundation of healthy bone may start to weaken, especially when a woman's nutrition and exercise regimens are lacking. You can maintain the collagen matrix in your bones and also help rebuild healthy bone in a variety of ways, which include getting adequate phytohormones from foods such as soy, from herbs, hormone replacement, calcium and magnesium supplements, getting adequate vitamin D from sun exposure or supplements, and by doing weight-bearing exercise. (See chapter 12, "Standing Tall for Life.")

Mood Swings

"I find myself crying during television commercials. Then I fly off the handle at my kids for no reason."

As I pointed out in chapter 2, many women experience an intensification of the kind of volatility in their moods that they once felt primarily before their periods, if at all. Part of the reason for this volatility, or for the increase in dark, negative moods, is hormonal. But it may also be a signal from your inner wisdom, trying to get your attention.

Insomnia

"I just don't seem to be able to get to sleep at night. When I do, I often wake up soaking wet and hot. So I throw off the blankets, and then get chilled!"

Many women wouldn't have insomnia if it weren't for their night sweats and hot flashes. For others, anxiety keeps them from sleeping soundly. And so does a refined-food, low-nutrient diet. If your sleep problems are related to hot flashes, they'll often resolve with hot-flash treatment. If they're due to anxiety, you may need to make some changes in your life that the anxiety is bringing to your attention. You may also need to clean up your diet. Other sleep problems may be related to the fact that perimenopause, like adolescence, is a time of transition in sleep patterns. Some of us, like teenagers, will suddenly start requiring much greater amounts of sleep than before. Typically, this changes again after menopause, when we need less sleep than during our twenties and thirties. Some women find daytime naps help during the transition. (See the sleep section of "How to Restore Your Adrenal Function" in this chapter, and also see chapter 10, "Nurturing Your Brain.")

Fuzzy Thinking

"I keep losing my keys. I walk into a room and forget why I'm there. Sometimes my head feels like it's filled with cotton."

Many women report a feeling of forgetfulness and "cotton head" during perimenopause. It's not unusual to have trouble concentrating or to do things like put the portable phone in the refrigerator. The same thing often happens postpartum when a woman comes home with a new baby and suddenly feels incapable of balancing her checkbook. The difference between the postpartum period and perimenopause is that during perimenopause you're giving birth to yourself. It often feels as though the logical side of the brain goes to sleep for a while as a way to force us to become more intuitive and more in tune with our emotions and inner wisdom. Herbs such as ginkgo and Saint-John's-wort can help keep your mind clear. So can following a diet that keeps blood sugar stable. (See chapter 7, "The Menopause Food Plan.") Some women find that soy isoflavones or hormones such as progesterone or estrogen are also helpful. The main thing to remember is that you're not getting Alzheimer's. You're just rewiring your brain for a whole new way of thinking. (See chapter 10, "Nurturing Your Brain.")

How Long Will My Symptoms Last?

Many women believe that the symptoms they are experiencing are what menopause—and life—will feel like from this day forward. The truth is that those symptoms, when present, are labor pains, as it were—part of our adaptation to the hormonal changes that take place as our biological focus switches from procreation to personal growth. In other words, the symptoms of the climacteric are temporary. How long they'll last depends on a number of factors, including the type of menopause a woman is experiencing (see page 112), what else is going on in her life at the time, and the ability of her body and soul to support her through this period of transition. In this culture the symptoms of perimenopause, in a natural transition, last anywhere from five to ten years, with a gradual crescendo in the beginning, a peak as the woman approaches the midpoint of the transition, and a gradual decrescendo toward the end as the body learns to live in harmony with its new hormonal support system.

Because all perimenopausal symptoms are interrelated, the treatment of one symptom may alleviate other symptoms as well. Since so many different treatments are effective, an individual woman will want to choose the ones that appeal to her most. Many women select several different treatments at the same time. An example of this would be taking bioidentical hormone replacement along with a soy product and a good multivitamin, and adding an exercise program. The bottom line is this: there's no need to suffer through perimenopause. As you read through the chapters that follow, choose the treatments that speak to you. Experiment. Your body is constantly changing. You can't really make a mistake.

5

Hormone Replacement:
An Individual Choice

The science of hormone replacement has been in continual evolution since estrogen replacement was first introduced in 1949 and the first birth control pills hit the market in the 1960s. The pill gave women a magic bullet that enabled them to go about their daily lives without being conscious of their natural hormonal and fertility rhythms. The downside is that these rhythms and the natural wisdom that created them have become pathologized, leading women to believe that synthetic, man-made hormones are safer and better than the "unpredictable" ones found naturally in our bodies. Conventional hormone replacement is an extension of this thinking: that the female body is deficient and needs to be fixed.

Today, however, there are new options that are much more respectful of the body's wisdom. To understand how they evolved, it helps to know where we're coming from.

A BRIEF HISTORY OF HORMONE REPLACEMENT

When I was doing my family practice training in a small Vermont hospital, I remember going to the library and taking down a book that caught my eye, way up on the top shelf. It was *Feminine Forever*

(M. Evans, 1966), by Robert Wilson, M.D. It described in graphic detail how the lack of estrogen at menopause led inevitably to the shriveling of a woman's body, leaving her old and decrepit.

His solution: estrogen pills to replace what her deficient body no longer produced. This was presented as a sort of magic potion that would leave her "feminine forever": youthful, resilient, moist, sexy, and desirable. The way Wilson described estrogen's benefits, I couldn't imagine a woman who would want to live without it at menopause— a life passage about which my medical training had taught me virtually nothing.

I was still unconscious about how embedded the devaluation of female bodies is within our culture, and how powerfully this devaluation influences the practice of medicine and the science that supports it. (At the time, anyone having her first baby at the age of thirty or older was referred to as an "elderly primigravida.") Like many of my peers, my own beliefs were clouded by my cultural legacy: just as male is superior to female, young is superior to old. Salvation would come through denying any differences between male and female, and endeavoring to stay forever young. Our better-living-through-chemistry society was poised to help us control our unruly female physiology through birth control pills during our reproductive years and estrogen during menopause. Not surprisingly, sales of Premarin— the first estrogen to be marketed—began to soar.

A Shadow Crosses over Premarin

When I was a third-year medical student, one of my mother's close friends confided to me that she had to stop taking her Premarin because she had started to have bleeding. She was later diagnosed with a condition known as adenomatous hyperplasia of the endometrium— indicating that her uterine lining was being overstimulated by the Premarin. Although she never resumed taking Premarin, her bleeding didn't return, and she didn't suddenly shrivel up, either. She was climbing mountains and going on long hikes with her friends right up to the end of her life at age ninety.

My mother's friend was not alone. In the mid to late 1970s, study after study appeared that proved beyond any doubt that taking estrogen resulted in an up to fourfold greater risk for developing uterine cancer. At about this same time, birth control pills were shown to increase the risk of stroke, pulmonary embolism, and heart attack— deadly complications in young women. Premarin sales plummeted.

Women grew afraid of the pill. It would take several years before new studies of lower-dose pills, and major marketing efforts, quelled these fears—though never entirely.

Premarin Sales Revive

Then studies began to appear showing that estrogen could help prevent osteoporosis. I was intrigued. My husband was doing his training in orthopedic surgery, and he spent many nights repairing hip fractures in older women, many of whom never walked or lived independently again.

I researched the link between estrogen and bone health and did a presentation on it for the OB/GYN staff at the hospital. Many of my professors were dead set against Premarin for any indication—they had been burned too badly by the uterine cancer findings. And although I was convinced that estrogen replacement could help prevent osteoporosis, I was far more interested in alternatives such as calcium supplementation and exercise. A colleague and I even discussed setting up a long-term study involving diet and exercise, but we were far too busy just trying to complete our residencies, and it would take another twenty years for those ideas to be proved and accepted by mainstream doctors.

Meanwhile, other studies showed that endometrial cancer could be prevented if a woman was given progesterone along with her dose of estrogen. Estrogen replacement slowly but surely made its way back onto the scene—this time in combination with Provera, a synthetic form of progesterone, which was given to all women on estrogen unless they had had hysterectomies. (In that case, doctors reasoned, there was no reason to give it.) Progesterone's role was thus reduced to that of a uterine vacuum cleaner—one that prevented excessive buildup of the uterine lining but had no inherent benefits of its own.

Premarin Becomes Synonymous with Hormone Replacement

Premarin is composed of estrogenic compounds derived from the urine of pregnant mares. Since its introduction in 1949, it has maintained its place as the queen of the hormone replacement world. In fact, when you say "hormone replacement," most people, including doctors, still think Premarin—end of discussion.

Its sales hit an all-time high during the 1980s and early '90s, when study after study (many supported by Wyeth-Ayerst, the maker of Premarin) began to support estrogen's role in keeping the cardiovascular system healthy. For example, it was shown to lower LDL cholesterol, which the famous Framingham study had identified as a risk for heart attack. Given that cardiovascular disease was also emerging as the number-one killer of women past menopause, doctors everywhere became convinced that all menopausal women needed estrogen to protect their hearts. Some even refused to care for women who wouldn't take it.

Other benefits were also touted. Premarin seemed to do everything: lift depression, thicken vaginal tissue, stop hot flashes, prevent heart disease, prevent osteoporosis, and even ward off Alzheimer's disease. Premarin was prescribed freely in a one-size-fits-all manner—the same dose for every woman, regardless of her size or her medical history. Provera was added for ten to twelve days of every month to protect the uterus. Later, Premarin and Provera were combined into one pill known as Prempro or Premphase. That was hormone replacement.

The End of the Premarin Empire?

But then a big fly found its way into the ointment. Multiple studies began to support an incontrovertible link between estrogen supplementation and breast cancer. This link makes biological sense, since estrogen is well known to stimulate the growth of estrogen-sensitive tissue, like that in the breast and uterus. Still, the cardiovascular benefits seemed so strong that many women were persuaded to override their fear of breast cancer and continue to take Premarin or Prempro.

At the turn of the millennium, however, several large prospective studies challenged the heart-protection gospel. In the large HERS (Heart and Estrogen/Progestin Replacement Study) trial of women who already had heart disease, hormone replacement in the form of Premarin and Provera not only *did not decrease* their risk of subsequent heart attack, it actually *increased* that risk significantly in the first year of use, after which the risk leveled off.

Then, in July 2002, one branch of the huge Women's Health Initiative, a long-term government-funded study of HRT, was stopped abruptly because the data showed that the risks of long-term Prempro use clearly outweighed the benefits. The study followed sixteen thousand initially healthy postmenopausal women randomly assigned to take either Prempro or a look-alike placebo. Those on the synthetic hormone combination were found to suffer more breast cancers, heart attacks, strokes, and blood clots than the women on placebo.[1] A second study from the National Cancer Institute, released on the same day, reported that women who used estrogen-only hormone replacement for longer than ten years doubled their risk for ovarian cancer.[2]

When this information was released, it created mass confusion for the millions of women and their doctors who had been convinced for over a decade that taking estrogen for life was the key to heart disease prevention, good skin, healthy bones, and a great sex life. Virtually overnight, there was a revolution in the way our culture views hormone replacement in general and Prempro in particular. Women stopped taking it in droves, and as a profession, we doctors realized that we needed to individualize our care.

Then in early 2006, a reanalysis of the data from the Nurses' Health Study and the Women's Health Initiative (WHI) study indicated that younger women who started HRT within ten years after menopause experienced an 11 to 30 percent decreased risk for heart attack—the kind of result that researchers had hoped to see when the WHI started. But those who started later (ten years or more after menopause—the majority of women in the WHI) experienced an increased risk for stroke, heart attack, and even Alzheimer's disease. Younger women on estrogen alone had a 44 percent decreased risk for heart disease as long as they started within ten years of menopause.[3] This new data certainly lines up with the well-documented beneficial effect of estrogen on blood vessels. No one knows for sure why HRT must be given earlier to get a good cardiovascular effect when the same drug given ten years later can be dangerous. I suspect it has something to do with preventing the kind of vascular damage that tends to result from years of stress, high blood sugar, a nutrient-poor diet, and not enough exercise.

At the end of the day, here's what we're left with. After decades of trying to convince all women that menopause was a deficiency state that could be "cured" by HRT, we finally realized the truth. There is no magic bullet, one-size-fits-all hormone prescription or drug regimen of any kind that is right and healthy for all or even most women to take indefinitely. And because each of us is an individual with differing needs, constitution, beliefs, and environment, there never will be—no matter how many studies are done. Quite frankly, I consider that good news.

On the other hand, there's no reason to throw out the baby with the bathwater. The science of hormone replacement is still evolving and the newest data from the reanalysis of the WHI and Nurses' Health studies is encouraging. HRT has some very real benefits. Even in the Women's Health Initiative study of older women, the women who were using Prempro (which I consider the least desirable form of HRT) were at decreased risk for bowel cancer and fractures compared to those who were on placebo. And no one would disagree that HRT offers many women one of the best ways to get relief from perimenopausal symptoms such as hot flashes. Thankfully, there are ways to get the benefits of HRT while decreasing the risks and side effects.

BIOIDENTICAL HORMONES: NATURE'S IDEAL DESIGN

In contrast to Premarin, Provera, and Prempro, the hormones that I recommend are exactly the same as those found in the female body. Though they are synthesized in the lab from hormone precursors found in soybeans or yams, their molecular structure is designed to be an exact match of the hormones found in the human body. Hence we call them *bioidentical*—a term that is far more precise than *natural,* which can be used in confusing and ambiguous ways—e.g., Premarin is said by some people to be a "natural" product because it is made from horse urine. As Joel Hargrove, M.D., a pioneer in the use of bioidentical hormones and the former medical director of the Menopause Center at Vanderbilt University Medical Center in Tennessee, has said, "Premarin is a natural hormone if your native food is hay."

Because bioidentical hormones are just like the hormones that our bodies were designed to recognize and utilize, their effects are more physiologic—consistent with our normal biochemistry—with less chance for unpredictable side effects at low replacement doses than with synthetic, non-bioidentical hormones.

To take advantage of these benefits, you first have to give up the notion that there is an easy, one-size-fits-all answer. There isn't. Some women need or want HRT, some don't. Some will need to use it for only a year or two. Some will want to stay on it longer. When it comes to hormone replacement, the science we look to for answers is inconsistent, influenced by market forces, and confusing to researchers, doctors, and patients alike. The blessing is that this dilemma forces us to tune in more fully to our inner wisdom, and to make our choices in full partnership with our intuition *and* intellect. This approach is the essence of feminine wisdom.

Moving Beyond Premarin

When Premarin was introduced, the technology to produce other types of estrogen was not yet available, so it became the gold standard. However, these equine estrogens aren't normally found in the human female body, and they are often associated with side effects such as headaches, bloating, and sore breasts. In addition, the metabolic breakdown products of Premarin in the human female are biologically stronger and more active than the original equine estrogens. A host of studies have shown that these breakdown products can produce DNA damage that is carcinogenic in tissue. Given this, it's no wonder that the incidence of breast cancer statistically increases when women are on this drug.[4] In contrast, the metabolic breakdown products of bioidentical estrogens are biologically weaker, so their effects on tissue do not last as long.

There's reason to believe that bioidentical estrogen at individualized low doses doesn't have the same carcinogenic effect on breast tissue as Premarin or Prempro. But until we have long-term studies of bioidentical estrogen to compare with the vast amount of data on Premarin, we won't have the scientific verification we need. Unfortunately, long-term studies are enormously expensive. The Women's Health Initiative study cost the American public well over $628 million.[5] It was also funded in part by Wyeth-Ayerst, the manufacturers of Premarin and Prempro, because the company hoped to be able to advertise its drugs as both preventives and treatments for heart disease, which is the leading cause of premature death among women.[6] Given the untoward results from the initial WHI study, what are the odds that a hormone manufacturer will take such a financial risk again? That remains to be seen. Nonetheless, many clinicians find that prescribing bioidentical hormone replacement for short-term relief of symptoms, such as vaginal dryness, hot flashes, and even mood swings, can work wonders for some women. The shifting news about Premarin and Prempro has actually opened the minds of many women and their doctors to these more physiologic and well-tolerated alternatives. Remember, this is all an ongoing process. So now, more than ever, you need to make the hormone choice in concert with your inner guidance.

HORMONE THERAPY: RESEARCH SUMMARY

Benefits of Estrogen

~ Hot flashes: Estrogen gives better hot flash relief than just about any other treatment. It can take up to four weeks to notice the effect.

~ Skin: Estrogen, either systemic or applied to the skin, can increase skin thickness and enhance the collagen layer in women whose estrogen is low. It can also help reduce wrinkling.

~ Sexual function: Estrogen can enhance sexual function by eliminating vaginal dryness and thinning which causes painful sex in many women. It works equally well either systemically or topically. Some studies suggest that estrogen enhances sexual desire. High-dose transdermal testosterone has been shown to increase desire in some women who've undergone surgical menopause.

~ Urinary tract: Locally applied estrogen may decrease the incidence of urinary tract infection. *Note:* Systemic estrogen has been shown to increase the risk of stress urinary incontinence.

~ Cognition: Estrogen (and other steroid hormones) have well-documented effects on nerve cells. However, estrogen does not prevent cognitive decline in older women nor does it improve already established dementia. Further studies are needed in this area.

~ Depression: Estrogen may have an antidepressive effect in some women but shouldn't be used as primary treatment. Synthetic progestins may have a depressive effect in some women. Menopause itself is not associated with an increase in depression.

~ Osteoporosis: Estrogen has a well-documented beneficial effect on bone density that is equivalent to the bisphosphonates (e.g., Fosamax). It definitely reduces fracture risk and probably does so in a different way than the SERMs (see page 152) or bisphosphonates.

~ Heart and blood vessels: Many studies have documented the positive effect of estrogen on the cardiovascular system. However, the WHI study released in 2002—a study of mostly older women who started HRT (estrogen plus synthetic progesterone) ten years or more after menopause—showed that Prempro increased the risk of heart attack and stroke. The 2006 reanalysis of the data on the WHI and Nurses' Health Study showed that estrogen decreases the risk of heart attack when women start it within ten years after going through menopause for reasons that aren't clear. More research needs to be done. But for now, most authorities don't recommend estrogen for the prevention of chronic diseases.

Risks of Estrogen

~ Breast cancer: Several randomized clinical trials and observational studies have shown that estrogen increases the risk of breast cancer. Once estrogen is discontinued, the risk quickly dissipates. The absolute risk of breast cancer with conventional HRT (estrogen plus synthetic progesterone) is very low (twenty additional cases over what would be expected per ten thousand women over five years). *Note:* Many well-designed studies do not show an increased risk of breast cancer with HRT.

~ Pancreatitis and gallstones: Women with high triglyceride levels are at increased risk for pancreatitis, which is sometimes fatal, when they take oral estrogen with or without progesterone. There is an increased risk of gallstones and biliary tract surgery with the use of estrogen in all women.

~ Blood clots and stroke: Estrogen appears to double the risk of blood clots. It also increases the risk of pulmonary embolism. Embolism is most likely to occur in the first year of therapy and especially in those with a history of blood clots. Randomized trials also show an increased risk for stroke with unopposed estrogen. This risk is greater in smokers and older women.

Neutral Effects of Estrogen

~ Weight changes and insulin resistance: Estrogen doesn't cause weight gain nor does it appear to affect blood sugar in those with diabetes.

~ Osteoarthritis: Estrogen doesn't help or hurt those with osteoarthritis.

~ Ovarian, endometrial, and bowel cancer: Some studies show an increased risk of ovarian cancer when estrogen is used for ten years or more. Estrogen therapy without the addition of progesterone increases the risk of endometrial cancer, but adding progesterone eliminates this risk. Estrogen definitely decreases the risk of colorectal cancer but experts agree that it shouldn't be prescribed solely for this purpose.

Source: American College of Obstetrics and Gynecology Hormone Therapy Task Force. (October 2004). *Obstetrics and Gynecology,* 104 (suppl. 4), 35–45.

The Balanced Approach:
Individualized Bioidentical Hormone Replacement

A full range of bioidentical hormones—either singly or in combination—is available by prescription from formulary pharmacies (pharmacies that make up preparations to order). The dosages can be individually adjusted. Hormones can be prescribed based on a woman's test results and symptoms, so she is taking only what she needs to maintain the optimal levels of hormones in her body. This approach is standard with thyroid hormone, but it wasn't applied to sex hormones until recently. (See Resources for how to locate a formulary pharmacy in your area.) It is also possible to create a bioidentical hormone replacement regimen using hormone preparations available in all conventional pharmacies. You just have to know which brands are bioidentical and which are not. (See the chart on page 165.)

These individualized hormones can be taken orally, transdermally, or vaginally, whichever route works best for the patient. Though most women are accustomed to taking pills, the transdermal route is the more physiologically appropriate way to take hormones because they go directly into the bloodstream from the skin. You can also keep the dose much lower with this route because absorption is more direct than through the GI tract. (The body's own hormones are secreted directly into the bloodstream by the endocrine organs.)

Oral preparations, on the other hand, have to first be absorbed from the gut and then transported to the liver, where they must undergo further metabolic breakdown before finally getting to the bloodstream. This process causes the liver to manufacture more clotting factors, which is one of the reasons that oral estrogen, especially at high doses, is associated with an increased risk of stroke, heart attack, and thrombophlebitis.

One popular form of HRT is to have a prescription created especially for you using a combination of one or more of the bioidentical estrogens (estradiol, estrone, estriol) combined with bioidentical progesterone and an androgen in the form of DHEA or testosterone, if needed. These hormones are mixed into a lotion, cream, or other base and applied to the skin.

Research has clearly shown that these bioidentical transdermal hormone replacement regimens provide adequate blood levels of hormone, protect the uterine lining from overstimulation, prevent breakthrough bleeding, and give very effective relief for perimenopausal symptoms.[7] Although the number of bioidentical hormone combinations is extensive, there are two formulations that I've found especially useful for relief of menopausal symptoms. These were developed by two pioneers in the bioidentical hormone field, Joel Hargrove, M.D., and Erika Schwartz, M.D. Dr. Hargrove was at the forefront of bioidentical hormone research for more than twenty years. His most recent and useful formulation combines estradiol, progesterone, and testosterone (when needed), mixed together in a dropper bottle so that you can easily apply them to your skin one drop at a time. The hormones are dissolved in a propylene glycol solvent that is absorbed almost immediately, so there's no residue. Each drop contains 0.25 mg of estradiol and 12.5 mg each of progesterone and testosterone (if needed). The usual dose is one to three drops per day. Any certified formulary pharmacy in the United States or abroad can create this formulation from your physician's prescription.

This method is particularly empowering because a woman herself can very easily adjust her dose as needed without danger of side effects. Dr. Hargrove notes, for example, that if a woman is having PMS symptoms such as water retention, headaches, and bloating, she's getting too much estrogen and needs to decrease her number of drops. The same is true if she develops vaginal bleeding. If she's getting hot flashes without PMS, she needs more estrogen and should

increase her dose. To date, thousands of very satisfied women are using Dr. Hargrove's approach, which is also highly cost-effective—
depending upon the pharmacy, many women spend as little as $70
per year total for their hormones.[8] (See Resources.)

Erika Schwartz, M.D., author of *The 30-Day Natural Hormone
Plan* (Warner Books, 2004) and *The Hormone Solution* (Warner
Books, 2002), is the founder of the International Hormone Institute,
which does research on natural hormones and educates the public
about their benefits. She offers online consultations in addition to
personalized three-month programs for balancing hormones. The
standard starting dose used by Dr. Schwartz is 0.3 mg of 17 beta
estradiol and 100 mg bioidentical progesterone—applied as a cream
to the inside of the wrists. A patient can gradually increase the dosage
to 0.6 mg estradiol and 200 mg progesterone daily. (For more information, call Dr. Schwartz at 866–373–7452 or visit her website at
www.drerika.com.)

Why So Many Hormones Are Synthetic

Though it should be intuitively and scientifically obvious that
bioidentical hormones in individualized doses would give the best results, many scientists and physicians have turned a blind eye to this
concept. The answer is simple: economics.

Bioidentical hormones cannot be patented, so there are no financial incentives for a pharmaceutical company to do the expensive
research and development necessary to develop new products containing them. (Unique delivery systems *can* be patented, however,
which is why patches such as Climara, Estraderm, and Vivelle, and
the vaginal ring Estring, all of which contain bioidentical estradiol,
can be profitable.)

Synthetic hormones, on the other hand, are made by altering the
molecular structure of a hormone enough so that it can be patented.
These maintain some of the activity of the natural hormone, but any
change in the three-dimensional structure of a hormone, no matter
how small, changes its biological effects on the cell in ways that are
not completely understood. (*Note:* Premarin is bioidentical for a
horse, not a human.)

Frankly, I trust the wisdom coming from Mother Nature's millions of years of experimentation much more than I trust fifty years
of biochemical wizardry from Father Pharmaceutical. But not all
women feel this way. Some feel far safer going with what their doctor

prescribes. And since beliefs affect biology, what you believe can shape your experience. It's your decision, and my approach is not meant to undermine any individual's positive experience.

What About Birth Control Pills?

Birth control pills are widely prescribed as a convenient way to put the perimenopausal body and its symptoms on autopilot until it's time to move to conventional hormone replacement. There's a currently popular trend to convince women that our menstrual periods themselves are dangerous and that going on the pill as early as our teenage years, and staying on it except to have children, will prevent long-term health problems. Please note, however, that all birth control pills consist of synthetics that mask our natural hormonal rhythms and the messages about our health that they convey. Birth control pills are also associated with a wide variety of side effects, including blood clots, headaches, and PMS. Although they are appropriate in some cases, I'd rather keep my hormones tuned in to the cycle of the moon and the planets—as opposed to the energy of a pharmaceutical company. You may not be prepared to use other birth control methods right now, or you may be using the pill to quell symptoms such as heavy or irregular periods—but just be aware that other options are available. Some women love how they feel on the pill. Others hate it. Make your choice based on how you feel!

A HORMONE PRIMER: ESSENTIAL INFORMATION EVERY WOMAN SHOULD KNOW

It's important to keep in mind that hormone replacement involves more than just estrogen. It also includes the other hormones produced by the ovaries: progesterone and androgens such as testosterone. Some women might be perfectly comfortable with no supplemental hormones; some might need progesterone only; some might need all three. Understanding their original roles in a woman's body, and the kinds of responses some women see when levels drop, can help you make your own very personal HRT decision.

Estrogen

For generations, estrogen has been the first (and often the only) hormone to be prescribed for women suffering from symptoms such as hot flashes, vaginal dryness, and mood swings. However, as I noted in chapter 4, estrogen levels don't fall until late in the menopausal transition, and the majority of perimenopausal symptoms in women with intact ovaries are related more to a lack of progesterone than to a lack of estrogen.

"Estrogen" actually encompasses three distinct estrogenic compounds produced naturally in the body: estradiol, estrone, and estriol. Estriol reaches its highest level during pregnancy; it has weaker biological effects on breast and uterine tissue than do estrone and estradiol. (Women with naturally higher estriol levels appear to have lower breast cancer rates than others, which has led some practitioners to prescribe estriol to decrease the risk of breast cancer.[9] Much more research is needed to establish the effectiveness of this approach.)

There is one area in which supplemental estriol is known to be particularly effective: urogenital symptoms. Applied locally in the

FIGURE 9: KINDS OF ESTROGEN

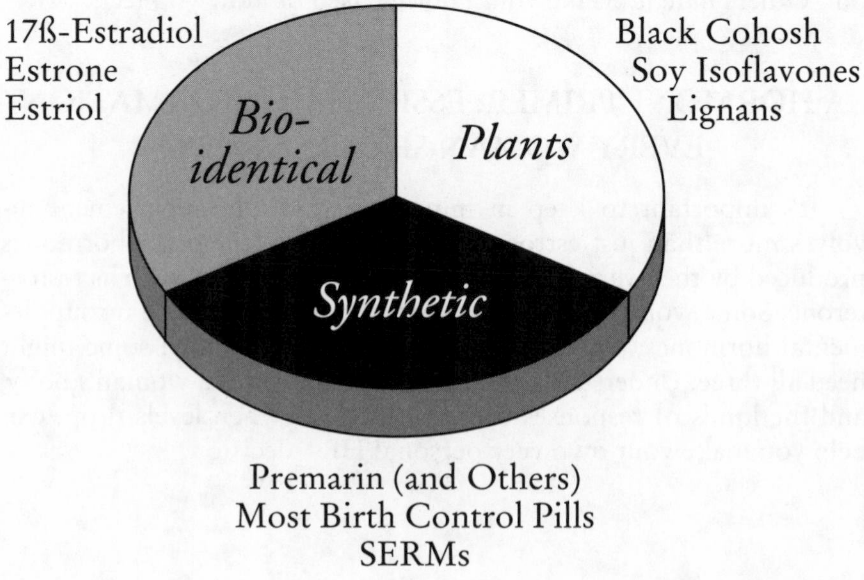

17ß-Estradiol
Estrone
Estriol

Black Cohosh
Soy Isoflavones
Lignans

Bio-identical

Plants

Synthetic

Premarin (and Others)
Most Birth Control Pills
SERMs

vagina, it relieves urinary frequency, vaginal dryness, and other conditions associated with thinning of these tissues.[10]

As I mentioned in chapter 4, there is reason to believe that estrogen's role during the childbearing years is quite different from its role after menopause. Before menopause, the primary role of estradiol is to stimulate growth in the breasts, ovaries, and uterus and to participate in the growth and maturation of egg-bearing follicles. It also is a major influence in stimulating maternal behavior. In other words, it promotes childbirth and child care. After menopause, estrone becomes the predominant estrogen. No one knows exactly why this happens, but obviously it has nothing to do with procreation. It is likely that estrogen's ability to protect heart and brain function, as well as bone strength, is part of its purpose in this phase of life.

Recall as well that the ovaries continue to produce small amounts of estradiol, as do the secondary hormone-production sites. As a result, it is biologically possible for a woman to produce enough of her own estrogen to support optimal health throughout the second half of her life. This is rarely taken into account, perhaps because stress, unmet spiritual needs, and cultural expectations conspire to impair a woman's natural ability to produce adequate levels of the estrogens.

The most obvious and immediate benefit of estrogen supplementation is relief from the symptoms of estrogen deficiency. (See box on page 152.) A longer-term benefit is estrogen's ability to help prevent excessive bone mineral loss leading to osteoporosis. Estrogen also helps maintain the thickness of the collagen layer in skin. Some studies have suggested that it may also help preserve mental function or at least delay the rate of so-called normal, age-related brain changes as well as dementia of the Alzheimer's type. However, a thorough review of all the major studies that have investigated this does not show a benefit—at least with Prempro or Premarin.[11] In general, there is not enough evidence to support prescribing estrogen for cognitive changes alone.

Estrogen is available in pills, skin patches, and vaginal creams. In low doses, even synthetic estrogen in vaginal creams has negligible systemwide absorption and is generally safe for women who need the local effect of estrogen but don't want any more exposure than necessary.

Symptoms of Estrogen Deficiency

- Hot flashes
- Night sweats
- Vaginal dryness
- Mood swings (mostly irritability and depression)
- Mental fuzziness
- Headaches, migraines
- Vaginal and/or bladder infections
- Incontinence; recurrent urinary tract infections
- Vaginal wall thinning
- Decreased sexual response

Symptoms of Estrogen Excess

- Bilateral, pounding headache
- Recurrent vaginal yeast infections
- Breast swelling and tenderness
- Depression
- Nausea, vomiting
- Bloating
- Leg cramps
- Yellow-tinged skin
- Excessive vaginal bleeding

A Note About "Designer Estrogens": SERMs

The selective estrogen receptor modulators (SERMs) are synthetic drugs such as tamoxifen and raloxifene. (These are the ones on the market at present; others are sure to follow.) They get their name from their ability to bind with estrogen receptors and selectively modulate the effects of estrogen in different body tissues. Tamoxifen (trade name Nolvadex) blocks the estrogen receptors on breast cells while maintaining some positive estrogenic effects on bone, uterine tissue, and the cardiovascular system. Raloxifene (trade name Evista) also promotes bone density while decreasing the stimulation of breast tissue by estrogen. This selective activity is possible because there are two different estrogen receptors, ER-alpha and ER-beta, each of which predominates in certain tissue. The same estrogen can produce different effects according to the receptor to which it binds.[12]

Tamoxifen, the most widely used SERM, was first approved by the FDA for the treatment of patients with estrogen-receptor–positive breast cancer in 1978. It is now prescribed for about half of all women diagnosed with breast cancer in the United States. It has been shown to reduce the risk of developing breast cancer in the remaining breast, as well as breast cancer recurrences and deaths. Tamoxifen is also approved for breast cancer prevention in women who are at high risk or perceived high risk for the disease. It helps prevent bone loss and also has a beneficial effect on LDL cholesterol but does not decrease the risk of heart disease.

Since the 2002 WHI study results underscored the risks of estrogen, especially in older women, raloxifene is being prescribed more than ever to protect women against osteoporosis. However, it doesn't protect bones as well as estrogen does. With or without estrogen, most women can get all the bone protection they need by doing weight-bearing exercise, getting enough vitamin D and minerals, and following the guidelines I've outlined for maintaining healthy bones in chapter 12. Why put yourself at risk with a relatively untested drug?

I'm very concerned about SERMs. They are not found anywhere in nature and have not been around long enough for us to truly assess their benefits and risks. Touted for their ability to stimulate the "good" effects of estrogen without the "bad" ones, these drugs are riding the current wave of panic about breast cancer and are being requested by women who really don't need them, or for whom there are far safer alternatives. If a young woman who fears breast cancer begins taking a SERM drug, she likely will be taking it for many years. This long-term blockage of some estrogen sites with stimulation of others is a double-edged sword. What if we find that these drugs actually increase the risk of Alzheimer's disease by blocking the estrogen receptors in the brain?

Troubling side effects of tamoxifen have already been documented, including an increased risk of certain visual disturbances, fatal pulmonary embolism, and endometrial cancer. Though studies indicate that raloxifene, unlike tamoxifen, can protect against endometrial cancer, both tamoxifen and raloxifene have been implicated in increasing the risk for colon cancer.[13] They also increase hot flashes in many women, the very symptom for which most perimenopausal women seek treatment in the first place.[14]

Even more disturbing is the finding that after five years of use, the anti-estrogenic effects of tamoxifen on breast cells appear to reverse. The drug now may become breast cancer–promoting, for reasons that are not clear.[15]

The bottom line is this: unless you have no other alternative, I recommend that you avoid SERMs or limit their use to five years or less. Better yet, stick with bioidentical hormones or the alternatives I outline in chapter 6.

Progesterone

A decline in progesterone is the first hormonal change to cause symptoms in a woman approaching menopause—sometimes years before she suspects she may be nearing the change. Because the body is designed for progesterone and estrogen to be present in a dynamic counterbalance with each other, the result is estrogen dominance, with symptoms of both progesterone deficiency and relative estrogen excess.

Progesterone comes primarily from the ovaries both before and after menopause, but it is also produced in both the brain and the peripheral nerves.[16] Its main job during the childbearing years is to prepare and maintain the uterus for its most important function: pregnancy. It also is a uterine muscle relaxant, preventing premature contractions. Progesterone levels rise in anticipation of pregnancy and stimulate the uterine lining to thicken with rich, well-vascularized tissue to support an embryo, then fall precipitously if pregnancy does not occur. This abrupt drop-off in progesterone is what signals the shedding of the "nest" (that thickened uterine lining) in the form of menstrual bleeding.

Progesterone also affects brain function. It produces a sense of calmness, and its sedating, antianxiety effect helps promote rejuvenating sleep.

Progesterone comes from a temporary yellowish gland in the ovary called the corpus luteum, formed quickly in the small cystlike structure left behind when a follicle ovulates. The corpus luteum produces increasing amounts of progesterone until the body sends the signal "We're not pregnant," at which point the corpus luteum is reabsorbed. As a woman reaches her mid-thirties to early forties, the follicle is more likely (at least in this culture) to fail to ovulate, which means the corpus luteum does not form.[17] Over time, this contributes to an increasing deficiency of progesterone.

Note: Our bodies are designed to accommodate very high levels of progesterone during pregnancy. For that reason, symptoms from excessive progesterone are rare. However, depression is a common side effect of synthetic progestins such as Provera. And a few women are so sensitive to progesterone that they become depressed even on very small doses of natural, bioidentical progesterone. Women who have this side effect should try using chasteberry (*Vitex agnus-castus*) to increase their body's progesterone naturally.

SYMPTOMS OF PROGESTERONE DEFICIENCY

~ Premenstrual migraine
~ PMS-like symptoms
~ Irregular or excessively heavy periods
~ Anxiety and nervousness

SYMPTOMS OF EXCESS PROGESTERONE

~ Sleepiness
~ Drowsiness
~ Depression

Bioidentical Progesterone

Bioidentical progesterone supplementation can help alleviate the symptoms of both progesterone deficiency and estrogen excess, restoring the body's balance.

This provides long-term as well as short-term benefits. As I've noted, a growing body of evidence points to estrogen dominance as a major factor in promoting breast or uterine cancer in susceptible women. Studies show that when estrogen replacement therapy (ERT) is taken in concert with an appropriate dose of progesterone (to form HRT), the incidence of uterine cancer does not increase. This is true whether the progesterone is synthetic or bioidentical. It is also clear

FIGURE 10: KINDS OF PROGESTERONE

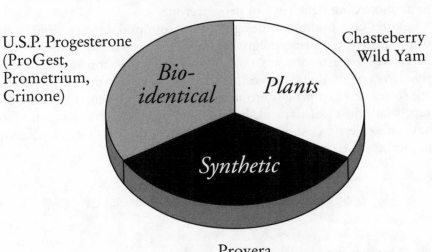

U.S.P. Progesterone
(ProGest,
Prometrium,
Crinone)

Chasteberry
Wild Yam

Provera
Norethindrone
Norgestrel (and Others)

that Prempro (Premarin and Provera) at the dosages used in the WHI study increases the risk of breast cancer. But we don't yet have long-term studies on the effects of bioidentical progesterone on breast cancer. (See chapter 13, "Creating Breast Health.")

Another advantage of progesterone supplementation relates to this hormone's relatively unique ability to be converted into other hormones as needed. If progesterone levels are adequate, for example, but testosterone levels are on the low side, supplemental progesterone can actually transform itself into testosterone. It also increases the levels of DHEA. (See Adrenal Replenishment Program, page 124.) Under the right circumstances, supplemental progesterone can even be metabolized into estrogen. This is one reason so many women enjoy symptomatic relief from using natural progesterone cream in early perimenopause, when there's a great deal of variation in the levels of all three hormones.

Progesterone cream is available over the counter in a 2 percent strength, and I've been recommending it for years. You can rub the cream anywhere on your body. One of the best places is right into your hands, because they are very well vascularized. But many women love the way progesterone cream works as a face or body cream. (I recommend ProGest Cream by Emerita and PhytoGest Cream by Kevala, available through Emerson Ecologics at www.emersonecologics.com.)

Natural progesterone is also available as a 4 to 8 percent gel (e.g., Crinone or Prochieve) or in an oral, micronized form (Prometrium). (Both require a perscription.) Though the manufacturer doesn't endorse this use, Prometrium capsules can be opened and the contents applied to the skin. I've found that this works very well for individuals who do not tolerate oral progesterone well but who require a higher dosage than is available with an over-the-counter cream.

THE YAM CREAM CAVEAT

Because bioidentical progesterone is often produced from wild Mexican yams, some women try to save money by buying one of a number of wild Mexican yam creams. The problem is, yam contains only a progesterone precursor, which remains inactive when it is absorbed through the skin. The conversion of wild yam into bioidentical (USP) progesterone can only occur in a laboratory setting. Yam creams may offer some beneficial phytoestrogens, but they certainly don't provide the documented benefits of laboratory-grade USP progesterone.

The Problem with Synthetics

Synthetic progestin is an altogether different story. The most commonly prescribed progestin is medroxyprogesterone acetate (MPA) (trade names Provera, Amen). Others include norethindrone, norgestrel, and norgestimate. Progestin actually causes or exaggerates many symptoms. (See list on page 158.) That's yet another reason why I don't recommend any of the HRT programs that employ synthetic progestins. Given the 2002 Women's Health Initiative findings, synthetic progestins are also implicated as a risk factor in strokes, heart disease, and breast cancer.

MPA has also been shown to attenuate some of estrogen's well-documented positive effect on blood vessels. It increases vascular resistance, inhibits blood flow, and increases cerebral artery resistance. A large study of women receiving continuous therapy consisting of estrogen plus MPA (Prempro is an example of this type of therapy) showed a marked increase in myocardial infarction, coronary artery disease death, and venous thrombosis (blood clots in the veins) during the first two years of therapy.[18] The 2006 reanalysis of the WHI and Nurses' Health studies data also supports an adverse effect from synthetic progestin. Younger women taking Prempro had a 30 percent decreased risk of heart disease when they started HRT within ten years of menopause. But those who were on estrogen only had a 44 percent decreased risk. I suspect that the difference in the two groups was due to the adverse effect of MPA.

Natural bioidentical progesterone contains no such risk and many benefits. In the famous PEPI (Postmenopausal Estrogen/Progestin Intervention) trial, oral natural progesterone in micronized form prevented the adverse effects on cholesterol that were seen in those women on Provera.

SYMPTOMS FROM SYNTHETIC PROGESTIN

~ Headache

~ Depression

~ Weight gain and bloating

~ Moodiness

~ Lack of sexual desire

~ Potential narrowing of blood vessels, causing chest pain and lack of oxygen to the heart

ELLEN: Too Much Estrogen, Too Little Progesterone

Ellen, a potter and yoga instructor in a college town, noticed a subtle, fuzzy-minded feeling and morning dizziness during the spring of her forty-third year. One day, as she was placing a bottle of aspirin in her grocery cart, she also realized that though she'd never had headaches before, she'd gradually begun experiencing them regularly— and attributing them to tension, or a weather change, or PMS. On a visit to her doctor, he drew a blood sample and tested her FSH level, which was high, convincing him she was menopausal. He told Ellen that her symptoms—the mental fuzziness, dizziness, and headaches— were consistent with menopause and that they'd improve if she took supplemental hormones. He gave her a prescription for Premarin to take daily, with some Provera for the last twelve days of every month.

Within days Ellen was miserable. What previously had felt like a tension headache now was a throbbing, splitting migraine; she felt depressed; she had restless legs that were keeping her awake; and most of her other symptoms persisted.

It's true that the symptoms Ellen experienced were consistent with the climacteric, but in light of her relative youth and the fact that she had not had these symptoms for more than a few months, it was probably early in the course of her perimenopause—which in many women is associated with low progesterone levels and a relative excess of estrogen. The blood test for FSH levels, upon which her physician based his diagnosis of menopause, is an inaccurate way to assess the big picture. It's like looking at a single frame in a very long movie. In fact, the symptoms Ellen experienced after taking the prescribed estrogen were consistent with estrogen overdose.

Even without knowing this, Ellen did the intuitive thing: she stopped taking her estrogen. Within twenty-four hours she started feeling better, and she vowed to "tough it out" without going back to the doctor. But her original symptoms persisted, and eventually a friend referred her to another doctor, who ordered hormone tests for estrogen, progesterone, and testosterone. The results confirmed that Ellen was in an early stage of perimenopause, with her primary hormonal change being low progesterone. Now using a natural progesterone cream to gently supplement her body's own dwindling supply, Ellen feels much better, and she understands a lot more about the transitional process. "I'm a work in progress," she wrote. "My hormonal status is changing, and I know that what works for me now might need to be tweaked a little in six months."

SAME DOLL, DIFFERENT DRESS

The latest wrinkle in the hormone replacement scene is prepackaged combinations. The synthetic hormones used in these preparations have been around for years; what is different is the packaging and the ways in which they are prescribed. The most commonly used, Prempro, a combination of Premarin and Provera, is the drug that was used in the WHI study. Others include Ortho-Prefest (a combination of bioidentical estradiol and the synthetic progestin norgestimate) and FemHRT (synthetic estradiol plus synthetic norethindrone). The advantage of these combinations is that they are convenient and women allegedly don't have any monthly bleeding on them. The problem is that many get spotting and intermittent bleeding for months before their bodies get used to the drug combos, causing many to stop taking them. The biggest drawback is that all of them contain synthetic progestin, which enhances a woman's chance of developing PMS-like side effects and also may increase her risk for heart disease and breast cancer. (To be fair, the 2006 reanalysis for the WHI and Nurses' Health studies data did, in fact, show a decreased risk of heart disease in younger women—even in those on Prempro, which contains a synthetic progestin. But why take any risk when other forms of progesterone are available?)

Testosterone

Testosterone is produced in both the ovaries and adrenal glands. Its primary job is to provide vital assertive energy and sexual drive. Testosterone and other androgens can increase the ease with which a woman becomes sexually aroused, as well as the frequency with which she follows through by initiating sexual activity. Testosterone also increases sensitivity of the erogenous zones, frequency of orgasm, intensity of sexual fantasies, and incidence of orgasmic dreams.

Not all women's testosterone levels drop perimenopausally—in fact, androgen levels actually increase in some. But if a woman is suffering from adrenal depletion due to chronic stress (see chapter 4), a precipitous drop in testosterone may occur, with symptoms of declining libido and overall energy depletion. Surgical removal of the ovaries, uterus, or both, as well as chemotherapy, radiation, or autoimmune disease, can also contribute to a drop in testosterone levels severe enough to cause symptoms.

For reasons that have yet to be clarified, some women experience a gradual decline in testosterone from early adulthood to old age, while other women continue to produce plenty of testosterone throughout life. The adrenals surely play a role, but whether there are other factors remains to be seen. Before you decide to try testosterone supplementation, it is essential to have laboratory confirmation of a deficiency via saliva or blood testing for free (unbound) testosterone. As with other menopause-related symptoms, there is considerable overlap among the three hormones. In many women, for example, a decline in libido is due to an estrogen deficiency, while testosterone may be normal. There is no benefit from taking supplemental testosterone if there is no deficiency to begin with. And many women with low testosterone levels have a normal sex drive! (See chapter 9.)

This bears emphasis because testosterone supplementation is now being requested by many women who think it will jump-start a flagging sex life. If there is a deficiency, the benefits may include heightened sex drive and sexual function, higher levels of energy overall, better muscle tone, and improved mood and outlook. There also is evidence that restoring normal testosterone levels can help improve bone mineral density. Incorporated into a vaginal cream, testosterone can also help restore normal vaginal wall thickness and lubrication. However, if there is no deficiency, supplementation will likely lead to overdose, which can produce symptoms most women find objectionable.

Bioidentical testosterone, or DHEA (dehydroepiandrosterone), an adrenal precursor for testosterone, is available from formulary pharmacies and can be used as a skin or vaginal cream by those women who require it. (Although DHEA is available over the counter, the quality varies considerably. I recommend pharmaceutical-grade DHEA, which is available from formulary pharmacies and Emerson Ecologics [visit www.emersonecologics.com]. I recommend 5 mg Sublingual DHEA manufactured by Douglas Laboratories; the suggested dose is one-half to one tablet daily, or as directed.) Testosterone is also available in a patch.

A synthetic, methyltestosterone is available in pill form or mixed with estrogen in a preparation known as Estratest, which I don't recommend.

SYMPTOMS OF TESTOSTERONE DEFICIENCY

- Decreased libido
- Impaired sexual function
- Decreased energy overall
- Decreased sense of well-being
- Thinning pubic hair

SYMPTOMS OF TESTOSTERONE OVERDOSE

~ Mood disturbances
~ Acne, particularly on the face and scalp
~ Increased facial hair growth
~ Deepened voice

HOW TO DECIDE WHETHER OR NOT TO TAKE HORMONES

Whether you should or should not take supplemental hormones at menopause depends on a number of factors, including your overall physical health, emotional and spiritual well-being, nutritional status, lifestyle, and so forth. All these factors can influence how well your secondary hormone-production sites are able to keep up with your body's new needs. For some women, just learning that the symptoms of perimenopause are temporary is enough reassurance; they become willing to experience those symptoms without masking them with medicine. And once we relax and allow our fears and resistance to fade, the symptoms themselves may lessen. This is the "placebo effect" in action, and it is a significant factor in menopausal treatments, as well. Knowing that we can ask for and receive help creates its own healing energy.

Taking Stock Before Making the Decision

Before deciding on hormone replacement, it is important to take an honest look at yourself and at your medical history—including that of your family members—so you can draw an accurate picture of your own goals and needs. Some women need hormones to feel their best. Others don't do well on them at all. Some women make enough hormones naturally in their own bodies to get through menopause without outside help. Others cannot make the biological conversions necessary to maintain the right hormonal balance. Still others have had their ovaries removed and need additional hormonal support, at least until they've reached the age when menopause would usually occur.

Despite the recent good news about HRT and heart disease, it's best to take an eyes-wide-open cautious approach to long-term estrogen use to prevent chronic disease. Few would disagree, however, that HRT can be very helpful for many women during the perimenopausal transition, when symptoms are at their worst. But for some women, the benefits of long-term HRT may outweigh the risks—for example, when there is a strong family history of osteoporosis, or when a woman clearly feels much better on hormones than off them!

Given the nature of science, medicine, and the pharmaceutical industry, you can expect that the conventional wisdom on HRT will continue to change. So stay tuned. If you have bothersome perimenopausal symptoms that aren't relieved by other methods, give HRT a try, stay with it for a year or so, and then taper your dose. See how you feel. If you feel fine, then taper some more until you've weaned yourself off it. If, on the other hand, you clearly feel your best on HRT, then stay with it and revisit your decision yearly.

The first step you need to take in making the HRT decision is to identify your risk factors and decide how much weight you intend to give them.

When I say "how much weight you intend to give them," I mean that only you have the power to decide how much influence your cultural and family script will have on your reality. Perimenopausal discomfort is a reality for most American women, while women in some other cultures have a different experience. Studies show that while 70–85 percent of North American women are affected by hot flashes, only 18 percent of Chinese factory workers in Hong Kong experience them.[19] I can assure you that the basic biology of the ovaries in China is not different than in North America. This speaks to the strength of expectations and how an entire culture can come to dictate what each individual will experience. Notwithstanding, each of us has the power to acknowledge this influence and then change our response to it.

Statistics predict what will happen to groups in general, not to specific individuals. Studies have shown that a woman's faith in (or rejection of) her cultural and genetic/familial script can play a significant role in how her reality plays out. People who are known in their families as "black sheep" are the least likely to fall victim to diseases that run in the family, perhaps because it is their own personal attitude and style to reject rules and color outside the lines. Since most health care providers are trained to look at statistics when making decisions and predictions about our health, it is crucial that each of us emphasize our innate ability to become "black sheep" when and if this stance can improve our health and outlook.

Although scientific studies may change how we think about something intellectually, our behavior and what we actually do with scientific information is shaped far more by our day-to-day relationships with friends and family than by any other factor. If, for example, you've watched your mother, sister, or best friend come alive again after going on some form of HRT, you're apt to feel very positive about the benefits of this approach. If, on the other hand, you've watched a family member suffer from headaches, sore breasts, and weight gain from taking too high a dose of estrogen, you're not going to be very eager to try it yourself. And if you are surrounded by aunts, grandmothers, or other older female role models who are vibrantly healthy, live well into their nineties in good health, and have never taken HRT of any kind, your inner blueprint for what is apt to happen after you go through menopause without medication will be quite positive.

My own personal legacy includes cardiovascular disease. My mother lost both her parents to heart disease, and my beloved father collapsed and died on the tennis court at age sixty-eight, a victim of a ruptured cerebral aneurysm, when my mother was only fifty-two and perimenopausal. She finished the climacteric as a widow, during an era when women were expected to fade physically and socially after menopause. Though my mother tends to avoid conventional wisdom in general and visits to the doctor in particular, her sister and her friends were told again and again that without supplemental Premarin they would become little old ladies with fragile skeletons and weak hearts. But my mother greeted that prediction with a dismissive wave of her hand. Now eighty, she climbs mountains wearing a heavy backpack and can ski rings around me on the slopes. She has an active social calendar, her mind is sharp, her blood pressure is 120/60, and no form of estrogen medication has ever entered her vibrant body. (She does use a natural progesterone skin cream, because it helps the "creakiness" in some of her joints.)

Which of my family's medical legacies will I inherit? I firmly believe that through the physical and emotional choices I make—and the expectations and beliefs with which I live my life—I shape my own future. My daughters and future grandchildren will do the same. Would I like to have the same level of health when I'm eighty that my mother now enjoys? Of course I would, but I believe it will happen because I have chosen it, not because I have inherited it.

SELECTED HORMONE OPTIONS

Product	Route of Administration	Estrogen	Progesterone	Bioidentical or Synthetic (for humans)
OGEN	Vaginal cream	Estropipate	None	Synthetic
ESTRING	Vaginal silicone ring	Estradiol	None	Bioidentical
AYGESTIN	Oral	None	Norethindrone acetate	Synthetic
PROVERA	Oral	None	Medroxyprogesterone acetate	Synthetic
AMEN	Oral	None	Medroxyprogesterone acetate	Synthetic
PROMETRIUM	Oral	None	Micronized progesterone	Bioidentical
CRINONE	Vaginal gel	None	Progesterone	Bioidentical
PROCHIEVE	Vaginal gel	None	Progesterone	Bioidentical
PREMPRO	Oral	Conjugated horse estrogens	Medroxyprogesterone acetate	Synthetic
FemHRT	Oral	Ethinyl estradiol	Norethindrone acetate	Synthetic
ORTHO-PREFEST	Oral	17-ß-estradiol	Norgestimate	Bioidentical estrogen synthetic progesterone
COMBI-PATCH	Skin patch	Estradiol	Norethindrone acetate	Bioidentical estrogen synthetic progesterone

What Are Your Goals?

Too many women see the HRT decision as an either/or, yes/no decision. I'd like to reframe it as a process. As a first step, it is important to define the goals you hope to achieve with HRT. Contrary to the message conveyed by pharmaceutical marketing efforts, HRT will not give you a means of moving backward, of denying the aging process and keeping you young forever. In fact, to do so would be counterproductive to your physical, emotional, and spiritual health. If you are determined to deny that you have passed middle age, HRT cannot put you at peace with that fact. However, a personally tailored program—with or without supplemental hormones—can help reduce physical symptoms and health worries so that you can focus your energies on finding your creative passions, which in and of themselves can stoke the flames of your life force. HRT can help mask the heart palpitations and irritability often associated with perimenopause. But it cannot resolve the underlying relationship problems that might be utilizing those symptoms to get your attention.

Every day more and more studies are showing how effective modalities such as dietary change, food supplements, exercise, and herbs can be in supporting a woman through her menopausal transition. Though some doctors still don't know about these approaches and may not mention them to you, they often work as well or better than hormone replacement. They can also be used in addition to hormone replacement, to reduce dosage levels, side effects, and potential risk. In other words, you don't necessarily have to choose between HRT and alternatives. Think of your perimenopausal support as a smorgasbord. You get to choose what appeals to you at the moment and leave what doesn't.

Becoming an Active Partner in the Decision

For our mothers and grandmothers, the decision to take HRT (or not) was very often a passive one, made by their doctors (or husband or best friend!) with their own involvement limited to "being good patients." Or they decided by not deciding and simply let time go by. In those days there were very few HRT preparations available, so the choices were only two: yes or no. And until very recently, the potential benefits were too often clouded by side effects from the wrong type of medications or fear of long-term consequences. As of the late 1990s, less than 20 percent of American women used hormone replacement, and those who did often discontinued it within six months.[20]

Today, many women (and their doctors) are more confused than ever about HRT. Part of this confusion arose because early reports on the Women's Health Initiative study seemed to indict all HRT. In fact, the women in the original 2002 WHI study were on the same dose of only *one type* of HRT—namely, Prempro. And the 2006 analysis of the WHI data showing a decreased risk of heart disease in women who started taking it early is a silver lining in a dark cloud. But there are still a lot of unanswered questions, plus the irrefutable increased risk of breast cancer with Prempro. One thing is clear: we need far more research on the role of hormones, particularly bioidentical hormones in low dosages.

At the same time, we also need to remember that medicine will always be an art, not an exact science. In the early 1990s, science seemed to indicate that the majority of postmenopausal women would benefit from HRT. Some were even dismissed from their doctor's office if they questioned that belief. Then the pendulum swung all the way in the opposite direction. Now it's coming back to center. In addition to the question "Do I want or need HRT, at least for right now?" we also have to ask: "What kind? What strength? What route of administration? In what combination? For what reason? For how long? At what risk?"

The number of options can be intimidating at first, but in the end you'll feel much better about your HRT decision if you're armed with facts, know your options, and are willing to listen to your inner guidance as well as to your doctor's advice. And although I discourage using HRT as a means of numbing oneself to what is happening in body and mind during perimenopause, there is nothing to be gained from suffering. Given the range of formulations and dosages now available—as well as the many alternatives to HRT—you can create an individual treatment program that supports you through the change, rather than helping you deny that it is happening.

EVIE: *Brittle Diabetes, Brittle Hormones*

Evie is an energetic, upbeat insurance saleswoman who steadfastly refuses to allow her diabetes—which she's had since the age of thirteen—to dominate her life. She checks her blood glucose levels regularly and gives herself two injections of insulin each day, but she's considered a "brittle" diabetic and still suffers at least one diabetic crisis each year.

Evie takes these episodes in stride, sometimes exasperating her friends and loved ones who wish she'd take her condition "more seriously," but she admits that she gets "prickly" when they dote on her. She has also begun to make the connection between the state of her diabetes and the state of her emotions. When she is upset with one of her children, her boss, or her husband, her insulin and dietary needs can change dramatically and quickly. It also came as no surprise to Evie's physician that because of her metabolic problems, her blood sugar levels went wild as she bumped and jolted through her menopausal transition. She wrote, "There's an amusement park nearby, with a really scary roller coaster. Let's just say I've got 'em beat. Estrogen, glucose, FSH—everything was bouncing all over the place."

Jerilynn Prior, M.D., a hormone researcher and professor of endocrinology and metabolism at the University of British Columbia and founder and scientific director of the Centre for Menstrual Cycle and Ovulation Research, calls this phase "estrogen's storm season" and has written a very helpful book with the same title (Centre for Menstrual Cycle and Ovulation Research, 2005). (For more information, see CeMCOR's website at www.cemcor.ubc.ca.)

Because Evie's levels were so erratic and sensitive, it was tough getting her regulated, but with trial and error Evie and her physician managed to arrive at a hormone replacement program that gently alleviated her discomfort, stabilized her metabolism (and therefore her glucose levels), and supported her body through the transition. "It was a pretty tough trip for a while there, but I noticed a difference within weeks of getting the right levels of hormones."

Clarifying Your Needs

In order to make the best choice for you, you need to clarify your needs, then become an active partner in getting them met. This may mean consulting more than one health care provider—an herbalist or acupuncturist in addition to your OB/GYN, for instance. It may also mean asking your physician to try an approach he or she is unfamiliar with—and sharing the responsibility for the results.

To begin, review the following eight health factors and determine which, if any, apply to you. This will help you focus your thinking about which replacement regimen to use, if any, and for how long.

FACTOR I: YOU WANT RELIEF FROM DISCOMFORT, PARTICULARLY HOT FLASHES THAT DISRUPT SLEEP. This is the most common reason why women choose HRT, especially estrogen. However, discomfort is also the most common reason for women to stop taking HRT—the formulation and/or the dosage prescribed may not be right for their particular metabolism, resulting in persistent medication side effects and/or symptoms of overdose.

If relief from symptoms is your sole reason for seeking treatment, treatment will probably be needed only until the perimenopausal transition is complete, which can be confirmed either by a lack of menstrual periods for at least a year or by the laboratory tests outlined in chapter 4. There might be a brief perimenopause-like adjustment when coming off hormone treatment, but if you are weaned off the hormones over a period of several months, the symptoms generally are mild. Many women come off HRT once they've become well established on regimens that include herbs, soy, exercise, or dietary supplements. This approach often smoothes the adjustment.

If you want symptomatic relief but your personal preference is to stay away from supplemental hormones, there are many non-hormonal treatments available over the counter or from health care practitioners such as naturopaths and acupuncturists. (See chapter 6.)

FACTOR 2: YOU ARE SUFFERING FROM UROGENITAL SYMPTOMS. The health of the vaginal lining and urethral tissues is highly influenced by the hormonal milieu in our bodies. Women may seek relief from stress incontinence (they leak urine when coughing, sneezing, laughing, or lifting heavy objects), urge incontinence (they have difficulty making it to the bathroom without leaking), recurrent vaginal yeast infections, vaginal dryness and/or discomfort during intercourse, recurrent bladder infections, or urinary frequency (they need to urinate more than eight times during the day, or one or more times during the night).

Taking estrogen (by mouth or applied locally) and/or androgen hormones (by mouth or applied as a skin patch or as a cream formulated for vaginal application) helps maintain healthy vaginal and urethral tissue, even when relatively small doses are used. As little as 1 to 2 mg of natural testosterone in a cream base, applied to the vagina two to three times per week, for example, is often all that is necessary. And sometimes the phytoestrogens found in herbs, soy, or flaxseed can restore vaginal tissue to its premenopausal moistness and resilience. (See chapter 6.)

Some studies from the late 1990s found that systemic oral conventional HRT actually increases the risk of urinary incontinence for reasons that aren't at all clear. What *is* clear is that urinary problems often clear up on their own with no treatment at all.

FACTOR 3: YOU CURRENTLY HAVE A HEALTHY HEART BUT
ARE AT INCREASED RISK FOR CARDIOVASCULAR DISEASE. A
woman's increased risk of heart disease is usually related to (1) a positive family history (heart disease or stroke in father younger than age
fifty-five, or in mother or other first-degree female relative at age
sixty-five or younger) and all the emotions that go with it, (2) lifestyle
factors such as smoking or lack of exercise, or (3) a predisposing factor such as low HDL cholesterol, high LDL cholesterol, or high
triglycerides.

Beginning in the late 1980s, doctors prescribed HRT liberally to
women to prevent heart disease because a large number of epidemiologic studies had shown a clear benefit. Estrogen decreases LDL (the
bad cholesterol) and increases HDL (the good cholesterol).[21] It also
has a positive effect on blood vessel walls that seems to involve nitric
oxide, a chemical produced in the body that helps keep blood vessels
dilated. (Viagra and other drugs for male impotence also exert their
effect through nitric oxide pathways.)

But then in 2002 the Women's Health Initiative study branch that
was testing Prempro against placebo in thousands of women was
abruptly halted because the drug caused an increase in strokes and
heart attacks, and the medical profession quickly backed away from
its original position on HRT and heart disease. The WHI was the first
long-term placebo-controlled trial of HRT, and it clearly showed that
the cardiovascular risks of Prempro outweigh the benefits. But the
2006 reanalysis of the data from both the WHI and Nurses' Health
studies has shown that when women begin HRT within ten years of
menopause, they decrease their risk of heart disease by at least 11
and as much as 30 percent. As it turns out, most of the women in the
original WHI study didn't start Prempro until they were in their sixties and well past the age of menopause. No one knows exactly what
to make of this data—but clearly estrogen can be heart healthy in
some women!

The problem here is that Prempro isn't synonymous with all
HRT. It contains synthetic progestin, which is known to partially
obliterate the beneficial effects of estrogen alone on blood vessels. In
addition, all hormones in the WHI study were given orally. This increases the risk of blood clots because oral hormones must be
processed in the liver, and increased clotting factors are the result—
especially in older women. There's still solid data to suggest that
low-dose, bioidentical estrogen, without synthetic progestin, given
transdermally and at physiologic levels, could be beneficial for the
cardiovascular systems of some women. Unfortunately, most of the

conventionally available combination hormone therapies contain synthetic progestins, including Prempro, Combipatch, FemHRT, and Activella. Studies of women who started HRT in early menopause have shown a decreased risk of death from heart disease. In the original 2002 WHI study on the other hand, the average age of the women on HRT was sixty-three.[22]

I feel strongly that estrogen would show a far greater potential benefit if women used individualized regimens consisting of natural, bioidentical hormones. Because of their deleterious effect on blood vessels, I believe that synthetic progestins (especially Provera or Amen) are more dangerous than taking no hormones at all. Tried-and-true methods to decrease heart disease risk also include avoiding smoking, regular vigorous exercise, taking supplements such as vitamin E, following a diet rich in fruits and vegetables, consuming soy foods, and keeping weight normal. (See chapter 14 for my heart health program.)

FACTOR 4: YOU HAVE ALREADY BEEN DIAGNOSED WITH HEART DISEASE. It is now clear that HRT, at least in the form of Prempro (Premarin and Provera), increases the risk of stroke and heart attack in older women—the ones most likely to have full-blown heart disease.

Many scientists feel that this is due to a hormone-stimulated increase in chemicals called "inflammation factors," such as C-reactive protein, which was found in the bloodstream in amounts that were 85 percent higher in women taking HRT. However, this is once again a case where you need to read the fine print. As I've said, I believe that the increased risk from conventional HRT boils down mainly to the adverse effects of medroxyprogesterone acetate (trade names Provera and Amen). It is also true that estrogens at high enough doses have long been associated with increased risk of blood clots that predispose to heart attack, especially in smokers.

Here's the bottom line: Women with or without heart disease should avoid synthetic progestins and keep their estrogen doses as natural and as low as possible. And no one should take estrogen as a way to treat already-diagnosed heart disease.

FACTOR 5: YOU ARE AT INCREASED RISK FOR OSTEOPOROSIS OR ALREADY HAVE BEEN DIAGNOSED WITH BONE LOSS. A woman whose mother or grandmother has osteoporosis is at increased risk for this potentially disabling condition, though it is unknown whether this is because of a genetic inheritance or because we tend to "inherit" habits, lifestyle choices, and life expectations, which may predispose us to less-than-optimal bone strength. (See chapter 12 for additional risk factors, many of which are under our control.) Estrogen replacement definitely helps prevent bone loss associated with menopause, and continuous use of estrogen decreases the risk of fracture by 50 percent or more. The bone-preserving effects of estrogen are maintained only as long as a woman stays on it.

Androgens such as testosterone also play a role in preserving bone health. Those women with naturally high testosterone levels have a decreased risk for osteoporotic fractures. Low-dose testosterone supplementation has been found to help maintain bone mass.

A number of drugs—calcitonin, the bisphosphonates such as alendronate (trade name Fosamax), and SERMs such as tamoxifen (Nolvadex) and raloxifene (Evista)—have also been shown to help prevent loss of bone and decrease fracture risk. As with hormone replacement, they are effective only as long as a woman is on them.

High doses of soy protein, regular weight-bearing exercise, and vitamin D are also very effective ways of maintaining bone density and decreasing fracture risk, both at perimenopause and beyond.

FACTOR 6: YOU ARE AT INCREASED RISK FOR ALZHEIMER'S DISEASE. At this point in our limited understanding of this organic brain disorder, a positive family history is the strongest predisposing factor, although most individuals who get it don't have any genetic predisposition. There is less consensus regarding some studies' suggestion that high levels of aluminum intake (from using aluminum cookware or consuming food from aluminum cans) might also contribute to an individual's risk of Alzheimer's disease.

It is clear that all hormones can affect brain function—androgens and progesterone as well as estrogen—and that many women continue making enough of these throughout life to protect their brains. In fact, a 2000 British study of postmenopausal women not on HRT found that those with the highest levels of endogenous estradiol were the least likely to have Alzheimer's disease.[23] But research has failed to show that estrogen decreases the risk of dementia. Some studies even suggest that estrogen, plus or minus progestin, may actually increase a woman's risk. There are many additional things a woman can do now to protect her mental functions in later life. (See chapter 10, "Nurturing Your Brain.")

FACTOR 7: YOU ARE AT INCREASED RISK FOR BREAST, UTERINE, OVARIAN, OR BOWEL CANCER. A positive personal or family history for one or more of these hormone-related cancers makes the hormone replacement decision particularly anxiety-provoking for many women. Here are the facts: Recent research has suggested that the dose and formulation of HRT are important factors in the cancer issue. All types of estrogen at high enough doses over a long enough period of time can potentially stimulate breast, uterine, and ovarian cancers because estrogen is a growth factor in these tissues. This includes the estrogens produced in your own body. Premarin, because of its association with DNA damage and because it has a stronger biological effect than bioidentical estrogens, may be more carcinogenic than bioidentical estrogens, especially when they are used in low doses. In other words, the increased risk of breast and uterine cancer shown by past studies may have been related to estrogen overdose or the wrong kind of estrogen, rather than estrogen per se. The addition of synthetic progestin further complicates matters. The 2002 Women's Health Initiative study clearly demonstrated that women taking the combination drug Prempro for five or more years had a higher risk for breast cancer than those on placebo. Not all studies show an increased risk for breast cancer with HRT. In fact, the estrogen-only branch of the WHI showed no increased risk. But these women had all had hysterectomies and were probably at a lower risk to begin with.

If estrogen is taken in a way that more closely mimics the way it is produced in the body—in physiological doses calibrated to the body's needs, in bioidentical formulation, and partnered with bioidentical, not synthetic, progesterone—it begins to lose its sinister profile. (See chapter 13.)

For the woman who is in the highest-risk category for breast, uterine, or ovarian cancer but who desires support through the symptomatic phase of perimenopause, there are two options that are unlikely to adversely affect that risk. First, she can take bioidentical hormones at the lowest possible levels during the five years or fewer when her symptoms are the most troubling. This may involve fine-tuning her doses with the aid of salivary or blood free-hormone testing, so she takes no more than the amounts necessary to achieve physiological balance and symptomatic relief. Second, she can opt for nonhormonal, herbal treatments. (See chapter 6.)

With regard to colorectal cancer, the picture is clearer. Colorectal cancer accounts for 11.2 percent of all cancers among American women—third after breast and lung. In both prevalence and mortality it outranks endometrial, ovarian, and cervical cancers. A summary of ten studies with information on the timing of estrogen use indicates a 34 percent reduced risk of colorectal cancer in current users. The 2002 WHI study confirmed this data. This protection is nearly lost within a few years of stopping hormone therapy. Though no one knows why for sure, it appears that estrogen causes a decrease in bile acids, substances manufactured in the liver that are associated with the promotion of colorectal cancer.[24]

FACTOR 8: YOU REACHED MENOPAUSE PREMATURELY (PRIOR TO AGE FORTY) OR ARTIFICIALLY AND ABRUPTLY (DUE TO SURGERY, ILLNESS, CHEMOTHERAPY, OR RADIATION). Women with this history are more likely to need systemic HRT, a program that provides physiologically appropriate hormone levels throughout the body, rather than more locally acting products, and rather than relying solely on herbal treatments and dietary approaches. This is because the physical and mental symptoms associated with a premature or abrupt cessation of natural hormone production are usually more severe than with a gradual perimenopausal decline. With premature menopause, the woman's body is left without endogenous hormone support for more years than if menopause had occurred later in life. I recommend using a combination of bioidentical hormones, with the dosage based on your symptoms and hormone levels.

SANDY: Surgical Menopause

Sandy had an "instant" menopause at age thirty-five, when her ovaries were removed because of severe endometriosis. This created the abrupt hormonal withdrawal characteristic of artificial menopause. Her symptoms were quite pronounced. Until her surgery, Sandy had believed that she would not take HRT when she reached her natural menopause. Now, to say the least, her discomfort was intrusive. And the fact that she would be without her normal complement of hormones for approximately fifteen extra years meant that her bone density, heart health, and mental functioning might suffer in the future. As a result, Sandy felt she had no choice but to start HRT. "Frankly," she wrote, "I was so miserable I couldn't give my full attention to the decision beyond that point." She and her doctor decided on a skin patch that delivered bioidentical estrogen (17-B-estradiol), along with natural progesterone oral capsules. With minimal tweaking, they arrived at the optimal dose for her, and her level of comfort vastly improved.

"At that point," Sandy wrote, "I could start applying myself to decisions that would affect my future. I really had not wanted to take

HRT after menopause, but I didn't want to increase my chance of os-teoporosis, so it felt right to take HRT under the circumstances. Then it hit me: I can have the best of both worlds! I decided I'll take these hormones until I'm fifty-five, when I'd probably have completed my menopausal transition naturally, and then I'll wean myself off the hormones and sail through my menopausal years au naturel. I feel much happier about this plan. I feel like the idea was a thank-you gift from my body for bending the 'rules' and providing it with hormones during these extra fifteen years of menopause."

When to Start HRT

Over the years I've watched scores of women left to "tough it out" during their stormy perimenopausal years because their doctors didn't want to prescribe hormones until they were definitely past menopause. There's no need for this. You should feel free to start what you need when you need it—and that includes hormones, herbs, foods, lifestyle changes, or a combination of all these. Because menopause is really a retrospective diagnosis, you won't know you're there until you're there! And symptoms are generally at their peak during perimenopause, not later.

For the woman who wants help with perimenopausal symptoms and finds that a nonhormonal approach does not provide sufficient relief but who is afraid that supplemental estrogen might increase her risk for breast or uterine cancer, HRT is not necessarily out of the question. (See chapters 8 and 13.) As I've said above, I'm not con-vinced that there is any significant risk from taking bioidentical estro-gen at a low dose only during the five years or less that menopausal symptoms are likely to be the most intrusive. After that, she can wean herself off some or all of the hormones or replace them with other al-ternatives. And if you feel your best on hormones, any increased risk might well be worth the benefits!

PRINCIPLES OF HRT

- Establish your natural hormonal levels by getting a base-line test in your late thirties or early perimenopause.
- Replace only those hormones that need replacing.

~ Use the lowest dose that does the job. Reevaluate your HRT decision yearly and plan to use alternatives when possible.

~ Use bioidentical hormones that are an exact molecular match to those naturally occurring in your body.

~ Support your HRT regimen with a healthy diet, the right nutritional supplements, and exercise.

~ Be realistic. The goal is not to turn back the clock. Rather, the goal is to optimize your comfort and overall health so you can live the second half of your life with maximal vitality and mental clarity.

RENÉE: Losing Control, Finding Compassion

Though many of us have fixed ideas about how we will negotiate menopause and what we will and won't do, we need to be willing to let go of all our preconceptions once we actually begin going through the experience. Renée's story is a beautiful example of this.

I'd decided a long time ago that I wasn't going to color my hair when it went gray and I wasn't going to take supplemental hormones when I hit menopause. Menopause for me was going to be a beautiful thing. I had it all figured out.

Then on my forty-seventh birthday my father died without warning, of a massive heart attack. My mother, confused and scared and in need of support, moved in with us. Then my husband, David, lost his funding and suddenly was faced with the prospect of being unemployed by the end of the year. And I was practically blindsided one week later with my first hot flash, which was so powerful it actually steamed up my glasses. Emotionally, financially, hormonally, and in terms of my overall sense of security, it felt like the proverbial rug was being pulled out from under my feet. My hot flashes became increasingly bothersome, particularly when they happened in the middle of the night and interrupted my sleep. I was feeling short-tempered with my mom and with David, and the house felt claustrophobic—I guess I just couldn't handle all the unexpected stresses that came up at what felt like the worst possible time in my biology. When my gynecologist suggested that I needed a little hormonal support, I sighed with relief and accepted it, and I feel much better now. In fact, just making the decision to accept help made a big difference in the way I felt, right away.

The lesson I learned from all this applies to more than just menopause: you can't control everything. I've always been a big control freak, but now I understand that in some ways we're all just along for the ride, and we need to be compassionate with ourselves and willing to change direction once in a while, in order to adjust to and accommodate what life throws our way, no matter what stage of life we're in at the time.

A DUSTING OF HORMONES

Okay, let's say that you've decided that you may want to try hormone replacement. You are still having periods, but you're getting hot flashes before they start. You also have occasional night sweats. I'd recommend that at this point you get your hormone levels tested. The ideal time is about a week before your period is due, because you'll be able to see what your peak progesterone level is at that time, and it will also give you an idea of how much estrogen and testosterone is normally circulating in your system. These levels will also give you an idea of what level you want to replace to once you start hormones.

The next thing you do, depending upon your hormone levels, is to start replacing the hormone that is lowest. In most cases, this will be progesterone, and maybe estrogen. Increasingly we're finding that many perimenopausal women also have an androgen deficiency. As already mentioned, natural progesterone in the form of a 2 percent skin cream has been shown to give good blood levels and is available over the counter. This alone may be all you need. Try it for two weeks before your period, then take two weeks off after your period starts. You can also use it for three weeks on and one week off. Most women notice a reduction of their symptoms within a month of starting this cream. Continue with this as long as you're getting good results.

If your estrogen level is too low or you're having lots of hot flashes, you'll want to start with the lowest level of estrogen available. Estrogen is available by prescription only, so you'll need to work with a health care practitioner to get the right dose and blood levels for you. Many women like the convenience of the estrogen patch, which comes in many different strengths and can be left on the skin for several days. Others prefer to take a pill. If you're taking estrogen, you have to be sure that you have enough progesterone to prevent excessive buildup of your uterine lining. This can be accomplished in some women with 2 percent progesterone skin cream. Others may need a higher amount of progesterone, available only by prescription. I recommend Crinone vaginal gel, Prometrium capsules orally, one of the formulations I mentioned earlier, or another one from a formulary pharmacy.

The good news is this: many health care providers are now familiar with bioidentical natural hormones and work closely with pharmacists who specialize in compounding individualized prescriptions to fit a woman's unique needs. Some health plans cover prescriptions for formulary pharmacies and others don't. If your plan doesn't, I'd recommend that you advocate coverage if your plan covers conventional hormone replacement. Your doctor may be able to assist you.

It's always best to call ahead and make sure that your doctor is open to discussing an individualized natural hormone approach before spending the time and money on an appointment. If your doctor doesn't know about this approach, either educate him or her or find someone who does. Many nurse practitioners are familiar with individualized hormone replacement and will work with you to find the right solution.

HOW LONG SHOULD YOU STAY ON HORMONES?

The length of time you continue to take hormones depends entirely on why you are taking hormones and what other things you are doing to achieve the same benefit. For example, if you originally started estrogen to maintain bone health but have since incorporated regular weight training into your lifestyle, you can probably taper off the estrogen and still maintain your bone density. If on the other hand, you are a confirmed couch potato, have been on steroids, or smoke and you know you are at risk for osteoporosis, then you may need a drug such as raloxifene (Evista) or alendronate (Fosamax) to help maintain bone density.

With bioidentical hormones at low levels, the benefits of HRT may far outweigh any risks—especially if you feel good on them, have risk factors that HRT is known to ameliorate, or have a health history that doesn't include a lot of healthy ninety-year-old relatives! The vast majority of women start taking hormones, herbs, or both for immediate relief of menopausal symptoms such as hot flashes or vaginal dryness and will need them for only a few years. Others are far more concerned about osteoporosis or sexual function. Taking hormones for short-term symptom relief is very different from taking hormones for long-term disease prevention. The majority of women experience most of their menopausal symptoms during a five- to ten-year period, after which the symptoms abate naturally.

IF YOU'VE BEEN TAKING HRT AND WANT TO STOP ALL HORMONES

Don't stop cold turkey. Wean yourself gradually and slowly, giving your body time to adjust. Here's a sample weaning schedule:

Week one: Skip Sunday's pill

Week two: Skip Sunday and Tuesday

Week three: Skip Sunday, Tuesday, and Thursday

Week four: Skip Sunday, Tuesday, Thursday, and Saturday

Week five: Skip Sunday, Tuesday, Thursday, Friday, and Saturday

Week six: Off hormones all together

During and after this tapering-off period, support your body by making sure you're getting enough plant hormones. Eat a wide variety of fruits, vegetables, ground flaxseed, and soy. (See chapter 6.) You'll also need a good multivitamin/mineral to help your adrenals and ovaries keep your hormones balanced.

Not Carved in Stone

Many women went into a panic after the initial Women's Health Initiative study results were announced and stopped their HRT cold turkey. Many also worried that they'd done irreparable damage to themselves by being on HRT. This simply is not true. To put matters into perspective, the vast majority of women in the WHI study did not experience any adverse outcomes from being on Prempro, and their risk of death was no greater than that for women taking placebo. The data indicate that if ten thousand women take Prempro for a year, eight more will develop invasive breast cancer compared to the ten thousand not taking Prempro. An additional seven will have a heart attack, eight will have a stroke, and eighteen will have blood clots. But they will also suffer six fewer colorectal cancers and five fewer hip fractures.[25] Unfortunately, we now face a situation in which many women who could truly benefit from HRT are so frightened by the risk of cancer that they are refusing it and suffering needlessly. Instead, every woman should know that she can decrease her risk of side effects from HRT by switching from synthetics like Prempro to low-dose bioidentical HRT. Or, if she chooses, she can wean herself gradually off HRT to avoid rebound symptoms.

Because every woman's body is a work in progress, your hormonal status—and your need for a particular type of support program—may well change. If you elect to take supplemental hormones, it is wise to have your hormone levels checked every six months during the first year of hormone use. Compare the results to how you're feeling. This can help indicate if, and where, your prescription needs fine-tuning. After you have reached a comfortable level, you only need to test every year or so.

If you've been taking Prempro or another type of synthetic HRT, feel good on it, but want to decrease any possibility of adverse side effects: I suggest that you switch to bioidentical hormones at the lowest possible dose. Your doctor can give you a prescription for bioidentical hormones, which include oral Estrace and some of the patches (Estraderm, Vivelle, and Climara). If you have a uterus, you'll also need a progesterone. Prometrium is available in all pharmacies. The usual dose is 100 mg a day, at least twelve days of the month. If you don't want to get a period, you may need to take it daily. These brands of bioidentical hormones are covered by most health plans that have prescription coverage.

Alternatively, you can have a formulary pharmacy make up a combination of estrogen and progesterone, and/or testosterone (if necessary), such as the formulations I've mentioned above.

Remember that formulations that work well for one woman do not necessarily provide optimal results for another. You may want to try a different formulation, a different delivery system, or a different dosage, or switch from hormone supplementation to nonhormonal herbal support or vice versa. Be calm and at peace about this decision process—you can always change your mind if what you've chosen falls short of your expectations.

6

Foods and Supplements to Support the Change

For thousands of years, long before our culture placed its trust in pharmaceuticals, women relied upon their intuition and Mother Nature to keep themselves and their families healthy. Guided by their inner wisdom, our ancestors plucked healing plants from nature's colorful pharmacy—fragrant chamomile for calming teas, fresh ginger to prevent nausea and calm the stomach, and foxglove to regulate the heartbeat.

It is remarkable that our herbalist ancestors, though separated by thousands of miles, often drew upon the same herbs to treat the same conditions. American Indian women and their Chinese counterparts, for example, both used angelica (dong quai) to treat menopausal symptoms.

Today this ancient, intuitive wisdom is being augmented by objective scientific studies confirming what wise women have always known: plants contain a wide range of ingredients, such as essential fatty acids, phytoestrogens, and antioxidants, that can heal and help keep us healthy at all stages of our lives, including perimenopause.

To use herbs and foods optimally requires an adjustment in thinking. Plant medicine and food do not work in the body the way drugs, or even bioidentical hormones, do. Modern pharmaceuticals and hormones usually consist of one purified active ingredient (often derived from a plant source and then altered biochemically) that is carefully standardized and measured for its biological effect.

Whole herbs and foods, on the other hand, contain many different active ingredients that act synergistically in the body. There is good reason to believe that to get the full range of benefits, you need to consume the whole plant—or a product made from part of the whole plant, such as leaves or roots—rather than a single ingredient. This is why some studies show that whole soy foods give better results than capsules or pills containing isolated soy isoflavones.

In allopathic Western medicine, we try to target a symptom or illness with a single drug—we give birth control pills, for example, to stop heavy bleeding or to regulate irregular periods. Birth control pills control symptoms, but they do nothing to treat the underlying imbalance.

Herbs and foods, on the other hand, with their exquisite combinations of interactive ingredients, work to balance the body at a number of different levels simultaneously. Accordingly, there are many different herbs or foods that one might use to regulate the menstrual cycle or as overall perimenopausal tonics, including soy foods, ground flaxseed, dong quai, or chasteberry, to name just a few. All contain substances that help balance the endocrine system in slightly different but synergistic ways.[1]

Herbs also work best when considered as part of an overall plan that includes a good diet, exercise, and improved relationships. In other words, we need to approach herbs and foods with a holistic mindset that asks, "What foods or herbs will best help me balance my body so that it can heal itself?" rather than the more dualistic "What pill do I need to take to remove this symptom?"

WHO SHOULD CONSIDER HERBS?

- ~ Your symptoms are mild but you'd like a little support.
- ~ You believe that herbs are simply more natural and beneficial than prescribed hormones.
- ~ You'd like to avoid HRT because of fear of breast cancer or another health concern.
- ~ You're on HRT of some sort but would like the added benefits of herbs.
- ~ You cannot tolerate HRT.

BASIC PRINCIPLES OF HERBAL THERAPY
AT MENOPAUSE

In order to use menopausal herbs well and wisely, you need to understand the following basic principles.

~ All plant foods contain what are known as phytonutrients. (*Phyto-* means "plant.") These are unique substances produced during the natural course of growth and are specific to a particular plant's genes and environment. In addition to providing taste and nutritional value, phytonutrients can play therapeutic roles by modifying physiological processes in our bodies. This is the basis for botanical medicine. An example of this is the phytochemical indole-3-carbinol, found in cruciferous vegetables such as broccoli. This substance appears to convert the most potent estrogens in the body into weaker, less carcinogenic forms. High consumption of cruciferous vegetables is associated with a decreased risk for breast cancer, breast tenderness, and bloating, all of which are related to estrogen levels that are too high.

~ The line between using herbs as foods and using them as drugs can be blurry. For example, ephedra (ma huang) can be an effective treatment for asthma and sinusitis, but it should be avoided as a daily supplement. (It was even taken off the market for a while because people were using it addictively to lose weight and suffered severe side effects from overdosing.) In general, the greater your intake of an herb, the greater the potential for druglike effects. For safety, keep doses moderately low, and follow the directions on the package or an herbalist's recommendation. It is also best to let your health care provider know what herbs you take regularly, because some herbs interact with some drugs in a way that either decreases the drug's potency or changes its effect. This is because both use the same metabolic pathways in the liver.

~ Recent advances in the standardization of herbal supplements have led to more consistent quality and potency. The most effective products are those that combine the whole plant (or plant part, such as the root) with a standardized percentage of the primary active ingredient.

~ The common menopausal herbs mentioned in this chapter have been used safely and effectively for thousands of years and rarely have side effects. However, a few people may react to some of them, some of the time—just as with any food or drug. There are also many herbs with known toxicity that shouldn't be used except under the care of an experienced herbalist. Examples include belladonna, blue cohosh, lobelia, and poke root.

~ Phytoestrogens, the natural hormones found in plants, are not the same as the hormones found in the female body, although they may have somewhat similar beneficial effects. Phytoestrogens are found in more than three hundred plants, including some that we routinely eat in the United States, such as apples, carrots, oats, plums, olives, potatoes, tea, coffee, and sunflower seeds. Soy and flaxseed are particularly rich in these substances.[2] Phytoestrogens can be divided into two main families: the *isoflavones,* which include substances such as genistein, daidzein, equol, and coumestrol, and the *lignans,* which include matairesinol, enterolactone, and enterodiol.

The estrogenic activity of phytoestrogens is lower than that of human estrogens—in the range of a hundredth to a thousandth that of estradiol. They also have antioxidant and antiproliferative activity that is still being elucidated. This means that they have the ability to prevent free-radical damage to cells, the number-one cause of premature aging of tissue, and they also help prevent abnormal cell growth.

Like other estrogens, phytoestrogens bind to estrogen receptors throughout our systems. (Research has shown that estrogen receptors are found on the surface of nearly every cell of our bodies, not just those of the vagina, uterus, and breast tissue.) When they bind, they exert a balancing, or "adaptogenic," effect.[3] This means that if your estrogen levels are low, the herbs will have an estrogenic effect, but if your estrogen levels are too high, they will block the stronger estrogens. That's why the same herb—dong quai, for example—can be used both for conditions in which there is too much estrogen (such as PMS) and for those in which there is too little (hot flashes).

Phytoestrogens do not stimulate the growth of estrogen-sensitive tissue such as in the breast and uterus; in fact, they have been shown to inhibit breast tumors in some animal studies, probably because they occupy estrogen receptor sites and prevent overstimulation of the cells.[4] Menopausal herbs have never been implicated in promoting cancer in humans, either, and indeed, some herbs are noted for their anticancer properties.[5] For this reason, menopausal herbs are an excellent choice for those who are concerned about cancer.

~ Many plant extracts exert a tonic effect on the female pelvic organs, and other organs as well. What this means is that they stimulate blood flow and sometimes even increase the weight of these organs.[6] Herbs such as black cohosh and chasteberry have also been shown to reduce menopausal symptoms by acting on the pituitary gland.

~ In general, herbs exert their influence in a much slower, more gradual way than drugs or even the bioidentical hormones that I often recommend. So be prepared to wait three or four weeks before noticing an effect from an herbal supplement.

~ Finally, menopausal herbs are often given in combination, since experienced herbalists have found that their actions are synergistic and produce better results when used this way. Chinese herbal formulations set the standard for this synergy.

Key Menopausal Herbs

The following are some of the best-studied herbs used for menopausal symptoms. They can be used singly or in combination. Please note that this list is far from comprehensive. Many others, such as peony, hops, motherwort, and false unicorn root, are also effective.

DONG QUAI (*Angelica sinensis*): Dong quai (also known as angelica, dang gui, and tang kuei) has excellent phytoestrogen activity and has been called female ginseng because of its ability to enhance energy and a sense of well-being. It is used for amenorrhea, irregular periods, and excessive uterine bleeding. My acupuncturist, who is from Taiwan, tells me that dong quai is one of the most widely used herbs in China and that many women take it throughout their reproductive and perimenopausal years.

Dong quai also has analgesic and antiallergy effects, is antibacterial, is a smooth-muscle relaxant, and can stabilize blood vessels.[7]

Dong quai is widely available over the counter. It is the foundation of almost all menopausal formulations and can be taken indefinitely. In Asia, women simmer the raw dried herb with chicken to make a soup or stew. Angelica root can be found in many herb shops or health food stores. It is also processed into capsules, tablets, and tinctures. (It is best to avoid alcohol-based tinctures.) The recommended dosages for most over-the-counter dong quai preparations are probably too low to be helpful (the usual dose is 4.5 g per day). Increasing the dosage on your own is unlikely to cause any problems, but it's always best to be under the supervision of a certified herbalist or practitioner of Traditional Chinese Medicine.

Note: Do not take dong quai if there's a chance you're pregnant.

CHASTEBERRY (*Vitex agnus-castus*): Chasteberry comes from the chaste tree, which is native to the Mediterranean. It is widely available at natural food stores, often under the name vitex. It has been shown to have a profound effect on pituitary function, increasing the secretion of LH (luteinizing hormone) and decreasing the production of FSH (follicle-stimulating hormone), which in turn shifts the production of hormones toward more progesterone and less estrogen.[8] This is thought to be the main reason why it helps balance the irregular periods that result from the hormonal swings of perimenopause. It also acts somewhat like the neurotransmitter dopamine. Chasteberry is particularly beneficial for women who are having PMS-like symptoms or are experiencing scanty, irregular periods. It has been shown to suppress appetite, relieve depression, and improve sleep. It can take several months to work.

The usual dose is 1 tsp of crushed fruit per cup of water one to four times per day, or 20–75 drops of the 1:3 liquid extract one to four times per day (or as directed on the bottle).

Note: Chasteberry can cause rashes in susceptible individuals. Don't take it with neuroleptic medicines such as haloperidol (Haldol) or thioridazine (Mellaril), or when pregnant or nursing.

BLACK COHOSH (*Cimicifuga racemosa*): Black cohosh has been used in this country for hundreds of years. Native Americans called it cramp bark. It is also a popular Chinese herb and is often used in formulations for perimenopausal symptoms. It binds to estrogen receptors, where it selectively represses the elevation of LH that occurs at menopause.[9] Its estrogenic effect decreases hot flashes, night sweats, and emotional lability. It is also helpful for PMS symptoms. A standardized extract of black cohosh sold under the trade name Remifemin is one of the most widely used herbs in Europe, where it is a well-documented alternative to HRT. Clinical studies show that it relieves menopausal symptoms such as depression, vaginal dryness, hot flashes, and menstrual cramps. Many women take Remifemin alone for relief of menopausal symptoms.

The usual starting dose for Remifemin is 1–2 tablets (20 mg per tablet) twice per day. Or take black cohosh in any of the following forms, three times per day: powdered root or as a tea, 1–2 g; solid, dry 4:1 powdered extract, 250–500 mg; fluid extract, 1:1 tincture, 4 mg (1 tsp, or about 5 ml).

Note: Black cohosh can interact with medicines for high blood pressure and may result in excessively low blood pressure in some women.

LICORICE ROOT (*Glycyrrhiza glabra*): Licorice is a perennial, temperate-zone herb that grows three to seven feet high. The parts used are the dried runners and roots. Licorice root is one of the most extensively used and scientifically investigated herbal medicines. The active constituents of licorice include both isoflavones and lignans. Licorice has many pharmacological actions, including estrogenic, anti-inflammatory, antiallergy, antibacterial, and anticancer effects. It helps regulate estrogen/progesterone ratios. It also helps replenish adrenal function, so it is very good for fatigue.

The usual dose is ¼ tsp of solid extract once or twice per day.

Note: Blood pressure should be monitored to be sure that it stays stable. The cortisol-like activity of this herb may cause a problem in those who are prone to hypertension. In those with low blood pressure, this herb can help correct and balance the problem.

Any of the key menopausal herbs above, either alone or in combination, often help to relieve a wide variety of symptoms, including vaginal dryness, hot flashes, and mood swings. My advice is to try one or more for at least a month. If you are still troubled by your symptoms, add another of the key herbs, or choose from the more specific remedies listed in other chapters.

MENOPAUSAL HEALING FOODS

Though many common foods contain vitamins, minerals, and phytoestrogens that are healthful for the perimenopausal transition, a few stand out as particularly helpful: soy, fresh ground flaxseed, and foods containing bioflavonoids. No matter what type of perimenopausal treatment you choose, if any, I'd suggest supplementing your diet with at least one of these "superfoods."

Soy

Soy, like menopausal herbs, can be used as a safe alternative to hormone replacement, offering most of the benefits of HRT without any of the risks or side effects. On the other hand, if you are taking hormones and are happy with your regimen, you can still enjoy the benefits of soy. In fact, a diet rich in soy and other phytoestrogens may allow you to decrease the total dose of hormones you are on and still maintain all the benefits.

Mainstream medical research is confirming that soy protein, as a regular component of the diet, can lessen both the frequency and the intensity of hot flashes and other perimenopausal symptoms. Soy protein appears to benefit just about every system in the body. Many perimenopausal women report that it helps their skin, hair, and nails, and after about two to three months on high doses of soy, many report a return of vaginal moisture to premenopausal levels. It also helps women with mood swings, PMS symptoms, migraine headaches, irregular periods, and weight gain, and has been shown to decrease calcium loss through the kidneys.[10] Studies also show that soy protein helps decrease fat and increase lean tissue in menopausal women.[11] It has also been shown to decrease the risk of breast and endometrial cancer because of its antiproliferative effects.[12]

Hundreds of studies are documenting the other benefits of soy. For example, one followed fifty postmenopausal women who consumed three servings of soy milk (7.5 oz each) or three handfuls of roasted soy nuts per day for twelve weeks, for a total daily dose of 60–70 mg of isoflavones.[13] The following benefits were reported.

HEART. Researchers measured a 5.5 percent increase in "good" HDL cholesterol and a 9 percent reduction in "bad" LDL cholesterol. Many other studies have also documented soy's ability to lower LDL cholesterol[14] as well as total cholesterol and triglycerides.[15] Soy has further been shown to reduce blood levels of C-Reactive Protein (CRP)[16] and homocysteine,[17] both markers for cardiovascular problems. In fact, on October 26, 1999, the FDA approved the health claim that soy protein reduces the risk of coronary artery disease.[18] It has also been shown to have a beneficial effect on blood vessel reactivity, which may be why it helps migraine headaches.[19]

BONES. The soy milk/soy nut study noted a 13 percent increase in osteocalcin, a marker of bone formation, and a 14.5 percent decrease in markers for osteoclasts, cells that cause bone loss. Soy protein revealed a bone-forming benefit that estrogen does not provide.

These same benefits have not been found with isolated isoflavones in tablet form, including a type of artificial isoflavone known as ipriflavone.[20] There are at least eight different brands of plant-based estrogen-mimicking pills on the market, but no controlled studies have been done that show the effects of the various doses. Nor are there any studies showing that the body can absorb isoflavones from the pill versions as well as from whole soy foods. This is probably because whole soy contains other known and unknown ingredients in addition to the isoflavones.

More recent studies show that the beneficial effect soy has on bone metabolism in postmenopausal women is especially true for those who already have low bone mass.[21]

COLON CANCER AND BOWEL PROBLEMS. Preliminary results of another study showed that a diet enhanced with soy protein may help reduce colon cancer incidence in people who have a history of the disease or who have had precancerous polyps removed. Based on these preliminary results, Dr. Maurice Bennink of Michigan State University suggests that there could be both a 50 percent reduction in risk in cancer incidence and an additional delay in onset of ten to fifteen years in patients taking soy.[22] Numerous animal studies also show that soy protein (not isoflavone pills) can reverse precancerous colon conditions. Animal studies show, too, that soy has an inhibitory effect on inflammatory bowel conditions such as Crohn's disease and ulcerative colitis.

SERMs. Many women on tamoxifen have reported relief of symptoms such as hot flashes and depression when they increase their intake of soy.

Is There a Soy-Thyroid Connection?
One of my newsletter subscribers wrote to me about her recently diagnosed thyroid disease and asked a question I hear frequently: "Does soy intake interfere with thyroid function?"

Based on a standard blood test, I have been told I am developing Hashimoto's thyroiditis. My doctor says it is not related to perimenopause, but I am a forty-five-year-old woman and you said in your newsletter that perimenopause and thyroid problems often occur together. I'd like to increase my intake of soy to help

with my perimenopause symptoms and protect my heart and
bones. But I've read that eating a lot of soy causes hypothyroidism. I'm confused. What should I do?

My reader may have seen a report on some studies done on animal cells in vitro, or on infants using soy-based formulas, that have
suggested the possible antithyroid effect of soy. However, a randomized, double-blind, placebo-controlled study was done at the Health
Research and Studies Center in Los Altos, California, on thirty-eight
menopausal women between the ages of sixty-four and eighty-three
who weren't on hormone replacement. Over the six-month period
during which these women took 90 mg of soy isoflavones per day, no
antithyroid effect was shown.[23] This correlates with the epidemiological evidence in Japan, a country whose inhabitants show no increased risk for hypothyroidism, even though the Japanese consume
an average of 100–200 mg of soy isoflavones per day.[24]

Here's the bottom line: there is no convincing evidence that soy
intake increases the risk of hypothyroidism during perimenopause.
However, women often begin increasing their intake of soy during
perimenopause, a time when they often get their thyroid function
checked for the first time as well. And given that fully 25 percent of
perimenopausal women have a thyroid problem, many believe that
soy is responsible. If you have any doubt about your thyroid function, get it tested. Make sure you test for TSH (thyroid-stimulating
hormone) along with T3 and T4, the two thyroid hormones. It's a
simple blood test, and it will put your mind at ease.

Soy Benefits Are Dose-Dependent

It is not always easy to compare soy foods, gram for gram, in
terms of effectiveness, because some soy foods contain more isoflavones than others. A lot depends upon where the crop is grown
and how it is processed. One serving of a typical soy food contains
20 g of protein and about 30 mg of soy isoflavones (genistein,
daidzein, etc.). In contrast, some supplements made from whole soy
are much more concentrated.

Most American research studies have been done with only 40–
60 g of soy protein per day (two to three small servings) because that
is the most American volunteers will eat! It is also the minimum
amount you'll need to eat to get any noticeable effect. At this level of
consumption, it takes about four to six weeks of consistent use to notice an effect. This is consistent with research that shows that when
women ate 60 g of soy protein per day in the form of a powdered

drink mix, they had a 45 percent reduction in hot flashes after twelve weeks.[25] Research and my clinical and personal experience suggest that most women need about 100–160 mg of soy isoflavones per day to get significant relief from other menopausal symptoms, such as vaginal dryness, as well as to protect their heart and bones. A randomized, double-blind, placebo-controlled three-month clinical trial conducted at the Johns Hopkins University in Baltimore showed that women consuming 160 mg of total isoflavones a day (in the form of Revival soy products) reported significant improvement in quality of life (including a reduction in mood swings, night sweats, hot flashes, and other menopausal symptoms).[26]

Each of the following servings contains approximately 35–50 mg of soy isoflavones:

~ 1 cup soy milk
~ ½ cup tofu
~ ½ cup tempeh
~ ½ cup green soybeans (edamame), available fresh or frozen
~ 3 handfuls of roasted soy nuts

Powdered soy protein can be mixed with water, milk, or juice. Various brands are available. This is a particularly convenient way to get the benefits of soy. Some brands, such as Revival, contain the equivalent of four to six servings of soy in one drink. (See Resources.)

Add soy foods to your diet gradually; otherwise you might experience gas, since your intestinal bacteria have to adjust to this new food. You can use digestive enzymes such as Beano to help.

SUE: *Depression Lifted, Breasts Healed*

I've heard many inspiring stories about how soy foods have changed women's lives. Here's a letter from a woman named Sue.

About a year ago my mom got me started on Revival, and I will be forever grateful. She herself had started taking Revival after she was diagnosed with breast cancer. She went through rigorous chemotherapy, radiation, and tamoxifen treatment. She is now doing well and is cancer-free.

I was on Prozac, Premarin, and Pravachol for years and had not been able to eliminate any of them. Cutting back on Prozac or Premarin left me unfit to live with. Two weeks after starting

Revival, I began cutting back the prescription medications and was off all the drugs and hormones within six weeks—with no ill effects. Now for the real surprise.

For years I have feared my regularly scheduled mammogram. I would usually get called back at least once for repeat views because I have severe fibrocystic breast disease and I've had two densities in my left breast that they've been watching closely. Yesterday I went for my regular mammogram and was absolutely shocked with the result. The left breast densities are almost totally gone—if you try really hard, you can see them. And the fibrocystic density has greatly diminished. On the old films the density could be seen throughout the breasts. Now there's about 30 percent normal breast tissue. I was told I no longer have to go for a mammogram every six months. I'm down to just once per year.

What to Expect When You Add Soy to Your Diet

Depending on the amount you're eating, you may notice a decrease in hot flashes within a few days of adding soy to your diet. The average woman in Japan (where hot flashes are relatively rare) eats four to six servings of soy per day, or the equivalent of 100–200 mg soy isoflavones.

Some perimenopausal women have found that their periods returned when they began taking soy or one of any number of menopausal herbal mixtures on the market. A patient came to me for a consultation after this happened, because her regular gynecologist was very worried that the herbs were having a dangerous adverse effect. However, the phytoestrogens in soy or menopausal herbs do not cause periods in women who are completely through menopause.

Irregular periods during the menopausal years are due, instead, to fluctuating hormonal levels. It is very common for a menopausal woman to go for months without having a period and then start menstruating regularly again for several months or even years. Soy intake won't prevent this. And the same is true of women who've reported that their fibroids began to grow when they started taking high doses of soy. Soy doesn't promote fibroid growth, though the highly fluctuating estrogen levels associated with perimenopause often cause very rapid fibroid growth. In fact, some women report a reduction in the size of their fibroids when on soy compared to when they take conventional hormones.

A woman taking Revival wrote: "I have been taking Revival for many months with great success (it reduced the size of my fibroid and slowed the bleeding). I started HRT and within a month my fibroid was growing again and I was bleeding again. I stopped. I am now back on Revival and here to stay."

Another of my patients told me that when she started to take a soy drink from her health food store, her hot flashes and hypoglycemia symptoms went away completely. Later, she said, "I began to doubt that something as simple as a soy drink could eliminate hot flashes. So I stopped. Sure enough, my hot flashes returned within a week. So I started taking my soy again. I wish I hadn't stopped it, because it took another two weeks for it to kick in again."

Soy Can be Used by the Whole Family

Making soy part of family meals can benefit everyone in your family. In men, soy protein has been found to help maintain healthy prostate tissue. In fact, many have found that they no longer need to get up at night to urinate once they start taking supplemental soy. A substantial body of research has documented the benefits of soy on prostate health, showing that eating soy can both help prevent prostate cancer as well as inhibit the progression of already established prostate cancer.[27]

Use Non-GMO Soy Products

It is estimated that about 20 percent of the American soy crop has undergone genetic modification to enhance drought resistance and other desirable traits. Such genetic engineering raises some disturbing ethical and health questions, and in Europe, unease about this development has led to the banning of genetically modified organisms (GMOs). The same movement is now becoming active in the United States. Until we know more about the possible health or environmental risks, stick with soy that is labeled non-GMO whenever possible.

Flaxseed: Super Source of Lignans, Fiber, and Omega-3 Fats

Flaxseed is the best available source of anticancer and phytoestrogenic compounds known as lignans—with a concentration more than a hundred times greater than other lignan-containing foods, such as grains, fruits, and vegetables. Lignans are plant substances that get broken down by intestinal bacteria into two chemicals, enterodiol and enterolactone. These substances then circulate through the liver and are later excreted in the urine.[28] Flaxseed is also an excellent source of fiber and of omega-3 fats.

There are a number of reasons why we all should be interested in incorporating more lignans into our diet. The following are some of the most compelling.

Lignans

LIGNANS HAVE POTENT ANTICANCER EFFECTS. An impressive number of studies have shown that flaxseed lignans help in both prevention and treatment of breast and colon cancer because of their ability to modulate the production, availability, and action of the hormones produced in our bodies.[29]

LIGNANS ARE POTENT PHYTOESTROGENS. In women who consume flaxseed, studies have shown significant hormonal changes, including alterations in estradiol levels, similar to those seen with soy isoflavones. This makes flaxseed oil or ground flaxseed a great choice for women who can't use soy or who simply want another source of phytohormones.[30]

LIGNANS ARE GOOD ANTIOXIDANTS. Like soy and many herbs, lignans have antiviral, antibacterial, and antioxidant properties, which means they help prevent free-radical damage to tissues—the cellular-level injury associated with aging and disease.

LIGNANS HELP PROTECT THE CARDIOVASCULAR SYSTEM. Studies have also found that lignans in the form of flaxseed significantly lower LDL cholesterol (the "bad" cholesterol), raise HDL cholesterol (the "good" cholesterol), and reduce the incidence of atherosclerosis.[31]

Fiber

Flaxseed is an excellent source of fiber. In addition to its phytoestrogenic properties, flaxseed is rich in both soluble and insoluble fiber. Adding a daily serving of ground flaxseed to your diet may eliminate any problems you have with constipation. (Just be sure you take it with enough liquid.) While the fiber in wheat bran is quite hard and can irritate the bowel, the fiber in flaxseed is much softer. When combined with fluid, flax fiber forms a mucilage in the body that can significantly help reduce the risk for diabetes and cardiovascular disease. Fiber has been shown to reduce both total cholesterol and triglyceride levels in the bloodstream.

The total dietary fiber content in 45 g of flaxseed (about ¼ cup) is 11.7 g. This is nearly four times greater than the fiber contained in a ½-cup serving of oatmeal.

Note: Ground hemp seeds are also an excellent source of high quality protein and fiber—⅓ cup contains 14 grams of fiber and 11 grams of protein. (For more information, see www.nutiva.com.)

Omega-3 Fats

Flaxseed is an excellent source of omega-3 fats. These fats are essential for the health of every cell in our bodies, including the cells in our brains and hearts. A deficiency of omega-3 fatty acids, which is quite common, can result in fatigue, dry skin, cracked nails, thin and breakable hair, constipation, immune system malfunction, aching joints, depression, arthritis, and hormone imbalances.

Omega-3 fats are found not just in flaxseed, but in fatty fish (especially salmon, bluefish, mackerel, sardines, and anchovies), fish oil, organ meats, egg yolk, and algae. Flaxseed meal is an excellent source of omega-3 fats if it's freshly ground. (Flaxseed oil also provides omega-3s, but it does not provide fiber. In addition, the oil must be kept refrigerated, or it will turn rancid.)

Fish, especially the cold-water fatty kinds, is a better source of DHA, the brain tissue building block that your body can't manufacture. That may be why studies show that individuals who consume fish exhibit a lower incidence of depression. If you can't or don't want to consume fish regularly, I think DHA (200–1,000 mg per day) is one of the best supplements you can take. (See Resources.)

How to Take Flaxseed

Not all flaxseed is created equal. I recommend buying golden flax grown in the northern Great Plains regions of North America (Manitoba and the Dakotas), where the rich soil and climate support flax that is high in omega-3 fats and flavor. (See Resources.) Although the brown flax found in most health food stores has all the nutritional benefits of golden flax, I personally prefer the taste of golden flax. For best results, use ¼ cup flaxseed three to seven days a week. Grind your daily serving in a coffee grinder and then stir the meal into soups and beverages, or sprinkle it on cereal or salad. I add half my daily dose to my morning soy drink and eat the other half with vanilla yogurt at the same meal. This combination makes a wonderfully fiber-full, phytoestrogen-rich, perimenopausal power breakfast. And it takes less than three minutes to prepare!

Bioflavonoids

Another rich food source for phytoestrogens are the bioflavonoids contained in many herbs and fruits. Bioflavonoids compete with excess estrogen for receptor sites and are therefore also helpful for balancing menopausal hormones and tonifying the pelvic organs. The white, spongy inner peel of citrus fruits is a very rich source, so eat some of it along with your orange or grapefruit. (I usually just take the orange peel and eat the inner white part directly—the same as I would an artichoke leaf.) Other rich sources of bioflavonoids include cherries, cranberries, blueberries, bilberries, many whole grains, grape skins, and red clover. In supplement form, 1,000 mg of bioflavonoids with vitamin C daily has been shown to relieve hot flashes.[32]

TRADITIONAL CHINESE MEDICINE AND ACUPUNCTURE FOR MENOPAUSE

Over the years I've referred hundreds of women for acupuncture and Traditional Chinese Medicine (TCM), a system of medicine that is over two thousand years old, for the relief of a wide variety of gynecological problems, including those related to menopause. I have personally used elements of Traditional Chinese Medicine, including various herbal formulas and acupuncture, to relieve menstrual cramps and hot flashes.

Traditional Chinese Medicine is by its very nature holistic, tailoring treatment to the individual's body, mind, spirit, and emotions. This system of medicine views our health as a balance between the two contrasting states of yin and yang. The following is a very simple explanation, courtesy of my own personal mother-daughter acupuncture team, of the most common pattern that occurs during menopause.[33]

According to Chinese medicine, the part of us that is referred to as *yin*—our vital fluids—begins to diminish as we grow older. This leads to an excess of *yang*—vital energy and heat—and/or stagnation of *chi* (life energy). Ideally, when our *yin, yang,* and *chi* are in balance, our body acts something like a kettle containing liquid (*yin*) heated by fire (*yang*). The resulting steam (the enhanced *chi* flow) circulates throughout the body, warming and nourishing it.

How much and to what degree *yin* becomes depleted depends

upon our lifestyle, diet, and genes. Depletion of *yin* causes the vital liquid in the kettle to burn off, so that the fire burns without producing the steam necessary to moisten and nourish.

Excess heat leads to hot flashes, the most obvious symptom, as well as to dryness of the skin, eyes, and vagina. Excess heat can dislodge the *shen* (spirit) from the heart, causing restlessness and insomnia. If excess heat enters the blood, it can cause heavy menstrual periods. *Chi* stagnation can cause pain anywhere in the body, as well as moodiness and emotional instability. A combination of excess heat and *chi* stagnation can lead to restlessness and anxiety.

Diet

According to Chinese medicine, diet is the most effective way to relieve many symptoms, and my experience bears this out. All heat-producing foods and substances should be eliminated. Caffeine, alcohol, refined sugar, food coloring, preservatives, and additives (including antibiotics and hormones fed to animals during the production of most meat, chicken, and eggs) will cause excess heat and *yin* depletion. Red meat should be consumed in small quantities, but being a complete vegetarian (vegan) is not recommended. You should eat at least 2–4 ounces of meat or fish every week or two, depending upon your size and lifestyle. It is also helpful to limit spicy, pungent foods, such as curries or chilies, and greasy, fried, or oily foods.

Foods should be lightly cooked, not raw or cold. (These days I microwave my salad greens for about thirty seconds with a little lemon juice on them.) The body has to work much harder to digest raw food, which creates heat and *chi* stagnation. Cold food, contrary to popular belief, doesn't cool the body in a balanced way. Instead, cold and ice create blockages in the *chi* channel, which creates *chi* stagnation. The following foods are especially cooling and helpful: melons, bean sprouts, tofu, white ocean fish, celery, apples, asparagus, and grapes.

Smoking obviously makes everything worse. When you smoke you are quite literally breathing in fire and toxins that enter the brain and bloodstream directly. It is also well documented that smoking poisons the ovaries, decreasing our estrogen levels about two years sooner than would normally occur.

Practitioners of Traditional Chinese Medicine also discourage the regular use of ginger and Asian ginseng (*Panax ginseng*) and Siberian ginseng during perimenopause because both are considered heat-producing.

Chinese Herbs for Menopause

An incredible variety of Chinese herbs and herbal combinations are available to treat every condition known to humanity—and the symptoms of perimenopause are no exception. While many individual Chinese herbs have Western counterparts, the most effective Chinese herbal combinations are unique to this system of medicine. Many of these so-called patent formulations have been tested and refined for thousands of years.

A full discussion of Traditional Chinese Medicine and Chinese herbs is beyond the scope of this book. The preparations mentioned below don't even begin to scratch the surface of what is available and safe for almost all people to take. Since most herbal prescriptions are based on an individual's unique constitution, it is best to work directly with a practitioner trained in this system.

If you are buying herbal formulations from a health food store, make sure that the ingredients are listed on the label.

The following are particularly useful for perimenopausal symptoms.

JOYFUL CHANGE is a safe, general perimenopausal herbal tonic. It consists of over a dozen different herbs, including dong quai and peony. It was especially created for the complex menopausal symptoms of women in our culture by knowledgeable practitioners of Chinese medicine. It is effective for symptoms such as hot flashes, insomnia, and dryness. It also addresses the cause of the symptoms by draining heat and nourishing *yin*. Joyful Change is helpful for balancing the menstrual cycle in those women whose periods have become irregular and scant because of skipping ovulations.

YUN NAN BAI YAO (also known as Yunna Pai Yao) is very helpful in controlling the heavy bleeding that is so common in perimenopausal women. It should not be used on a long-term basis (more than a month) because it is not a cure. In other words, you should also take measures to address and treat the underlying cause of your bleeding, such as estrogen dominance or a fibroid.

CHAI HU LONG GU MULI WANG moves the liver *chi* and sedates the spirit. It is helpful for moodiness, anxiety, emotional instability, and outbursts of anger and feelings of frustration. It is also used to treat insomnia. This herbal combination can be taken indefinitely; it is widely used by the general population in China, not just menopausal women.

Acupuncture

Acupuncture is an essential part of Traditional Chinese Medicine. Because it works to normalize the flow of life energy or *chi* in the body, it is particularly appropriate for perimenopause, a time when our energy is completely renewing itself. It is extremely effective for relieving hot flashes, insomnia, night sweats, anxiety, restlessness, emotional instability, moodiness, menstrual cramps, and excess bleeding.

Though most people resort to acupuncture only after conventional Western drugs and surgery have failed, and though it is often effective even in these difficult situations, acupuncture is best used as preventive health care or at the onset of symptoms. It can unblock stuck *chi* long before the problem manifests in actual illness.

When I was in my thirties, I was able to eliminate my menstrual cramps with acupuncture treatment. They have never returned. I have also referred patients for acupuncture who have had illnesses ranging from migraine headaches to chronic urinary tract infections. Acupuncture can help regulate menstrual periods, control heavy menstrual bleeding, stop seizures, and even in some cases help shrink fibroids. Research has shown that acupuncture improves cortisol balance in the body, enhances immune function, and helps quell addictions to cigarettes and alcohol.

Acupuncture works by redirecting the flow of *chi* along energy pathways in the body known as meridians. Because the meridians have no known anatomical counterparts, allopathic medicine dismissed acupuncture's effectiveness for years, until the presence of meridians was definitively demonstrated in a French study. Researchers injected a radioactive tracer into both traditional acupuncture points and into random sham points. The tracer that was injected into the genuine acupuncture points could easily be tracked as it ran up the meridians.[34] The clinical evidence of acupuncture's effectiveness has also become too compelling to ignore.

START SOMEWHERE

Don't let all these choices overwhelm you or become another heavy list of "shoulds." The wisdom in nature is user-friendly, and you have a lot of it within you already. To tap into it, just pick the herb, the formula, or the foods that seem to jump out at you and say "Try me." Because all of the herbs and foods I've mentioned contain phytohormones of some kind and have virtually no side effects, feel free to experiment.

7

The Menopause Food Plan: A Program to Balance Your Hormones and Prevent Middle-Age Spread

Over the years, countless women in their late thirties or forties have come to me with one or more of the following complaints: "Where did this spare tire around my middle come from?" "Why can't I lose that last five to ten pounds I used to be able to shed within a few weeks?" "Why is it that although I weigh the same as I did in college, my body seems different?"

Some women find themselves gaining weight at midlife even if they are eating no more than before. Others simply change shape: their waistlines thicken, and fat accumulates on their abdomen, flanks, and shoulders. Most of us have to make changes in our diets and exercise regimens if we expect to negotiate menopause without ten to twenty pounds or so of extra baggage, weight that, in addition to wreaking havoc with our appearance, is also a well-documented health risk.[1]

Midlife weight gain results from a series of metabolic changes that actually begin decades before but then reach critical mass (no pun intended) during perimenopause. Rapid changes in hormonal levels along with increased stress hormones also exacerbate midlife weight gain.

Thankfully, there are ways to negotiate the metabolic shifts that manifest at midlife and rebalance your hormones without any significant weight or fat gain. I know this path from the inside out, not only professionally but also personally.

MAKING PEACE (ONCE AGAIN) WITH MY WEIGHT

My weight has been an issue for me since I was twelve years old, when I went on my first diet. In my teens and early twenties I was always trying to weigh ten to twenty pounds less than I should have, given my rather sturdy frame and large muscles. (No one understood at that time that weight could be a very misleading measure of health.) Throughout my teens, I struggled to weigh 115, a weight I achieved only for a month or so when I starved myself in college. In my twenties, I ran regularly and was able to maintain my weight at around 125 with a great deal of effort, which included fighting constant cravings for sweets.

After my pregnancies I, like so many other women, was never able to get my weight back to 125 no matter what I did. I had run headlong into another aspect of Mother Nature's wisdom, which has set up postpartum weight gain so that we new mothers will be likely to stay alive during lean times to nurse and care for our children.

In my thirties, after I had nursed my two daughters for a total of nearly four years, my weight stabilized between 137 and 140. During these years I added weight training to my fitness regimen, and I figured that my weight gain was as much muscle as fat. (Muscle weighs more than fat, but it also burns calories far more efficiently.)

Finally, in my early forties, I came to a place of peace with my weight and size, even though my skeleton will never be a size 4! Through careful attention to my diet—which had consisted mostly of whole foods, healthy fats, lots of fruits and vegetables, and lean protein—and consistent exercise including weight training, I managed to maintain my body fat percentage at a healthy 22 to 25 percent and my weight at about 140, plus or minus (mostly plus) a few pounds. Yes, I still wanted to lose five to ten pounds, but I wasn't willing to further change my lifestyle—or give up my regular, though modest, servings of chocolate brownies or pie—to lose them. I was certainly following my own recommendations and keeping my blood sugar stable!

My Metabolism Takes On a Life of Its Own

But then a month or so after turning fifty—about the time my periods became irregular—I began, inexplicably, to gain weight. Every day the scale showed another pound, even though I wasn't eating or exercising any differently. I was horrified. Yes, horrified. Lest you think that this is too strong a word, let me explain. I have the kind of body shape and metabolic rate that could very easily lead to obesity if I were not so disciplined about my diet and exercise routine. There was an upper limit on the scale beyond which I would not allow myself to go, and that number was 144. But now I stood by helplessly and—in the space of a few weeks—watched the scale climb to 149, one pound less than I had weighed at the end of my pregnancy with my first daughter!

I knew that a new plan of action was called for. But what should it be? I'd been so sure I'd finally won the battle of the bulge and found a comfortable way to eat that would work for me for life. Now what?

Ketosis and Me

I decided to try a more extreme form of carbohydrate restriction. Maybe I'd let too many carbs creep into my diet. I went out and bought a copy of *Dr. Atkins' New Diet Revolution*. The cover said two million copies had been sold; could that many people be completely wrong?[2] In any case, given the connection between carbohydrates, insulin, and weight gain (which I will discuss in more detail below), Atkins's research and clinical expertise made sense to me.[3]

I had also researched ketosis, the metabolic state that results when you cut down carbohydrates enough to begin burning body fat for fuel. Although critics cite ketosis as a danger of high-protein diets, I knew that this metabolic state was safe for people with no kidney problems, at least for the limited amount of time recommended by Atkins and quite probably for much longer periods. More than that, it appeared to be associated with consistent and relatively fast weight loss.

I decided to follow the Atkins "induction" diet to the letter for at least fourteen days. I bought some urine testing strips at the drugstore to test for ketosis. (Ketone bodies, which result from the breakdown of body fat, are excreted in the urine and can be easily tested for at home.) According to Atkins, the presence of ketones in the urine is a virtual guarantee that you're burning fat for energy. Then I cut my carbohydrate intake to less than 20 g per day, a level of restriction I'd never tried before.

According to Atkins, the vast majority of people reach a state of ketosis within forty-eight hours. That is how long it takes the liver's glycogen stores to be depleted so that the body begins to use its fat for energy. So I cut the carbs, waited forty-eight hours, and then began to test my urine two to three times every day. Nothing. The strips didn't turn purple. Though I actually felt good and had a lot of energy, I didn't go into ketosis until I began to add relatively high doses of the supplement L-carnitine.

After a full ten days of carbohydrate restriction, I managed to produce just a little bit of ketosis—the urine strips measured "trace." But even then I failed to lose weight or inches. In fact, I gained three pounds on the induction part of the Atkins diet. I had now plateaued to a new high. Talk about frustration! Here I was, exercising regularly, eating a very limited amount of carbohydrates, keeping the rest of my food portions normal, and following a diet that has helped millions lose weight. But it didn't work for me. Like many other perimenopausal women, I had hit a metabolic wall; our midlife bodies seem to hold on to fat for dear life until we learn the secrets of releasing it!

I finally did. Within four months, I got back down to 140 pounds and after menopause was able to get down to 132 again, a weight I've maintained through consistent dietary discipline and regular exercise.

The following program is based on my own experience, reports from thousands of my newsletter subscribers, and leading-edge research on the effect of food on blood sugar. It is designed to help you tame your midlife fat cells, balance your hormones, and safeguard your health on all levels.

SIX STEPS TO MIDLIFE WEIGHT CONTROL

Step One: Maintain Normal Blood Sugar and Insulin Levels

Like many women (and doctors), I used to operate under the delusion that the reason we tend to gain weight at midlife is because our metabolism slows down, our bodies become more efficient at storing energy in the form of fat, and falling estrogen levels result in increases in appetite.[4] As it turns out, these metabolic changes, though real enough, are not the result of menopause, per se, but are instead the natural progression of a process that begins much earlier: glycemic stress (from blood sugar that is too high) and resulting insulin abuse. Here's what happens.

When you eat too many refined carbohydrates (in the form of french fries, mashed potatoes, cookies, ice cream, soda pop, white bread and rolls, etc), you get an immediate and substantial increase in blood sugar. This excess sugar in the blood is converted to triglycerides in the liver. At the same time, however, excess blood sugar actually causes inflammation in the lining of blood vessels throughout your body, starting in the skeletal muscles. This is known as "glycemic stress," a term coined by family physician Ray Strand, M.D., whose research has documented how glycemic stress, if left unchecked, eventually results in syndrome X, which is characterized by central obesity (too much belly fat) and an increased risk for type 2 diabetes, male pattern baldness, and heart disease.

Excess blood sugar over long periods of time eventually leads to insulin resistance. Let me explain: Insulin is produced in the pancreas and is responsible for ferrying glucose from the bloodstream into our cells, where it is used for fuel. Good health depends upon our body's ability to make and utilize just the right amount of insulin to keep our blood sugar at optimal levels and our metabolism working normally. Consumption of refined carbohydrates results in an immediate surge in blood sugar. This triggers the pancreas to secrete large amounts of insulin to process the blood sugar. Every cell in the body has insulin receptors on the surface. These allow insulin to "open the door," so that glucose can enter the cell.[5] But over time, when blood sugar levels continue to be too high, the insulin receptors lose their ability to respond to this abnormal metabolic burden. The excess blood sugar is also stored as fat, which in turn contributes to insulin problems. Over time our cells become insensitive to insulin's effect and a condition known as insulin resistance develops, in which more and more insulin is poured out, to less and less effect. Eventually neither the body tissues nor the pancreas can keep up with the blood sugar load. Virtually every cell in our bodies is adversely affected by this abnormal metabolic state. In severe cases, an individual with this condition may be diagnosed with type 2 diabetes and require insulin injections to meet the demand.

About 25 percent of the population appears to be genetically resistant to the adverse effects of overproduction of insulin and insulin resistance. These individuals usually manage to stay very slim no matter what they eat. But 75 percent of the population is not so lucky, especially during perimenopause.

Most perimenopausal symptoms, such as heavy bleeding, cramps, fibroids, and PMS, will respond to a diet that keeps your blood sugar and insulin levels stable—a diet that will also help prevent cellular inflammation. In general, insulin and blood sugar levels stay normal on a diet of unrefined whole foods that include carbohydrates with a low to moderate glycemic index, such as fruits, vegetables, and whole grains. The glycemic index is simply a measurement of the rate and degree to which a given carbohydrate-containing food raises blood sugar levels. High-glycemic-index carbohydrates—including alcohol, starchy and sugary foods such as cookies, candies, soda pop, alcohol, and white bread, and almost all refined, processed foods—are quickly metabolized into sugar, triggering a rush of insulin into the blood.

On the other hand, carbohydrates with a low glycemic index break down slowly, raising blood sugar to relatively low levels over a longer period of time. This allows them to be metabolized with only a small amount of insulin.

Evolutionarily speaking, most of the high-glycemic-index carbohydrates are "new" foods that have been rapidly increasing in our diets only over the last century. Up until then, for millennia, our food supply and metabolism evolved side by side along with the active lifestyles that also keep insulin levels normal.

INSULIN RESISTANCE (SYNDROME X)

The medical conditions associated with insulin resistance are collectively known as Syndrome X, a term first coined by Gerald Reaven, M.D., a world-renowned endocrinologist at the Stanford University School of Medicine.[6] They include:

~ Increased risk for type 2 diabetes[7]

~ Abnormal cholesterol levels[8]

~ Hypertension

~ Heart disease: coronary artery disease and peripheral vascular disease[9]

~ Obesity

~ Anovulation[10]

~ Overstimulation of ovarian testosterone[11]

~ Polycystic ovary disease

~ Excess hair on the face, hair loss on scalp (male pattern baldness in women)

~ Adult acne

~ Increased risk for breast cancer and endometrial cancer[12]

A diet high in refined carbohydrates makes all perimenopausal problems worse because of its adverse effect on hormone balance. It reinforces the tendency toward excess fat around the waist and belly (central obesity), which in turn favors production of estrogen and androgens. Central obesity and high insulin levels—which can occur even in women of normal weight and BMI—are also associated with higher blood triglyceride levels and low HDL cholesterol. (A low HDL level is one of the first signs of insulin abuse. I had this in my early thirties!) This, of course, has a negative effect on heart health, but it also interferes with the normal mechanism by which the body deactivates free estradiol. A relative increase in the amount of metabolically active estradiol in the bloodstream can target estrogen-sensitive breast and endometrial tissue, resulting in possible excessive growth of these tissues. This is one of the reasons why hyperinsulinemia (excess insulin in the blood) with insulin resistance is a significant risk factor for breast cancer as well as polycystic ovary disease.[13] High insulin levels also increase tissue sensitivity to a protein known as insulin-like growth factor (IGF-1), which is known to stimulate the growth of breast and other tissues.[14]

Skeletal muscles are designed to burn blood sugar effectively, which is why maintaining adequate muscle mass and exercising regularly are important keys to maintaining stable blood sugar. But as women age, they often stop exercising as much as they did in their teens and twenties. Lifestyles become increasingly sedentary, so by the time they hit perimenopause, many women have replaced their muscle mass with fat and years of insulin abuse have stored excess energy as fat—particularly abdominal fat. (Fat weighs less than muscle but takes up more space. This is the reason why so many midlife women notice that their clothes don't fit well anymore even though they haven't gained any weight!) One of the earliest signs of insulin resistance is increased belly fat—that spare tire around the middle.

Body fat is loaded with insulin receptors, and the fatter you get, the more insulin it takes to get blood sugar into the cells. Type 2 diabetes will often disappear simply with weight loss alone.

Glycemic stress and insulin resistance are also associated with heartburn, insomnia, swelling, sugar cravings, fatigue, and excess daytime sleepiness—all of which are associated with tissue inflammation that is the result of the complex interaction between insulin, blood sugar, stress hormones, and essential fatty acids. People with excess body fat, from years of eating high-glycemic meals, actually produce high levels of inflammatory chemicals such as IL-6 (interleukin 6) from their body fat. They are prone to aches and pains, estrogen dominance, and PMS as a result. Ultimately, glycemic stress leads to insulin resistance and, later, diabetes and/or heart disease, if left unchecked.

Step Two: Measure for Health—Waist/Hip Ratio, Body Mass Index, and Body Fat Percentage

Years of eating too many refined carbohydrates and exercising too little finally catch up with us at midlife. Slowly but surely, our lifestyles predispose us to central obesity (excess belly fat), which *is* a problem. Abdominal fat cells are more metabolically active—and potentially more dangerous—than the fat cells on your hips and thighs. Abdominal fat increases blood triglyceride levels and is a sign of insulin resistance.

And belly fat cells also pump out too much androgens and estrogen. The classic apple-shaped figure is associated with an increased risk for heart disease, breast cancer, uterine cancer, diabetes, kidney stones, hypertension, arthritis, incontinence, polycystic ovary disease, urinary stress incontinence, gallstones, stroke, and sleep apnea.[15] Your waist/hip ratio is a quick way to gauge your risk. Measure around the fullest part of your buttocks. Then measure your waist at the narrowest part of your torso. Divide your waist measurement by your hip measurement. A healthy ratio is less than 0.8. The ideal is 0.74. A ratio greater than 0.85 is associated with all the health risks listed above.[16] Dr. Strand, an expert on diagnosing and reversing the effects of insulin resistance, prefers using your waist measurement in inches because it directly measures belly fat. If your waist measurement is more than 34.5 inches, there's a strong likelihood that you already have insulin resistance and metabolic syndrome.

The body mass index (BMI) is another way to measure your health risk. To determine your BMI, simply find your weight and your height on the table on the following page. A BMI of 24 or below is ideal. For people who don't smoke and aren't chronically ill, a BMI of 30 or higher (considered obese) is associated with a 2 to 3 times greater risk of dying prematurely compared to a person with a BMI of 24 or less. For those with a BMI between 25 and 29 (considered overweight, but not obese), the risk of premature death is still 20 to 40 percent higher than for those at normal weight.[17]

Percentage of body fat is the final number you'll need. This can be measured by your doctor, at a health club, or at your YMCA. Though it's possible to purchase over-the-counter devices that measure body fat, I have not found them to be very accurate. It is possible to have a healthy body fat percentage (between 20 and 28 percent for women) and have a BMI that is higher than 24. This is especially true in athletes who have a great deal of muscle mass.

If your waist/hip ratio, BMI, and body fat percentage are all in the healthy range, then you simply have to fine-tune what you are already doing to maintain your weight and balance your hormones. If not, then do whatever you can to lower your risk. A 1999 study from Harvard Medical School found that women who gain approximately twenty pounds in adulthood experience a decline in physical function and vitality even greater than that associated with smoking. Weight gain was also associated with an increase in bodily pain, regardless of a woman's baseline weight. The reason for this is that excess fat produces inflammatory compounds, e.g., cytokines and interleukin 6 that cause tissue damage and pain. Happily, this is all reversible. Once the overweight women lost weight, all characteristics of health and vitality improved.[18] This is very good news. You don't have to reach your ideal weight; even a modest five- or ten-pound fat loss— or achieving a BMI that is one number lower than your current number—can dramatically improve your health, lower your blood pressure, and balance your hormone levels.

Step Three: Check Out Your Metabolic Stressors

In her book *Fight Fat After Forty* (Viking, 2000), Pamela Peeke, M.D., a researcher with the National Institutes of Health, documents the connection between toxic stress and toxic weight gain—the kind of weight that accumulates in the abdomen and puts women at risk

FIGURE 11: BODY MASS INDEX CHART

Height (Feet and Inches)

Weight (Pounds)	5'0"	5'1"	5'2"	5'3"	5'4"	5'5"	5'6"	5'7"	5'8"	5'9"	5'10"	5'11"	6'0"	6'1"	6'2"	6'3"	6'4"
100	20	19	18	18	17	17	16	16	15	15	14	14	14	13	13	12	12
105	21	20	19	19	18	17	17	16	16	16	15	15	14	14	13	13	13
110	21	21	20	19	19	18	18	17	17	16	16	15	15	15	14	14	13
115	22	22	21	20	20	19	19	18	17	17	17	16	16	15	15	14	14
120	23	23	22	21	21	20	19	19	18	18	17	17	16	16	15	15	15
125	24	24	23	22	21	21	20	20	19	18	18	17	17	16	16	16	15
130	25	25	24	23	22	22	21	20	20	19	19	18	18	17	17	16	16
135	26	26	25	24	23	22	22	21	21	20	19	19	18	18	17	17	16
140	27	26	26	25	24	23	23	22	21	21	20	20	19	18	18	17	17
145	28	27	27	26	25	24	23	23	22	21	21	20	20	19	19	18	18
150	29	28	27	27	26	25	24	23	23	22	22	21	20	20	19	19	18
155	30	29	28	27	27	26	25	24	24	23	22	22	21	20	20	19	19
160	31	30	29	28	27	27	26	25	24	24	23	22	22	21	21	20	19
165	32	31	30	29	28	27	27	26	25	24	24	23	22	22	21	21	20
170	33	32	31	30	29	28	27	27	26	25	24	24	23	22	22	21	21
175	34	33	32	31	30	29	28	27	27	26	25	24	24	23	22	22	21
180	35	34	33	32	31	30	29	28	27	27	26	25	24	24	23	22	22
185	36	35	34	33	32	31	30	29	28	27	27	26	25	24	24	23	23
190	37	36	35	34	33	32	31	30	29	28	27	26	26	25	24	24	23
195	38	37	36	35	33	32	31	31	30	29	28	27	26	26	25	24	24
200	39	38	37	35	34	33	32	31	30	30	29	28	27	26	26	25	24
205	40	39	37	36	35	34	33	32	31	30	29	29	28	27	26	26	25
210	41	40	38	37	36	35	34	33	32	31	30	29	28	28	27	26	26
215	42	41	39	38	37	36	35	34	33	32	31	30	29	28	28	27	26
220	43	42	40	39	38	37	36	34	33	32	32	31	30	29	28	27	27
225	44	43	41	40	39	37	36	35	34	33	32	31	31	30	29	28	27
230	45	43	42	41	39	38	37	36	35	34	33	32	31	30	30	29	28
235	46	44	43	42	40	39	38	37	36	35	34	33	32	31	30	29	29
240	47	45	44	43	41	40	39	38	36	35	34	33	33	32	31	30	29
245	48	46	45	43	42	41	40	38	37	36	35	34	33	32	31	31	30
250	49	47	46	44	43	42	40	39	38	37	36	35	34	33	32	31	30

☐ Underweight ▨ Weight Appropriate ☐ Overweight ■ Obese

for premature death. Toxic stress can come from any daily challenge, but a number of circumstances make it especially common in women over forty: the resurfacing of childhood trauma, perfectionism, relationship changes such as divorce and caregiving, job stress, acute or chronic illness, dieting, and the effects of menopause.

This explanation clicked with me because my initial perimenopausal weight gain coincided with new stresses in my life. The scale started to climb just before Thanksgiving, when my older daughter arrived home for her first vacation from college and we officially launched our first holiday season as a "broken" family. My daughters were scheduled to split their holiday time between my house and their father's, a situation I had always been sure would never happen to us.

I was also caring full time for a friend, who was recovering from major spine surgery. I was preparing her meals, trying to anticipate her needs, watching her go through excruciating pain unrelieved by narcotics, and generally trying to provide a safe place where she could heal. For well over a month I was basically on call twenty-four hours per day, with only an occasional break. In retrospect, no wonder the pounds piled on.

Get out your calendar, do some detective work, and see if you, too, have a stress pattern that could be leading to weight gain. Be particularly aware of the danger of the late-afternoon hours when the main hormones that allow us to mount a response against stress—serotonin and cortisol—tend to fall, leaving us feeling more vulnerable to our underlying emotions. In particular, when serotonin, the "feel-good" neurotransmitter, is depleted, we are apt to eat anything in sight—particularly refined carbohydrates—to bring it back to normal.

The effect of stress on weight also works in the opposite direction. One of my perimenopausal physician colleagues recently went on a trip with one of her grown children, who is in medical school. They went to a stimulating medical meeting and then explored the Grand Canyon together. Though she paid no attention to her diet and ate whatever she wanted, she arrived home six pounds lighter! She told me, "I think that my cortisol levels returned to normal because for ten days I got to sleep through the night and not worry about being called in for an emergency. And besides that, my serotonin was up from all the exciting conversation and healthy sunshine I was getting!"

Step Four: Exercise

If you don't already exercise, there is no time like the present to start. Your muscles are loaded with insulin receptors. The more muscle mass you have and the more heat you generate from your muscles on a regular basis, the more efficiently you'll burn carbohydrates and body fat. You'll also be protecting your bones and your heart. In fact, of all the lifestyle changes that best predict permanent weight loss, regular exercise is number one. I recommend at least thirty minutes of sustained exercise at least five times per week.

If you already exercise, change your routine. Perhaps you've found yourself, like me, stuck at a metabolic roadblock, even though you've already changed your diet and are exercising regularly. When this happens, it is usually because your body has adjusted to your current level of activity—just as it's possible to maintain your weight on as little as 1,000 calories per day—the body's metabolic rate simply decreases to accommodate its perception of starvation.

In order to get your stubborn fat cells to release their load, you have to confuse them a little. Try a different exercise routine that recruits other muscles. If you've been walking, try a stair-stepper, an elliptical trainer, weight training, or a cross-country ski machine. The idea is to get your body out of its metabolic rut.

I personally had to increase the intensity and length of my weight-training sessions while cutting back on my walking—something that had become so easy I barely even broke a sweat. The weight workouts were much harder. Over time this switch worked.

Step Five: Get Your Thyroid Checked

About 25 percent of women develop or have preexisting thyroid problems by the time they reach perimenopause. Excess levels of estrogen relative to progesterone can lower thyroid function and so can excess stress-hormone levels. These conditions are very common during perimenopause. Low thyroid function is associated with a decreased metabolic rate. If you have any symptoms of thyroid problems (fatigue, weight gain, cold hands and feet, thinning hair, or constipation), get your thyroid checked. I finally did this during my own metabolic slowdown and found out that my thyroid hormone levels were consistent with what is known as subclinical hypothyroidism, which is characterized by normal thyroid hormone levels in the blood but a slightly elevated level of TSH (thyroid-stimulating hormone). I had no symptoms other than the weight gain. I started on a very low dose of thyroid hormones—levothyroxine (T_4) and tri-iodothyronine (T_3)—which I used for about two years, after which things returned to normal. (Though most doctors prescribe only levothyroxine, many women do better on a combination of T_3 and T_4, which is available through formulary pharmacies.) It's difficult to say whether the thyroid hormone replacement is what finally turned my weight gain around, because I also changed my exercise routine and cut down on all refined carbohydrates. In addition, the stress I was under decreased dramatically when the holidays ended and my friend recovered fully. I was eventually able to get off the thyroid replacement altogether.

Step Six: Quell Cellular Inflammation

The number-one reason for cellular inflammation—and all the diseases and symptoms associated with it—is a refined food, high-glycemic diet, which has the following characteristics.

~ Too many refined carbohydrates, resulting in the overproduction of insulin. Too much insulin favors the production of the pro-inflammatory substances, like prostaglandin F2-alpha and the cytokines.

~ Deficiencies in the polyunsaturated fats known as omega-3 fats. Omega-3 fats are necessary for the function of nearly every cell in the body, particularly those of the nervous system, brain, eyes, and immune system. Omega-3 fats also decrease cellular inflammation. Currently levels of the especially important omega-3 fat DHA (docosahexænoic acid) are 40 percent lower, on average, in American women than in European women.

~ Too many trans fats, usually from margarine and shortening, which increase cellular inflammation. (See page 222.)

~ Deficiencies in the micronutrients that are necessary for combating cellular inflammation. Too little vitamin C, vitamin B_6, and magnesium, for example, favor the overproduction of pro-inflammatory substances.

Unremitting stress is also a factor in cellular inflammation. It results in the overproduction of epinephrine and cortisol, stress hormones that promote cellular inflammation. Caffeine, which is often used to alleviate the effects of stress and fatigue, has the same effect. When you follow the hormone-balancing food plan below, supplement your diet with additional antioxidant nutrients (see page 226), and consciously decrease stress through meditation, relaxation, and regular exercise, you will be well on your way to quelling cellular inflammation.

THE HORMONE-BALANCING FOOD PLAN

Given the average lifestyle of today's perimenopausal women, it's not difficult to see why insulin and estrogen become unbalanced, putting us at increased risk for everything from heart disease and high blood pressure to arthritis and breast cancer. Fortunately, when you follow the food plan I suggest here, you won't have to wait long to feel better. In a matter of days, you'll probably notice that your sleep improves, you begin to lose excess fat, various troublesome symptoms begin to disappear, and your skin takes on a healthy glow. At the same time you'll be reducing your risk for the diseases of aging.

Eat at Least Three Meals a Day

Many women skip both breakfast and lunch, saving up their calories until dinner. The problem with this approach is that the metabolic rate naturally peaks at noon and decreases after that. So the food you eat at night is far more likely to be stored as excess fat compared to the food eaten earlier in the day. Here's another reason why you can't afford to skip meals for weight control: it is well known that yo-yo dieting and periodic starvation lower your overall metabolic rate over time, resulting in a body that is so metabolically efficient that it is possible to remain at the same weight despite a very low calorie diet. That's why, when I faced my own midlife weight gain, severe calorie restriction was not an option. I had starved myself too many times in my teens and twenties, including fasting. I've always had a relatively slow metabolic rate, and now midlife was lowering it further. I couldn't risk another slowdown. It is also clear that severe food restriction often results in a decrease in beneficial lean body mass but not necessarily a decrease in body fat. That means that after severe food restriction, you might end up with a higher percentage of body fat than when you started.

Most perimenopausal women do best when they keep their blood sugar stable throughout the day by eating frequent, smaller meals. I highly recommend a snack at around four in the afternoon, right during the time when blood sugar, mood, and serotonin tend to plummet. This snack can keep you from overeating at night when you get home. (If you don't, you're apt to begin your evening meal the minute you get home and then end it when you go to bed, in a desperate attempt to make up for a full day's worth of deprivation.)

To successfully negotiate the metabolic challenges of midlife, you need to be patient. And you also need to rethink your "diet" mentality. In other words, you need to think of your new metabolism as something that will require a new way of living and eating, not another quick-fix diet. (I certainly learned that when I tried the Atkins induction program.)

Focus on Portion Size, Not Calories

Instead of calorie counting, concentrate on eating the highest-quality food available, in smaller portions. Cup your two hands in front of you. That's how big your stomach capacity is. Limit your intake to no more than that at each meal or snack. Overeating in general—regardless of the food—is associated with overproduction of insulin. In general, the food portions in U.S. restaurants are much bigger than in Europe, which is one of the reasons Americans are so overweight compared to Europeans. (That is changing, however, and obesity has become a global problem!) At one local restaurant, for example, the chicken dish I usually order comes with two halves of a chicken breast. I always eat just one and take the other one home with me for another meal.

In order to keep my weight stable, I've had to cut down on my total food intake, eliminate grain products most of the time (see below), reduce my consumption of desserts to no more than once per week, make lunch the biggest meal of my day, eat very lightly at dinner, and increase my exercise time.

Eat Protein at Each Meal

That means eggs, fish, lean meat, dairy food, or a vegetarian alternative to animal protein, such as soy protein powder, whey protein powder, whole soybeans, tofu, or tempeh. Beans contain protein, but they also contain a considerable amount of carbohydrate. Though the carbohydrate in beans tends to be on the low end of the glycemic index, beans can be too high in carbohydrate for some peri-menopausal women. They work very well for others. You have to judge this for yourself.

Protein needs vary depending upon your size and physical activity. The bigger and the more active you are, the more you need. In general, if you have any tendency toward weight gain at midlife, your diet should be about 40 percent protein, 35 percent low-glycemic-index carbs, and 25 percent fat. You don't have to adhere to this rigidly at every meal and snack, but it's an average to shoot for over about a week's time.[19]

If you are at risk for any condition, including cancer, stimulated by excess estrogen, you might want to increase your protein even more. Protein can actually decrease your risk. Here's how it works: When the liver, body fat, and ovaries metabolize estrogen, they use an enzyme system known as cytochrome P450. A diet rich in protein increases the activity of the entire P450 system, thus helping to protect your body from overstimulation by estrogen. In one study, for example, individuals who were fed a diet that contained 44 percent protein, 35 percent carbohydrates, and 21 percent fat experienced a profound shift in their body's ability to deactivate excess estrogen.[20]

Cut Down on Refined and High-Glycemic-Index Carbohydrates, Including Alcohol

Remember, not all carbohydrates are created equal. One gram of carbohydrate from table sugar has a different metabolic effect than the same amount of carbohydrate from blueberries.

Keep your blood sugar stable and you'll experience:

~ More energy

~ Ability to sustain exercise

~ Clearing of brain fog

~ Ability to build muscle

~ Less hunger—ability to control portion sizes *and* cravings

~ Fewer PMS symptoms

~ Fewer hot flashes

~ Better-looking skin

~ Clear eyes without puffiness or dark circles

~ Deeper, more restful sleep

~ Stable moods and more optimism

Your success will be contingent on eating foods with a low glycemic index. The glycemic index was created to measure how much
the blood sugar rises after you eat a carbohydrate meal, using white
bread as the benchmark. White bread has a glycemic index of 100,
whereas the glycemic index of corn is 54, an apple is 38, and an avo-
cado is 0. The rule of thumb is white and processed foods have a very
high glycemic index, whereas whole foods and those high in protein
typically have a low glycemic index.

Eliminate as many refined carbohydrates from your diet as possible. That means cutting out white rice and pasta and other foods
made with white flour, such as muffins, rolls, bagels, biscuits, French
bread, bread sticks, crackers, snack foods, and pretzels. (*Note:* When
you plan to indulge, know that white rice is better than pasta because
it raises insulin much more slowly.) You also need to eliminate soda
pop, which is nothing but sugar water. An occasional diet soda is
okay if you're not sensitive to aspartame. (See chapter 10.)

It also means eliminating or cutting way back on alcohol in every
and any form, including wine coolers, wine, beer, and hard liquor.
Alcohol is nothing but sugar in a form that is so absorbable that its
effects are felt within minutes in the brain. One of the first things
women notice when they eliminate the empty calories found in alcohol is that they lose weight very quickly. Many also notice that their
hot flashes go away as well. That's because alcohol significantly interferes with estrogen metabolism and causes an almost immediate hormonal imbalance, with too much estrogen in the blood relative to
progesterone.

You also need to eliminate or cut way back on sweets: candy,
cookies, cakes, pastries, and ice cream. You may still want to have
them on special occasions, but as your blood sugar stabilizes, you'll
find that your craving for these foods will decrease dramatically and
you won't like the way you feel after eating them.

Remember, your body will be able to burn stored fat and keep
your insulin and blood sugar levels normal only when you don't eat
or drink excessive amounts of the wrong kinds of carbohydrates.
Otherwise excess blood sugar will be stored as fat, which will accumulate not just on your belly and hips but also in other places, like
your arteries and in your heart and brain.

IF YOU ARE A TRUE CARBOHYDRATE ADDICT

Women who grew up in alcoholic or chaotic family systems may have brain and body chemistry that is overly sensitive to the effects of food, and particularly to the neurochemical known as serotonin. Serotonin is released in the brain quite rapidly when you eat refined-carbohydrate-rich foods, such as most breakfast cereals or cookies. True carbohydrate addicts cannot stop after eating a few cookies or potato chips. They don't seem to have a normal satiety mechanism in place, most likely because food is being used as a drug to soothe emotional pain. If this describes you, I recommend consulting one of the following books:

> *Potatoes, Not Prozac* (Simon & Schuster, 1999), by Kathleen DesMaisons
>
> *The Sugar Addict's Total Recovery Program* (Ballantine, 2000), by Kathleen DesMaisons
>
> *Holy Hunger: A Memoir of Desire* (A.A. Knopf, 1999), by Margaret Bullitt-Jonas

Consume Grain Products with Caution

Even if you have eliminated refined grains in all forms, you can still get into trouble with whole wheat, whole rye, whole oat, or millet flour. A fascinating line of research now suggests that the degenerative diseases that currently plague the human race didn't arrive on the scene until agriculture became widespread. Paleoarcheological studies show that many of the ancient Egyptians were fat and had dental caries—diseases associated with a grain-based diet and virtually absent in hunter-gatherers.

Many carbohydrate-sensitive individuals find that eating grain products triggers binge eating. I've certainly seen this happen with brown rice—a "health food" that I used to consume regularly but have had to virtually eliminate. I've also had to eliminate nearly all whole-grain bread products, even the unleavened ones. (One line of thinking suggests that yeast bread is difficult to digest because of the potential for yeast overgrowth in the intestines. Unleavened bread is better tolerated by many, but not everyone. Even a whole-wheat un-leavened tortilla wrap sandwich at lunch tends to make me feel groggy and bloated.) Looking back, I can see that eating too much bread has been a problem with me for years. But at perimenopause, my body finally said, "Enough!"

Eat a Wide Variety of Fresh Fruits and Vegetables Daily

You want to shoot for at least five servings a day, but it's easy, at least in the summer, to get in more. Remember that a serving is small, as little as 4 ounces or ½ cup in many cases. The healthiest fruits and vegetables are the ones that are the most colorful. That's because the pigments in these foods, such as the carotenes or carotenoids, are very powerful antioxidants. Go for broccoli; red, yellow, and green peppers; dark green leafy vegetables such as collards, kale, and spinach; and tomatoes. Pigment-rich blueberries have been found to have the highest concentration of antioxidants compared to forty other fruits and vegetables.

Studies suggest that the carotenoid content of tissue may be the most significant factor in determining life span in primates, including humans.[21] Though beta-carotene (the vitamin A precursor found in carrots, other yellow-orange vegetables, and dark leafy greens) has received the most attention and is the carotenoid most commonly found in multivitamins, other carotenes that have little or no vitamin A–type activity exert much greater antioxidant protection. Alpha-carotene (usually found in the same foods as beta-carotene) is ap-proximately 38 percent stronger as an antioxidant and ten times more effective in suppressing liver, skin, and lung cancer in animals.[22] Even more powerful is lycopene, the red pigment found in tomatoes. Some studies have shown a 50 percent reduction for all cancers among elderly Americans reporting a high tomato intake.[23] Food pro-cessing doesn't destroy lycopene, so tomato juice and canned tomato products also offer protection.

Every day the list of benefits from the natural antioxidants found in pigment-rich foods grows. They help balance hormones, protect the skin from sun damage, keep the skin and eyes radiant, maintain the lining of the blood vessels, and help prevent varicose veins. They also boost the immune system and help the body resist cancer and other degenerative diseases.

In addition to being good sources of cholesterol-lowering fiber, fruits and vegetables are also good sources of lignans, which are metabolized into phytohormones that help balance hormones and metabolize excess estrogen. Flaxseed is by far the richest source of lignans and is also very rich in essential omega-3 fats (see pages 221–222).

High-glycemic-index fruits and vegetables such as potatoes, corn, and bananas have a lot of nutrients in them, though their antioxidant content isn't as rich as that of the foods I've mentioned previously. You don't have to eliminate them completely. Just remember that the more processed they are, the higher their glycemic index. A baked potato is an entirely different food from a potato chip or french fry, and it is far healthier. And fresh corn on the cob in season is a better choice than canned creamed corn, which is often processed with added sugar in the form of corn syrup. Though fresh vegetables are always the best choice, research has shown that even canned and frozen varieties still contain many nutrients.

HOW TO QUELL YOUR SUGAR CRAVINGS

While you're changing to a diet that is lower in sugar, you can help balance your brain biochemistry and quell your sweet cravings simultaneously by taking the amino acid L-glutamine, which appears to help prevent the mental fatigue that can result from sugar withdrawal. (Take 1 g per day with lunch.) Some research also suggests that L-glutamine helps alcoholics avoid alcohol—the ultimate sugar buzz.[24]

Artificially sweetened products may also help with sugar cravings for some women. For others, they can make the problem worse. The sweetener I like best is stevia. Stevia is a natural sweetener made from an extract of the leaves of the South American plant *Stevia rebaudiana*. It is usually sold in health food stores as either a liquid or powdered leaves, and it tastes bitter if you use too much. (I use it to sweeten the cranberry sauce every Thanksgiving and no one has noticed yet.) Stevia is also stable in liquid or when heated. Though I feel that some other artificial sweeteners are quite safe, they have not yet stood the test of time. It's probably best to use them sparingly.

Some women find that using artificial sweeteners results in an increase in food binges. I haven't found this to be true for me. Though some authorities suggest we should eliminate all artificial sweeteners, I'm not ready to do that and may never be. In any case, I know they're far healthier than the cookies and other desserts I used to consume regularly.

Eat Healthy Fats Each Day

Back in the 1980s and early 1990s, when the low-fat craze reached its peak, I watched patient after patient come in complaining of sallow skin, brittle fingernails, weight gain, difficulty fighting infections, inability to concentrate, and fatigue. None of these women was getting enough healthy fat in their diets, having been brainwashed into thinking that all fat was the enemy. Now we know differently.

Essential fatty acids (EFAs) are indispensable for human development and health. Our bodies cannot synthesize EFAs, so we need to consume them in our foods. There are two essential types of EFAs: omega-6 fats and omega-3 fats. Omega-6 fats occur in relative

WHAT SHOULD I DRINK?

The answer is water, pure and simple. Too many women avoid water in the mistaken belief that they will put on weight if they drink too much. Then they end up dehydrated, and it shows in their skin. In fact, you need lots of water to help your body eliminate the breakdown products of fat if you are trying to lose weight.

If you can't stand the regular flat kind, go with designer waters with lime or another flavor. Iced tea is another healthy choice. I keep a pitcher of decaffeinated green tea in the refrigerator at all times. It's loaded with antioxidants, and it contains phytohormones that have been shown to build bone. You can also drink diluted fruit juice occasionally (watch the carbs—it's easy to drink too many). It's nice mixed half and half with sparkling water and is a good alternative to a cocktail. An occasional diet soda won't hurt unless you are sensitive to aspartame.

abundance in the foods we eat. However, the current American diet is woefully deficient in omega-3 fats. This is partially a result of our food choices, with trans fats and refined carbohydrates often displacing omega-3 fats. In addition, because of agricultural practices, the fats in eggs and meat do not contain nearly the percentage of omega-3 fats that they used to. Farm animals raised on wild grasses instead of grain have a healthier, leaner body composition. Animals, like humans, get fat on diets composed mostly of grain, especially if they aren't allowed to roam.

Omega-3 deficiency often begins in utero, when our only source of these fats is our mothers, who are likely to be deficient in them already. Ideally, the omega-3 fats, particularly a fat known as DHA, are found abundantly in human breast milk, but DHA is absent in the baby formulas used in the United States and Canada. Research is rapidly accumulating that implicates DHA deficiency in the epidemic of attention deficit disorder in both children and adults. This essential fat is also one of the reasons why children who were breast-fed as infants have been found to have higher IQs than formula-fed babies.[25] Gratifying improvements in learning ability and mood stabilization have resulted when both children and adults have had their diets supplemented with omega-3 fats.

In addition to their role in nervous system and brain function, omega-3 fats also favor the production of substances known as series 1 and 3 eicosanoids that help block the effects of cellular inflammation. It's not surprising, then, that supplementing the diet with omega-3 fats in either foods or pills has been shown to alleviate conditions associated with eicosanoid imbalance, including arthritis, PMS, eczema, breast tenderness, acne, diabetes, brittle fingernails, thinning and brittle hair, psoriasis, dry skin, and the sex hormone imbalance so common during perimenopause.

Good sources of omega-3 fats include pumpkin seeds, sunflower seeds, flaxseed or flaxseed oil, hempseed or hempseed oil, organ meats, cold-water fish or fish oil supplements, and docosahexænoic acid (DHA) supplements. Nuts are also a good source, and they make a very satisfying low-carb snack—I take them to the movies in lieu of high-carb popcorn. Just make sure you enjoy them in moderation— no more than a handful once or twice per day.

Trans Fats: The Bad Actors of the Fat World
The most dangerous fats by far are the trans fats—the partially hydrogenated fats and oils that aren't found anywhere in nature.

They are present in shortening and margarine, which are made by blowing hydrogen into liquid vegetable oil at very high temperatures and pressures. Trans fats contribute directly to the overproduction of pro-inflammatory eicosanoids and have therefore been found to contribute to the development of cancer and heart disease.

Unfortunately, trans fats are added to just about every type of packaged baked good because they don't get rancid nearly as quickly as unprocessed fats. This prolongs the shelf life of the product. Since such products are also invariably high in refined carbs, it's best to simply eliminate them from your life. (If you have them once in a while, pray over them first.) The good news is that food manufacturers must now add information about trans fat content to labels.

Saturated Fat: An Overrated Threat

Saturated fat is not the culprit we've made it out to be as far as heart disease is concerned. If you're following a diet that keeps your insulin and blood sugar levels normal, then saturated fat isn't likely to become a problem. After all, the epidemic of heart disease didn't start in this country until margarine and shortening—which are trans fats, not saturated fats—were added to the diet back in the 1940s. Before that, lard and butter were widely used, and heart disease was rare. Some women, however, are sensitive to the arachidonic acid found in dairy foods, eggs, and beef, which contributes to cellular inflammation, and in turn to menstrual cramps and arthritis. The symptoms go away when they eliminate these foods. Other women have no problem. As with all things, I'd suggest that you enjoy saturated fat in moderation.

You don't have to count fat grams if you are keeping your carb level relatively low. In the absence of excess insulin, it appears that fat in your diet is not stored as fat. But the minute that fat is combined with sugar or starch—as in a doughnut, for example—the pounds pack on.

Cooking and Salad Oils

Most salad and cooking oils contain omega-6 fats, and since an excess of omega-6 fats can lead to the overproduction of pro-inflammatory chemicals in cells, I suggest that you limit their use. Substitute flaxseed oil or olive oil whenever possible. (Olive oil is a monounsaturated omega-9 fat with metabolic effects that are neutral when it comes to eicosanoid balance.) You can also use a little clarified butter—also known as ghee—for cooking, since it won't burn.

My favorite salad dressing is made by mixing a little balsamic vinegar with some high-quality olive oil. For variety, try light sesame or nut oils.

EDUCATE YOURSELF

All of the following books contain meal plans and recipes that have helped thousands of women lose or maintain their weight. All of them will help balance hormones as well as insulin and will help decrease cellular inflammation. I recommend that you go to a library or your local bookstore and look through a few of them. Then choose the one that speaks to you.

The Midlife Miracle Diet (Viking, 2003), by Adele Puhn

Healthy for Life: Developing Healthy Lifestyles That Have a Side Effect of Permanent Fat Loss (Real Life Press, 2005), by Ray Strand

Schwarzbein Principle Cookbook (Health Communications, 1999), by Diana Schwarzbein, Nancy Deville, and Evelyn Jacob Jaffe

Recipes for Change: Gourmet Wholefood Cooking for Health and Vitality at Menopause (Dutton, 1996), by Lissa DeAngelis and Molly Siple

The No-Grain Diet (Dutton, 2003), by Joseph Mercola with Alison Rose Levy

The Glucose Revolution: The Authoritative Guide to the Glycemic Index (Marlowe and Co., 1999), by Jennie Brand-Miller, Thomas Wolever, Stephen Colagiuri, and Kaye Foster-Powell

Eating Well for Optimum Health: The Essential Guide to Food, Diet, and Nutrition (Knopf, 2000), by Andrew Weil

Fat Flush Plan (McGraw-Hill, 2002), by Anne Louise Gittleman

The RESET Program

For a quick but scientifically sound program that will help you get off the sugar roller coaster, I recommend the RESET program by USANA. This five-day, high-fiber cleanse is designed to decrease tissue inflammation, eliminate glycemic stress and reset your metabolism. I've personally found it to be very effective and so have thousands of others.

Here's how the program works: You drink three shakes a day at mealtimes, eat a nutrition bar for a mid-morning and a mid-afternoon snack, and you eat one serving of fruit and one serving of vegetables anytime during the day. (All the low-glycemic shakes and nutrition bars you need for the five-day plan are included in the RESET kit, as are enough high-potency vitamins for the five days of the program—the same vitamins I take as part of my daily regimen.) You also need to drink eight to ten glasses of water daily, in addition to getting moderate exercise (such as walking for 20–30 minutes or following the routine on the 30-minute exercise video included with the program). Although some women experience tolerable hunger, most don't feel hungry or have food cravings because the shakes and bars provide the perfect balance of high-quality proteins, fats, and low-glycemic carbs to keep blood sugar levels stable. The fat you eat on this or any other low-glycemic food plan will not be stored in the body as fat—unless your body is overproducing insulin because of the effects of stress or an excess of food.[26] The average weight loss for the five-day period is five pounds, mostly from losing the excess fluid so common in people with high insulin levels; even better, this weight loss tends to be most noticeable in the abdominal area, where insulin-resistant women commonly gain the most fat! Many women also find the program gives them more energy than usual. (For more information, visit www.usana.com.)

After the initial five days, if you decide to continue the plan to lose more weight, USANA recommends that you keep using the meal-replacement shakes and bars for two meals and two snacks a day, having one low-glycemic meal and snack on your own. Once you reach your weight-loss goal, use the

shakes and bars for one meal each day as a maintenance program. (Revival soy shakes and bars are another excellent
source of low-glycemic meal replacement products that I also
use myself and recommend highly. For more information,
visit www.revivalsoy.com.)

Ray Strand, M.D., has created a twelve-week, online program called Healthy for Life for those who would like further
support (including individualized guidance) in reversing
glycemic stress and insulin resistance and starting to release
body fat. In one trial of this program, participants lost an average of 15.2 pounds, decreased their cholesterol by an average of 9.8 percent (dropping their level by 60 or 80 and some
even by 100 points!), and decreased their systolic blood pressure by an average of 12 points and their diastolic reading by
an average of 6 points. More importantly, they reported feeling great and having no hunger. (For more information, visit
Dr. Strand's website at www.releasingfat.com.)[27]

Protect Yourself with Antioxidants

Every day, more and more research is showing the benefits of vitamins and minerals, especially those known as antioxidants. Antioxidants combat cellular damage from free radicals, which is one of
the key underlying mechanisms leading to chronic conditions such as
heart disease, cataracts, macular degeneration, and many cancers.

Free radicals are highly reactive unstable molecules that have lost
one electron and are aggressively seeking a replacement—a process
that, in your body, results in damage to everything from your DNA
to the collagen layer of your skin. You can't escape from free radicals
completely, because they are a by-product of normal metabolism.
They are formed in our bodies when, for instance, molecules of fat
react with oxygen in a process similar to the one that turns fat rancid
or makes iron rust. But free radicals are also formed by exposure to
ozone, tobacco smoke, car exhaust, chemicals outgassed from new
carpet, and other pollutants. Exposure to radiation, insecticides, and
excessive amounts of sunlight can also lead to the formation of free
radicals. Free-radical damage results in cellular inflammation and the
release of too many of the "bad" eicosanoids that appear to be involved in virtually every disease process known.

The body was designed to fight off free-radical damage in the same way that your immune system is designed to fight viruses and bacteria. One mechanism that your body uses to fight free-radical damage is to repair the damage once it's done. Another mechanism is to "scavenge" the free radicals before they cause harm: to supply the extra electron they need before they can grab it from vulnerable tissue. This is what antioxidants do.

Antioxidants are found abundantly in fresh fruits and vegetables, especially the brightly colored ones. The amount of antioxidant in a given fruit, vegetable, grain, or protein source depends upon the soil in which it is grown or on which its food source is grown. Organically grown fruits and vegetables that are picked and eaten when ripe have the highest amounts of antioxidants and minerals in them.

Food is the best source for our antioxidants. They seem to work synergistically—that is, they're more powerful in balance with one another and with other nutrients as they occur naturally. However, if you don't manage to consume five servings of fruits and vegetables a day, supplements can still provide significant protection.

PERIMENOPAUSE SUPPLEMENT PROGRAM

Over the years I've seen hundreds of patients who have been helped by a good supplement program such as the one below.

Following this program means that you'll have to give up the idea of getting everything you need in one tablet. You'll probably end up taking ten or more capsules or tablets per day. Think of them as food, not medicine.

Antioxidants

Vitamin C	1,000–5,000 mg
Vitamin D_3	800–5,000 IU
Vitamin A (as beta-carotene)	25,000 IU
Vitamin E (as mixed tocopherols)	400–800 IU
Glutathione	2–10 mg
Alpha-lipoic acid	10–100 mg
Coenzyme Q_{10}	10–100 mg

Omega-3 Fat

DHA   200–2,500 mg
EPA   500–2,500 mg
                                   (total of 1,000–
                                   5,000 mg)

B Complex Vitamins

Thiamine (B_1)   8–100 mg
Riboflavin (B_2)   9–50 mg
Niacin (B_3)   20–100 mg
Pantothenic acid (B_5)   15–400 mg
Pyridoxine (B_6)   10–100 mg
Cobalamin (B_{12})   20–250 mcg
Folic acid   400–800 mcg
Biotin   400–500 mcg
Inositol   10–500 mg
Choline   10–100 mg

Minerals

Calcium   500–1,200 mg
                                   (amount depends
                                   on calcium
                                   content of diet)
Magnesium   400–1,000 mg
Potassium   200–500 mg
Zinc   6–50 mg
Manganese   1–15 mg
Boron   2–9 mg
Copper   1–2 mg
Iron   15–30 mg
Chromium   100–400 mcg
Selenium   50–200 mcg
Molybdenum   10–20 mcg
Vanadium   50–100 mcg
Trace minerals—usually from marine mineral complex

OPTIMIZING MIDLIFE DIGESTION

Digestive problems, especially in the form of bloating and gas, are very common in women. Sometimes they begin at midlife and sometimes they develop only later, when you are in your sixties or seventies. I recently talked with one of my mentors from childhood, a woman who at the age of ninety still teaches yoga at a nursing home. Two of her biggest problems are constipation and heartburn, but she is otherwise doing well.

Being a Gut Reactor: Digestion and Your Third Emotional Center

One of the first things you need to do in order to heal your digestive problems at midlife is to shore up your third emotional center. The third emotional center is located in the solar plexus area, and the health of this area affects all our organs of digestion, including the stomach, liver, gallbladder, pancreas, small intestine, and upper large intestine. Women with substantial weight problems usually have unresolved issues in the third emotional center.

The health of the third emotional center depends on a balance between responsibility to ourselves and responsibility to others, and also on our sense of self-esteem. It is adversely affected whenever we feel overly responsible for the welfare of others or when we avoid taking responsibility altogether. Gloria, a patient I've followed for years, illustrates the conflicts in the third emotional center very well. Gloria is the oldest of four children. Her mother always told her that she was responsible for her siblings because she was the oldest and should "know better." Whenever any of her siblings was injured or got into trouble, she was blamed. As a result of having this responsibility placed on her at a relatively early age, Gloria developed a very acute "gut feeling" about when things were about to go wrong. This ability has served her well in her job as an executive assistant at a large hospital. Nevertheless, she still suffers from digestive upsets whenever there are conflicts at work—conflicts for which she always feels responsible. She once told me that she always seems to be caught in the middle between her boss and a coworker, and this conflict quite literally goes into the middle of her body. It is not surprising that Gloria has problems with her weight and her blood sugar, and that she tends to overeat whenever she feels bad about herself for not doing enough at work. In fact, she does far more than most, but she still feels as though she hasn't done enough.

At midlife our job is to learn how to take care of ourselves instead of everybody else. If we don't learn how to do this, we soon learn that no one will do this for us. But as we begin to go about learning this important skill, we often find ourselves feeling guilty. Who will do everything around the house or the office if we don't? This feeling of guilt hits us right in our solar plexus, which is also the body center associated with self-esteem and personal power.

Self-esteem comes from feeling good about ourselves in the world. It is effectively created by developing skills in the outer world of work—one of the reasons why so many midlife women heal their lives and their digestion when they go back to college and get the degree they didn't finish after high school. Our third emotional center is also related to how good we feel about our relationships, our bodies, our homes, and our lives in general. Sometimes a lifetime of weight and self-esteem problems are solved at midlife as we finally learn the self-acceptance and self-celebration that is part of self-esteem.

WHAT TO DO ABOUT BLOATING

During perimenopause there is a shift toward fat-accumulating hormones (cortisol and insulin) and away from fat-mobilizing hormones (estrogen and growth hormone). If your body is under stress of any kind, this shift will worsen. In addition, your abdominal fat cells have more cortisol receptors on them at midlife, so fat is preferentially directed toward them. This often results in fluid retention and bloating.[28] Try the following to reduce bloating.

~ *Decrease consumption of high- to moderate-glycemic-index carbohydrates.* Yet another symptom of cellular inflammation and too much insulin is excess stomach acid. A diet lower in carbohydrates and higher in fat and protein very often results in complete and fast relief of heartburn and indigestion.

~ *Eat three to five small meals per day.* Consuming large quantities of food elevates insulin levels and makes bloating worse—even when the foods are healthy.

~ *Include some protein, healthy fat, and low-glycemic-index carbohydrates in every meal or snack.* However, fruit is best eaten alone. Consuming it with fat causes bloating and indigestion in many women.

~ *Eliminate all breads and baked goods for at least a week.* See if this makes a difference. Many women are sensitive to gluten.

~ *Drink plenty of water.* It helps the body rid itself of toxins.

~ *Leave at least three hours between your last meal and bedtime.* Going to bed on a full stomach can cause acid reflux.

~ *Stop or cut way back on alcohol.* Alcohol is a gastric irritant.

~ *Use enteric-coated peppermint.* This supplement can be very soothing for digestion problems. Take 2–3 capsules between meals. If rectal burning occurs, reduce the dose.

~ *Take digestive enzymes.* Digestive enzymes are naturally occurring catalysts that help the body process sugars, starches, proteins, and fats. Taking the proper enzymes can dramatically improve bloating and gas as well as a host of other health problems stemming from faulty digestion. Look for a ph-balanced full spectrum formula such as Wobenzym (www.wobenzym.com). For more information on this important topic, read *MicroMiracles* (Rodale, 2005) by Ellen Cutler, D.C., an authority on digestive enzymes, or visit Dr. Cutler's website at www.bioset.net.

MELBA: Stress and Antacids

Melba was forty-two and perimenopausal when she first came to see me. She had worked for ten years at the registry of motor vehicles. Every morning she had to face lines and lines of disgruntled drivers awaiting renewal of their licenses, getting new license plates, and the like. After several months of working in this job, Melba began to feel abdominal pain, bloating, and indigestion. After a routine check at her doctor's office, she was told to "reduce stress" and eat a high-carbohydrate, low-fat diet. Her problem became worse, but a coworker introduced her to the world of antacids. Soon she would not travel without a few rolls of Tums in her purse. At first she noticed immediate relief upon taking antacids, but then after a while she began to take them earlier and earlier in the day, until she was popping antacids from nine until five, when she left her job. Over time, however, she noticed that she began to feel weak and tired, and she lost her appetite. In addition, her bowel movements became all messed up. When she first came to see me for a routine annual GYN checkup, I suspected that some of her problems were related to both her diet and her excessive use of antacids. Within a week of eliminating refined carbohydrates and grain products, and also learning some stress-reduction skills, Melba was able to cut way back on her antacid use. Some days she didn't need them at all.

Avoiding Antacid Addiction

Many women are addicted to antacids and acid medications such as ranitidine (Zantac) or the popular proton pump inhibitors such as Prilosec, Nexium, and Prevacid. Antacids have been known for many decades to be useful for indigestion, and even in the treatment of gastroesophageal reflux and ulcers. There are several types of antacids, but all of them work by either blocking the production or function of stomach acid. Conventional over-the-counter antacids such as Tums and Rolaids contain either aluminum hydroxide or magnesium hydroxide. Neither of them is without side effects. Aluminum hydroxide neutralizes stomach acid but tends to produce constipation. Prolonged and regular use may reduce the body's phosphate levels, with resultant fatigue and loss of appetite. In addition to this, the jury is still out about whether aluminum consumption contributes to Alzheimer's disease, so it's best to avoid it whenever possible. Magnesium hydroxide, on the other hand, produces loose stools or diarrhea in some individuals. Although some antacids combine both aluminum and magnesium, there may still be side effects.

Other antacids, such as Tums, have calcium carbonate as their main ingredient. (Tums is also being heavily marketed to women as a way to prevent osteoporosis.) Though these can help with indigestion, over time they cause acid rebound, a condition in which the excess calcium actually stimulates increased acid secretion. In addition, chronic excessive calcium carbonate intake is associated with a pattern of abnormal blood chemistry known as milk alkali syndrome, producing elevations of blood calcium, phosphate, bicarbonate, and other abnormalities. Over time, kidney stones and even progressive kidney disease may result.[29] The irony is that while many people believe that indigestion and heartburn are due to excessive stomach acid, which is why they are led to take antacids in the first place, chronic indigestion results, in part, not from excessive stomach acid, but from *deficient* stomach acid. It's no wonder that the most common side effect of the heavily promoted proton pump inhibitors is diarrhea and nausea—classic signs of digestive problems! And if stomach acid is chronically deficient, it can lead to nutritional deficiencies of vitamins such as B_{12}, which can set the stage for both chronic anemia and dementia over time.

If you have an imbalance of protein and carbohydrate in your diet, with refined carbohydrates predominating, this diet may be promoting a decrease in the production of gastric acid and overproduction of inflammatory substances, which may be (1) suppressing your immune system, (2) increasing inflammation in the stomach lining, and (3) increasing stomach discomfort and other pain. Since it is well documented that high blood sugar results in a decrease in gastric acid secretion, it's not surprising that refined carbohydrates are a setup for indigestion. Hundreds of individuals who switch to a low-glycemic diet have noted a complete disappearance of gastritis, reflux, and indigestion. I have personally experienced this myself since changing my diet. I used to have to take Tums or Di-Gel after dinner sometimes, and I never connected it with the bread I was eating until my problem disappeared along with the bread and rice (and cookies, I might add). This diet has been shown to improve the quality of the protective mucus in the stomach lining and also to normalize muscular control, preventing reflux and spasm.

If you find yourself popping antacids regularly, here's what I'd suggest.

~ GET OFF THE ANTACID MERRY-GO-ROUND. If you need to take one, use one without aluminum. And use it for as short a time as possible.

~ TAKE YOUR ANTIOXIDANTS. Low levels of vitamin C, vitamin E, and other antioxidant factors in gastric juice have been shown to encourage the growth of *Helicobacter pylori,* a bacterium whose overgrowth is associated with ulcers. Higher antioxidant intake may prevent these bacteria from growing and also improve the healing of the stomach and intestinal lining.

~ TRY DEGLYCYRRHIZINATED LICORICE (DGL). DGL may also help reduce *H. pylori* and stimulate the body's natural internal defenses. Unlike antacids, DGL does not reduce acid in the stomach.

DGL improves both the quality and quantity of protective substances that line the intestinal tract, increases the life span of intestinal cells, and improves the blood supply to the intestinal lining.[30]
DGL is available in most natural food stores.

~ TAKE THE RIGHT CALCIUM SUPPLEMENT. Though the calcium in
Tums is better than no calcium at all, you're much better off taking
a calcium supplement that also contains magnesium and vitamin
D, which help the body efficiently utilize calcium.

~ TRY SEACURE. SeaCure is a polypeptide supplement made from
predigested whitefish; it appears to nourish the bowel well directly
during the absorption process. It can be very easily absorbed by
anyone who can take food by mouth, no matter how ill they are.
SeaCure has helped many of my patients recover from a broad
range of digestive problems, including chronic indigestion, irritable bowel syndrome, and ulcerative colitis, as well as the side effects of chemotherapy. It also provides the many well-documented
benefits of eating fish. The recommended dose is three capsules in
the morning and three capsules in the evening.

~ TRY DIGESTIVE ENZYMES. (See "What to Do About Bloating"
box on page 230.)

THE FINAL FRONTIER: ACCEPTING OUR BODIES

Ultimately, our digestive, food, and weight problems will not be
healed completely until we have accepted our bodies unconditionally.
Part of creating health at midlife is to regain the body acceptance and
self-esteem that most of us lost when we entered adolescence. This is
not inconsistent with wanting to make changes—and in fact may facilitate them. May the following story from one of my newsletter
subscribers inspire all of us about what is possible when we cultivate
enough compassion and self-acceptance and resolve to heal our third
emotional center at last.

*TRACEY: Reconnecting with Body Acceptance at
Menopause*

I disconnected from my body when I became pregnant at eighteen, an unmarried freshman in college who dropped out for my
"shotgun wedding." I hated being pregnant—it was a daily re-

minder of my guilt and shame at having had sex before marriage, out there for the whole world to see and know. I never caressed my big belly, rubbed my aching feet or back, felt the wonder and magic that was going on inside me. I looked at myself totally nude only once and felt nothing but shame and disgust.

From that point onward, Tracey was anywhere from fifty to a hundred pounds overweight and at war with her body. In retrospect, she reasoned that the extra weight was a way to keep herself safe from sexual relationships, since the negative self-image it created kept intimacy at arm's length. Over the years, with maturity and years of self-discovery and therapy, Tracey slowly realized that she no longer needed such protection. Now, at the age of forty-seven and in the midst of perimenopause, her insights have clarified. She wrote:

I remembered something I said to my therapist many years ago. We were talking about what I liked about my body, and I honestly couldn't say there was anything I liked. I said, "Well, look at me—I look pregnant!" And it's true. In varying degrees of heaviness since my pregnancy, my body has always looked pregnant, patiently waiting for me to love it, which I never did when I was actually pregnant. Now I can mourn the loss of enjoying the real experience and move on. I love my essence. I'm very happy with who I am inside. I've come to understand that my physical body is the way my essence can have presence in this world. Therefore I can celebrate it now—I can reconnect my essence with my body. I can celebrate that my hands and senses allow me to express creativity and my body allows me to express my love.

No matter what your size, shape, percentage of body fat, or BMI, you and I, like Tracey, can start right this minute to express gratitude to our bodies for being home to our souls and allowing us to express our uniqueness on the earth at this time. The best way to do this is to stand in front of the mirror, look deeply into your eyes, and say, "I love you. You are beautiful." Over time, this will change every cell in your body!

8
Creating Pelvic Health and Power

Perimenopause is the most common time for women to develop problems with their pelvic organs, ranging from heavy bleeding to fibroids and urinary incontinence. It is also the most common time for women to undergo hysterectomies or other surgical procedures to treat these conditions.

Though numerous approaches help alleviate midlife pelvic symptoms, women can heal fully only when they acknowledge the message behind the symptoms. The emotional and energetic reason that so many women have midlife pelvic problems is associated with the rising need to undergo individuation at midlife and to transform the relationship struggles that tend to make themselves known in the organs of the second emotional center: the genitals, lower bowel, lower back, and bladder. As the transforming kundalini energy rises through us, it often stops in our pelvic organs to create symptoms that will nudge us to address the money, sex, and power issues that are related to this area of our bodies. Whether or not we need surgery or other treatments, perimenopause is a crucial time to develop pelvic power by claiming and shoring up our boundaries, and by assuming more dominion over our creative energy.

WHAT IS YOURS, WHAT IS MINE, WHAT IS OURS? RECLAIMING OUR BOUNDARIES

The health of the second emotional center is tied in to our creative drives: how well do we balance going after what we want in the world with spending time and energy on our relationships? As I've pointed out, young women are both biologically and culturally predisposed to funnel a great deal of creative energy into maintaining relationships. Men, on the other hand, are biologically and socially programmed to focus on the outer world. However, as the energy in our bodies shifts during perimenopause, many women begin to turn their focus toward more worldly accomplishments. Men of the same age often turn inward and become more interested in relationships and nurturing.

Given both our cultural heritage and our shifting creative drives, it is not surprising that boundary conflicts often emerge as we begin, sometimes for the first time, to go after what we really want. This always requires us to claim or reclaim the healthy personal boundaries that allow us to access our power and autonomy.

BETTY: Unmet Creative Needs

Betty was forty-two when she first came to see me for recurrent urinary tract infections. She seemed surprised when I asked her what was going on in her life and what gave her life meaning, but she clearly welcomed the chance to talk.

Betty had graduated from college over twenty years before and had made her living as a freelance writer before her marriage. She clearly had a keen mind and lots of ambition. When she was thirty-two Betty met a wonderful man named Ralph who was supportive of her writing. Ralph's dream was to run his own business, a family restaurant.

In the first year of their marriage, Betty became more flexible with her usual productive writing schedule. After all, Ralph needed help interviewing personnel for his restaurant. And could she help set up the accounting books?—it would take just a week or so, he said. But what started out as a week expanded into a month, and so on, until it became a nearly full-time job.

Despite Ralph's stated support for her writing, Betty's projects invariably took a backseat to the needs of his restaurant. As she started missing due dates, referrals began to dry up. More and more of her waking hours were spent on his business—which he was now calling "their" restaurant. Somehow, inexorably, "his" had turned into "theirs." And "hers" (Betty's writing career) had nearly disappeared.

As midlife adults, it is imperative that we assume responsibility not only for our current circumstances, but also for the often outmoded beliefs that created them—beliefs that usually result from childhood programming. When I asked Betty about her family history, she told me that her father had been very demanding and invasive when she was growing up. He had a finger on every detail of their lives, and he kept after her about how she spent every minute: "You should be working on your homework now." "When are you going to do the dishes?" "Why aren't these clothes being put away as soon as you get home?"

Betty's body had registered this invasion of her second emotional center at an early age. She was only eight when she started to have bladder infections. They continued intermittently until she left for college, after which they cleared up for nearly twenty years. Five years into her marriage, they began again.

As she told her story, Betty realized that her bladder and its symptoms were part of her inner wisdom letting her know that her life was out of balance. She had been overrun by her father as a child, and she had re-created a similar pattern with her husband. In addition to checking out her urinary system thoroughly, I suggested that it was time for Betty to begin shoring up her leaky boundaries.

How Healthy Are Your Boundaries?

Every single one of us has experienced some violations of our personal identity—attempts to control how we think, dress, spend our money or our time, use our creativity, pursue a career. As children, we do not have the ability to form our own boundaries, and we need our parents to help us make healthy choices. But as we get older, we need more and more distance between our own choices and those of our parents. Individuation actually begins when we are two or three years old, which is why toddlers delight in saying no. In many cases, however, this process is incomplete, leaving us with less-than-ideal boundaries—which we may not even be aware of until the wake-up call of perimenopause.

Whatever our history, we must learn to live with healthy respect for our own boundaries—and for those of others. When we do, we'll have an easier time creating health in our second emotional center.

Become Aware of Ongoing Boundary Problems

What events seem to make your symptoms worse? What makes them better? When was the last time you felt really healthy? Betty noticed, for example, that her UTIs disappeared completely when she was in college and during the first few years of her writing career—times when she did not feel required to compromise her creativity to meet the needs of a loved one.

A boundary violation may be so unconscious or subtle that you do not notice it. For example, one of my patients couldn't buy shoes without checking with her husband first. When I questioned her about this, she said, "Well, he's paying for them, isn't he?" I pointed out that the shoes were for *her* feet, not his. Consider the following questions.

Can you buy an article of clothing without asking your partner's opinion or permission? Do you feel guilty if you do so?

Have you ever made a major purchase (such as a camera or appliance) without first running it by your mate? Does your mate make such decisions without consulting you?

Does your mate have the right to veto your decisions? Do you have an equal right to veto his/hers?

If you bring a purchase home and your mate doesn't like it, do you feel you must return it?

At election time, do you and your mate decide together for whom you are both going to vote? How do you resolve any differences of opinion?

Do you find yourself eventually giving in to your mate's preferences for how to spend time and money?

Do you defer your career development needs for the sake of your mate's business or well-being?

If your mate makes more money than you, does that automatically mean that his/her career is taken more seriously and gets more support than yours?

Are you constantly on the receiving end of criticism or unsolicited advice from your mate or family about how you should live your life?

Sometimes awareness alone can help create healthier boundaries. However, if you think your boundary problems are affecting your physical health, it is almost always helpful to discuss your situation with a trusted friend or counselor. He or she can help you get clear on what healthy boundaries look and feel like in a relationship, and, most important, whether you are likely to be able to create them in your current relationship.

HORMONAL IMBALANCE: FUEL TO THE FIRE

The emotional imbalances that demand our attention at perimenopause are fueled by—and in turn contribute to—hormonal imbalance at a cellular level. This hormonal imbalance is characterized by a relative excess of estrogen, not enough progesterone, and, often, too much insulin, all of which can also result in the overproduction of androgenic hormones. Stress of all kinds, emotional, physical, or nutritional, also leads to an imbalance in the evanescent cellular hormones known as eicosanoids, such as prostaglandins and cytokines, which govern every aspect of cellular metabolism and are responsible for cellular inflammation. These same midlife metabolic imbalances also contribute to physical conditions such as fibroids, cramps, endometriosis, adenomyosis, and heavy bleeding. Some women have all of these simultaneously.

Whether your problem is an asymptomatic fibroid or heavy bleeding, the dietary and nutritional supplement approach to these conditions is identical, because both estrogen dominance and eicosanoid imbalance are related to the same dietary factors. Follow the guidelines in chapter 7 with regard to refined carbohydrates, protein, types of dietary fat, and essential vitamins and minerals. In the sections that follow, I will discuss additional medical approaches to each pelvic condition.

MENSTRUAL CRAMPS AND PELVIC PAIN

Starting in the teenage years, about 50 percent of all females suffer from menstrual cramps (dysmenorrhea). During perimenopause, the tendency toward cramping may worsen because of hormonal imbalance and the conditions associated with it, such as fibroids and adenomyosis. My own menstrual cramps started when I was about fourteen and occurred on the first two days of each cycle until I had my first child. They went away for a couple of years (which is very common because of the changes that pregnancy makes in the uterus) but came back in my mid-thirties. My cramps responded to acupuncture and dietary change, and by the age of forty I had recovered from them completely.

Too Many "Bad Eicosanoids"

Cramps result when the uterine muscle and the endometrial produce too much of the eicosanoids called prostaglandin E2 and F2-alpha. When these prostaglandins are released into your bloodstream (usually within an hour or two after the onset of your period, but sometimes even before) you begin to experience the effects of these hormones: spasm in the uterine muscle, sweating, hot flashes, feeling cold alternating with feeling hot, loose stools, and possibly feeling faint. A gel made of prostaglandin E2 (one of the eicosanoids) is used to induce labor, and it can produce exactly the same symptoms you get when your period starts. However, in the case of cramps, the eicosanoid imbalance starts in your own body and is affected by the food you eat and the amount of stress you're under, among other factors.

The Wisdom of Cramps

Are your cramps trying to get you to slow down, rest, and tune in to yourself? Slowing down and resting can help balance eicosanoids. How do you view your menstrual cycle? Is it merely a biological inconvenience for you—or do you see it as part of your wisdom?

The menstrual period is a natural time for rest and renewal. It's nature's way of slowing you down so that you can replenish your body for the next lunar cycle. In many ancient cultures, and even in some contemporary societies such as parts of India, women were expected to take it easy during their periods. But in this society all of us have been taught to try to be efficient, upbeat, and at 100 percent energy all the time. No wonder our wiser bodily processes try to get our attention! Women are lunar. Our bodies and our energies quite naturally follow the phases of the moon. Though this has been considered a sign of female weakness, once you begin to listen to your body, you will find that your cyclic energy shifts are a source of inspiration. If we have not been doing this regularly in our twenties and thirties, our pain can become particularly acute during perimenopause, when the wake-up call to health becomes louder. As one of my perimenopausal patients said, "If I just slow down, take a long bath, and take care of myself, I rarely suffer during my cycle. But when I try to bull my way through and ignore my needs, my body—and my cramps—really try to get my attention."

As you learn to slow down during your premenstrual and menstrual times, not only will your cramps diminish, you'll often find that your intuition is at an all-time high. Insights may come to you more easily. And you'll begin to look forward to this special time.

Keep the following in mind: Whenever the majority of a population—in this case, the majority of women—suffers around a perfectly normal function like menstruation, you can be sure that there is a cultural blind spot in operation. Waking up and seeing the blind spot—and how it might be related to your cramps—is part of embracing your woman's wisdom.

Treating Pelvic Pain and Cramping

~ FOLLOW A HORMONE-BALANCING DIET. (See chapter 7.)

~ ELIMINATE ALL DAIRY FOODS (CHEESE, ICE CREAM, CREAM, MILK, YOGURT) FOR TWO MONTHS. Though I do not have any statistics on this, I've seen many women get rid of their menstrual pain altogether (even in cases of severe endometriosis) by eliminating dairy foods, which are high in arachidonic acid, from their diets. Some are able to prevent cramps by avoiding dairy just for the two weeks before their periods. During perimenopause, when periods so often become irregular, you may need to stop dairy altogether for a few months to experience the benefits.

~ ELIMINATE RED MEAT. Red meat, like dairy foods, is high in a fatty acid eicosanoid precursor known as arachidonic acid, which results in symptoms such as cramps and arthritis in susceptible individuals. Eliminating it from your diet can cut down on the inflammatory eicosanoids associated with cramping and endometriosis pain.

~ TAKE ADDITIONAL SUPPLEMENTS. Follow the supplement program outlined in chapter 7, with special attention to the following.

> *Magnesium:* 100 mg taken as frequently as every two hours during times of actual pain has been shown to help relax smooth muscle tissue and therefore decrease cramping. Do

not exceed 1,000 mg per day, otherwise stools may become too loose.

Omega-3 fatty acids: Omega-3 fats are precursors for series 1 and 3 eicosanoids. Consume at least one of the following:

~ Fatty fish (3–4 oz) three or four times per week, or fish oil, 1,000 to 2,000 mg per day

~ DHA, 100–400 mg per day

~ 4 tbsp ground fresh whole organic flaxseed per day

~ 1 tbsp fresh flaxseed oil daily

Vitamin C: 1,000–5,000 mg per day. Increase when cramping occurs.

~ ACUPUNCTURE AND CHINESE HERBS. Acupuncture has been scientifically shown to alleviate menstrual cramps and pelvic pain.[1] I have seen its benefits hundreds of times in my practice, and I personally found it extremely helpful for severe cramping in my early forties. I also took individually prescribed Chinese herbs for about a year. If you cannot locate a trained practitioner of Traditional Chinese Medicine near you, it is safe to try Bupleurum (Xiao Yao Wan, also known as Hsiao Yao Wan). This patent medicine is widely available, and many of my patients have done very well with it. (See Resources section.) Take four or five of the tiny tablets four times per day during the two weeks before your period is due, and continue through the first day of bleeding. It may take two to three months to see full results. Yun Nan Bai Yao is a traditional Chinese medicine that can stop heavy bleeding within one to two weeks— sometimes sooner. Take one to two capsules, four times daily.

~ TOPICAL TREATMENT. The active ingredient in Menastil (an over-the-counter, topically applied, homeopathic product) is calendula oil—an essential oil extracted from marigold petals. The United States Food and Drug Administration and the Homeopathic Pharmacopoeia U.S. recognize this pure grade of essential oil for the temporary relief of menstrual pain. This all-natural product, which comes in a small roll-on applicator bottle, is designed to relax the uterine muscle, which increases the flow of blood and oxygen to the uterus, which in turn reduces pain. Claire Ellen Products manufactures and distributes Menastil; for information, call the company at 508–366–6311 or visit www.menastil.com.

~ CASTOR OIL PACKS. Lying down with a castor oil pack on your lower abdomen for sixty minutes two to four times per week is often very helpful for both treatment and prevention of cramps and pelvic pain. Edgar Cayce, the renowned medical intuitive of the early to mid-1900s, recommended this immune-system-enhancing treatment for all kinds of conditions. (See Resources section.) *Note:* Do not use these if they increase your pain or if you are bleeding heavily.

~ NONSTEROIDAL ANTI-INFLAMMATORIES (NSAIDS). Nonsteroidal anti-inflammatory drugs such as ibuprofen (Motrin, Advil), naproxen sodium (Anaprox, Aleve), and ketoprofen (Orudis) work by partially blocking your body's production of prostaglandin F2-alpha. (So do aspirin and acetaminophen [Tylenol], but through a slightly different mechanism.) For best relief, NSAIDs must be taken *before* you get uncomfortable. If you take them only after the pain has begun, the prostaglandin will already be in your bloodstream. The drug stops production of prostaglandin F2-alpha, but it cannot stop the effect on your cells once the prostaglandin has been released.

~ BIRTH CONTROL PILLS. All pelvic conditions tend to quiet down when the natural hormonal cycles are put to sleep by the steady-state synthetic hormones in birth control pills. Take the lowest-dose pill available. Avoid birth control pills altogether if you are a smoker.

HEAVY BLEEDING

Many women develop heavy and irregular bleeding in the years before menopause because estrogen dominance causes the lining of the uterus to overgrow. Emotional stress of all kinds can make this worse. Instead of the normal monthly buildup and shedding of the uterine lining, too much endometrial tissue builds up and then breaks down in a disordered way that results in spotting or irregular heavy bleeding.

What do I mean by heavy bleeding? Many women experience a heavier flow on the first or second day of their periods, which slows them down a bit, but I consider this within the realm of normal. (You may still wish to try some of the gentler treatments listed.) However, if your bleeding prevents you from leaving the house or participating fully in your life for more than two days per month, if you routinely soak through a couple of tampons and a pad all in place at the same time and then through your clothes or your nightgown, or if you've been diagnosed with iron deficiency anemia, you need to take action.

The Wisdom of Bleeding: Are You Leaking Life Energy?

I always ask my patients with heavy bleeding if they are leaking their life's blood into any dead-end job or relationship that doesn't fully meet their needs. Are you giving more than you are receiving in return? Is someone or something draining your energy by being a kind of Dracula? Take some time alone, sit right down on the earth, and pray for guidance and a boost of energy for yourself.

Physical Causes of Heavy Periods

In addition to hormonal imbalance, physical conditions may impede the normal uterine contractions that help stop menstrual blood flow each month.

Fibroid tumors are the most common physical reason for excessive bleeding. Whether or not a fibroid causes bleeding depends upon its location in the uterine wall. Bleeding is most often caused by submucosal fibroids, which are located right under the endometrium, the mucous membrane that lines the uterus.

Adenomyosis is another condition that can cause heavy bleeding. Adenomyosis results when the endometrial glands that line the uterus grow into the uterine muscle (the myometrium). When this happens, little lakes of blood form in the uterine wall that do not drain during menstruation. Over time, the uterus enlarges and becomes boggy, spongy, and engorged with blood, disrupting the normal uterine contraction patterns.

Since both fibroids and adenomyosis are associated with excess estrogen, minimal progesterone, too much prostaglandin F2-alpha, and frequently too much insulin, hormonal and physical factors are often present at the same time.

Treatment Choices for Heavy Bleeding

Before you start any treatment program for heavy bleeding, I recommend that you get a physical exam and a Pap smear if you haven't already had one within the year. Though the vast majority of cases of heavy bleeding are benign and can be treated with the advice I'm about to give you, you want to be sure that you don't have some other condition that is contributing to your problem.

~ DIET AND VITAMINS. Follow the hormone-balancing diet outlined in chapter 7, with special attention to supplemental antioxidants and B vitamins. These help strengthen your blood vessel walls and help your liver break down and clear excess estrogen from your body.

> *B complex:* Take the mid to high range of the B vitamins on page 523. These help neutralize excess estrogen.
>
> *Vitamin E* (mixed tocopherols): 400 IU, twice per day.
>
> *Vitamin C complex with bioflavonoids:* 1,000–5,000 mg per day.
>
> *Vitamin A* (as beta-carotene): 25,000 IU per day.
>
> *Supplemental iron:* In many women with heavy bleeding, the primary symptom is fatigue from iron deficiency anemia. Get your blood count checked. If it's low, take iron. The recommended daily allowance is 15 mg per day. You may need to take three to four times this amount until iron levels are restored. (Iron supplementation itself has been shown to decrease menstrual flow in some women.)

The best, most absorbable iron supplement I've found is ANR Iron 27+. (See Resources.) It is time-released, doesn't cause stomach upset or constipation, and is easily and readily absorbed. It has helped many women in my practice keep their blood counts normal—something they were previously unable to do with other iron supplements. It has even saved some women from needing surgery.

~ ACUPUNCTURE AND TRADITIONAL CHINESE MEDICINE. See discussion on pages 196–199.

~ CASTOR OIL PACKS. See the discussion on page 244.

~ NATURAL PROGESTERONE. A nonprescription cream that contains 2 percent natural progesterone can be used to decrease heavy bleeding. Rub ¼–½ tsp into your palms or on the soft areas of your skin two times per day starting two to three weeks before your period is due. Stop when your period begins, then start again one to two weeks later. If this approach is going to work, you should see results after about three months. For some women, 2 percent natural progesterone isn't strong enough to counteract their own estrogen. In this case, ask your doctor for a stronger prescription, such as Crinone gel, which comes in 4 percent and 8 percent strengths, or micronized oral progesterone tablets (brand name Prometrium). The usual dose of Prometrium is 100–200 mg once or twice per day for the two weeks before your period is due.

~ NSAIDS. Take a nonsteroidal anti-inflammatory drug, such as ibuprofen (Motrin, Advil), naproxen sodium (Anaprox, Aleve), or ketoprofen (Orudis), daily starting one to two days before your period, and continue it regularly through your heaviest days. Use the lowest dose that gives you results. The NSAIDs have definitely been shown to decrease menstrual blood loss because of their ability to interrupt excess prostaglandin F2-alpha.

~ SYNTHETIC PROGESTERONE. When natural progesterone doesn't work, it is sometimes necessary to use a strong synthetic progestin such as medroxyprogesterone acetate (Provera). (This is the only circumstance in which I recommend the synthetic.) This is especially true if you have a fibroid that bleeds and you haven't been able to stem your problem with gentler approaches. Provera for heavy periods is prescribed at a dose of 10 mg once or twice per day for the two weeks before your period is due. Then you give your body a rest for two weeks and start over. Usually a three-month cycle of two weeks on and two weeks off will result in a significant decrease in excessive bleeding. Though Provera can have side effects, these are usually acceptable compared to losing your uterus.

~ BIRTH CONTROL PILLS. Many women who are having heavy, irregular periods due to fibroids, lack of ovulation, excess estrogen relative to progesterone, or a combination of these conditions often do well on birth control pills. Although they do not result in a true cure, they are a good option when the alternative is surgery.

~ D&C (DILATATION AND CURETTAGE). This standard surgical treatment for heavy bleeding involves scraping the uterine lining and removing excess tissue. It frequently decreases the problem, for reasons that aren't entirely clear. It is often used also to diagnose the specific condition causing the bleeding.

~ ENDOMETRIAL ABLATION. In this surgical procedure, the lining of the uterus is obliterated with a laser or with cautery. Because the procedure destroys the endometrial lining, it often results in complete cessation of periods or very light periods. It should never be used by anyone who wants to maintain her ability to have children.

Endometrial ablation works very well for many types of intractable bleeding and is usually done as an outpatient surgery. The procedure should be done by someone highly skilled, with extensive previous experience. For a referral, consult a university medical center or teaching hospital. You can also call your local hospital and ask who does the surgery. Make sure the surgeon you choose is a board-certified OB/GYN.

I've referred a number of women for this procedure. For some it provides great relief. One of my newsletter subscribers wrote to me: "Three months ago I underwent an endometrial ablation and tubal ligation. At age forty-four this sterilizes me two ways, for which I'm grateful, and has remedied the constant bleeding and clots for weeks on end. I now have no more periods! Yeah!"

MARTHA: *Intractable Heavy Bleeding*

Martha wrote me the following about her midlife bleeding problem.

I am forty-two years old. I weigh about 190 on God-given big bones, exercise regularly, and am generally healthy. My problem has been described as flooding. I have seen several doctors about this. They prescribed a double dose of birth control pills that I took for four months with no result. I have had a biopsy done, with negative results. My Paps are normal.

My periods last twelve days and are very heavy with lots of clots. There is constant bleeding in between. I consulted a herbologist, who thought that because of my forty excess pounds, my fat cells could very well be overproducing estrogen. That is why the pill and the progesterone cream that I have used have not helped the constant bleeding.

I have read Susun S. Weed's book *Menopausal Years: The Wise Woman Way.* In it she suggests using homeopathic remedies such as lachesis. I am also drinking raspberry leaf tea and using shepherd's purse. I am taking iron, as that has been low. Also *Lactobacillus acidophilus,* calcium, magnesium, and a good multiple vitamin.

The bleeding still has not stopped. I am becoming pretty tired of all of this, and as you can well imagine, my desire for sex is low with me having to constantly wear a pad. The bleeding has been going on for four months. Do you have any suggestions that may help?

I suggested to Martha that she seek help from an acupuncturist right away and also continue taking iron. I also recommended a Chinese patent medicine called Yun Nan Bai Yao, which is superb for helping flooding problems. (See Resources.) It generally works within a week or two. I also suggested that she lose 10–20 pounds, which could significantly reduce her excess bodily estrogen production.

It is possible that Martha has an undiagnosed submucosal fibroid. The diagnosis is made with ultrasound, MRI, or with a procedure known as hysterosalpingogram, in which dye is injected into the uterine cavity under X-ray visualization. If this is the case, she may need a surgical approach such as endometrial ablation or fibroid removal done via the vagina. I've also seen her type of problem respond well to a D&C done in the operating room.

The main point here is that there are many, many approaches to controlling heavy bleeding during perimenopause. In every case, it's helpful to have a diagnosis and treatment plan with alternatives to hysterectomy. Here is the bottom line: Every perimenopausal woman who is experiencing heavy bleeding needs to know that there are many safe and effective treatment options. Hysterectomy, which amounts to killing the messenger, should be a last resort.

FIBROIDS

Benign fibroid tumors of the uterus are present in 30–50 percent of women in the United States. They occur in women of all races and backgrounds, but they are more common in women of African-American or Caribbean descent. Fibroids arise from the smooth muscle and connective tissue of the uterine muscle itself. Though they can occur in women as young as their late teens or early twenties, they are most often diagnosed when a woman is in her thirties or forties.[2]

The majority of fibroids do not cause any real problems. In other words, they are just there. Sometimes, depending upon their location, you will be able to feel them. They feel like a smooth lump in your lower abdomen, just above your pubic bone. Because the female

FIGURE 12: TYPES OF FIBROIDS

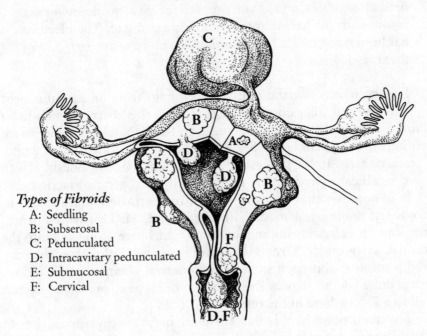

Types of Fibroids
  A: Seedling
  B: Subserosal
  C: Pedunculated
  D: Intracavitary pedunculated
  E: Submucosal
  F: Cervical

pelvis can accommodate growths the size of a newborn baby, it is obvious that small and even large fibroids don't necessarily lead to any problems. In other words, you may not even be aware that you have one unless you have a pelvic exam or pelvic ultrasound. Your periods may not be any different, and chances are you won't experience any pain or other symptoms. Fibroids may grow dramatically during perimenopause because of estrogen dominance (their growth is stimulated by estrogen), but they often shrink just as dramatically after menopause—nature's treatment.

The Wisdom of Your Fibroids

Though there are well-established dietary and hormonal reasons why so many women have fibroids, the baseline energetic patterns that result in fibroids are related to blockage and stagnation of the energy of the second emotional center. Women are at risk for fibroids (or other pelvic problems) when we direct our creative energy into dead-end relationships that we have outgrown. When my own fibroid appeared at age forty-two, for instance, I knew that it was related, in part, to my staying in a one-on-one direct patient care practice for several years longer than I really wanted to. I was afraid that I wouldn't be respected as a "real" doctor if I wasn't doing surgery regularly and maintaining a full office practice. Though I longed to channel my creativity into more writing and teaching, I also feared my colleagues would resent me if I worked only part time. This is the classic second emotional center double bind. Our simultaneous ambition and need for love and approval create a logjam in the creative center of our bodies that, under the right circumstances, becomes a fibroid.

ELLEN: Birthing Her Creativity

Ellen, thirty-eight, was married with two children and worked as a research associate at a local university. She loved everything about her job, from the subject matter itself to the people she worked with daily. She was proud of the fact that her colleagues sought her out when they needed help with their own projects. But as the years progressed, Ellen found herself drawn to working more independently. Unfortunately, because she had become "indispensable," it was very difficult for her to set those other projects aside to birth her own individual creation. Her fibroid tumor was diagnosed at about this time.

Over the next several years, her fibroid continued to grow as she found herself torn between the needs of her own particular research and the needs of her colleagues, children, and husband. During an office visit in which she consulted me about possible surgery for the fibroid, I asked her to consider where she was "leaking" her energy. She said that a large part of her identity and sense of self-esteem came from being there for others. She told me that if she was to go off and work by herself, she was afraid that she wouldn't feel as useful—and that others would think she was selfish. As we talked about this, she realized that she had to make some long-overdue changes in her schedule and in her priorities. Then she told me that she wanted to give herself another six months before having any surgery.

The next time I saw her, her fibroid hadn't grown any further and was even a bit smaller. But more important, Ellen had told her colleagues what she was and was not willing to do for them—and had simultaneously made some big steps toward pursuing her own projects. In other words, she had started to birth her own creativity.

If you have or have had a fibroid, ask yourself the following questions: What are the creations within me that I want to put out in the world before I'm no longer here? If anything at all were possible, what would my life look like? If I had six months to live, what relationships would I release from my life immediately? What relationships would I give more of my time and attention to? What relationships truly feed and nourish me? Which ones drain my energy? Write your answers in a journal. Discuss them with supportive friends. Deep within you, you have all the answers you need. You just need to be open to hearing them.

Treatment of Fibroids

The first thing to consider is that a fibroid may not need to be treated. A watch-and-wait attitude is not unreasonable in many cases; you can live with fibroids for years with no adverse health consequences if they are not bothering you. What may well bother you, however, is simply knowing that you have them. Given our cultural inheritance about our pelvic organs, the perception that something *will* go wrong is often a bigger risk to a woman's well-being than the fibroid itself.

It would do most women a world of good to lighten up about their fibroids. At the time your fibroid is diagnosed, you usually will not know what has caused your second-emotional-center imbalances. Understanding comes retrospectively. Instead, commit to learning from the process, whatever course of treatment you decide upon.

An essential element of this learning experience is to release self-blame. It is never helpful to hold the idea that you have a particular illness or symptom because you are "doing something wrong." If you knew ahead of time what the condition was trying to bring to your attention, you wouldn't have had to manifest it. And in fact, all physical conditions have genetic, dietary, environmental, and emotional components simultaneously.

On the other hand, there are times when you may wish to seek treatment for a fibroid. Though most fibroids will shrink after menopause is complete, you may not want to live with a growth that makes you look pregnant until that time comes. If you find, as I did, that you are dressing to disguise your fibroid, and your menopause is six or more years away, then you may want to take action. And, of course, if your symptoms include pain, heavy bleeding, cramping, or backache, you'll definitely want relief. Thankfully, the treatment options are extensive.

Dietary Change and Supplements

Any dietary or alternative approach that works to balance excess estrogen or enhance the flow of energy *chi* through the pelvis often works for fibroids as well as for heavy bleeding or menstrual cramps. These include acupuncture and Chinese herbs, phytoestrogens from sources such as soy or flaxseed, dietary change, and estrogen-balancing supplements. (See chapter 6.) Exercise such as yoga is also helpful.

Such approaches are always worth a try, as this letter from a newsletter subscriber attests.

I have been suffering for years with multiple uterine fibroid tumors, approximately twenty-five to thirty in number in the wall of my uterus. For two weeks out of every month I had excruciating, unbearable pain. I was unable to sleep, would lie down curled up in a ball, and literally sweat in agony. In 1991 and 1992 I had laser surgery through the laparoscope twice, and the surgeon was only able to remove three or four of the larger fibroids. Then I read your book and have been religiously following your advice to cut out dairy products and take B complex vitamins as well as 800 mg of magnesium. As a result, if I could, I would give you my firstborn child in gratitude! My pain is gone! Though I was planning reconstructive surgery, I changed my mind when I realized that your suggestions were working. I feel like a completely new woman—reborn, revitalized, and empowered.

Hormonal Treatments

~ BIOIDENTICAL PROGESTERONE. Progesterone skin cream helps to counter estrogen dominance. It is available over the counter in a 2 percent strength (trade names Emerita, PhytoGest). The usual dose is ¼–½ tsp rubbed into your palms or on the soft areas of your skin once or twice per day, three weeks on and one week off. If you are having regular periods, time the application so that your week off corresponds to the week of your period. If your periods are irregular, I suggest coordinating use of the progesterone cream with the phases of the moon, to which every human life is attuned. Plan to be off the progesterone during the dark of the moon—the time when women were most apt to have their periods before the advent of artificial lighting. Some women do best using the cream every day, with no week off.

Some women may need a higher dose. Stronger natural progesterone creams are available by prescription from a formulary pharmacy. (See Resources.) Natural progesterone is also available as a vaginal gel (trade name Crinone or Prochieve), which is available by prescription from all pharmacies.

Most women do well on transdermal or transvaginal progesterone, which is absorbed into the bloodstream directly. Oral progesterone must be metabolized by the liver, and the breakdown products that result sometimes cause excessive sleepiness or even depression in susceptible women. However, some women find that they do best on an oral preparation. The dose is 100–200 mg once or twice per day for at least two weeks per month. Some women need to take it daily.

⁓ BIRTH CONTROL PILLS. Birth control pills are a combination of synthetic estrogen and progestin that can smooth out the estrogen dominance that so often causes fibroids to grow or become symptomatic. Because they consist of synthetic hormones, I'd suggest that they be used only after more natural approaches such as dietary change or acupuncture and herbs have failed, or in situations in which a woman is unwilling or unable to try a more natural approach.

⁓ GNRH AGONISTS. GnRH agonists such as nafarelin (Synarel) or leuprolide (Lupron) act at the level of the pituitary gland and put the body into a state of artificial menopause. This lowers estrogen levels and shrinks fibroids. Side effects include all the symptoms of late perimenopause, such as bone loss, hot flashes, and vaginal dryness, but these can sometimes be effectively countered with low-dose hormone therapy that doesn't cause fibroids to grow.

GnRH agonists can be quite effective as alternatives to surgery for some women. I do not recommend them if you have a family history of Alzheimer's disease, because the rapid withdrawal of estrogen from the brain may not be advisable in susceptible women.

Surgical Treatments

⁓ MYOMECTOMY. Fibroids can often be removed surgically. The size and location of a fibroid will determine the surgical route. Fibroids that are located just under the uterine lining deep within the uterus, for example, can sometimes be removed vaginally. Others can be removed via laparoscopy (sometimes known as belly-button surgery). Large ones, such as the one I had, usually require abdominal surgery.

If you decide to have your fibroid removed surgically, the procedure should be done by a pelvic surgeon who is trained in the repair and preservation of the pelvic organs and who philosophically is aligned with your desire to keep your uterus. When he was finished with my surgery, my pelvic surgeon told me, "Well, I'm happy to report that you now have completely healthy and normal pelvic organs. I didn't have to remove a thing except the fibroid!" That's exactly what I wanted to hear.

Having your fibroids removed can be a very empowering experience. As one of my newsletter subscribers wrote me:

> After having fibroids surgically removed, I also removed most negative issues from my life. It is wonderful! No headaches, no cramps, no backaches. I am still working on more dietary changes, but the ones I have already made have made me more positive, stronger, and carefree. I am also a praying person. So with this, and lifestyle changes, I am well on my way to healing and growing up at the age of forty!

- FIBROID EMBOLIZATION. Uterine artery embolization (UAE) is a relatively new treatment for fibroid tumors that involves injecting a substance (usually polyvinyl alcohol particles) into the uterine artery. This causes clotting of the blood supply to the fibroid, which then shrinks over time. The procedure is done by interventional radiologists specifically trained in the technique. To reach the uterine arteries, a catheter is threaded into the femoral vein of the thigh. Most centers report good outcomes, with a worldwide success rate of about 85 percent. All types of fibroid symptoms, including heavy or irregular bleeding, uterine enlargement, and symptoms related to the size of the fibroid, such as urinary frequency, have responded.

The average patient who undergoes this procedure can expect a 40–60 percent decrease in uterine size after about six months, but even those women who have no reduction in uterine size report improvement in symptoms such as heavy bleeding. Although no long-term follow-up data are yet available, UAE has a low risk of complications compared with myomectomy or hysterectomy. However, some serious complications, such as renal failure or an allergic reaction to the clotting agent, have been reported.[3] If this procedure appeals to you, seek out the advice of a specialist at a center where UAE is frequently done or call the Society of

Cardiovascular and Interventional Radiology at 800–488–7284 or visit their website, www.scvir.org.

~ EXABLATE: ULTRASOUND TREATMENT FOR FIBROIDS: A new FDA-approved device combines MRI imaging to map out uterine fibroids with high-intensity focused ultrasound to heat up and destroy fibroid tissue. Because the blood vessels in fibroids help the body to dissipate the excess heat generated during this procedure, it's particularly well suited for treating fibroids. Called ExAblate, this noninvasive, outpatient procedure leaves the uterus and ovaries intact. It involves lying on your abdomen in an MRI tube for up to three hours. Side effects may include blisters on the abdominal skin, cramping, nausea, and some pain (that's easily treated with over-the-counter pain medication).

About 70 percent of patients report that this treatment successfully reduces their fibroid symptoms, although 20 percent require additional surgery within a year. The FDA reports that though the ExAblate treatment successfully reduces symptoms in most women, those symptoms—and the fibroids—may return. (Because of this, I recommend that *all* women suffering from fibroids also adopt lifestyle changes that alter hormone metabolism and reduce fibroid symptoms naturally.) Even so, I feel that ExAblate is an exciting use of technology and a major step forward; in fact, if it had been available when I had my fibroid (which was very large), I would have strongly considered this treatment. *Note:* Women who want to get pregnant should not use ExAblate because there's not enough data yet to determine what happens to the uterine wall and lining following the procedure. For more information, call InSightec, the company that developed the technology, at 866–392–2528 or visit the company's website at www.uterine-fibroids.org.

~ HYSTERECTOMY. Hysterectomy should be the last resort for fibroid treatment, reserved for those women who, in addition to their fibroids, also have intractable bleeding or pain problems that simply have not responded to other measures. When this is the case, hysterectomy can be a real blessing, dramatically enhancing the quality of a woman's life.

CAROL: *The Need to Let Go*

Carol was forty-six when she first came to see me for a second surgical opinion. Carol had multiple fibroids in her uterus that were causing her to bleed heavily each month, resulting in chronic anemia and fatigue. For the past four years she had tried desperately to keep her uterus, clinging to the hope that she'd be able to have a child of her own someday. Carol's condition had deteriorated to the point that keeping her uterus had become her career. In fact, she had even lost her job because of constant absenteeism due to doctors' appointments and episodes of heavy bleeding that required her to leave work. Though Carol had tried birth control pills, synthetic hormones, and multiple D&Cs to control the bleeding, nothing had helped. Her condition was too dangerous to suggest alternative treatments such as diet or acupuncture. I suggested that her health and overall well-being would best be served by a hysterectomy. (If I were to see her now, I would suggest uterine artery embolization or ExAblate.)

Carol's uterine condition was preventing her from actually living her life. She was stuck in a holding pattern consisting of pouring her life's blood (literally) into unrealized hopes and dreams that had little or no chance of manifesting. Like all of us at midlife, Carol needed to let go of an unrealized dream from her past (having a biological child), allow herself to grieve fully, and then finally move on. Though this is never easy, sometimes it is the most healing choice.

AN EMPOWERED APPROACH TO SURGERY OR INVASIVE PROCEDURES

When you feel that you have been involved with the choice to have surgery, UAE, or ExAblate and really know your options, then you've stepped out of the victim role and into the partnership model. This shift alone improves your chance for a good outcome. You can continue that partnership mode by reading *Prepare for Surgery, Heal Faster* by my colleague Peggy Huddleston. Peggy has written the definitive manual for how to have a healthy and empowering surgical experience. I personally used her approach when I had my own fibroid surgery. (See her website at www.healfaster.com.)

Hysterectomy for the Wrong Reasons

Make sure that you get a second opinion if someone gives you one of the following reasons for having a hysterectomy for a fibroid.

1. *"You should have surgery before your fibroid gets any bigger. If you don't, your fibroid may grow and make the surgery much more difficult in the future."*

Unless a small tumor is causing intractable bleeding or fertility problems, it does not need to be removed. Not all fibroids are destined to grow, and even if they do, studies have shown that surgery to remove a uterus with large fibroids poses no increased risk to the patient. If necessary, the fibroid can be removed (see the section on myomectomy on page 254) leaving the uterus, and the blood supply to the ovaries, intact.

2. *"Your fibroid may become cancerous"* or *"We cannot be sure it is not cancerous unless it is removed."*

It is extremely rare for a fibroid to be cancerous (the incidence is less than one in a thousand). If a fibroid tumor does become cancerous, it is called a uterine sarcoma, and currently the prognosis for this condition is very poor, which means that diagnosing it via surgery will not greatly increase your chances for survival. In fact, the chances of dying from complications of hysterectomy, though small, are statistically a little greater than the chances of having a uterine sarcoma.

3. *"Your ovaries can't be seen on ultrasound."*

If you have had an ultrasound examination (or even an MRI) to confirm the diagnosis of a fibroid, one of your ovaries may not be visible because it's hidden behind the fibroid. Since doctors can be held liable for failing to diagnose an ovarian problem if it's present, they may suggest surgery to be absolutely certain that your ovary is okay.

However, if you have no reason to believe that your ovaries are diseased, you can ask simply to be followed by your doctor. Remember, inability to see an ovary on ultrasound doesn't mean that something is wrong with it—it just means that there are limits to technology! In this situation, some women will want to schedule laparoscopic surgery so that the pelvis can be examined from the inside with a light. (The uterus and ovaries can also be biopsied during this procedure.) Others will feel comfortable trusting that they are okay. Make whichever choice brings you the most peace of mind.

Should You Have a Hysterectomy?

Fibroids and heavy and irregular bleeding are the most common reasons why women have hysterectomies at midlife. Though hysterectomy is sometimes necessary, far too many women have them when they could have resolved their symptoms more easily and naturally using other means, including the newer technologies, such as uterine artery embolization. In addition, there is great value in keeping our pelvic organs intact when possible.

In an ideal world, every girl and woman would be taught the value of her pelvic organs from an early age; their benefits would be as well studied as those of the male organs, research on safe and effective natural alternatives to bleeding and pain would be common, and hysterectomy with or without removal of the ovaries would be a very rare operation performed only when all other alternatives fail. This mindset is currently in place when it comes to male sexual organs. As a result, orchiectomy, the removal of the testes, is performed only as a last resort, though it is a very effective treatment for prostate cancer. And removal of the penis is just about unheard of, even in cases of penile cancer.

Unfortunately, the uterus and the ovaries have been the target of bad press for so long that many women have internalized a fear of their pelvic organs. Recently I overheard a woman I'll call Jane talking to her friends at a party about her upcoming hysterectomy. Her fibroid was the size of a small orange, she told them, and she wasn't having symptoms. But, she explained, "I'm fifty, and at my age it's just a matter of time before something happens in that area. I might as well get it out now." Many physicians reinforce these fears. A patient who came to me for a second opinion to avoid hysterectomy for a fibroid had been told by her gynecologist that her uterus (which had produced a healthy baby girl only seven months earlier) was "not her friend."

The Greek word *hystera* (womb) was used in ancient times to describe all manner of women's suffering, both psychological (hysteria) and physical, believed to be caused by the uterus. In the 1800s after the advent of anesthesia, hysterectomy became an enormously popular cure for women's ailments and was performed for just about anything that a woman's husband, father, or doctor thought was wrong with her: overeating, painful menstruation, psychological disorders, and most particularly masturbation, promiscuity, or any erotic tendency.

FIGURE 13: PELVIC ORGANS WITH SUPPORTING MUSCLES

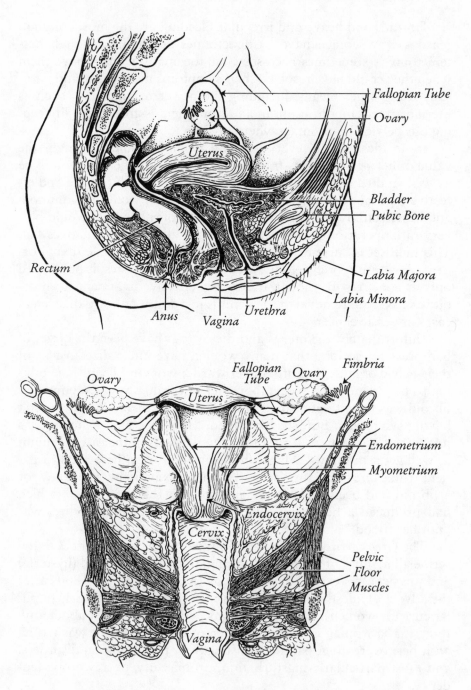

Surgical removal of the uterus remains one of the most commonly performed operations in the United States—both doctors and their patients have been taught that these organs are dangerous at worst or expendable at best, though this stance is now changing rapidly! One in three women in this country has had a hysterectomy by the age of sixty. This is a staggeringly high number. Not surprisingly, hysterectomy rates are very high among doctors' wives. And about 43 percent of women have their ovaries removed at the same time as their uterus, to prevent the possible development of ovarian cancer, despite the fact that the vast majority of us will never get ovarian cancer, but could definitely benefit from the hormones produced by our ovaries throughout our lives.

Good Reasons to Keep Your Uterus, Cervix, and Ovaries

~ Your uterus, cervix, and ovaries all work together to provide your body with hormonal support throughout your entire life. They also share much of the same blood supply. When the uterus is removed, the function of the ovaries is affected even if the ovaries are left in. Up to 50 percent of women who have had hysterectomies lose the function of their ovaries earlier than they normally would—and they go through menopause earlier, thus increasing their risk for heart disease and osteoporosis.[4]

~ Ovaries are the female equivalent of the male testes. As such, they are an important producer of androgens, the hormones that are involved in normal sex drive. Some studies have shown that up to 25 percent of women have decreased sex drive following removal of the ovaries. Removal of the ovaries literally castrates the female—and it is called that in the medical literature.[5]

Many doctors routinely remove the ovaries at the time of hysterectomy in order to prevent ovarian cancer. If a woman has a strong genetic risk for ovarian cancer, this may be a sound decision. But the vast majority of women will never get ovarian cancer, and the routine removal of normal ovaries as prevention is a very high price to pay.

~ Natural menopause, with ovaries and uterus intact, is a normal physiological event that takes place over a period of six to thirteen years. As your ovaries gradually shift function, the adrenal glands naturally take over some hormone production, as does the body fat. When a woman has her uterus, or uterus and ovaries, removed, her body goes through an instant menopause, which can be a shock to the hormonal system.

~ The uterus itself undergoes rhythmic contractions during orgasm, which contribute to the depth of sexual pleasure that many women experience during lovemaking. Some women who have had a hysterectomy complain that orgasm is not as satisfying anymore.

~ Hysterectomy with ovarian removal decreases pheromone secretion, which may decrease a woman's sexual attractiveness.[6] Fortunately, pheromone preparations are available to remedy this. (See chapter 9.)

~ The cervix (the lower portion of the uterus that protrudes into the vagina) is part of the normal pelvic floor and helps to support the bladder. The nerves that go to the bladder are intimately connected to the cervix. When hysterectomy with removal of the cervix is performed, these nerves can be damaged, resulting in an increased risk for urinary incontinence.[7]

~ Only 10 percent of hysterectomies are done because of cancer. That means that up to 90 percent of the time, a woman's pelvic organs are removed for benign disease—disease that can often be treated effectively by nonsurgical approaches.

Unearthing Your Hysterectomy Legacy

Over the years I've found that all the education and information in the world won't change a woman's life as long as she's operating from old, unconscious, and unexamined beliefs. Each of us carries a unique personal legacy passed down to us from family members. This is especially true when it comes to women's pelvic organs, a subject that has been shrouded in secrecy and misinformation for generations. Here are some questions to help you uncover your hysterectomy legacy.

Which of your family members, if any, have had hysterectomies? Why? Do you know what was going on in their lives at the time? Do you know what their diagnoses were and what symptoms they were having? Would it be possible to find out? Do you feel that you can't ask because this information is "too personal"? Does a belief in "better living through surgery" run in your family?

One of my patients believed that she would need a hysterectomy sometime during her forties because "all my sisters had them then." As a result, she became overly focused on her pelvic organs at midlife, noting every irregular or heavy period and every twinge. Ultimately, her mind/body connection—plus her unhealthy lifestyle—created enough symptoms so that she actually wanted a hysterectomy "for relief."

If, after going through these questions honestly, you still believe that hysterectomy is the best solution for you, then it well may be.

If You've Already Had a Hysterectomy

If you've had a hysterectomy and didn't know that you had any other choice, I know that it's upsetting to hear that the surgery may not have been in your best interest. One of my newsletter readers said:

> After reading your article on the benefits of keeping your ovaries and uterus, I wept. I was only forty-five when I had my hysterectomy for a fibroid that wasn't really bothering me at all. They took my ovaries, too. But that was twenty years ago. I didn't know that I had any other choice. And I also realized that I had never fully grieved for the loss of my pelvic organs. I have now completed that process, and I can let it go and move on.

The first step to healing after hysterectomy is to appreciate any benefits you've experienced from having the surgery. In a landmark study here in Maine, it was found that hysterectomy for noncancerous conditions of the uterus, such as bleeding and pain, was positively associated with improving the woman's quality of life in the vast majority of cases.[8] I want to stress that in this particular study, all of the women were given a choice: to have the surgery or to not have it and be followed. I referred many women to this study and even performed some of the hysterectomies that were included in the data. Many of the women who chose surgery were convinced that they'd be better off with a hysterectomy. Some had lived with pelvic discomfort or heavy bleeding for years that was cured by the surgery. Others actually had an improvement in their sex lives following the surgery. The moral is this: hysterectomy can be a healing surgery under the right circumstances.

Yes, your uterus and ovaries are important, but always remember that you are more than the sum of your organs. Your spiritual body, the field of electromagnetic energy that surrounds and nourishes your physical body, is always whole and intact. You cannot destroy this essential part of yourself, no matter what happens to your physical body.

Appreciate the fact that your body has the ability to rebalance your hormones and maintain its health if you follow a healthy diet, exercise regularly, and use natural hormone replacement strategies that match as nearly as possible what your body normally produces.

If you had a hysterectomy that you now regret, realize that you probably made the best decision you could have under the circumstances that were present at the time. Give yourself credit for that. Our medical care system and its beliefs simply reflect those of the culture we're all a part of. And we can't help but be affected by these beliefs, at least to some degree. Maybe you would have avoided your hysterectomy if you had known more—but you didn't have that knowledge. Let any emotions you have around this issue come to the surface, even if they aren't pleasant ones. (One of my patients had a recurrent fantasy that she wanted to injure or even kill the surgeon who did her surgery. When she allowed herself to feel these unladylike revenge fantasies fully and express them out loud, she was able to release herself from the past and get on with her life, eventually forgiving herself and the surgeon.)

You can heal from anything—even events as life-changing as losing some body parts to surgery. And when you heal, your story can help someone else on her journey toward health. One of the most helpful things you can do to improve your health right now is to look back on the events leading up to your hysterectomy and see if you had any issues with boundaries or creative drive at the time. Making this link can be very empowering and will also give you greater appreciation for the wisdom of your body. Remember, too, that your second-emotional-center power and passion is still there. It doesn't get removed with your uterus.

STRENGTHEN YOUR URINARY HEALTH AND PELVIC FLOOR MUSCLES

At midlife, the loss of hormonal support in the vagina and lower urinary tract is often accompanied by the loss of muscle tone in the pelvic floor. As a result, many women experience urinary problems, ranging from loss of urine when coughing or sneezing to recurrent urinary tract infections, as well as uterine prolapse (a condition with a hereditary component that is often exacerbated during midlife).

While you're learning how to create healthy boundaries in your personal relationships, I also highly recommend that you develop the muscles in your pelvic floor by doing Kegel exercises or using vaginal weights regularly. This not only strengthens the pelvic floor, but also increases blood flow to the vagina, bladder, and urethra, making the tissue more resilient. This will greatly improve both your sex life and your bladder control.

Keeping Dry: Maintaining or Regaining Bladder Control

Urinary incontinence, the involuntary leakage of urine, is a major health problem that affects approximately thirteen million people in the United States. Though 10–30 percent of women age fifteen to sixty-four experience urinary incontinence at least some of the time, the condition tends to increase in frequency with age. It often makes itself known during perimenopause, when a great deal can be done to make sure it doesn't progress. By the time women reach age sixty-five and over, the overall rate of incontinence increases to about 15–35 percent.[9]

Though the problem does affect men, it affects women five times as often. Many women feel too embarrassed to bring it up with their doctors and therefore don't know about many of the new and effective treatments that are available. To compound the problem, many physicians aren't up on the latest treatments, either. In an editorial in the *Journal of the American Medical Association,* Dr. Neil M. Resnick wrote, "Most physicians have received little education about incontinence, fail to screen for it, and view the likelihood of success as low."[10]

This doesn't mean that you should suffer in silence. Urinary incontinence is easily diagnosed and often treatable with excellent results. Read through the treatment options outlined below and see which ones speak to you. Then discuss them with your health care practitioner. If possible, seek out someone who specializes in the evaluation of female urological problems. Determining exactly what type of incontinence you have will allow you and your provider to create an individualized plan of action. Many gynecologists are now trained in urogynecology and routinely do this evaluation in their offices.

Stress urinary incontinence (SUI) is the most common type of incontinence. It is diagnosed when a woman loses urine while performing any activity (such as laughing, standing up quickly, or exercising) that increases her intra-abdominal pressure and thus overrides the ability of her urethral sphincter to stay closed. This may result from problems with the sphincter muscle itself or from the fact that the angle of the urethral tube has changed, becoming too mobile to function properly—a condition known as urethral hypermobility. A number of factors that are increasingly common in perimenopause lead to the following situations.

~ Weakened pelvic floor muscles. Unless you work out regularly and include your pelvic floor muscles, then these muscles, like your biceps, may be weaker than they should be.

~ Thinning of the tissue of the outer urethral area, from estrogen deficiency.

~ Nerve damage resulting from childbirth, major pelvic surgeries, a history of radiation, smoking, or excess intra-abdominal fat that pushes the urethra out of the proper position every time you urinate. Innervation of the urethral sphincter also tends to decrease with age, but age alone does not inevitably lead to loss of function. (Research has shown that nerve density in this area varies widely in perimenopausal women.)[11]

~ Underlying neurological disorders such as multiple sclerosis can result in other types of incontinence.

Whatever the exact cause of your problem, there are a lot of solutions besides spending the rest of your life wearing adult diapers!

Nonsurgical Incontinence Solutions

~ KEEP A RECORD. Keeping a record will help both you and your health care practitioner learn which substances and situations may be contributing to your incontinence. Record how often you experience the problem, any activity that precedes it, how much urine actually leaks, whether or not you experience a warning beforehand, if it wakes you up at night, and whether it follows the ingestion of certain foods, drinks, or medications. Sometimes you can alleviate your problem just by becoming aware of when it happens and making adjustments.

Many women also have an increased urinary output on the first day of their period, when they get rid of all that premenstrual fluid. On these days, stress incontinence will always seem worse because your bladder fills more quickly.

⌐ REDUCE OR ELIMINATE CAFFEINATED DRINKS. Many women have stress incontinence only when urine output is increased from drinking coffee or tea. Even decaf coffee is a diuretic—and so is cold weather (I never drink a cup of coffee in the morning if I'm going skiing, otherwise I'll have to stop at the lodge after every other run). Coffee is also a known bladder irritant. I've been able to help some women resolve their incontinence problem completely just by providing them with this information.

⌐MEDICATION. Since there is a great deal of overlap between pure urinary stress incontinence and urge incontinence, many women are also offered medication to relax the bladder muscle. (See section on urge incontinence, page 273.)

⌐STRENGTHEN YOUR PELVIC FLOOR. Many women are able to resolve or greatly improve their incontinence by strengthening the muscles of the pelvic floor and urethra, so that they can withstand increases in intra-abdominal pressure without giving out. Strong muscles in the pelvic floor also increase blood flow and innervation of the pelvic organs. That is exactly what Dr. Kegel had in mind in 1948 when he told his patients to practice vaginal contractions in preparation for childbirth. Ideally, every pregnant woman should be doing Kegels regularly both before and after birth so that these muscles will be strong enough to withstand the rigors of childbirth. When Kegel exercises are done properly and consistently, they work very well, and improve your sex life as well. Kegel exercises actually condition the PC (pubococcygeus) muscle for sexual arousal. They also increase the flow of blood to the genitals, which enhances the ability to reach orgasm and also improves vaginal lubrication. Some studies report that up to 75 percent of women are able to overcome stress incontinence with Kegels alone.[12]

Unfortunately, the vast majority of women who are told to do Kegel exercises are not instructed in how to do them properly and they also give up too soon—which is why so many women think they don't work and why the reported results are so variable.

DEVELOP LIFETIME PELVIC POWER BY STRENGTHENING YOUR PC MUSCLE (KEGEL EXERCISES)

1. Identify the PC muscle. Sit on the toilet with your legs spread apart. See if you can stop the stream of urine without moving your legs, your abdomen, or your buttocks muscles. The muscle used to stop the flow of urine is the PC muscle. This is the only muscle that should be contracting. Your PC muscle will not become stronger if you contract your abdominal, thigh, or buttocks muscles at the same time that you are doing a PC contraction. Check yourself by inserting two fingers in your vagina while contracting. You will feel the muscle tighten around your fingers.

2. Learn the exercises.

   Slow clenches. Squeeze your PC muscle and hold it clenched for a slow count of three. Work up to slow count of ten after a couple of weeks or so. Though it's not necessary to hold your breath while counting, it may be helpful at first to establish your concentration. Release and exhale.

   Quick contractions or flutters. Now contract your PC muscle quickly. Once per second.

   Push-outs. Clench your PC muscle and then push out as though you are bearing down to move your bowels. Hold for a count of three to ten. Note that your abdominals will contract when you do a push-out. Your anus will also contract.

3. Train your PC muscle gradually. Begin training your PC muscle with ten slow clenches, ten flutters, and ten push-outs (one set) three to five times every day. After one week, add five slow clenches, five flutters, and five push-outs to the original ten. That's a total of 15 reps for each set. Continue to do three to five sets a day.

   Add five of these the following week until a set equals 20 reps. Continue doing three to five sets per day to maintain optimal pelvic tone, urinary continence, and sexual function. In as little as a week's time you will definitely notice a difference in your ability to strengthen these muscles. It may take three to four weeks to notice a change in urinary symptoms. You will probably notice a change in sexual responsiveness in a couple of weeks if you do Kegels properly.

Note: You can do Kegels anywhere and anytime: driving, watching TV, cooking, sitting in the bathtub, riding the lift while skiing, etc.

When you start training your PC muscle, you'll probably find that it doesn't want to stay contracted for the entire count of ten. It may also be difficult to do the flutters. That's because the muscle is weak. Don't worry about it. Take a rest during a set if needed. But be persistent. Like all muscles, the PC responds beautifully to resistance training. You'll be amazed by how fast you'll get results if you stick with it. Also, every time you do the exercises, you'll be giving yourself a powerful reminder that you have the strength and stamina to create and maintain healthy boundaries (while also enhancing your sex life! What could be better!).

There's another way to do Kegels that doesn't require counting to ten or focusing on which muscles to contract. In this method, which is based on ancient Chinese techniques (see jadegoddess.com), you insert a weighted cone into your vagina and simply hold it in place for at least five minutes twice a day, gradually working up to fifteen minutes twice a day. You start with the heaviest cone that you can easily hold in for one minute, gradually move on to the heavier cones, and finally shift to a maintenance program. (Cones range in weight from 15 to 100 g.) Holding the cone in the vagina automatically uses just the right muscles. I have been recommending these cones for years and my patients have had excellent results with them, provided there are no complicating factors such as infection, neurological damage, or use of diuretic medications or caffeine. About 70 percent of women can expect improvement or cure within four to six weeks of consistent use.[13] (See Resources.) You can also purchase a highly effective pelvic floor exerciser called the FPT (Feminine Personal Trainer), a stainless steel vaginal weight (see www.aswechange.com, product AG211). I also recommend a progressive resistance vaginal exerciser known as the Kegelmaster 2000, which is inserted into the vagina. (See www.kegelmaster2000.com.)

~ HIGH-TECH PELVIC FLOOR REHAB (BIOFEEDBACK AND EMRT). Biofeedback-assisted behavioral treatment provides immediate audio and visual feedback to reinforce your control of your pelvic muscles. It has shown excellent results, ranging from 50 percent to 89 percent improvement after six to eight weeks. It has been shown to be far more effective for incontinence than medication, and it is generally available from physical therapists specially trained in the technique.[14] The disadvantage is that it requires the use of rectal or vaginal probes. Another technique known as extracorporeal magnetic resonance therapy (EMRT) has recently been approved by the FDA. This device, known as Neocontrol, uses a magnet built into a special chair. Magnetic energy is targeted on the pelvic floor muscles and increased slowly to create a magnetic field. The resonating magnetic flux will, in turn, induce electrical depolarization of nerves and muscles, resulting in contraction and exercise of exactly the right muscles. Studies have shown a 77 percent improvement in patients tested so far.[15] For more information, contact the manufacturer, Neotonus, Inc., at 800–895–4298 or visit the company's website at www.neocontrol.com.

~ ESTROGEN CREAM. The outer third of the urethra is estrogen-sensitive, just as is the vaginal tissue. In post- or perimenopausal women with stress urinary incontinence, estrogen cream placed on the top surface of the outer third of the vagina has been shown to enhance nerve function and blood supply to the urethra, which in turn increases muscle size and strength. About 50 percent of women who have incontinence associated with estrogen depletion will be cured or greatly improved simply by re-estrogenizing their urethral area. This success rate increases for women who also strengthen their pelvic floor simultaneously.

While systemic HRT also works to relieve urinary symptoms, I recommend estriol vaginal cream for this purpose. It is extremely effective when applied locally, and it doesn't result in any appreciable absorption into the bloodstream. That makes it ideal for any woman who is worried about the risks of estrogen, including those with a history of or risk factors for breast cancer. Estriol vaginal cream is available by prescription from any formulary pharmacy that carries natural hormones. The usual strength is 0.5 mg/g.

~ ALTERNATIVE DEVICES. The FDA has approved a variety of urethral prosthetic devices over the past few years. These devices are very useful for stress incontinence caused by urethral hypermobility and are especially good for those women who have incontinence only during specific activities such as golf or aerobics.

The Impress Softpatch (from UroMed) is a single-use soft foam patch that is coated with an adhesive. It is placed over the urethral opening to create a seal that stops mild to moderate leakage.[16]

The Reliance Urinary Control Insert (also from UroMed) is a small, soft balloon-tipped catheter-like insert that is fitted inside the urethra. The balloon is inflated with a small amount of air, so it stays in place. It is removed at the time of voiding by pulling a small string. The device is very effective, although there is a risk of urinary tract infection in some patients.[17] It is not meant to be used during intercourse, though many women find that it works well to prevent incontinence during sex.

Fem-Assist (from Insight Medical) and CapSure Shield (from Bard Urological) are silicone devices that fit over the urethral opening like a suction cup with the help of an ointment that helps seal them in place. The mild vacuum that results gently supports the surrounding tissue and squeezes the urethra shut. Once in place, these devices are concealed within the labia, so they can be worn with leotards or bathing suits. When you wish to urinate, you simply pull the device by the edge to remove it. It can then be washed with hand soap and warm water and reapplied. A single device can be used for a week before disposal. They are available by prescription only.[18]

Some urinary incontinence devices work by stabilizing the bladder base and reestablishing a normal angle between the bladder and urethra. Products available include the Incontinence Ring, Incontinence Dish, and Incontinence Dish with Support (from Milex). Introl's Bladder Neck Support Prosthesis is a silicone vaginal device designed to elevate and support the bladder neck. (You may have noticed that it's more difficult to urinate with a tampon in. This is because the tampon elevates the bladder neck.) This device is meant to mimic the effect of a minimally invasive surgery known as urethropexy, which permanently tacks the bladder neck into place. The device has to be fitted by a physician (there are sixteen different sizes). It also has to be removed and cleaned every twenty-four hours.[19]

Many users of these devices report a heightened sense of self-confidence and freedom. The devices can be used on an as-needed basis and are virtually risk-free. They can also be used temporarily while you're strengthening your pelvic floor muscles.

Surgical Techniques to Relieve Bladder Symptoms

If you've strengthened your PC muscle maximally and still have incontinence problems, then a surgical solution may help.

⁓ STANDARD SURGICAL PROCEDURES. There are a variety of tried-and-true surgical techniques for treating stress urinary incontinence that give long-term success rates of 80–95 percent in the hands of an experienced surgeon. In all of these procedures, sutures are placed in the tissue near the urethra to elevate the bladder neck so that it functions properly. The disadvantage of these approaches is that they require an abdominal incision and a fairly long recovery period.[20]

⁓ MINIMALLY INVASIVE PROCEDURES. A whole host of new surgical techniques have recently been developed to help permanently reposition the bladder neck so that urethral function is restored. They are done laparoscopically on an outpatient basis. Short-term results with the new techniques are also favorable, with a cure rate of about 82 percent. Long-term results are not yet available.[21] In addition, several surgical techniques have become available in the last ten years to suspend the uterus—including laparoscopic suspension—thus "curing" prolapse without removing the uterus. (See Resources.)

⁓ INJECTABLES. A variety of agents, including body fat or bovine collagen, can be injected around the urethra under local anesthesia. These injections increase the volume of urethral tissue, allowing it to close properly and prevent the passage of urine during times of increased intra-abdominal pressure such as coughing, laughing, or change of position. They are effective immediately and can be done as an office procedure. A skin test is necessary four weeks prior to the procedure to be certain that there will be no allergic reaction to the material. It usually takes two or three injections over time to get the desired result, and they may eventually have to be repeated. The improvement or cure rate ranges from 82 to 96 percent, depending upon the type of incontinence being treated.[22]

Irritable Bladder: Urge Incontinence

Some incontinence is caused by involuntary contractions of the bladder muscle (the detrusor muscle). These involuntary contractions cause strong, sudden urges to urinate and the feeling that you might be about to wet yourself—which sometimes happens. Women with an overactive bladder often find themselves missing out on normal activities because they have to go to the bathroom so often and worry whether or not one will be available.

Urge incontinence is commonly treated with drugs such as tolterodine (Detrol) that inhibit detrusor contractions. Side effects include headache, dry mouth, dry eyes, constipation, and indigestion. Though this type of medication can be very helpful, there are other options.

Sometimes bladder irritation is caused by the localized lack of estrogen in the bladder and urethral area associated with perimenopause and menopause. The problem resolves with local or systemic estrogen therapy. Caffeine is also a bladder irritant. As little as one cup of coffee per day can result in bladder symptoms.

Irritable bladder syndrome can also be associated with stressful psychological situations such as taking an exam, being evaluated at work, or worrying about some aspect of your life that isn't working. Many perimenopausal women find that they repeatedly have to get up at night to urinate when their sleep is interrupted by chronic worry or anxiety. In my experience, there is an exquisite connection between the worry-and-obsess area of the brain and the bladder. Happily, we each have the ability to interact consciously with this area and get it to cooperate with us.

Biofeedback-assisted behavioral training, for example, has been shown to reduce involuntary incontinence episodes by about 80 percent (drug therapy results in a 68 percent reduction).[23] In one controlled study, women were asked to keep a voiding diary in which they recorded the time of day of the urgency and what they were doing at that time, so that their voiding patterns and the circumstances surrounding them would become clear. They were then taught how to identify their pelvic muscles and contract and relax them voluntarily while keeping abdominal muscles relaxed (the same as with

Kegels)—a procedure that took only one session. Women were then taught to respond to the sensation of urgency by pausing, sitting down if possible, relaxing their entire body, and then contracting their pelvic muscles repeatedly to diminish urgency, inhibit detrusor muscle sensation, and prevent urine loss. When the urgency subsided, they were taught to proceed to the toilet at a normal pace. Women were encouraged to practice pelvic muscle contraction at home in various positions and also during activities when urge incontinence is most apt to occur. Finally, they were taught to practice interrupting or slowing their urine stream during voiding once per day.

Recurrent Urinary Tract Infections

Urinary urgency and frequency are often the result of recurrent urinary tract infections.

- Get a medical evaluation to be sure that you don't have some anatomical problem that is contributing to your infections. Make sure that the outer third of your urethra is well estrogenized. Your doctor should be able to evaluate this during a pelvic exam, because the urethra runs right under the top part of the vagina and is easily felt and observed. If there is any evidence of thinning of the outer urethra, get a prescription for estrogen cream. (See page 299.)

- Stop all caffeine, even decaf, for two weeks. Caffeine is a bladder irritant. Reintroduce to see if symptoms recur.

- Drink copious amounts of water or unsweetened (or artificially sweetened) cranberry juice the minute you feel any bladder symptoms. The extra liquid helps encourage frequent urination, which tends to flush out any bacteria lurking in the system, and cranberry juice renders bacteria less able to establish an infection in the lining of the urethra or bladder.

- Try cranberry capsules available at natural food stores. Take as directed. Cranberries contain a substance that prevents bacteria from sticking to the bladder wall, thus decreasing the risk for recurrent infection.

- Take a probiotic regularly to help recolonize your gut with "friendly" bacteria. Because the anus and urethra are so close anatomically, encouraging the growth of favorable bacteria in one area of the body also helps the other. My favorite probiotic is PB 8, which doesn't have to be refrigerated.

~ If these approaches don't work, consider a course of acupuncture and Chinese herbs. This treatment works very well for recurrent UTIs.

There you have it. I hope this information has given you hope and some peace of mind about the problem. Don't resign yourself to using adult diapers the rest of your life when so many other solutions are available. You are not alone—incontinence is more common than diabetes. It is also often easier to treat! But you have to take the first step. Ask for help.

9

Sex and Menopause:
Myths and Reality

R emember the first time you fell in love? You thought you had
discovered the moon and the stars. The lyrics of the songs on
the radio seemed as though they had been written especially
for you. And chances are you felt so high and full of life that you
didn't even feel much like eating. When a woman falls in love, she begins to experience an almost overwhelming influx of energy, filling
her with exhilaration, benevolence, vigor, creativity . . . and an eager,
often insatiable sexual desire. She is, quite literally, turned on!

This can't-eat-can't-sleep feeling is not limited to young women
experiencing their first love. It can be experienced at any age, any
time we are able to connect at a deep emotional and spiritual level
with ourselves or another person. Our life force—our desire—is what
makes us magnetically attractive to uplifting people and circumstances. When that kind of connection is made with another, we bask
joyfully in the knowledge that we are two people seeing, and being
seen, as our truest selves. It is intoxicating. But to feel it we must begin with ourselves.

This wonderful feeling of connection is something we have been
led to believe can be experienced only by those in love. Our culture,
through its books, movies, and media images, promotes love and sex
as the major, if not exclusive, route to happiness. But this is only part

of the truth. When we are fully open to the energy that created the universe in the first place—which is another way of saying when we are in love with our own lives—then we can re-create the chemistry of being in love simply by tuning in to the vitality of the world around us and in us. It's everywhere—in the beauty of nature, the pursuit of a cause we believe in, the exercise of our creative powers. Falling in love with and getting turned on by life itself, whatever form it takes, is an experience so powerful that I've known it to cause even women who were well past menopause to start getting their periods again.

In other words, if we think of sexual energy in the largest possible context—as life force, or as Source energy—then the relationship between the two becomes clear: the health and vitality of our sexuality is inexorably linked to the health and vitality of our lives.

THE ANATOMY OF DESIRE

By the time we reach midlife, the challenge for each of us is to be able to access that in-love feeling in other ways besides looking to another person for fulfillment and gratification. The call goes out for each of us to expand our personal repertoire for accessing Source energy in our lives.

Many women who are in the midst of negotiating this step for themselves find that in order to tap into their Source energy directly, they first have to withdraw their energy from the outer world of relationships and work for a while while they do the inner work of reassessing their goals, boundaries, and relationships. With this more inner focus, the sex drive of many wanes for a while.

Though a menopause-related deficiency of hormones most often gets the blame for a drop in sex drive at menopause, the most recent research of sexual function at midlife (which is increasingly being carried out by women) has found that menopausal status, per se, is not related to most aspects of sexual functioning. Though some women report a decrease in desire, less interest in sex, and changes in arousal, research on healthy nonsmoking menopausal women with partners shows that there's no change in sexual satisfaction, frequency of sexual intercourse, or difficulty reaching orgasm.[1]

Researchers have also demonstrated that a woman's perceptions of "being menopausal" may also affect her sexual functioning, especially if she has been led to believe that her sexy years are finished! For years and years, women have been brainwashed into thinking that menopause is the end of their sexual attractiveness. When you have been led to believe that you are no longer desirable or attractive, this belief itself certainly can affect sex drive—not to mention one's body image and self-esteem! Older studies done on women seeking treatment for menopausal symptoms have reinforced this cultural bias. It is well documented, for example, that women who seek treatment for menopause tend to report more life stress, and they suffer from more clinical depression and anxiety and also psychological symptoms than women who don't seek care. And of course, these factors are all strongly related to sexual functioning.

The Truth About Sexual Functioning and Menopause

Sexual function is a complex, integrated phenomenon that reflects the health and balance not only of the ovaries and hormones, but also of the cardiovascular system, the brain, the spinal cord, and the peripheral nerves. In addition, every factor that affects sexual function has underlying psychological, sociocultural, interpersonal, and biological influences of its own. Happily, current research on women and sex is finally taking into account how complex female sexual arousal really is. Consequently the entire concept of so-called female sexual dysfunction is being updated. New research (much of it done by women) is shedding increasing light on how seamlessly psychological states affect biological responses. Finally research has begun to validate what women already know: a woman's experience of sexual arousal is more influenced by her thoughts and emotions than by feedback from her genitals. In other words, her emotions and thoughts must be in sync with the goal of sexual satisfaction for her body to perform sexually.[2] This is very good news! When you learn how to change your thoughts, you can change your sexual response.

~ The truth is that a woman's relationship satisfaction, attitudes toward sex and aging, vaginal dryness, and cultural background have a much greater impact on sexual functioning than does menopause, per se.[3]

~ What was previously called a woman's sexual "dysfunction" may well be a logical adaptation to such things as past negative experiences, pain with intercourse, fatigue, depression, and medication. Or lack of emotional intimacy with a partner.[4]

~ There is nothing about the menopausal transition, per se, that results in decreased libido in healthy, happy midlife women. In fact, the number-one predictor of good libido at menopause is a new sexual partner—even in those women who previously had sexual problems in prior relationships.[5]

~ Genital sexual responsiveness of premenopausal and postmenopausal women doesn't differ significantly.[6]

~ Male sexual function is an issue for many midlife women. More studies need to address the effect of a male partner's erectile dysfunction on a woman's sex life. Many midlife men experience this problem and some are not comfortable talking about it or seeking treatment. (For crucial information on this, see *The Male Biological Clock: The Startling News About Aging, Sexuality, and Fertility in Men* by Harry Fisch [Free Press, 2005].)

~ A woman's overall mental and physical health are more important to sexual functioning than menopausal status.

~ Smoking has a much greater impact on a woman's sexual functioning than her menopausal status. Smokers have decreased blood flow to the genitals and other organs. Toxic substances in cigarettes also poison the ovaries, changing hormone levels.

~ Vaginal dryness is more common at midlife because of the effect of lower estrogen levels on the vagina. As a result, midlife women suffer from painful intercourse more often than younger women unless they are fully aroused or adequately lubricated prior to intercourse.

~ There are significant ethnic and cultural variations among menopausal women. Compared to white women, studies have shown that African-American women have a higher frequency of sexual intercourse, Hispanic women report lower physical pleasure and arousal, and Chinese and Japanese women report more pain and less arousal.[7]

Resolving problems in an existing relationship can have an effect on sex life that's comparable to that of a new sex partner—when a woman makes a decision to have more fun and pleasure with the man (or woman) she loves, she experiences a boost in her life energy, which translates to an equivalent boost in sexual energy. Hanging on to old anger and resentment, on the other hand, quells libido rapidly.

In turn, an active and joyful sex life can have amazingly restorative effects on life force. Nothing illustrates the parallel circuitry between sexual energy and life energy better than the power of sexuality to heal when it is able to express itself freely. In her 1999 book, *Reclaiming Goddess Sexuality: The Power of the Feminine Way,* Linda Savage writes about her experience of recovering from Crohn's disease, a chronic disease involving inflammation of the gastrointestinal tract that can result in weight loss, bloody stools, bloody diarrhea, and an increased risk of bowel cancer. Her weight had dropped to eighty pounds when she met a man with whom she began a very remarkable relationship. Within a few weeks all traces of her Crohn's were gone. She attributes her recovery entirely to the healing power of sexual energy, which is simply one of the many forms the life force takes.

This doesn't mean I'd recommend running right out and having sex in order to heal yourself of a disease. The only way sexual energy can act as a healing force is if you experience it in the context of an unconditionally loving relationship in which your body, your soul, and your psyche are all cherished by another—or by yourself. *Remember, you do not have to have a partner to experience the rejuvenating energy of your own sexuality. You simply have to start thinking of yourself as a sexually desirable woman!*

With all this in mind, it is also important to remember that as a woman traverses the perimenopausal transition and all the changes it invites, her libido may seem to go underground for a time, while she reprioritizes her life and the manner in which she uses her energy on a day-to-day basis. This is a perfectly normal diversion of life energy— an investment that can yield great dividends—but it is only temporary. There is no reason for a diminished sex drive to become a permanent feature in the life of a menopausal woman.

MIDLIFE CHANGES IN SEXUAL FUNCTION

All of the following changes in sexual function have been associated with perimenopause. Reading through the list, you can quickly appreciate that change itself—and not the nature of the change—is one common theme.

- Increased sexual desire
- Change in sexual orientation
- Decreased sexual activity

~ Vaginal dryness and loss of vaginal elasticity

~ Pain or burning with intercourse

~ Decreased clitoral sensitivity

~ Increased clitoral sensitivity

~ Decreased responsiveness

~ Increased responsiveness

~ Fewer orgasms, decreased depth of orgasm

~ Increase in orgasms, sexual awakening

SEXUALITY AT MENOPAUSE: OUR CULTURAL INHERITANCE

Like it or not, our sexuality has been, and continues to be, influenced by a male-dominated culture with an inherent double standard. In a recent best-selling book on how to slow the aging process, for example, the quality of a man's sex life and its purported effect on his health was determined solely and meticulously by the annual number of orgasms—with a figure over three hundred being considered the most healthful. When it came to women, the author never bothered to tabulate or quantify how many orgasms a year could promote longevity. We got points only for being "satisfied with quantity and happy with quality" of orgasms. Happily, the data on women is starting to catch up to the data on men!

Still, the double standard is also apparent in the fact that men can buy Viagra at any of hundreds of Internet sites without seeing a doctor, while women still can't get birth control pills anywhere without a doctor's visit and a prescription. There are even television ads addressed to the one-third of men who allegedly suffer from erectile dysfunction, letting them know they can buy themselves a cure in the perfect form: take a pill and get a reliable erection without having to connect your heart with your penis in any way. It's no wonder the most notorious side effect of this medication is sudden cardiac arrest.

Along those same lines of phallocentric reasoning, I once read about an ongoing study testing Premarin vaginal cream as a kind of "female Viagra" for women whose husbands are already on Viagra. The premise is that women's sex drive decreases at midlife because of vaginal thinning and dryness. Inserting Premarin cream in the vagina, the researchers posit, would result in a re-estrogenization of the vagina, making the experience of sex more comfortable for the woman (who, we assume, is already having intercourse regularly with a Viagra-enhanced penis). When I discussed this study with Dr. Mona Lisa Schulz, her response was: "Applying vaginal estrogen cream to the vagina and expecting this to be the female Viagra is a joke. All you're doing is reducing the vagina and female sexuality to a runway that requires deicing for the plane to be able to take off more comfortably." For most women, sexual desire is related to far more than the estrogenic state of the vagina (though estrogen cream certainly helps some women). First of all, female sexual response depends on adequate and reliable stimulation of the clitoris and its 8,000 nerve endings. This usually cannot be accomplished with intercourse alone. Second, a woman's sexual desire is related to a woman's total being: emotional, psychological, and spiritual, in addition to physical and hormonal. And we are profoundly affected by touch, taste, and smell, as well as emotions. All are part of our sexuality.

I am reminded that our word *vagina* is derived from the Latin word meaning "sheath for a sword." It would appear that we have not come very far in this respect since the ancient Romans. Too many women still see female sexuality predominantly in terms of how well our bodies meet and satisfy the needs and desires of males, rather than ourselves. That attitude, and the beliefs associated with it, finds its way into every aspect of our lives, including the medical research upon which women's health treatments are based.

In a study entitled "Vaginal Changes and Sexuality in Women with a History of Cervical Cancer," the authors note that women who had been treated for cervical cancer experienced changes in their vaginal anatomy and function that had negative effects on their sexual function, including decreased lubrication, decreased elasticity, and decreased genital swelling during arousal. The authors said that the women experiencing these changes reported them to be "distressing," and then went on to make the following observation.

Although numerous studies have documented the distress associated with the loss of a breast, changes in the vagina have been neglected in this respect. A [literature] search performed in mid-1998 with the combined terms "cancer," "breast," and "distress" yielded 197 references. In contrast, a search in which the term "vagina" was substituted for "breast" yielded only 2 references. One might assume that vaginal changes would affect sexual function at least as much as the loss of a breast. An obvious reason for the predominant interest in the breast is that, in developed countries, breast cancer is more common than cancer of the female genital organs. Nevertheless, the paucity of literature on the effect of vaginal changes is noteworthy, and it may not be irrelevant to speculate about nonscientific reasons. For men, female breasts have aesthetic as well as sexual value, which may influence research policies in academic medicine, where male investigators predominate.[8]

Overcoming Cultural Barriers:
The First Step Toward Waking a Sleeping Libido

Although progress is being made, change in our culture's attitude about women and sexuality is slow in coming, and many women have never felt as though they had permission to explore their own sexual energy on their own terms. In *Reclaiming Goddess Sexuality*, Linda Savage writes:

> [Women] want the beauty of the context of sexual encounters to be more important than the act. They want to be touched in slow, sensual ways. They want to be ravished with intense passion that demonstrates how much their partners need them, rather than just needing an orgasm to relax. All in all, women want to be adored as precious feminine beings.[9]

The fact that this need is incompletely met for women in our culture is what drives the multimillion-dollar romance novel industry, with books that have increasingly explicit and very erotic sexual content. Many women are absolutely addicted to these stories, because they invariably show women being adored for who they are, not just for their bodies.

LORI'S STORY: *What I Did for Love*

Over the years, Lori had become gradually aware that her sex life with her husband, Roy, was not meeting her needs. "There was never any cuddling, caressing, nothing to get me in the mood. And he wanted it at least once a day—the harder his day had gone at work, the more he needed it. For him it was a tension reliever. For me it had become mechanical and pretty much unsatisfying." With the help of a marriage counselor, Roy became aware of Lori's needs, and together they learned techniques that opened up a whole new world for them both. "The sex became great," Lori wrote. But Roy's needs for regular "pressure release" after work didn't go away, and to engage in that sort of sex seemed to Lori like a step backward. "To be honest, it made me mad," she reported. "I felt like screaming, 'Haven't you been listening?' " Their counselor, in subsequent sessions, led Lori to believe that to be in a fair partnership, she must be willing to meet Roy's needs, too.

Generally speaking, Lori's counselor was correct. All couples must learn how to compromise in order to satisfy the needs of each person, and sex is no different from any other area of need. But there were parts of Lori and Roy's story that deeply concerned me when I first spoke to Lori, who came to see me about hormone replacement at the age of forty-five, when she started skipping periods.

I wanted to be sure Lori didn't believe that it was her "job" to relieve Roy's tension and stress by allowing her body to be used in this way every day. I validated her anger at this and told her that it was her barometer, letting her know that the problem it signaled was real and needed to be addressed. Second, I suggested that when an individual needs that much sex to medicate his (or her) stress, something is wrong in his (or her) life. I asked if their therapist had suggested that Roy examine his life, his job, and his stress levels. Lori said that she had raised this in therapy but had been told that this was an individual, not a couples, issue. Since Roy had refused individual therapy, there was nothing further she could say on this subject during their sessions.

This is a perfect example of what can happen when couples therapy goes awry. Fully 96 percent of all couples therapy involving heterosexual relationships is initiated by the woman, who usually holds it over her husband's head as a last-ditch effort to save the marriage. He goes in, usually reluctantly, often feeling, "It's her problem, but I'll go along," and unable or unwilling to understand that his own issues are part of the couples dynamic.

Candidly, many therapists have told me that if the man's issues were addressed directly, he'd be sufficiently uncomfortable that he'd probably terminate therapy altogether. So the therapist tries to keep him engaged with so-called couples issues. Too often, the woman's individual concerns also get subverted to the needs of the "couple." This kind of therapy can go on for years, relieving the relationship tension just enough so that the couple stays together, while the fundamental power dynamic of the relationship never changes because key individual behaviors never change. When this happens, there's no chance for the transformational power of true partnership.

To create a true partnership, Roy needed to see that he was using

Lori sexually as an opiate, to medicate himself for stress. There was no way Lori could have a sense of true communion or of being cherished by him as long as stress relief was the main energy driving his lovemaking. Though it would be perfectly reasonable for them to compromise with a "quickie" now and again, for Roy to make a daily pattern of using sex to self-medicate for stress sounded like sexual addiction and dysfunction to me. It was certainly undermining Lori's ability to feel good about their sexual relationship. Roy needed to take responsibility for his own stress reduction needs, and he needed a wider repertoire of behaviors to accomplish this. This might include exercise, meditation, or even masturbation. Though wives have been expected to serve their "wifely duty" in this way for centuries and have acquiesced for fear that he might go elsewhere to "get his needs met," there is no place for these assumptions today if a couple is to reach the joyful communion that's possible at midlife.

At the time of her next annual exam, Lori told me that over the past year Roy had begun to realize he needed to change his job if he didn't want to follow in the footsteps of his father, who had died at age sixty, only one year after retiring from a job he had hated. He had also found several ways of achieving stress reduction, including going to twice-weekly yoga classes and joining a basketball league at work. Thanks to these changes, Roy's blood pressure and cholesterol dropped to normal, and he began to feel better about himself, knowing that he had been able to assert this kind of control over his life and free himself of the pattern that had probably helped bring about his father's premature death. Once Lori saw that he had become more emotionally self-sufficient, she found him more sexually attractive— to the point that she was actually initiating sex.

What Viagra Tells Us About Our Sexuality

Viagra and the enormous publicity surrounding it speak volumes about the values of our culture. There is no question that Viagra and related drugs can be a boon to quality of life for many couples in which the male partner suffers from erectile dysfunction. (Note, however, that new reports link these drugs with an increase in a condition called ischemic optic neuropathy [ION], which leads to vision loss. In October 2005, Public Citizen petitioned the FDA to immediately require a black-box warning on the labels for each of the three erectile dysfunction drugs. If your partner relies on these drugs, take heart—there are all kinds of ways to treat erectile dysfunction with nutrition, herbs, and exercise!) There are also other ways to enjoy sexual fulfillment besides intercourse. Enhanced sexual performance through medical manipulation of the male's genitals only cannot heal a relationship that needs more love and attention or may need to end.

Our culture is quick to forget the holistic nature of sexual function and how profoundly it is enhanced when a couple is truly connected via their hearts and minds. It is well documented, for example, that the excitement and plateau phase of the sexual response can be prolonged if the connection between the man and woman is not only genital but also related to heart and mind. In fact, both men and women are capable of experiencing far more sexual pleasure and fulfillment than most currently enjoy. A first step toward experiencing this pleasure is knowing that it's possible and health-enhancing.[10] At midlife many couples find that they have the time and the desire to be fully present to each other in this way, and as a result they experience the best sex of their lives. This is in part because older, more experienced women tend not to be as inhibited as when they were younger. They know their bodies better. I've heard their stories repeatedly in my office. But for some, making love is just another task on the to-do list. Sex therapist Dr. Patricia Love wrote:

> Sensuality, the ability to be comfortable in one's body, suspend time, and communicate through the skin is what is missing in many marriages. . . . All too often husbands and wives go to bed feeling distracted and numb, reflexively groping for each other's genitals. The unspoken goal is to go from neutral to orgasm in 15 minutes like a car zooming from zero to sixty.[11]

This results in what sex therapists call "spectatoring," which is a mental disconnection during lovemaking, thinking more about work or household chores than about the partner beside them. For the man, this may translate to erectile difficulties; for the woman, difficulty reaching orgasm. The man who looks first to Viagra to "save" him may be discounting the importance of making a deeper connection with himself and his lover. A woman involved with a man who feels he needs Viagra for psychogenic impotence would be wise to ask herself about the quality of their connection. Those things that remain unspoken between them, the issues and feelings that are too uncomfortable to talk about, may be blocking full erection and orgasm, and may also be putting their health at risk in other areas.

VICTOR AND VIAGRA: Ginny's Lament

Ginny and Victor had been married for thirty years and had a pretty happy relationship. Victor had always prided himself on his virility, and he and Ginny had enjoyed a vigorous sex life for years, making love about three times per week. When he turned fifty-five, however, Victor noticed that his erections were not as hard as they used to be, and it sometimes took him longer to achieve them. Occasionally he even found that he was unable to sustain an erection long enough to bring Ginny to orgasm. He and Ginny had gradually slowed down in their lovemaking to about once every two weeks. This didn't bother Ginny, particularly because she was very busy starting a new catering business—something she'd always dreamed of. Her business was taking off, and now that their youngest child had left home for college, her life was no longer focused solely on the needs of her husband and children. But Victor, who was planning to retire in a year or two, was not nearly as happy with his life. It seemed that just as he was starting to slow down, Ginny was taking off in the outside world.

Victor sought a consultation with his doctor, who prescribed Viagra. Victor was elated with the results. Ginny wasn't. The Viagra introduced a "mechanical" element to their sex life that had never been present before. She didn't like having to be sexually available just because Victor had taken his pill, and she began to spend more and more time away from home, partly because she was having so much fun at work, partly because she didn't want to have sex "on demand." When asked how she felt about Viagra, Ginny replied, "I think we were better off without it. I love Victor and it really didn't bother me when it took him a little longer to get hard. I usually knew how to help. Now I feel as though a vital emotional component of our lovemaking has been replaced by a pill."

Their situation is not unusual. Victor's change in sexual function is, in part, related to his sense of decreasing power in the outer world, even though it is his own choice to retire from work. Though Viagra is probably a relatively safe solution for him for a time, I would strongly recommend that he also find a new life's purpose into which to pour his energy. Otherwise he won't be able to keep up with his wife, in the bedroom or otherwise, without resorting to a drug for support. That doesn't mean there aren't valid indications for Viagra. Rather, it is to point out that sexual function is related to much more than the size and duration of an erection. There is also a great deal that men can do to improve their health, circulation, and erectile function. Exercise, an inflammation-reducing diet, and a good supplementation program are the first places to start.

MENOPAUSE IS A TIME TO REDEFINE
AND UPDATE OUR RELATIONSHIPS

Before writing the first edition of this book, I would have written all of this while thinking it did not apply to me. Similarly, many of you may be thinking, "That's interesting, but my relationship with my significant other is good," and you may be right, overall. For many of us, the relationships we have maintained over the years have served us well and have been mutually beneficial, even passionate. But it is very often necessary to renegotiate some of the terms of the old relationship as you enter the transformative years of midlife. No matter how good that relationship may have been, what worked for you in your "previous" life will, in all likelihood, need some updating in order to serve the person you are becoming.

One area in which the necessity for change may become apparent is in the waning of a woman's libido. Just as wild animals refuse to breed in captivity unless everything is in balance in their environment, a woman and her significant other may notice problems in their sexual intimacy if their relationship is in need of rebalancing. Menopause is also a time when what a woman wants from a relationship begins to change. And that change has to start with her relationship with herself.

As we have seen, it has usually been the woman who sacrifices career and personal growth for the sake of maintaining and nurturing the family, even if she works full-time outside the home. Not only the unwritten rules of society but the hormones flowing through her veins encourage her to give high priority to family, nurturing, nesting, and protection of loved ones. At menopause the hormonal changes are only part of a woman's ongoing transformation, which begins at an energetic level and triggers changes not only in her biology but also in her perception, intuition, neural pathways, emotions, creative drive, and overall focus. While she spends the first half of her life giving birth to others (literally and figuratively), everything about her menopausal transition suggests that the second half of life is when she is meant to give birth to herself.

If, through the lens of your transforming self, you discover that you are not in love with your life, your libido may suffer as a result. The same thing may happen if you've given too much of yourself away in your relationship. In fact, a fading sex drive may be one of the first places a red flag will pop up, as a signal of a fading love of life—a waning life force. Only if both you and your significant other are willing to question what is no longer viable in your relationship and work together on the necessary remodeling can you open the door to rejuvenation of your life energy and the rekindling of your passion, sexual and otherwise. Healing will require a bilateral effort—both you and your partner must be willing to ask, and hear the answers to, some difficult questions in order to restore and renew your relationship.

Terminal Busyness Leads to Exhaustion and Waning Libido

Someone sent me the following anonymous posting from the Internet. This one paragraph summarizes the plight of many midlife women—and the difference between their lives and those of their husbands.

> Mom and Dad were watching TV when Mom said, "I'm tired, and it's getting late. I think I'll go to bed." She went to the kitchen to make sandwiches for the next day's lunches, rinsed out the popcorn bowls, took meat out of the freezer for supper the following evening, checked the cereal box levels, filled the sugar container, put spoons and bowls on the table, and started the coffeepot for brewing the next morning. She then put some wet clothes into the dryer, put a load of clothes into the wash, ironed a shirt, and secured a loose button. She picked up the newspapers strewn on the floor, picked up the game pieces left on the table, and put the telephone book back into the drawer. She watered the plants, emptied a wastebasket, and hung up a towel to dry. She yawned and stretched and headed for the bedroom. She stopped by the desk and wrote a note to the teacher, counted out some cash for the field trip, and pulled a textbook out from hiding under the chair. She signed a birthday card for a friend, addressed and stamped the envelope, and wrote a quick note for the grocery store. She put both near her purse. Mom then creamed her face, put on moisturizer, brushed and flossed her teeth, and trimmed her nails. Hubby called, "I thought you were going to bed."
> "I'm on my way," she said. She put some water into the dog's dish and put the cat outside, then made sure the doors were

locked. She looked in on each of the kids and turned out a bedside lamp, hung up a shirt, threw some dirty socks in the ham-
per, and had a brief conversation with the one still up doing
homework. In her own room, she set the alarm, laid out clothing
for the next day, and straightened up the shoe rack. She added
three things to her list of things to do for tomorrow.

About that time, the hubby turned off the TV and announced to no one in particular, "I'm going to bed," and he did.

MARY: *Overcare and Burnout Send Libido Underground*

Mary was a registered nurse. As the eldest of five children from
an Irish Catholic family, she had always been expected to take care of
her parents and younger siblings. When her mother died suddenly,
Mary's alcoholic father, a man in the early stages of dementia, came
to live with Mary and her husband, Jeff, a police officer. Despite having four other siblings, Mary had never questioned her role as the
designated family caregiver. But the increased need for "alone time"
so many women experience at menopause led Mary to feel not only a
total loss of sexual desire, but also complete emotional burnout. She
had recently been diagnosed with hypothyroidism and was suffering
from weight gain, depression, lethargy, fatigue, dry skin, and the desire to sleep all the time. Though her family doctor had prescribed
thyroid hormone replacement, Mary saw little improvement in her
depression. And despite normal estrogen, progesterone, and testosterone levels, her sexual desire remained nonexistent.

When a woman is experiencing caregiver's burnout, her body is
often, quite literally, running on empty. She may have insufficient levels of many nutrients, such as the B vitamins and magnesium, which
contribute to her fatigue. And her adrenal glands may be producing
too much adrenaline and either too much cortisol or, after years and
years of unabated stress without replenishment, too little cortisol.
Either way, the end result is physical exhaustion. Sleep, not sex, is what
women like Mary find themselves fantasizing about. Interestingly,
sleep is often the best way to restore hormonal balance.

I prescribed a program for Mary that focused on her rejuvenation
from the inside out. I told her that she needed to get help at home at
least two days per week. She also needed to improve her eating
habits, cutting way back on refined carbohydrates like cakes, candy,
and cookies and increasing her intake of protein, essential fatty acids,
and fresh fruits and vegetables. I also suggested a high-potency multivitamin and told her she needed to go to bed by ten o'clock every

night and get at least eight hours of sleep per night—preferably ten! Mary had known all along that her life needed to change, but, she told me, she was relieved to finally have a medical authority supporting her in the changes she would have to make if she was going to resume optimal functioning—which would include the rekindling of her libido. If she didn't stem the chronic draining of her life force by getting adequate rest, exercise, and nutrition, then her libido, like every other aspect of her health, would pay the price. It's too bad that so many women who have taken on the caretaker role need a doctor's "prescription" to give them permission to live more healthfully.

HORMONE LEVELS ARE ONLY ONE PART OF LIBIDO

One of my colleagues underwent a hysterectomy (uterus removed, ovaries left intact) at the age of forty-eight, a procedure that is associated with measurable declines in estrogen and testosterone because the surgery compromises the blood supply to the ovaries. This is the reason given for the fact that many women experience some sexual problems following hysterectomy. But my colleague, who had started a new relationship just prior to her surgery, couldn't wait to get out of the hospital and back into bed with her new love. She told me, "When you have someone waiting for you whom you're madly in love with, you can bet you're not likely to have much problem with desire or lubrication, or anything else." And that is exactly what the new research shows. On the other hand, if you are in a relationship that has been problematic for years, a relationship in which you have had little or no interest in sex (perhaps because you didn't know how to get your sexual needs met) but put up with it anyway, you can bet that your body will do anything it can to keep you from having to get back into that position again. It is well documented, for instance, that unassertive women in dysfunctional sexual partnerships experience limited genital arousal and few if any orgasms. Sexually assertive women, on the other hand, report higher levels of sexual desire, orgasmic frequency, and greater satisfaction with both their sexual and marital relationships.[12]

Psychiatrist and neuroscientist Mona Lisa Schulz points out that sexual impulses and desire are controlled, in part, by the frontal lobes of the brain, and anything that changes frontal lobe activity can affect libido—in either direction. Frontal lobes are areas of the brain involved in choosing and directing conscious thought. Frontal lobes can also inhibit unbridled desire, channeling it into socially appropriate behavior. In the frontal lobe dysfunction known as depression, libido is often decreased. But in the frontal lobe dysfunction known as dementia, sexual impulses can run rampant, sometimes resulting in socially embarrassing behavior. An example of this is a nun I once treated who had developed an uncontrollable urge to masturbate all the time. Although she was not distressed by this, her community was. She eventually ended up under the care of a neurologist, for dementia.

Changes in libido can, of course, be triggered by declining hormone levels, especially in women who have undergone medical or surgical menopause.[13] In my professional experience, however, fading life force is equally likely, if not more so, to be at the root of declining sexual desire. Two influences are universally underestimated in terms of their potential impact on libido: the state of a woman's relationship with her sexual partner, and her overall emotional and spiritual love for life. And, interestingly, both of these factors may well have the potential to change hormone levels in and of themselves.[14]

A woman with a strong current of life force, who is in love with her life, who feels sexy, and knows how to turn herself on, can continue to have a strong libido regardless of what her hormones are doing. This fact is supported by research that shows that the hormonal changes of menopause, per se, are not the cause of decreased libido. In fact, the relationship between hormones and libido may be a chicken-and-egg question, as it seems equally plausible for a faltering life force to be the result, rather than the cause, of a dying sex life.

Therefore I want to encourage every woman to consider the health and vitality of her connection with life—her connection to Source energy—along with the more conventionally accepted hormonal issues as she evaluates her sex life and the possibility that it may need help at this stage of her life. I also encourage every woman to update her thoughts about her sexual desirability. It's important to think of yourself as sexy and desirable, even though you may not even be in a relationship right now. Remember, the vibrational quality of our thoughts creates a magnetic field around us that attracts our circumstances to us. A woman who is tapped into Source energy has the power to transform her body-mind-spirit and sexual experience starting with how she feels about herself.

SECONDARY LIBIDINAL SUPPORT:
ESTROGEN AND PROGESTERONE

With all that said, it is possible for a woman to experience a fading libido during and after menopause even if she is involved in a true partnership, one that supports her life force rather than drains it. If a woman is in love with her life, if her life force—a repository for sexual energy—is free-flowing and vigorous, then a weakening libido may be due to secondary, hormonal, or nutritional factors. Factors such as hysterectomy, ovarian removal (or decreased ovarian function), and premature menopause (before age forty) may also have an adverse effect on hormone balance.[15]

As we learn more about the roles of estrogen and progesterone in the maintenance of bodywide functions such as circulation, nerve transmission, and cell division, it becomes clear how declining levels of these hormones may contribute to changes in sexual response in some women.[16]

~ The entire nervous system is surrounded with estrogen-sensitive cells.[17] It stands to reason, then, that a decrease in estradiol levels can have a dampening effect on nerve transmission during sex for some women. Research has shown that estrogen deprivation can lead to actual peripheral neuropathy—a form of nerve dysfunction that makes a woman less sensitive to touch and vibration. Estradiol replacement can restore this sensitivity to levels that approach those seen in women who are still menstruating.

~ Declining levels of estradiol and progesterone can have an effect on a woman's potential for sexual arousal, sensitivity, sensation, and orgasm, because at optimal levels these hormones increase the flow of blood to the sexually sensitive areas. In other words, a woman's physical response to sexual stimulation may be slower and less likely to build to orgasm because of decreased speed and volume of blood supply to the sexually sensitive areas, which may in any case be less sensitive than before because of the nerve dysfunction sometimes caused by estrogen deprivation.[18] It is also completely possible to learn how to maximize sensation in these areas by consciously spending time learning how to pleasure oneself through genital stimulation.

~ Estrogen levels that are too low can lead to cell atrophy in the genital region, which can cause thinning of the vaginal and urethral tissue, with the result that intercourse becomes painful. Women with estrogen depletion may also experience urinary problems such as recurrent urinary tract infections or even stress urinary incontinence.

~ Vaginal fluid production during sexual arousal and intercourse is also an estrogen-dependent process. If estrogen is low, there may be a reduction of vaginal fluid, resulting in vaginal dryness and painful intercourse. Because a woman's level of sexual arousal tends to be judged by the amount and ease of vaginal lubrication achieved, lack of vaginal fluid can lead to the perception that she has low sexual arousal. While sexual arousal may be negatively influenced by the anticipation of pain, libido is not the real issue in these circumstances. Because of the powerful mind/body connection, some women can teach their bodies to lubricate well just by turning themselves on.

~ Progesterone has additional effects on libido that have not been as well studied as those of estrogen but are no less important. Its effect seems largely to be one of maintenance, valuable in keeping a woman's existing libido from declining. Moreover, as a precursor of estrogen and testosterone, progesterone is important for maintaining high enough levels of these other hormones for optimal sexual pleasure. A normal balance of progesterone also acts as a mood stabilizer and supports normal thyroid function, thereby enhancing the libido both emotionally and metabolically.

The bottom line is this: a deficiency of estrogen and/or progesterone can decrease a woman's libido by orchestrating physical changes that, quite simply, make the sex act less pleasurable. Dryness and thinning of the vaginal wall can result in physical discomfort during intercourse, as can vaginal muscle spasms. Changes in nerve function can numb ordinarily sensitive body parts, and changes in blood circulation can decrease the physical response when stimulation occurs, making it ever more difficult to reach orgasm.

Research has shown that libido-dampening effects are most likely to occur when a woman's blood levels of estradiol (our body's most biologically potent natural estrogen) drop below 50 pmol/l. Salivary estradiol levels can also be used, with 1 pg/ml being the lower end of the threshold for normal sexual function.[19] Blood flow to the vulva and vagina is dramatically increased when supplementation brings estradiol back to these levels, and often this is enough to restore sexual response. With the help of a woman's health care provider, achieving this level is simple. Depending on the individual woman, a transdermal estradiol patch (usually the 0.1 mg strength) or 0.5 to 1 mg oral estradiol taken twice daily is adequate, gentle, and consistent in restoring estradiol levels to that comfortable threshold. And in the early stages of perimenopause, when many women have declines in progesterone levels but estrogen levels that are still within the normal range, ¼ tsp of natural progesterone cream massaged into the hands or soft skin twice a day can have a restorative effect on a subtle downturn in libido.

JEANNETTE: Where Did My Sex Drive Go?

"Dave and I have been through some rough times," Jeannette said, "but I really feel our relationship has grown along with us— we're better than ever. The trouble is, I just don't have any desire to make love. I love Dave, I really do, but I could go the rest of my life without having sex and I wouldn't care."

Now forty-five years old, Jeannette had noticed some early signs of perimenopause. She hadn't had any hot flashes or vaginal dryness, but her periods, which used to come "like clockwork," were more erratic, and she thought she might have had some night sweats ("either that or I just had on too many covers").

Hormone testing revealed that Jeannette's estrogen levels were still well within the rather broad limits of the normal range, but her progesterone level was on the low side, and her testosterone level was significantly below normal for a woman her age. After some discussion, we decided to boost her progesterone levels with a 2 percent natural progesterone cream, ¼ tsp massaged into her hands and wrists twice a day. For her testosterone supplementation, Jeannette opted for an oral testosterone pill. Her prescriptions were filled at a formulary pharmacy. "It made all the difference," she reported. "I find that I'm in the mood more often, and even if I'm not in the mood, I can get aroused a lot faster than before."

TESTOSTERONE: THE HORMONE OF DESIRE?

Although much has been written in the popular press about testosterone's role in sex drive, a deficiency of testosterone is probably the least common cause for a woman's waning libido, coming in at a distant fourth place behind relationship issues and progesterone and/or estrogen decline. Part of the reason testosterone has gotten so much attention, however—aside from the fact that testosterone is universally thought of as a male hormone—is its very specific effect.

While estrogen and progesterone play a supportive role in a woman's healthy libido, supplemental testosterone can directly and quickly stimulate the sex drive in both men and women if the reason for the diminished libido has to do with lowered testosterone levels.

Contrary to popular belief, however, testosterone levels do not fall appreciably after menopause. In fact, in most (but not all) women, the postmenopausal ovary secretes *more* testosterone than the premenopausal ovary. Still, testosterone levels do undergo a gradual decline in some women, beginning in their late twenties and continuing through midlife, and it is possible for levels to dip low enough to quash libido.

Sometimes the decline in testosterone—and hence in libido—is sudden, rather than gradual. This can occur following removal of, or loss of function of, the ovaries. The same can happen if the adrenal glands are exhausted. (See chapter 4.) That's because the ovaries and the adrenals (as well as the liver and the body fat) all produce the steroid hormones collectively known as androgens, one of which is testosterone. If you've had a loss or sudden decrease in ovarian function secondary to chemotherapy, radiation, or surgery, then you may find that your libido dramatically decreases because your body has not had time to shift androgen production to the other body sites that make it. Women with this problem often complain of "not feeling like myself anymore . . . it's as if my life energy has somehow gone." And they lose their libido—their sex energy—as well. The reason this doesn't happen to *all* women who lose ovarian function is that some women's bodies *are* able to make the move to other androgen production sites without much interruption in the hormonal output. But for those whose bodies don't adjust as easily, prescription supplemental hormones may be required to restore their androgen levels.

In women with testosterone levels that have declined significantly, for whatever reason, supplemental testosterone often does have the desired effect on libido. Some studies have shown that 65 percent of menopausal women with depleted testosterone who received testosterone supplementation experienced an increase in libido, increased sexual response, increased frequency of sexual activity, increased sexual fantasies, and increased sensitivity of erogenous zones.[20]

However, in my experience, results are completely satisfying only if a woman has a positive view of herself and her sexuality and a healthy relationship. This is particularly true at midlife, when a woman is less likely to sweep resentments under the rug. When her significant relationship is in trouble, testosterone supplementation is much less likely to be effective in stimulating her sex drive.

If, however, you think your decline in libido may be related to lowered levels of testosterone or one of the other androgens, you may want to have your unbound (free) testosterone and/or DHEA levels checked. This can be done through either blood or saliva testing. Ask your physician to submit blood or salivary samples for you, or submit a salivary sample on your own. (Salivary testing is available through a number of different laboratories; see Resources.)

If your levels turn out to be low, your physician can prescribe natural testosterone, available through a formulary pharmacy. Natural testosterone can be used either as a capsule or as a vaginal cream. The usual starting dose is 1–2 mg every other day, gradually increasing if necessary. Another option is to take the nonprescription supplement DHEA at a dose of 5–10 mg once or twice per day. In some women this hormone, which is a precursor for testosterone, will raise testosterone levels sufficiently to improve a waning sex drive. Currently a great deal of study is being done in this important area.

AIDS TO LUBRICATION

Some women at midlife find that, although the spirit is willing, the body is not. Their libido is unchecked, but for reasons they don't understand, they no longer get sufficiently lubricated. There are a variety of treatments that can help with this problem.

NATALIE: Sustaining Ongoing Relationships

Natalie first came to see me when she was fifty-two. Her husband, Brad, accompanied her on her visit. Natalie's health was good, but she had been having problems with intercourse. She couldn't seem to get lubricated before intercourse, which made lovemaking difficult. And she had also had a couple of episodes of urinary burning and frequency that felt like urinary tract infections (UTIs).

As I watched Brad and Natalie interact, it was clear that although Brad was uncomfortable talking about the situation, he was genuinely concerned about his wife. He didn't want to hurt her, but he couldn't understand what had gone wrong with their lovemaking. And both expressed fear that their sexual problem could spread, causing them to become distant from each other in general. I performed a pelvic examination on Natalie and found that her vaginal wall was significantly thinned, which would make it less resilient and more sensitive to irritation and discomfort from the stretching and friction inevitable during intercourse. Her vaginal thinning also explained the UTI symptoms, given that vaginal thinning is associated with thinning and irritation of the outer third of the urethral passage as well. Natalie's exam also showed an obvious lack of natural lubrication, which would make intercourse more traumatic for her and less pleasurable for both partners. Suspecting that Natalie was in perimenopause, I took a vaginal sample and sent it to the lab for what is known as a "maturation index," a test to see how many cells are well estrogenized and how many aren't. I also had her estrogen, progesterone, and testosterone levels tested. Her testosterone was well within normal range, but her estrogen and progesterone were low. Her maturation index confirmed that she had what is called atrophic vaginitis, a term that simply refers to a lack of estrogen in the cells of the vaginal lining, making it thin and inflamed.

I explained to Natalie her treatment options and ultimately prescribed estriol cream for the vagina, plus progesterone cream to be applied anywhere on her skin. By retesting her levels and adjusting her dosage according to how she felt, over a three-month period we established optimal baseline estrogen and progesterone levels for that particular stage of Natalie's life. In a follow-up visit within a month, Natalie reported that their sex life was "back to normal." This is exactly what I had expected would happen. Treating bona fide perimenopausal vaginal dryness and thinning is safe, easy, and very effective.

GRACE: Beginning a New Relationship

Grace was fifty-five when she came to see me for a checkup. Her husband, with whom she'd enjoyed a monogamous relationship for twenty years, had died five years before. Her marriage had been a happy and fulfilling one, and she did not actively look for a new partner after his death. She enjoyed a busy life teaching tennis, gardening, and traveling. But then she was reintroduced to a man who had been one of her boyfriends in high school and whom she hadn't seen for many years. He, too, was widowed—his wife had died several years before. Since he lived in Utah and she in Maine, they began writing letters and calling each other. Her visit to me was prompted by his invitation to come out to his ranch to spend a few weeks. He had told her he wanted her to consider marrying him. Though she wasn't exactly planning on having sex with him during her visit, she wanted to be prepared. Like many women, Grace was worried that her vagina had "shriveled up" from so many years of disuse. I assured her that her vagina was designed to be functional for her entire life, even though it might need some initial help after years of abstinence. (This is not always the case. Women who pleasure themselves in ways that involve vaginal penetration often maintain excellent vaginal function even when not in a relationship that involves sexual intercourse. And of course, many women achieve orgasm and good vaginal lubrication without penetration.)

Grace had been postmenopausal for five years and had decided not to take hormone replacement therapy because her bone density was excellent, and she wanted to avoid any increased risk for breast cancer.

On pelvic exam, however, Grace's vagina looked a bit reddened, and the lining, called the vaginal mucosa, appeared somewhat thin. Sometimes this condition is associated with painful intercourse, and sometimes it is not—it depends on the individual. When women are fully aroused, lubrication is often adequate without hormonal assistance. It was entirely possible that Grace would be able to have intercourse with no problem at all, but on the other hand, given the newness of her situation, I felt it was best if she had a couple of options. Grace agreed that she didn't want to take chances. Though she had not experienced any sensation of vaginal dryness or discomfort for the past ten years, she wanted to be sure that she'd be able to have comfortable intercourse.

I offered three options: vaginal estrogen cream, the Estring vaginal ring, or a very effective and safe nonhormonal lubricant. Grace chose the vaginal estrogen (estriol) cream so that by the time she got to Utah three weeks later, her vaginal tissue would be very well estrogenized and thicker than it now appeared. She also wanted to come back to see me just before leaving so that I could assess her progress. The hormone estriol is a natural estrogen that does not stimulate the growth of breast or uterine tissue as strongly as the other estrogens, estrone and estradiol. It can be given orally as a pill or locally to relieve vaginal dryness. Given locally in the vagina only, it is safe to use even if you've had breast cancer, uterine cancer, or ovarian cancer, or are concerned about getting these estrogen-related problems. Estriol is available by prescription from a formulary pharmacist and has a very beneficial local effect on the estrogen-sensitive tissues of the vagina. All conventional estrogen creams, such as Premarin or Estrace—or estradiol in the vaginal ring called Estring—also work well for vaginal thinning and dryness, but the estrogen in these can act as a growth factor in breast and uterine tissue, which may be of concern if you've had cancer in one of these organs. However, at low doses they don't appear to cause any appreciable problem. Like estriol, these creams can also be very helpful in treating urinary incontinence that stems from localized lack of estrogen.

I prescribed daily use of the cream for one week, to build up what is called the cornified layer of epithelium in the vagina, then one to three applications per week afterward, to maintain the suppleness, resilience, and moistness of her vaginal tissues. I also told her that if she began having regular intercourse, the blood supply to her vagina would increase. This, combined with the repeated stimulation and stretching of her vagina, would result in a much decreased need for the cream—possibly to the point of being able to eliminate it completely, with just a touch of a nonprescription lubricant as needed.

Nonprescription Help with Lubrication

With or without the use of prescription estriol, there are several choices of lubrication available that work just fine for relieving vaginal dryness. Good old K-Y Jelly is available at every pharmacy, though this water-soluble lubricant may not be enough for some, and for others it can form an annoying residue. Other lubricants that work very well are Crème de la Femme (available from Amazing Solutions, www.amazing-solutions.com/creme.html), Albolene (available in pharmacies), and Emerita's Personal Lubricant, which contains a number of soothing herbal extracts such as *calendula* (available at health food stores or Emerson Ecologics, www.emersonecologics.com). A number of herbal remedies taken systemically can also help restore vaginal lubrication: black cohosh, wild yam, dong quai, or chasteberry are good examples. Vitamin E suppositories are effective, too. And many women find that their vaginal resiliency and moisture are restored when they start eating whole soy foods regularly—the higher the daily dose of isoflavones, the more effective. (Note, however, that oil-based lubricants may weaken latex condoms and diaphragms, making them less effective.)

Another approach to vaginal health is to do Kegel exercises regularly to stimulate and strengthen the muscles of the vaginal floor. They're easy to do, and they can be done anytime, anywhere; nobody can tell what you're doing. Studies have shown that in addition to increasing blood supply (which will increase vaginal wall thickness as well as lubrication), these exercises can improve libido by increasing clitoral tumescence and sensitivity and increasing the strength of orgasm. As a happy side effect, Kegel exercises also can help prevent, or reverse, urinary incontinence (leakage). (See chapter 8.)

TELLING THE TRUTH

At midlife, more and more women become comfortable with telling the truth about their sexuality—to themselves and to others. Here are some areas you might want to reevaluate.

- COME TO TERMS WITH YOUR OWN SEXUALITY. All humans are sexual by nature—it's part of being human. Women undergo vaginal lubrication at regular intervals during sleep, and men get erections. But how you choose to express your sexuality when you're awake will depend upon many factors, including your upbringing, your hormone levels, your general overall health, and your level of satisfaction with your sexual partner, if you currently have one. The most important thing I'd like all women to know is that through the power of their thoughts and emotions, they can learn how to turn themselves on and feel more sexually desirable. This change alone can be revolutionary.

- STOP KEEPING SCORE. What is a normal sex life? Only you can answer that question for yourself. To help you find your personal truth about this issue, let me remind you that we live in a society that often confuses quantity with quality. Even the medical profession equates the quality of one's sex life with the frequency of intercourse. This is a gross disservice to couples everywhere, many of whom will inevitably feel they don't measure up. For perspective, you may find it comforting to know that a recent study from the University of Chicago pointed out that it's pretty common for couples to have intercourse three times per month and be completely satisfied with that. Ask yourself the following question, and answer it honestly: if your life were ideal, how much time would you like to devote each week to being sexual—either with yourself or with a partner? Like anything else, what we pay attention to expands. You can always improve your sex life by intending to do so!

- RESPECT YOUR INHERENT SEX DRIVE. Sex therapist Dr. Patricia Love notes that people can be divided into three different categories when it comes to innate sex drive: high, moderate, and low.[21] Individuals with relatively high testosterone levels (high T's) tend to have a higher sex drive than those with lower levels (low T's), while those with low T levels often find that after the initial honeymoon period of a relationship wanes, it takes a lot of energy for them to initiate or become interested in being sexual. Because it's not uncommon for a high-T individual to be attracted to a low-T person, there's a good chance that a couple's sexual appetites may differ from time to time. But this doesn't make either of them "wrong" or "abnormal."

And although our culture teaches us there is something wrong with us if we can't keep our sex life at its original fever pitch, the truth is that the initial emotional and physiological high of a new sexual relationship eventually needs to be replaced by a more consciously created and sophisticated form of passion and intimacy.

~ PRACTICE SAFE SEX. Many of today's perimenopausal women came of age during the 1970s, when, for many, having multiple sexual partners was common. And many were married or in monogamous relationships by the time the AIDS epidemic emerged in the early 1980s. If you've been divorced or widowed since then, you may have little awareness of the risk you face from unprotected sex. You need to know that 11 percent of new HIV infections are among people over fifty, and that from 1991 to 1996 HIV in that population rose more than twice as fast as among young adults.[22]

It is all too easy to assume that anyone you would partner with is probably not infected. You may be a good judge of character, but a sexual partner is only as safe as every partner he or she has ever had. Remember also that there are many other STDs out there, including genital herpes, genital warts, and hepatitis B. Perimenopausal and postmenopausal women are at greater risk for contracting all STDs than are younger women. The decrease in vaginal lubrication and the thinning of the vaginal walls make it easier for microscopic tears to occur during intercourse, creating an entry point for bacteria and viruses.

Safe sex means keeping your partner's body fluids out of your vagina, anus, and mouth until you are certain you are safe together. Body fluids include semen, vaginal secretions, blood, and the discharge from STD lesions, such as herpetic sores. Though most people reduce the concept of safe sex to the use of a condom, it is really much larger than that. It includes being honest with yourself about the risk you face from unprotected sex with a partner whose STD status is unknown to you. It also includes waiting to have sex with someone until you know each other well enough to discuss your sexual history, and such issues as using a condom and/or getting a blood test. Though this kind of conversation is rarely easy, it is a good test of the intimacy that is possible between you and your partner.

~ USE CONTRACEPTION IF REQUIRED. I've seen all too many change-of-life pregnancies in women who were absolutely sure they could not get pregnant and who thought diapers and car seats were out of their lives for good. Even if you are skipping periods regularly, you can still be ovulating. The general rule is that you should use contraception for a full year after your last menstrual period. Obviously, you won't know exactly when that is until you have reached the one-year mark.

TEN STEPS TO REKINDLING LIBIDO

Psychiatrist Helen Singer Kaplan, a pioneer in the field of human sexuality, originated the term "hot monogamy," using it to refer to the potential for enduring sexual passion in a committed, monogamous relationship. Dr. Patricia Love has identified several factors that can help sustain that state of desire. As she explains in her book *Hot Monogamy*, they all interconnect with each other, so that progress in one area will have beneficial effects in the others.[23]

I. COMMUNICATION. Even if you and your partner haven't talked much about your sexual relationship until now, being able to talk easily about sexual changes will become increasingly important. Simply letting your partner know what is going on with you is a good first step, and it can pave the way to discussing adjustments you'd like to make. I also recommend that you read *Mama Gena's School of Womanly Arts* (Simon & Schuster, 2002) and also *Mama Gena's Owner's and Operator's Guide to Men* (Simon & Schuster, 2003), both by Regena Thomashauer. Both books are filled with wonderful, uplifting, and practical advice for accessing your feminine power in a relationship.

2. MOOD. At midlife, women must take responsibility for getting in the mood, even if desire doesn't arise as spontaneously as it used to. A fifty-six-year-old colleague told me that for her, "getting older means *deciding* to have a sex life, instead of being *driven* to it." (For

help in this regard, see "Sensuality," below.) The good news is that getting in the mood is a choice that begins in your mind!

3. INTIMACY. Take time to make the personal connection. There is nothing more conducive to a good sex life than the ability to share one's thoughts and feelings with one's partner on a regular basis. One of the really nice things about midlife is that we often have more time to spend with our partners than ever before. That time can translate into a second honeymoon. One of my male colleagues and his wife went on a prolonged European vacation recently—their first significant time away since their four children were born. When I asked him about the trip, he told me, "We got acquainted all over again. I remembered why I had married her in the first place." Another one of my patients described how rejuvenating it was to be able to make love without children in the house. She laughed and said, "We can be loud!"

4. TECHNIQUE. It takes skill and practice to learn what arouses your partner and what arouses you. Learning to pleasure yourself to the point of orgasm is an invaluable skill when it comes to making love with a partner, because you've already discovered, and can teach, what works for you and what doesn't. If you don't know how to do this, I suggest you read more about the process. There's a great section in the book *Extended Massive Orgasm* (Hunter House, 2000) by Drs. Steve Bodansky and Vera Bodansky. You might also find that a device known as an eroscillator can help (www.eroscillator. com). But in general, I find that overuse of vibrators actually decreases one's sensitivity over time.

5. SEXUAL VARIETY. Both you and your partner need to explore your willingness to add creativity, fun, and novelty to your lovemaking. To help you, I recommend the DVD *10 Secrets to Great Sex* (www.bettersex.com).

6. ROMANCE. You and your partner need to learn how to show love for each other in concrete ways. Flowers, cards, special nights out, and so forth are all part of what it takes to keep romance alive.

7. BODY IMAGE. Patricia Love describes body image as "your inner image of your outer self." Many of us don't feel good about our bodies because we've learned to compare ourselves with the airbrushed, perfect models we see in the media. This is especially true when our bodies start changing at midlife. When we feel bad about our bodies, it is very difficult to be fully present for lovemaking. If

body image is a problem for you, use my mirror exercise: stand in front of a mirror twice a day for thirty days, look deeply into your own eyes, and say out loud, "I accept myself unconditionally right now." Spend time admiring yourself in the mirror. The more you do this the more illuminated you will feel. This may sound silly, but it works—and it can instantly point out to you the areas in your life that need love and compassion. The more you enjoy your body yourself, the more erotic you'll feel. Feeling sexy starts as an inside job with your thoughts and beliefs.

8. SENSUALITY. To enhance your libido, you must be willing to relax and involve all your senses in your lovemaking.

Sight. According to feng shui, the Chinese art of placement, the bedroom should be a place of rest and relaxation, not a place to pay bills or watch television. The bedroom should also be a sensual place. To help make it so, choose bedroom wall and sheet colors with your partner that will enhance the romance of your surroundings.

Many couples enjoy watching sensual movies together. Most women, including me, find that sensual movies need a good sound track, a good story, and good lighting. Some suggestions include *Emmanuelle I* and *II, Delta of Venus,* and *Two Moon Junction.* Many women also like erotic literature, which tends to leave more to the imagination than graphic movies. I personally like the erotic stories compiled by Lonnie Barbach, such as *Pleasures* and *The Erotic Edge.* Anaïs Nin's erotica (*Delta of Venus* and *Little Birds*) has also stood the test of time. Romance novels can also help get you in the mood. Here are two of my favorites, both of which have great erotic sections: *The Valley of Horses,* by Jean Auel, and *Outlander,* by Diana Gabaldon. *Note:* Be selective when it comes to erotic material and make sure that the movies, photos, or books you look at are not degrading to women in any way. Nothing is a bigger turnoff. Lovemaking should be an activity that enhances the well-being and self-esteem of both partners. If you are currently with a partner whose sexual demands feel degrading to you in any way, get outside help.

Smell. Women are more attuned to the sense of smell than men are, and we often prefer different odors than men do. You and your partner will need to be honest with each other about odors one of you might find offensive, such as sweat, bad breath, and the like. Aromatherapy can be wonderful—but you must agree on a scent. Speaking of scent, the science of pheromones, though just in its infancy, is fascinating. It has been well documented by the research of

Winnifred Cutler, Ph.D., and others that pheromones are important sexual attractant molecules secreted by glands in the armpits and pubic areas. When women are ovulating, they secrete a pheromone that increases their attractiveness to men. Men also secrete pheromones that make them more attractive to women. Women who've had hysterectomies may have a decreased amount of pheromone secretion—and midlife women who are no longer ovulating may have the same thing. But the good news is that commercially available pheromones can be added to your perfume or just applied to your skin. Though more studies need to be done, there's enough information (and anecdotal evidence) on the effectiveness of pheromones that I wouldn't hesitate to give them a try and see what happens with your sex life and sex appeal. (See the Athena Institute at www.athenainstitute.com; or Love Scent at www.love-scent.com.) Just remember, feeling sexy is the most powerful sex attractant there is.

Touch. Practice giving each other foot and shoulder rubs. Learn to *receive.* You'd be amazed at how many women have difficulty lying still and receiving pleasure in this way. Practice telling your partner what feels good and what doesn't. Don't forget the clitoris! More than 60 percent of women don't reach orgasm through intercourse. Instead, oral sex or manual sex is necessary, or try the woman-on-top position.

Taste. Many options are available in this area if it appeals to you, such as flavored oils.

Sound. Use sensual music to set the mood. Turn on the answering machine to intercept the phone, make sure that the children aren't around or that the door is locked, and so on. Nothing is more distracting for most women during lovemaking than the fear that one of the children might walk in at any minute.

9. PASSION. Dr. Love notes that it is not possible to be passionately in love with a person you don't know. She describes passion as the "ability to combine intense feelings of arousal with love for your partner." However far we may have strayed from this state, it is certainly a destination to which we can all aspire—an example of what is possible at midlife as our kundalini energy rises to our hearts and we achieve a fusion of sexuality and spirituality not just in our genitals, but in our hearts and souls as well.

10. TAP INTO THE POWER OF PLEASURE. Never forget that the brain is the biggest sex organ in the body. Your ability to choose how you think about sex and your sexuality are your most powerful allies in reinventing yourself sexually at midlife. A woman's desire—her

ability to get turned on—is one of the most potent aphrodisiacs in the world. A woman who feels irresistible and desirable has the ability to turn herself on and thus enjoy a far more pleasurable life. Her life force and enthusiasm are contagious. If you don't currently have a partner, cultivate a sensual relationship with yourself. The sexier and more attractive you become (for yourself) the happier and healthier you'll be.

The two things that block us from feeling our natural desire for all kinds of pleasure, including sexual pleasure, are anger and self-doubt. At midlife, when all the unfinished business of the first half of our lives rises up to be cleansed, it takes great courage to own our anger and use it as fuel to burn through years of self-doubt and self-limitation—whether sexual or otherwise. Deciding to see ourselves as irresistible, sexy, beautiful, and deserving of pleasure is an act of power. Deciding to tell our mates and our children what we want without undue anger and resentment is also an act of power. This is an inside job. We don't need a white knight to rescue us, a new job, or breast implants. We need to know, deep in our cells, that we are worthy of the best that life has to offer—and that we have the power to attract it by making time for and concentrating on what brings us pleasure. The crucible of menopause is the ideal time to allow our self-doubts and anger to be burned away so that we may truly reclaim the erotic—the life force—in our lives.

10

Nurturing Your Brain:
Sleep, Depression, and Memory

T he changes that go on in women's brains at midlife prepare us for living with more wisdom than ever before. This new wisdom gets wired in our brains as we move from the alternating current of our menstruating years to the more direct current available after menopause. As this natural adjustment takes place, we may find ourselves experiencing disturbing symptoms, ranging from insomnia and depression to forgetfulness. Rather than succumbing to the common cultural view that we are about to begin the long, slow glide into senility and depression, we need to realize that the brain changes we are experiencing are usually normal—temporary bumps in the road that can be alleviated when we have the courage to see them as messages from our inner wisdom. No study has ever shown that menopause per se increases one's risk for any mental disorder, whether depression, forgetfulness, or anxiety, unless we are already predisposed to them. Perimenopause *amplifies* our brain and thought patterns, highlighting the areas that need support and change.

Fighting or trying to control mental symptoms with denial, drugs, or even overdependence on mental techniques such as meditation is ultimately doomed to fail. Instead we need to heed the messages behind our symptoms, support ourselves fully with sound information, and, when necessary, be willing to take life-changing action.

Given our culture's love affair with control, this approach takes a great deal of courage and faith. Some women have to go through painful breakdowns before they are ready to relinquish this struggle for control.

PRUDENCE: *The Anxious Siren*

Prudence, a corporate attorney married to a college professor, first came to see me when she became pregnant with her first child, at the age of thirty-four. Prudence and her husband appeared to be the perfect couple, with the kind of dual-career lifestyle to which many of us aspire. Prudence's pregnancy, labor, and birth were normal, but postpartum she fell into a dark depression that lasted for about six months. During this time she sought help from a psychiatrist and went on antidepressant medication for about a year. She subsequently remained stable except for rather severe PMS symptoms such as anxiety, mood swings, and cravings for sweets that lasted from mid-cycle through the first day of her period. Prudence was able to control these symptoms with progesterone cream, diet, and exercise. I never pressed her further to see what was going on in her life that might be precipitating her PMS symptoms. Her program was working, she was satisfied, and I intuitively felt that Prudence was not interested in looking more deeply into her life or her psyche. That all changed at perimenopause.

When Prudence began skipping periods in her mid-forties, she couldn't seem to get a handle on her PMS symptoms anymore. She didn't know exactly when to use the progesterone cream, and her former self-discipline when it came to diet and exercise disappeared. In addition to this, she often found herself unable to get to sleep at night. But Prudence had another worry that completely surprised me: every time she skipped a period, she worried that she might be pregnant. Since her husband had had a vasectomy after their child was born, I knew that something had definitely changed in her life.

When I asked Prudence if there was anything unusually stressful going on, she admitted to me that she was having an affair with a coworker. She said, "I don't know what has come over me. I never thought I'd ever do anything like this. But I feel possessed. When I'm with David, I feel young and wild—as though a part of me has awakened that I didn't even know existed. I'm interested in sexy black underwear for the first time in my life. I sit at my desk, and when I should be going over legal briefs, I fantasize about my next business trip with him. I feel higher than a kite when we're together or even just thinking about him. But when I have to be home and we can't see each other for a while, I crash. I feel anxious and depressed and I can't sleep."

At first Prudence simply wanted my opinion about contraception and also whether or not she should go back on antidepressants or start using sleeping pills. She also wanted to know what effect medication might have on her newly recharged sex drive. Though I agreed that drug therapy of some sort might be an option to help her symptoms, I also wanted to help Prudence make the link between her perimenopausal mental symptoms and her life.

Why was she having the affair now? At first she told me that her marriage was fine and that her husband was a good man. But after a few minutes she broke down in tears and told me that he had not been given tenure at his university and had become more difficult to live with over the past year or so. As is so often the case, Prudence's husband was also going through a midlife crisis of sorts, but he preferred not to talk about it. This was especially difficult for Prudence because her own work life was better than ever. In fact, given her husband's discouragement and apparent depression, she increasingly preferred being at work to being at home.

I asked Prudence what the affair had done for her. She thought it over for a moment and replied, "It makes me feel alive, powerful, and sexy in a way I haven't felt before." Prudence's uncharacteristic affair allowed her to move into a part of her brain—the temporal lobe—that had probably been relatively shut down since her late teens or early twenties but which, as we've already seen, becomes increasingly activated during perimenopause. Neuroscientist Mona Lisa Schulz, M.D., Ph.D., points out that this area of the brain is associated with ecstasy, sensuality, and creativity and that its messages are often overridden by our frontal lobes—the centers in our brains associated with rules, regulations, and conventional morality.

At midlife our bodies and brains cry out for balance. Those who have been overly intellectualized and controlled need to break free and become more fluid and spontaneous, while those who have lived in the moment, pursuing pleasure and creative self-expression with abandon, now need to rein themselves in with more structure and self-discipline if they are to stay healthy.

Though I don't prescribe midlife affairs, I do recognize how therapeutic a passionate out-of-control experience of some kind can be for women like Prudence. Unfortunately, an affair rarely provides a healthy structure for relinquishing the need for control and learning how to trust and work consciously with ecstasy and creativity. Ultimately it becomes another means of controlling joy by allowing yourself to feel it only through sex, and only within contrived, secretive parameters.

I suggested to Prudence that she spend a few months thinking about the following questions, either alone or with the help of a therapist or other professional: Did she love her husband? Did she intend to stay married to him and grow old with him? What were the circumstances that led to the affair? What feelings had it brought up for her? Did she believe that it was possible to feel the ecstasy of the affair in other parts of her life? Was her affair important enough to her to risk losing the life she had built with her husband? Was she willing to see the link between her symptoms and her life?

Prudence told me she'd think about what I had said. She then went to see a psychiatrist for her depression, anxiety, and insomnia. Over the next two years she went through a series of medications, none of which worked for very long and all of which gave her side effects. After having been given prescriptions for Prozac, Celexa, Effexor, Xanax, Valium, Elavil, and Desyrel, Prudence was finally offered Nardil, a monoamine oxidase inhibitor (MAOI), which required her to be on a special diet. After all these attempts at trying to find peace through pills, many of her symptoms were still present.

Prudence did not return to my office for an exam until two and a half years later. Her affair had come to an end, she told me, and she was still married. When I asked her how her husband was doing, she told me that he had found another teaching job but seemed to be just marking time until retirement. When I performed the physical exam, I found a small but distinct lump in her left breast that concerned me. I referred Prudence to a local breast care center for diagnosis and possible treatment. Before she left, Prudence began to sob. Through her tears, she said, "I feel as though my body is totally out of control. The more I try to control my symptoms, the worse things get. I have no idea what to do next." I told Prudence that she had finally reached "breakdown to breakthrough"—a place that, while uncomfortable, is usually the first step toward living more fully.

Prudence is finally working with a therapist to work through the aspects of her life that require changing. Her breast lump turned out to be carcinoma in situ, and she is being followed regularly by a breast surgeon. Her diagnosis leaves her with uncertainty about the future: medical science still can't identify which cases of carcinoma in situ will become invasive cancers later on and which won't. Prudence's body had presented her with a dilemma that simply couldn't be solved with more control or more information. She finally surrendered and knew that she had to take her life and her health one day at a time.

Midlife teaches us a liberating truth: Many aspects of our lives, including our mates, our families, our children, and our jobs, are simply not under our control. True mental health always involves striking a balance between certainty and ambiguity. At midlife the kinds of certainty and control that often served us well earlier in our lives must now make way for another way of being in the world. We must learn to trust our inner wisdom, a reality that we cannot see, taste, touch, or measure—let alone control.

ENHANCING MIDLIFE SLEEP

Midlife women often go through changes in their sleep patterns, not unlike those we experienced at adolescence. Some of us find ourselves needing more sleep than ever, some suffer from insomnia, and some find that sleep simply isn't as refreshing as it used to be.

Unfortunately, insomnia makes the entire midlife transition harder. Insufficient sleep increases our levels of corticosteroids and catecholamines, stress hormones that can, over time, throw off our hormonal balance and depress our immune system. Studies show that 20–40 percent of women have sleep disorders and are far more likely than men to have insomnia after the age of thirty-five.[1] Perimenopausal women often need more sleep than do men of the same age.[2]

Sleep restores both physical and mental energy. Experimental animals have been shown to die from sleep deprivation. Insufficient sleep leaves us obviously drowsy, fatigued, and irritable. We also suffer from decreased concentration, lowered efficiency, decreased work motivation, and a higher rate of errors in judgment. This is why the Federal Aviation Administration has strict rules about how much sleep flight crews require. When we are sleep-deprived, we are more accident-prone, since our brains will fall into "micro-sleeps" that may not be apparent to those around us.

Insomnia Is Often a Message from Our Inner Guidance

At menopause, insomnia and fatigue are frequently the result of unprocessed and unresolved emotions such as anger, sadness, or anxiety, which often accompany the enormous changes of midlife. The brain chemicals that are important for sleep undergo changes in many women at menopause, and they are also profoundly affected by our feelings.

For example, it is not uncommon to be so exhausted emotionally after a fight with a spouse that despite going to bed early and sleeping for ten hours, you still feel tired. One of my patients realized that her insomnia was associated with chronic worry about her daughter's seeming inability to find a career and a living situation that suited her. Her sleep problem resolved when she decided to stop enabling this twenty-three-year-old by allowing her to live at home without making any contribution to the household. She insisted that her daughter find a job—any job—and learn how to support herself in the world.

One of my perimenopausal patients could not understand why she was having trouble sleeping. She said she was not having hot flashes or sweats, did not drink coffee, and wasn't really stressed. I asked her if she slept better when she was not in the same bed as her husband. She said, "Yes. I've noticed that I do." I told her that this was a sign from her inner wisdom. She replied, "But what am I supposed to do? You can't not sleep with your husband." I told her that although I couldn't tell her what to do about her sleeping arrangements, she still needed to be aware of the connection. She might consider sleeping separately for a while. She would learn a lot by how her husband responded to this suggestion. And a new arrangement could open the door to even more intimacy later on.

How Much Sleep Is Enough?

Our inherent biological rhythms are also taxed by the demands that modern life makes on our sympathetic nervous system, which is responsible for keeping us alert. We forget that the electric lightbulb has only been around for a very short time, evolutionarily speaking, and most of us weren't meant to stay up until midnight every night. Taking naps, sleeping late on dreary mornings, or going to bed at sunset are regarded with disdain in our culture. Instead, we worship hyperactive individuals who work sixteen hours a day, and we even brag about how little sleep we get!

In medical school, particularly after lunch as I was sitting in lectures, I would fantasize that there was a bed up on the podium, where I could sleep while the lecturer droned on. Some of this fatigue was from low blood sugar; I was eating too many carbohydrates. But even with a better diet, I couldn't have stayed alert on only five to six hours of sleep a night. Whenever I get too little sleep I feel extremely groggy in the morning and have difficulty getting motivated to do my work. It's important to be flexible and compassionate about our needs when life makes extra demands. Like it or not, what we really need during those times of unusual demands is to get into bed and let our parasympathetic nervous systems restore us. The much-maligned midday nap can be profoundly rejuvenating. Some corporations have even found that the productivity of their employees goes up when they are allowed to nap. Sleep is an indispensable bodily function, as important as breathing and eating. Although physicians and scientists don't really know exactly why sleep is so important physiologically, most agree that it is critical for bodily rest, for consolidation of learning and memory, and also as a way to help us sort out in our minds and bodies the things we have learned and experienced during the day. You've probably noticed how a good night's sleep helps you integrate new information or even new physical skills, like exercise or dance moves that you may have struggled with the day before. When we allow ourselves to "sleep on" something, we're actually allowing ourselves to make connections in our sleep that we couldn't have made before.

Research has shown that our most restful sleep takes place when we are following our internal biological rhythm. For some that means getting up with the sun and going to bed relatively early, between nine and ten at night. This takes discipline, and it may not be your natural rhythm. Think back on a time in your life when you felt clearest and most rested. What time did you go to bed and what time did you wake up? In other words, synchronize your daily clock with your biological one.

Many of my menopausal patients have been dismayed when they find that the amount of sleep that sustained them a year or two earlier seems inadequate now. I personally found that I needed much more sleep during perimenopause than I did a few years before. I knew that this was my body's way of getting the restoration it needed, given all the changes that were happening in my life. During both adolescence and perimenopause, it is a biological truth that we need more sleep than at other times in our lives. It is important for a woman to recognize this, honor it, and get the rest she needs, any way she can. For many, this means eight to ten hours a night. When I've been traveling or in times of stress, I often sleep for twelve hours! And I no longer feel guilty about it.

Tips for Better Sleep

The following are some suggestions for better sleep during peri-menopause. What works for one person may or may not work for another, so you should expect to go through some trial and error. Experiment with such sleep aids as meditation, deep relaxation exercises, listening to soothing music, or sipping a mug of warm chamomile tea. Whatever your routine, be sure to keep it free of "performance anxiety"—don't think about how few hours of rest you'll get if you don't fall asleep right away, don't look at the clock, and above all don't give in to your mental to-do list and get busy. You might end up establishing a night-owl habit that will be that much harder to break in the long run.

~ COOL YOUR HOT FLASHES. Hot flashes and night sweats are by far the most common reasons for sleep deprivation during menopause. Unless you're able to grab a nap during the day, your first priority should be to cool your hot flashes so that you can get the rest you need at night.

As I've explained, hot flashes and night sweats are triggered by neurotransmitter changes in the brain that result, in part, from erratic estrogen levels or by wide deviations in the balance between estrogen and progesterone levels (even when total estrogen is normal). In addition to maintaining hormonal balance, progesterone also has a calming effect on the central nervous system, particularly on the brain.[3] It follows, then, that unbalanced estrogen can be a cerebral irritant, affecting the body in much the same way as adrenaline.

Sleep disturbances are one of the most common reasons that I recommend natural progesterone cream, estrogen replacement, acupuncture, or herbal remedies (alone or in combination) to help a woman stabilize her hormone levels. But keep in mind that erratic hormones are not the only factor in sleep disturbances. Hot flashes are also exacerbated by underlying unresolved stress and anxiety and the unfinished business that fuels these symptoms.

~ EAT FOR BETTER SLEEP. High blood sugar and insulin are often associated with poor sleep because they result in cellular inflammation throughout the body—including the brain. Following the diet outlined in chapter 7 (and adding foods like soy) will often result in a good night's sleep. The number-one rule of thumb is: do not go to bed on a full stomach. Lying horizontal when your stomach is full can cause gastric reflux, which occurs when pressure from the stomach's contents overwhelms the lower esophageal sphincter and food (or stomach acid) comes back up the esophagus. The result is heartburn, sour stomach, a bad taste in the mouth, and, possibly, asthma-like respiratory distress. The ideal is to wait three hours after eating before going to bed (or reclining on the couch).

On the other hand, a carefully chosen snack before going to bed can be good for you. A snack that is relatively high in protein and low in carbohydrates, or high in complex (unrefined) carbohydrates, is usually well tolerated. This would include fresh fruit, cheese, brown rice, a baked potato, lean meat, tofu, or cottage cheese. Notice what this list does not include: a Ring Ding, cookies, leftover pie, brownies, pizza, ice cream, Oreos, or potato chips. Refined and processed foods simply do not promote rest, relaxation, and the sort of deposits that need to be made in your health bank while you're rejuvenating yourself for the next day.

Taking antioxidant supplements twice a day can also support refreshing sleep.

~ AVOID CAFFEINE. Even one cup of coffee in the morning can disrupt sleep that night. Caffeine is cleared from the system much more slowly in women than in men. In addition to its effects on the central nervous system, caffeine, especially in coffee, is a bladder irritant: it will wake you up at night to urinate.

~ AVOID ALCOHOL. Alcohol is a sedative, but it also disrupts the brain-stem sleep mechanism, resulting in rebound insomnia—meaning that you are more apt to awaken in the middle of the night because your body will need more sedative to get back to sleep.

~ GET REGULAR EXERCISE. Among a host of other benefits, regular exercise improves one's ability to get a good night's sleep. However, vigorous exercise within three to six hours of bedtime is counterproductive. The increased activity boosts the metabolism and stimulates the central nervous system, making restful sleep more difficult to achieve. Relaxation exercises, on the other hand, such as hatha yoga and meditation, can be very helpful. Experiment with your own body's response to before-bed activities. As a general rule, the hour or two prior to bedtime is best spent winding down.

~ SLEEP IN THE DARK. Electric lights, headlights of passing autos, even moonlight streaming through your window can disrupt a good night's sleep. If lack of pure darkness is disturbing your sleep, pull your shades down and make sure that you can't read the face of your alarm clock. Seeing what time it is can cause anxiety if you have a tendency toward insomnia. You might want to try wearing an eye pillow, as I do, if I'm in a place where I can't make the room dark. For added comfort, I scent mine with calming lavender oil.

~ COVER YOUR BEDROOM MIRRORS AT NIGHT, OR REMOVE THEM. If you have mirrors in the bedroom that you can see when lying down, they can be a deterrent to sleep. The reflections in them can make you feel jumpy and unsafe. According to the principles of feng shui, the ancient Asian art of working with the environment, mirrors enliven a room and increase the energy flow in it. Obviously, this is exactly the opposite of what you want in a place designed for sleep and relaxation. One solution is to put curtains over your mirrors that can be drawn back during the day.

~ DEVELOP, AND ADHERE TO, A GOING-TO-SLEEP RITUAL. Sleep aids such as melatonin, valerian, and other natural remedies (see page 319) can be great for getting you through several restless nights, but you also need to establish and adhere to a going-to-sleep ritual based on good overall sleep habits. This is known in the trade as "good sleep hygiene."

First, count backward from your preferred wake-up time to establish a bedtime that gives you sufficient sleep. Keep to this bedtime every day, even on weekends, so that your body clock can stabilize.

Get out of your regular clothes and into something more comfortable (even your pajamas) up to a half hour before sleep, to give your body the signal that it's time to start winding down. Do your bathroom rituals at least half an hour before bedtime, too, including brushing your teeth, washing your face, and taking bedtime medications, so you can go straight to bed without reawakening yourself with these tasks.

~ BE YOUR OWN EDITOR. Don't read, watch, or listen to anything that might be disturbing before bedtime (especially the 11:00 P.M. news), because this can activate your sympathetic nervous system, thereby taking the rest-and-rejuvenation functions of the parasympathetic nervous system offline. (When I went to see the movie *Titanic* with my kids, I couldn't sleep that night because of visions of freezing, drowning victims.) Also, please get the television out of the bedroom. On an energetic level, even having a television hooked up in your bedroom means that you are only a switch away from all the worries of the world.

~ AVOID EMOTIONALLY STRESSFUL DISCUSSIONS OR POTEN-TIALLY DIFFICULT PHONE CALLS NEAR BEDTIME. For some, however, an urgent unresolved issue with a loved one will result in a sleepless night. The point here is to know yourself and consciously decide which approach works best for you.

~ GET THE GERBIL WHEEL OUT OF YOUR HEAD. One of the most common sleep detractors is the gerbil-wheel-in-the-head syndrome: stewing over worries, things not said, things not done, or things on the docket for tomorrow. When I get into one of these states, I get out of bed, take a couple herbal tinctures known as Amantilla and Babuna (see page 319), step into a warm bath, and read a good book. Then, when I am sleepy, I consciously send God's love into my sleep and into my dreams. After about a half hour I go back to bed, and I don't look at the clock.

~ PUT YOUR WORRIES TO BED. Another way to get rid of the gerbil wheel is to write down everything that is bothering you just before you turn out the light. Then turn your worries over to the higher power of your choice, asking this power to guide you toward solutions to your problems while you sleep. Then imagine that when you wake up the next morning you'll have a healthier perspective and be inspired to the right action to change your situation for the better.

~ IMPROVE YOUR SLEEPING SURFACE. Many people try to get a good night's sleep using mattresses that have lost their support years before. You spend about one-third of your life asleep. Make sure you support yourself well when doing so.

Prescription Sleep Medications: Caution

Use prescription sleep medication sparingly if at all. Many health care practitioners prescribe sleep medications such as Lunesta and Ambien very freely. (Ambien was the 26th most commonly prescribed drug in 2003.) Other sleep medications are of the benzodiazepine class of drugs, such as diazepam (Valium), lorazepam (Ativan), and temazepam (Restoril). All of these drugs work in conjunction with the GABA receptors in the brain to produce a calming effect. All are habit-forming and lose their effectiveness over time as the brain builds up tolerance, so that you need more and more to get the same effect. I've seen many older women who were prescribed Valium for anxiety and insomnia during their perimenopausal years and who were still addicted to it thirty years later. These drugs have their place, but don't use them for longer than 7 to 10 consecutive days.

Other medications that can initially help sleep problems include the SSRI antidepressants such as fluoxetine (Prozac), venlafaxine (Effexor), and sertraline (Zoloft). Like the benzodiazepines, these can also lose their effectiveness over time.

Over-the-counter sleep remedies such as diphenhydramine (Sominex or Benadryl) interfere with the production of the brain chemical acetylcholine, which is very important for memory. Over time, the use of these drugs can cause serious memory problems and confusion.

Natural Sleep Aids

NATURAL PROGESTERONE: Try ¼–½ teaspoon 2 percent natural progesterone skin cream at bedtime. Natural progesterone also binds to the GABA receptors in the brain and has a calming effect. Addiction to its brain effects is very rare but has been reported; I've only seen it in one patient in more than twenty years of practice.

AMANTILLA AND BABUNA: Amantilla and Babuna are natural medicines, originating from the valerian plant (*Valeriana officinalis*) and the flower of the manzanilla plant (*Matricaria recutita*, commonly known as chamomile) respectively. In a double-blind, randomized, placebo-controlled multicentered study of these two herbal medicines, patients received 15 drops of each or of both together, administered thirty minutes before sleep. Amantilla was 82.5 percent effective in helping patients sleep, while Babuna was 68.8 percent effective.[4] I personally take Babuna (15 drops) thirty minutes before I go to sleep when I'm keyed up or anxious, and then I follow it with Amantilla (15 drops) just before turning off the lights. What I like about these tinctures is that they have no side effects. (See Resources.)

VALERIAN: Studies comparing valerian to small doses of the benzodiazepines and barbiturates have shown that it is just as effective in inducing sleep and preventing nighttime awakening, but without inducing morning sleepiness.[5] Valerian has a very bad taste, so I recommend taking it in capsule form. Dosage is 150–300 mg of a product standardized to 0.8 percent valerenic acid at bedtime.

MELATONIN: The hormone melatonin is secreted by the brain's pineal gland in response to cycles of light and darkness. It produces drowsiness. Our natural melatonin secretion is affected by depression, shift work, seasonal affective disorder, and jet lag, and supplemental melatonin can often help the sleep problems associated with these conditions. The usual dose is 0.5–3.0 mg taken an hour before bedtime. If you are a shift worker, you can maintain a normal sleep pattern by taking melatonin about an hour before going to bed—even if bedtime occurs in the middle of the day. Melatonin also helps reset your biological clock if you have to go on a new sleep/wake cycle.

5-HTP: Melatonin is made from the precursor molecule 5-HTP (5-hydroxytryptophan), which has also been found to be very effective for treating sleep disorders, as well as PMS and seasonal affective disorder. It is safe and widely available. The starting dose is usually 100 mg three times per day. This can be very gradually increased over several months' time to a dose of 200 mg three times per day.[6] *Note:* Even natural substances such as valerian and natural progesterone may eventually lose their effectiveness over time, because they bind to the same place in the brain as prescription sleep drugs. It's best to use them sparingly, and only after you've tried other routes to a good night's sleep.[7]

DEPRESSION: AN OPPORTUNITY FOR GROWTH

Twenty-five percent of women will suffer from at least one major depression in their lifetimes. Women receive the vast majority of prescriptions for drugs like Elavil and Prozac.

But contrary to popular myth and medical opinion of the past, depression is *less* common among middle-aged women compared to women of other ages.[8] Having said that, there are still a significant number of women who experience midlife depression or an exacerbation of underlying depression when they enter midlife. Dr. Gladys McGarey, a family physician and friend of mine who has been in practice for over forty years, told me that before hormone replacement and antidepressant medication, she sometimes saw women who negotiated the change by closing the door and taking to their beds, leaving their families to care for all the details of daily life. Months later, many emerged from the chrysalis of depression rejuvenated and ready to face the second half of their lives. By then, of course, their families' expectations about their roles and duties had also been transformed.

Fortunately, there's now a great deal more that can be done to support women's bodies through midlife depression. If you are depressed, it is crucial that you take action to get help. Depression can rob you of the pleasure of your achievements or the initiative to make changes for the better. It is also an independent and highly significant risk factor for both coronary artery disease and osteoporosis.[9]

Remember that depression, sadness, or anger often accompanies the emotional growth spurt that our psyches are undergoing. Just knowing this is sometimes all that is necessary to get you past the dark days. Sometimes outside help in the form of diet, herbs, or even antidepressant medications is needed. Before you can decide what action to take, you need to ask yourself the following questions.

- Am I depressed? (Depression often is masked as unexplained symptoms such as chronic pain, constipation, headache, mood swings, or backache.)
- What is my depression related to?
- Would medication help me?

The discussion below may help you to answer them.

The Anatomy of Depression

Depression exists on a spectrum, from the blues, which go away on their own, to the normal grief following a loss, to a more persistent and dangerous disorder. In major depression, as defined by psychiatric handbooks, a person not only suffers from depressed mood, but also has changes in appearance, behavior, speech, perception, and thoughts. When you are depressed, your insight and judgment can be affected, as can your ability to work, take care of yourself, and function in society. Depressed people may appear sad or have an expressionless face. Poor posture and grooming are sometimes evident. If you are depressed, you may derive very little enjoyment from normal daily activities, and you may begin to complain about numerous physical aches and pains that never bothered you before. (Statistics gathered at centers for chronic pain show that up to 90 percent of those with chronic pain have emotional stress factors such as depression that contribute significantly to their pain syndromes.)[10] Depression is often accompanied by sleep disturbances: you may be unable to get out of bed, or you may suffer from insomnia or early-morning awakening. Appetite disturbances—either overeating or loss of appetite—can result in significant weight gain or loss. Your thoughts can be affected by depression, and you may have difficulty concentrating and remembering things. (Many midlife women blame their memory loss on aging when it's really caused by depression.)[11] Your mind can go around and around in circles, and you may dwell on thoughts of guilt, self-blame, hopelessness, helplessness, and worthlessness. As depression deepens, thoughts of death and suicide can occur.

If you recognize yourself in this description, I urge you to consult a physician or licensed mental health practitioner without delay. You and your practitioner will be able to evaluate whether or not you are suffering from a major depressive disorder and whether or not you need medication and professional assistance to work through the backlog of unfinished emotional business that may be contributing to it. Now is the time to address your unmet needs. Treatment can be lifesaving.

Depression and Hormone Replacement

All sex hormones, including progesterone, estrogens, and androgens, can affect mood, memory, and cognition in complex and interrelated ways. Receptor sites for these hormones are found throughout the brain and nervous system, and nerve tissue itself has been found to produce them. Estrogen, the hormone that predominates during the first half of the menstrual cycle, has been shown, for example, to increase mood-enhancing beta-endorphins in menopausal women as well as in cycling women.[12] It has also been shown to boost levels of serotonin and acetylcholine, neurohormones that are associated with positive mood and normal memory.[13] Though androgens such as testosterone have not been as well studied as estrogen, they, too, appear to be associated with improvements in mood and vitality in some cases.[14] Given this, it's not surprising that many women report they feel better when they take some kind of hormone replacement. One of my colleagues tells me that she needs just a small amount of estrogen (less than 1 mg of estradiol twice per week) to keep her from getting the blues. As a physician, she swears by this. When the dosage of estrogen or androgen is too high, however, women often report adverse CNS effects such as headache and increased anxiety. Synthetic progesterone is frequently associated with depression in women. Bioidentical progesterone only rarely has this effect. The general consensus at this time, given the WHI study results, is that there's not enough data to recommend HRT as a primary treatment for depression. But I feel it is definitely worth considering in many women.

IRIS: A Cloud Descends at Midlife

Iris first came to see me when she was fifty-one. She had not had a period in six months. Iris was a very slim, attractive, healthy woman who exercised regularly, took nutritional supplements, and had a fulfilling career. She told me that starting about a year previously, a cloud had come over her mood, and she couldn't shake it. She couldn't pinpoint any particular life crises or other changes that might have precipitated her dark mood. Since her estrogen and progesterone levels were low, we decided to give estrogen replacement with natural progesterone a try.

When Iris came back two months later, she looked like a different person. She told me, "Within a few days of taking the estrogen and progesterone I felt like the lights went back on in my head."

Iris continued to feel better for the next two years. But then her depression returned despite the hormone therapy. Iris told me that she had begun to have flashbacks and memories of sexual abuse from early childhood. In retrospect, she realized that these memories had begun to surface during perimenopause. Though she had tried to ignore them and get on with her life, she felt that they had finally culminated in depression, which she was initially able to quell with estrogen and progesterone. When even that stopped working, she realized that "the only way out was through." She had to be willing to allow her body to feel and her brain to know what had happened to her as a child so that she could finally release the pain she'd been holding on to for a lifetime.

Iris consulted a skilled art therapist, who helped her work actively with her dreams and the creative process. She also signed up for a series of weekly full-body massages, which helped her release muscle tension. She later told me, "I was so surprised when the tears came the first time the massage therapist touched me. But I felt safe and secure, and she intuitively knew enough to simply let me do what my body needed to do. I just lay there and let myself feel everything. I let myself sob."

Within six months, Iris's depression lifted completely and has not returned. She continues with her hormone replacement because it feels right for her. Many times, depression lifts only when a woman gets in touch with her anger, anger that may have been suppressed by "niceness" for years. Anger is always preferable to depression because it mobilizes us and leads to change. It's a stage, not a destination. But I can assure you, it's a very powerful stage that can be liberating and life-giving!

Treating Depression: The Conventional Approach

Today, antidepressant drugs are usually the first treatment offered if you are suffering from depression. The popular drugs fluoxetine (Prozac), citalopram (Celexa), escitalopram (Lexapro), paroxetine (Paxil), and sertraline (Zoloft) work, in part, by increasing the availability of the neurotransmitter serotonin in your brain. (Together with a number of related drugs, they are classed as selective serotonin reuptake inhibitors, or SSRIs.) Another commonly prescribed group of drugs, the tricyclic antidepressants, have been used successfully for many years. Tricyclics include imipramine (Tofranil) and amitriptyline (Elavil).

Despite their helpfulness, however, you need to know that antidepressant medications, like any drug that alters brain chemistry, may have side effects that can be quite troublesome. Prozac and other SSRIs can cause nausea, loss of appetite, headache, nervousness, insomnia, restless leg syndrome, and difficulties with libido and sexual dysfunction. The tricyclic antidepressants can cause blurred vision, dizziness, dry mouth, heart rate disturbances, constipation, and difficulties with memory. You may have to try a different drug or dosage level in order to find the one that works best for you.

Despite these difficulties, a six-month trial of antidepressant medication is worth considering if you feel miserable and stuck. Optimally, the medicine will result in a gradual lifting of your depression. This will give you the energy to mobilize your own resources to make positive changes in your life.

To support your treatment, I recommend the following.

~ STOP DRINKING. Alcohol consumption can make depression particularly persistent. This is partly because alcohol is itself a depressant, and partly because women too often use alcohol as a way to suppress their feelings.

~ ENGAGE IN REGULAR EXERCISE. Exercise changes brain chemistry by increasing beta-endorphins, lowering catecholamines, and increasing monoamines, and both aerobic and nonaerobic forms have been shown to be helpful in individuals with mild to moderate depression. (In some studies, 50 percent of people with depression were cured with exercise alone.)[15] Exercising twenty to thirty minutes per day four to five times per week can have a significant positive effect on your mood. It doesn't matter what you do—even dancing around the house to the radio will help.

~ GET OUTSIDE IN THE NATURAL LIGHT AS MUCH AS YOU CAN. This helps combat seasonal affective disorder (SAD) and raises your brain levels of serotonin naturally. In the winter, you may need a light box or full-spectrum lightbulbs to get enough light. (See Resources.)

~ TAKE A GOOD MULTIVITAMIN THAT SUPPORTS YOUR BODY AND BRAIN, AND MAKE AN EFFORT TO EAT WELL. If you are to function optimally, it is important that your brain gets balanced levels of serotonin, essential fatty acids (particularly omega-3 fats), and glucose. Avoid refined carbohydrates, eat protein at least three times a day, and be sure to include a source of omega-3 fat in your diet regularly. Eating balanced amounts of complex carbohydrates (with protein) provides the body with appropriate amounts of tryptophan, a building block of serotonin. (See chapter 7.)

~ AVOID FREQUENT CONSUMPTION OF CAFFEINATED BEVERAGES AND REFINED SUGAR. There is evidence to suggest that they may play a role in recurring depression.

~ BE SURE TO GIVE YOUR MEDICATION A CHANCE TO WORK. Half of those who stop their medication within three months of starting get depressed again. To avoid this, it's a good idea to stay on your medication for a minimum of six months, if your depression is severe enough to warrant this approach in the first place.

~ TRY HEALTHY ALTERNATIVES TO PSYCHOTROPIC DRUGS. (See "Supplements to Combat Depression," page 328.)

Antidepressants Do Not Cure Depression

Many experts believe that depression is a recurrent disease. Of the patients who experience a major depression, 50–85 percent have additional episodes after they are successfully treated. Studies have shown that about 80 percent of people on antidepressants have a recurrence within three years after stopping medication.[16] Though these statistics seem grim, they would be much less so if all of us were willing to take a good look at what depression really is.

All too often antidepressants are given in a vacuum, as though depression were just a "Prozac deficiency." But depression is not a simple chemical disorder that lands on you when you least expect it. And depression is not a natural human condition. Studies have shown that depression is virtually nonexistent among many indigenous peoples. Depression is a consequence of how we live our lives. To get over it, we must be willing to make some changes that will support healthy brain biochemistry. Otherwise, depression is likely to recur. Antidepressant medication and getting help are associated with a very significant placebo effect. When you feel you are getting help, your body naturally gets better. I have never prescribed antidepressants of any kind unless my patient was also willing to enter some kind of therapeutic relationship with a counselor to help her sort out the aspects of her life that needed improvement. In other words, we, as a society and as individuals, need to understand that getting on the right medication does not guarantee a cure for depression.

Like all symptoms, depression is one way your body's inner wisdom tells you that something in your life is out of balance. Often its message is that a part of you has ceased to grow or has stagnated, or that you have lost the passion for living that is a natural part of being alive. It may also be a hint that you are angry with someone but do not feel free to express that anger directly. Depression may result from unresolved loss and grief over the loss of a loved one through separation or death.

The best cure for depression that I know is to be completely honest with yourself about everything you are feeling—even, and especially, those feelings you've been told you shouldn't have, such as jealousy, anger, guilt, sorrow, and rage. All of these feelings are part of being human. They will never hurt you if you simply acknowledge them, express them safely, and, ultimately, accept yourself for having them. Then you must take action. I've never seen depression lift without the sufferer taking some kind of positive action to help herself. This could be as simple as volunteering at an animal shelter.

In my experience, staying in dead-end jobs and/or relationships is a major factor associated with unremitting, chronic depression in women. If you feel depressed and "dead," and this has been going on for six months or more, it is probable that either you have unresolved grief about an important loss in your life or you have anger or resentment or resignation about continuing to participate in relationships or jobs that do not replenish you at the deepest levels. Many women at midlife finally have enough ego strength, life skills, and support systems in place to safely feel and release the unacknowledged pain of their pasts. For those who are finally willing to do this kind of work, depression and other symptoms may be alleviated rather quickly. There is no medication, supplement, exercise, or herb that will cure this problem. However, they *can* be a valuable support as you work on the problems that are preventing you from moving forward in your life.

I'd suggest that you consider an antidepressant medication if any of the following describe you.

~ You've had three or more episodes of depression.

~ You have suffered from low-level depression your whole life and have also had a major depressive episode (called double depression).

~ You have leftover symptoms after going off an earlier course of antidepressants.

~ You are having your first depression at midlife or later.

Are Antidepressants Safe?

There are apt to be side effects from the long-term use of any drug that alters brain chemistry, and many of the popular psychotropic drugs on the market today are too new for anybody to say with authority that they are safe in the long run. Candace Pert, the scientist who discovered the receptor sites for many important chemicals in the brain associated with mood, commented:

I am alarmed at the monster that Johns Hopkins neuroscientist Solomon Snyder and I created when we discovered the simple binding assay for drug receptors 25 years ago. Prozac and other antidepressant serotonin-receptor-active compounds may also cause cardiovascular problems in some susceptible people after long-term use, which has become common practice despite the lack of safety studies.

The public is being misinformed about the precision of the SSRIs [Prozac, fenfluramine (part of fen-phen), Zoloft, Paxil, Zyban, etc.] when the medical profession oversimplifies their action in the brain and ignores the body as if it exists merely to carry the head around.[17]

I couldn't agree more, especially in light of a PMS drug that has been heavily marketed to women. This drug, Sarafem, *is simply Prozac under a new guise* and with a new indication—an indication guaranteed to support women's continued mistrust of their body's wisdom.

Think of psychotropic drugs as a bridge to help you cross a particularly rough stream in your life. But don't plan to live on that bridge for good. The true cure for depression lies in learning the skills associated with full emotional expression and then taking positive action.

Supplements to Combat Depression

If you prefer to try alternatives to prescription medications, the following vitamins, herbs, and other supplements have demonstrated clinical effectiveness. (Remember to follow the lifestyle suggestions on pages 324–325, as well.) Do not combine them with prescription medications without consulting your physician.

VITAMINS AND OTHER NUTRIENTS: Deficiencies of biotin, folic acid, vitamin B_6 (pyridoxine), vitamin B_{12}, and vitamin C have all been linked to depression. Vitamin B_6 deficiency, for example, has been shown to lower levels of serotonin. Vitamin B_6 has a role in the production of the monoamine neurotransmitters, which are important for mood stabilization. Deficiencies of calcium, copper, magnesium, and the omega-6 fatty acids may also relate to depression. For preventive and/or therapeutic benefits, consider adding the following nutritional supplements to your program.[18]

~ *Pyridoxine (B_6):* recommended dose, 50–500 mg per day (Pyridoxine should be taken with the other B complex vitamins listed on page 523.)

~ *Vitamin C:* recommended dose, 1,000 mg per day

~ *Omega-3 fats:* EPA and DHA 1,000–2,000 mg twice per day

~ *Magnesium:* Magnesium deficiency is associated with anxiety in many women. Taking 400–1,000 mg a day can often work wonders and is, along with a good multivitamin and omega-3 fat source, the first thing I'd recommend.

SAINT-JOHN'S-WORT: This herb, which contains the active ingredients hypericin and hyperforin, has been very well researched, with some studies indicating that it is as effective as Prozac in treating mild to moderate depression. The usual dose is 300 mg of herb standardized to 0.3 percent hypericin and 3 percent hyperforin, three times per day.

VALERIAN: If you have an anxiety component with your depression, add valerian to your Saint-John's-wort. The usual dose is 100–300 mg standardized extract containing 0.8 percent valerenic acid.

GINKGO: If your depression is associated with attention and memory problems and you are age fifty or older, consider *Ginkgo biloba* in addition to Saint-John's-wort. The usual dose is 40–80 mg three times per day.

INOSITOL: Inositol is an effective over-the-counter alternative to many commonly prescribed antidepressants.[19] The exact mechanism of action is unknown, but it appears to be linked with the serotonin system, affecting the same pathways of brain chemistry as do the tricyclic and SSRI antidepressants, but without the side effects. I've prescribed inositol for several patients, who have tolerated it well. One, a person with a very significant family history of depression, used it following the loss of a loved one. She reported, "In the past, before inositol, I would have gone through my grief and then fallen into a black hole. This time I could still feel all of my feelings deeply, but I was able to move through them without a depression hangover." Usual therapeutic starting dose is 12 g per day; however, inositol has been shown to be well tolerated in doses as large as 18–20 g per day. (See Resources.)

5-HTP: 5-hydroxytryptophan is a compound naturally produced in the body from the amino acid tryptophan, which is an important precursor to serotonin. Although tryptophan is found in many foods, it can be difficult to consume enough tryptophan in the diet to overcome serotonin deficiency. (Tryptophan supplements were once widely used as sleep aids, but they were taken off the market after some products were found to be contaminated.) 5-HTP can be extracted from plants and is now available as a nutritional supplement. It has been used for decades in Europe as an approved treatment for both depression and sleep problems. The side effect of nausea is sometimes reported, but an enteric-coated formulation should help avoid this. The usual dose is 100–200 mg three times per day. (See Resources.)

SAM-e: S-adenosyl-L-methionine has been found to be instrumental in promoting cell growth and repair. On a molecular level, it also contributes to the formation of key neurotransmitters, the basis for its mood-stabilizing activity and the promotion of mental clarity. Additionally, SAM-e has antioxidant and anti-inflammatory properties, and thereby supports immune function and joint health, mobility, and comfort.[20] The usual dose is 800–1,600 mg per day. (See Resources.)

If mild depression and/or anxiety is your primary problem and you're already taking a good multivitamin plus omega-3 fats and magnesium, then the next thing I'd add is Saint-John's-wort. It has a history of hundreds of years of safe use. If after two months you've not noticed any difference, switch to 5-HTP. Reports on 5-HTP use have been particularly positive from people suffering from weight problems and insomnia in addition to depression. Be sure to get it from a reliable source, because of the possibility of contamination. If you also suffer from symptoms of panic disorder, obsessive-compulsive disorder, or anxiety plus depression, then I'd recommend a trial of inositol.

Remember, each of the suggestions above works well in some people but not in others. This is true whether you opt for medication, exercise, psychotherapy, nutritional supplements, or another approach. You need to be willing to experiment in order to find the approach that seems to beckon to you. For a very comprehensive approach to depression, anxiety, and memory problems, I recommend that you consult *The New Feminine Brain* (Free Press, 2005) by neuropsychiatrist Mona Lisa Schulz, M.D., Ph.D.

MEMORY LOSS AT MENOPAUSE:
IS THIS ALZHEIMER'S?

Many women experience "fuzzy thinking" or "cotton head" during perimenopause. They complain of forgetting names or misplacing objects or having difficulty balancing their checkbook. This is not the beginning of Alzheimer's disease. It is a fairly normal state that many women go through as our hormones change and our brains rewire. Some become terrified of this fuzzy-headed feeling because of their need for a high degree of intellectual control. Others find themselves willing to trust the process once they're reassured that it's normal—part of the wisdom of perimenopause that focuses our attention inward. The same thing often happens both premenstrually and during the postpartum period.

Memory problems at midlife are also due to temporary overload from the many external demands on your limited time. It's like trying to make a phone call on Mother's Day: you can't get through because all the circuits are busy. If you can't remember something instantly, just relax, do something else for a while, and give yourself the time, space, and respect that allows your brain to retrieve stored information. Getting anxious and putting yourself down for forgetting only makes the problem worse.

But Aren't We Losing Brain Cells?

A woman's brain reaches its peak size at about age twenty, followed by a gradual decline in size throughout the rest of her life. If bigger is better, that would mean that we also reach peak wisdom and intelligence by age twenty. That this is a completely ridiculous notion is made immediately obvious if you watch much MTV.

In fact, studies have shown that throughout our lifetime, as we move from naïveté to wisdom, our brain function becomes molded by our experience. Think of your brain as a tree that requires regular pruning if it is to acquire its optimal shape, size, and function. Brain cell loss with aging is akin to pruning the nonessential branches. In addition, while the number of neurons may decline, the interconnections among them continue to grow. These connections—created by dendritic and axonal branching—actually increase with age, as our capacity to make complex associations increases. In short, the older and more experienced you become, the more efficient and sophisticated your brain.

Dementia of all types, including Alzheimer's, is associated with free-radical damage to brain tissue, which results from the overproduction of inflammatory chemicals at the cellular level, eventually leading to the damage or death of brain cells. Free-radical damage and the resulting tissue inflammation are the final common pathway by which emotional, physical, and environmental stressors of all kinds adversely affect every tissue in our bodies, including our brains.[21]

Studies also show that those who are well educated, in good health, and financially secure, with above-average intelligence and social status, and who actively pursue their interests as they age, have a very good chance of preserving their memory as they grow older. In fact, they may even improve it, whether or not they're on estrogen.[22]

Preventing Alzheimer's: Some Lessons
from the Nun Study

Even with reassurance that it's normal to go through some transient changes in thinking and focus during perimenopause, many women still fear becoming demented and unable to live independently as they get older. Alzheimer's disease currently affects about four million Americans and is the leading cause of dependence and institutionalization in the elderly. It appears at an earlier age in women than in men, and up to two-thirds of cases reported have been in women—in part simply because women live longer. Currently about 5 percent of women have dementia of some type at age sixty. This climbs to 12 percent after age seventy-five. After age eighty-five, between 28 and 50 percent of all people suffer from some form of dementia, depending on what studies you believe. (This 50 percent figure is felt by many authorities to be an exaggeration.)[23] Given these numbers, each of us will want to do everything we can to care for and enhance our brain function at perimenopause—long before memory problems or dementia have a chance to develop.

Alzheimer's disease was named after Alois Alzheimer, a German neuropathologist who, in 1906, looked under a microscope at the brain tissue of a fifty-five-year-old woman who had spent the last years of her life in a mental institution, where she was prone to paranoia and fits of anger. Alzheimer identified two substances in her brain that have come to be associated with the disease: dense *plaques* formed by the protein beta-amyloid outside the brain cells, and stringy *tangles* within the nerve cells themselves. Whether these plaques and tangles are the cause of Alzheimer's dementia is controversial. We do know, however, that there's a great deal of overlap between the senile dementia caused by cerebrovascular insufficiency and stroke and that which is associated with the plaques and tangles of Alzheimer's disease.

Alzheimer's also has a genetic component.[24] But even if Alzheimer's runs in your family, that does not mean you will inevitably get it. Brain function is multifactorial, meaning that it is affected by many different aspects of our lives, from the amount of antioxidant-rich vegetables we eat to the level of education we've attained. It is also shaped by events and behaviors that begin in childhood and continue into old age. That's why there will never be a hormone or magic bullet that can guarantee brain protection for life. However, you can affect your brain health by the lifestyle choices you make.

Nowhere has this been more convincingly demonstrated than in the famous study of a group of hundreds of nuns belonging to the School Sisters of Notre Dame, who have donated their brains for study after death.[25] Because these women have spent much of their lives in the order, there is a wealth of data about each woman, often spanning many decades. One surprising finding was that a greater or lesser capacity for complex thought—known as "idea density"—in early life was correlated with the likelihood of developing Alzheimer's disease in later life. Upon entering the convent (usually in her early twenties) each of the nuns was required to write an autobiography. When linguistics experts analyzed these years later, they found a startling correlation between the nuns' language skills and the eventual occurrence of Alzheimer's. The lower their idea density, the higher their risk.

Another fascinating finding from the Nun Study is that the presence of plaques and tangles in the brain does not always predict the mental status of an individual. One of the nuns had strikingly good mental status and attitude before her death in her late eighties; researchers were startled to find severe loss of neurons and multiple amyloid tangles in her brain at autopsy. This evidence supports a great truth: that the physical body and the spirit are inextricably linked. For people who are optimistic, lively, and engaged, as this particular nun was, anatomical limitations often seem not to result in disability.

On the other hand, the Nun Study has shown that small-vessel disease, in the form of mini-strokes, is strongly predictive of dementia. Chronic depression also seems to be correlated with Alzheimer's.

When we shut off the circulation of blood to an area of our body, we are shutting off life force. Similarly, depression is a shutting down of the life force within us.

ESTROGEN AND ALZHEIMER'S

An impressive number of studies have shown an association between estrogen use and the delay or even prevention of Alzheimer's.[26] This wasn't the case with the 2006 WHI study, however, which showed an increased risk with Premarin and Prempro. Nevertheless, estrogen (as well as progesterone and testosterone) has been shown to stimulate the regeneration of damaged neurons. Estrogen also appears to increase the production of the neurotransmitter acetylcholine, which regulates memory, learning, and other cognitive functions. In fact, estradiol (a type of natural estrogen) binds to the areas in the brain that are associated with memory: the cortex, the hippocampus, and the basal forebrain. Estrogen has also been shown to enhance nerve cell branching.[27] Research also shows that women with the highest endogenous levels of estradiol have the lowest risk for Alzheimer's disease.[28]

Despite the results of the WHI study, there is still convincing evidence of the beneficial effect of hormones—not just estrogen—on brain function.[29] For example, women who have undergone premature menopause have a slightly higher risk of early dementia. And there is evidence that small baseline amounts of estrogen are essential for certain memory functions. Many women's bodies produce enough throughout life, while some do not. The research of Barbara Sherwin, Ph.D., has shown that women's verbal memory decreases following hysterectomy with removal of the ovaries, but then returns to normal following hormone replacement.[30] Dr. Sherwin used only estrogen replacement, but other studies support a role for progesterone and probably androgens as well.[31]

Ovarian hormones also bind to areas of the brain that are important for mood regulation. This helps to explain research findings indicating that estrogen has significant antidepressant effects and that progesterone decreases anxiety and promotes restful sleep. While the research on estrogen and memory is not conclusive, a small amount of bioidentical estrogen (and/or progesterone or testosterone) definitely helps the brain function of some women. But hormones shouldn't be prescribed simply for this reason.

NONHORMONAL WAYS TO PROTECT YOUR BRAIN

Consider the following brain-health-enhancing practices.

~ FEED YOUR BRAIN WITH NUTRIENTS. A diet high in refined sugars and including partially hydrogenated fats is associated with depletion of many nutrients necessary for optimal brain function. For brain function as for every other aspect of your health, I recommend a relatively low-fat diet that contains lots of fruits, vegetables, and whole grains. Studies have shown that demented and depressed patients often have inadequate levels of zinc, B vitamins (especially vitamin B_1 or thiamine), selenium, and antioxidants such as vitamins E and C, compared to patients with normal mental function.

Zinc, for example, is necessary for optimal transport of the B vitamins into the cerebrospinal fluid. This fluid bathes and nourishes the brain and spinal cord. Many women do not get adequate levels of zinc in their daily diets.[32] In one study of severely demented patients, ten patients were given vitamin supplements for two months, while a control group was not. After one month, the patients who received the supplements showed clinical memory improvement.[33] Some authorities also feel that Alzheimer's is associated with the inability of some elderly people to absorb enough minerals, vitamins, and essential trace elements from their food.[34] They may also have problems with transporting these nutrients from the blood to the brain. Since nutritional supplementation improves memory in people who are already demented, imagine the preventive potential of feeding your brain right!

~ QUELL POTENTIAL FREE-RADICAL DAMAGE TO YOUR BRAIN TISSUE. A great deal of brain health is affected by free-radical damage. Get serious about antioxidants. Make sure your diet is rich in vitamins C and E, the B vitamins (including folic acid), and selenium.[35] Another class of powerful antioxidants is the proanthocyanidins found in pine bark and grape pips. (The dosage ranges for these are given in chapter 14.) Studies have shown that the risk of stroke is very low in those women who eat at least five servings of fruits and vegetables per day. Clearly, brain protection is yet another reason to eat plenty of these nutrient-rich foods.

~ AVOID SMOKING AND EXCESSIVE ALCOHOL INTAKE. Cigarettes are well-known factors in causing cardiovascular disease and small blood vessel changes that decrease oxygen to your brain, among other areas. And excessive alcohol intake affects the basal fore-brain, an area associated with memory.

~ EXERCISE. Researchers at the Aging Research Center of the Karolinska Institute in Sweden found that those who exercise at least twice per week reduced their risk of dementia by more than 50 percent and of Alzheimer's by 60 percent. The study, which is the first to show a long-term relationship between physical activity and dementia later in life, examined 1,449 participants at midlife and again twenty-one years later at ages 65 and 79. At the follow-up exam, 117 showed evidence of dementia and 76 had Alzheimer's. But those who exercised had a greatly reduced risk of dementia and Alzheimer's even after adjusting for other lifestyle factors. Interestingly, the greatest benefit was seen in those with a genetic susceptibility to dementia and Alzheimer's.[36] Exercise definitely turns on a whole-body mechanism that helps to keep the brain healthy. It also increases blood flow.[37] Basically, any activity that increases heart rate and results in sweating will work!

~ ENHANCE YOUR BRAIN'S ACETYLCHOLINE LEVELS. Many factors can affect your acetylcholine levels and, subsequently, your memory. If you're already on estrogen or other hormones to treat other symptoms, stick with them—though I wouldn't recommend hormones solely for Alzheimer's prevention, be reassured that they are probably helping your acetylcholine levels. And avoid drugs that are known to decrease acetylcholine levels.[38] You'd be amazed by how many of these there are and by how few doctors realize their adverse affect on brain function. Check the label of any medication used for sleep, colds, or allergies to see if it contains di-phenhydramine. Examples of such medications include Sominex, Benadryl, Tylenol PM, Excedrin PM, Contac Day & Night, and Tylenol Flu PM. The cough suppressant dextromethorphan also affects acetylcholine and has other anticholingeric effects that can impair memory. It is found in Robitussin DM and a wide range of other cough and cold remedies.

~ BOOST YOUR DHEA LEVELS. Studies suggest that DHEA (and related hormones progesterone and pregnenolone) act as neuro-transmitters in the brain and can promote the same kind of dendritic and axonal branching between brain cells that is seen with estrogen. The best way to enhance levels of DHEA is to follow the adrenal restoration program on page 124.

Other Brain Food Choices

The food supplements listed below have been shown to help memory in many people. Try just one at a time, so that you know if it works for you. Use your intuition to pick one to start with. Your first impulse will usually be the right one.

GINKGO: *Ginkgo biloba* is the number-one prescription herb in Europe, with more than forty double-blind studies demonstrating its benefits. It appears to work by increasing blood flow to the brain, and it is widely used to treat arteriosclerotic blockage of the small arteries in the brain. The usual dosage is 40–80 mg three times per day.

GOTU KOLA: Widely known as a "memory herb," gotu kola (*Hydrocotyle asiatica*) also increases circulation to the brain. The usual dosage is 90 mg per day. *Note:* Gotu kola is a stimulant and should not be taken at bedtime.

OMEGA-3 FATS: Nerve fibers throughout your body are coated with a fat called myelin. For good brain and nerve function, you need small amounts of high-quality (not partially hydrogenated) fat in your daily diet. Two studies on rats (and one on mice) have shown that a diet supplemented with the omega-3 fatty acid DHA (docosahexænoic acid) significantly improves memory—one study showed dramatic improvement after only four days![39] Dutch researchers who tracked more than 1,600 adults between the ages of forty-five and seventy for six years concluded that those who ate more omega-3 fats regularly scored higher on a battery of tests involving brain health, including memory.[40] I recommend consuming fatty fish, such as salmon or sardines, ground flaxseed, or fish oil in supplement form. DHA, made from algae, at a dose of 100–400 mg per day, is a good choice for taking oil in supplement form, particularly for vegetarians. Mercury-free fish oil supplements (including USANA BiO-omega-3 and Vital Choice Alaskan Sockeye Salmon Oil) are also available. (See Resources.)

SOY: In Japan, where consumption of soy is far higher than it is in the United States, the incidence of Alzheimer's and other dementias is much lower than it is here. The Bowman Gray School of Medicine at Wake Forest University was recently awarded a patent based on their research of the use of soy to prevent Alzheimer's disease.[41] Preliminary research has shown that soy phytoestrogens affect the brain like estradiol, but not as strongly.[42] Soy isoflavones also act as antioxidants in the brain.[43] Several studies indicate soy can help boost memory as quickly as six weeks after adding it to your regular diet.[44] One recent study showed that postmenopausal women consuming 60 milligrams of soy isoflavones a day for six weeks improved their nonverbal short-term memory, mental flexibility, and planning ability.[45] Another study of postmenopausal women showed consuming soy isoflavones improved verbal memory.[46] And since soy definitely helps the cardiovascular system, it may also help prevent the strokes that are so common in dementia.

Substances Your Brain Doesn't Need

ALUMINUM: Aluminum has been found in the brains of Alzheimer's patients, and this disease has been associated with increased tissue levels of aluminum along with decreased levels of zinc and selenium. Although the nature of the link is not clear, there is evidence to suggest that aluminum is, indeed, a brain toxin in individuals who are genetically predisposed to Alzheimer's. If you have any Alzheimer's sufferers in your family, I'd recommend that you avoid aluminum cookware, antiperspirants containing aluminum, soda from aluminum cans, and baking powder containing aluminum. (Use Rumford's, for example, rather than Calumet or Clabber Girl.)[47]

EXCITOTOXINS: Aspartame, with the proprietary names Equal and NutraSweet, is an excitotoxin, which means that it causes nerve cells to overfire. In susceptible people this can lead to the death of brain cells. This is one of the reasons aspartame has been associated with a multiple-sclerosis-like syndrome in some women.[48] The aspartame in diet colas seems to cause the worst problems in susceptible women.

Many women are addicted to diet cola, drinking several liters per day without taking in much else in the way of other nutrients. This is a setup for a wide range of neurological symptoms in susceptible individuals, including headache, dizziness, anxiety attacks, memory loss, slurred speech, numbness, muscle spasms, mood swings, severe depression, personality changes, PMS, insomnia, fatigue, hyperactivity, heart palpitations, arrhythmia, chest pain, hearing loss, ringing in the ears, blurred vision, decreased sense of taste, skin lesions, nausea, digestive disturbances, water retention, and seizures. If you have a history of such problems, avoid this artificial sweetener, especially in the form of diet colas. (Aspartame-induced symptoms go away when consumption is stopped.) The herb stevia is a safe sweetener. MSG (monosodium glutamate) is another excitotoxin that not only adversely affects the brain, but is also added to junk food to stimulate appetite. You don't need it!

SERMs (Selective Estrogen Receptor Modulators): Given the role of ovarian hormones in brain function, the anti-estrogen drugs tamoxifen (to prevent breast cancer) and raloxifene (to prevent osteoporosis) stir up some legitimate concerns about the whole-body effects of estrogen deprivation over time. Just as tamoxifen blocks the effects of estrogen on the breasts, there is also compelling evidence that it blocks some of the effects of estrogen on the brain.[49] Raloxifene (Evista), a drug prescribed to women to prevent osteoporosis, also affects the brain. This is one of the reasons hot flashes (which are mediated in the hypothalamus) are listed as one of the side effects of SERMs. Depression is also among a host of other side effects. Though these drugs have their place and may be appropriate for some women who are truly at very high risk, the very real potential drawbacks of these drugs are not getting enough attention.

If you're currently taking tamoxifen or raloxifene, it's doubly important for you to follow some of the suggestions outlined above to protect your brain function. Many women report alleviation of their tamoxifen-associated depression, for example, when they take high doses of soy. This may be because of soy's hormonal effects. (For a fuller discussion of SERMs, see chapters 5 and 13.)

MAXIMIZING MIDLIFE WISDOM

Your brain is like your muscles. If you want it to stay in peak form, you have to use it regularly. Brain function is also profoundly affected by our expectations and attitudes about life. While there is no formula—hormonal or otherwise—to "cure" aging, there are many things you can do to preserve your mental vitality.

STEP ONE: Catch yourself indulging in any stereotypical thinking about the aging process. For example, if you forget something, don't say "I'm having a senior moment." Don't ever allow yourself to make comments such as "I'm too old for this!" I've seen this kind of thinking in women who are only in their early thirties! My mother told me that when she turned sixty, her mailbox was suddenly full of ads for all kinds of health aids, ranging from incontinence diapers to hearing aids. She simply "recycles" this information in the wastebasket at the post office. Instead, start viewing yourself as a younger person, unfettered by the age-related problems the media tells us all to expect. When I use an exercise machine, for example, I always program in my age as forty! Though "thinking young" may seem simplistic, it is one of the most important health behaviors you can adopt. In fact, buying into negative stereotypes about aging (which tends to happen in childhood, e.g., as you age you become useless) actually translates into an increased risk of premature death.

Consider this: a study of six hundred people age fifty and older by Yale researcher Becca Levy, Ph.D., showed that those who had a more positive view of aging as relatively young adults lived an average of 7.5 years longer than those with less positive views—even after factoring in such variables as age, gender, socioeconomic status, loneliness, and overall health. How the subjects viewed aging had a greater effect on their longevity than having low blood pressure and low cholesterol (each of which is associated with living up to four years longer), or having a lower body mass index, no history of smoking, and a tendency to exercise (each of which can add up to three years to your life). "Our study carries two messages," the study reports. "The discouraging one is that negative self-perceptions can diminish life expectancy; the encouraging one is that positive self-perceptions can prolong life expectancy."[50]

One of the ways that I routinely "program" my own mind for youth and vigor is with affirmations. Here are a couple of my favorites (I say these out loud every morning when I'm working out on the elliptical trainer).

"My body is now radiantly healthy, beautiful, flexible, strong, and eternally youthful. The spirit of Divine Love and Power now manifests throughout my entire body as radiant health, radiant beauty, and radiant youth."

"I give thanks that my body, mind, spirit, and behavior now align to easily maintain my ideal size and weight."

STEP TWO: Stay mentally active and socially connected. Continuing to expose yourself to new ideas, new people, and new environments is as necessary to staying mentally healthy as physical exercise is to maintaining the health of your heart, muscles, and bones.[51] Remember that learning causes actual growth of new neurons, even in an older brain.[52] Step outside the comfort of familiar territory. Cultivate a wide social network of individuals from diverse age groups. Take classes, get together with friends, learn a new sport or activity, start a new career or business, engage in volunteer work. Tone your brain cells and neural pathways with new ideas, new connections, and new thoughts every day. I started taking Argentine tango classes this year and I love it!

I've noticed that some of my older friends tend to get a vacant look on their faces when they are with a group of new people or in an unfamiliar setting. Although they seem fine in their own homes, they can't seem to keep up with the conversation when challenged with a new situation. They've spent so much time screening out any newness from their environment, digging themselves deeper into the safety of their day-to-day ruts, they've lost the ability to adapt to change. It's tragic to witness what happens to the faces, bodies, and minds of these formerly vital people as they begin this downhill slide.

The famous brain researcher Marian Diamond says, "There's a very simple principle when it comes to the brain. Use it or lose it." When our nervous system no longer receives new input, it atrophies, a phenomenon that has been demonstrated clearly in the laboratory. In one study of aging rats, Diamond added new toys and other novel items to enhance the environments of some rats, while leaving the other rats in their familiar surroundings. At the end of the study, the rats in the enriched environments had more cortical brain tissue than those with the standard environments. Interestingly, this change in brain structure occurred even in old rats that were 75 percent of the way through their life spans.[53]

STEP THREE: Develop an optimistic attitude toward life. Optimism—the ability to perceive the glass as half full instead of half empty—is a natural protectant against depression. Also, an impressive body of research has documented that optimists are healthier and live longer. In one study of individuals with no risk factors for heart disease, for example, depressed people were four times more likely to suffer from heart attacks than their optimistic, non-depressed counterparts; since heart disease is also associated with dementia, you can see the connection between a healthy attitude and a healthy brain.

STEP FOUR: Actively work with your thoughts and behaviors to modify those personality traits—such as hostility, pessimistic thoughts, and the tendency to isolate yourself socially—that are known to be associated with premature death and disability. If necessary, seek help from a therapist. Cognitive behavioral therapy (CBT) can make you more aware of your negative, self-limiting thoughts and help you find ways to redirect them in a more positive, empowering direction. This does not mean denial of life's difficulties. CBT also teaches you how to accept your situation and validate it, but at the same time deal with it more constructively. As a result, you learn to worry less. To help you use your own power to change your thoughts, I recommend that you read *I Can Do It!* (Hay House, 2004) by Louise Hay and *The Amazing Power of Deliberate Intent* (Hay House, 2006) by Esther and Jerry Hicks.

STEP FIVE: Develop and express a healthy sense of humor. Get "humor aids," such as Loretta LaRoche's video *How Serious Is This?* or her book, *Relax—You May Only Have a Few Minutes Left* (Villard, 1998). Or watch reruns of comedy programs you loved years ago.

STEP SIX: Eat healthfully and exercise regularly. A large body of research has demonstrated that almost all dementia is due, in part, to small-blood-vessel disease in our brains. The number-one reason why so many of us get these blood vessel changes is because we eat poorly and avoid exercise. Get moving, every day. This includes walking, aerobics, sports, swimming, or lifting weights. Movement keeps the blood flowing to all your organs, including your brain, and brings more nutrients and oxygen to your tissues. If you want, you can get your movement and social needs met at the same time by taking up a sport with a group of people who are noncompetitive and just enjoy the fun of moving.

STEP SEVEN: Practice full emotional expression and heal your life as you go along. The emotional pattern associated with heart disease, including hardening of the arteries in the brain, is a tendency to avoid feeling your emotions fully—whether those emotions are positive or negative. One of my perimenopausal patients once told me:

> I grew up in a household in which we were taught to be afraid of strong emotions. You weren't allowed to feel too good—or too bad—about anything. If we needed to cry, we were told to go into the basement and bury our face in a pillow so that we wouldn't disturb the rest of the family. If we shouted with joy about a good grade or winning a game, we were told not to "blow your own trumpet." So I learned to distrust an entire

range of feelings—basically anything except bland and boring pleasantness. Not surprisingly, dementia, depression, and heart disease run very strongly in my family on both sides. At midlife I feel as though I have to completely relearn how to feel. Often I have to tune in to symptoms in my body and just sit with them until I start to feel the emotion associated with them.

If you find yourself feeling sad, for example, just allow yourself the fullness of your feeling. What you will find is that it dissipates. But if you instead try to make yourself feel something else, and put yourself down for having an "unpleasant" emotion, then that emotion will get locked in your body and may be expressed later as a disease.

Hostility, on the other hand, is a stuck chronic emotional pattern. It can be self-destructive to loiter in this space for very long, and the best way to get out is to find something to appreciate about every situation you are in, no matter how small it is, until appreciation begins to replace hostility as a mental and emotional pattern.

STEP EIGHT: Never retire. Don't allow yourself to start thinking about "retirement" at midlife, the way so many people do. Instead, do what Dolly Parton does: find out what you love to do for work, and you'll never work a day in your life! You may wish to retire from working for a company or for another individual, but you need to have something that you're interested in doing—for pay or not—every day of your life.

In conclusion, consider the following experiment: In a famous study at Boston's Beth Israel Deaconess Hospital, researchers Dr. Jeffrey Hausdorff, a gerontologist, and Harvard graduate student Becca Levy tested the effect of subconscious beliefs on walking speed. Walking speed often declines with age, and that in combination with balance and coordination problems as well as other factors, such as medication, produces the stereotypical elderly "shuffle." The researchers tested healthy individuals ages sixty-three to eighty-two by first having them walk down a hall the length of a football field. They measured both speed and "swing time"—the time the foot spends off the ground. After that, the participants played a brief computer game. On half of the computers, upbeat words like *accomplished, wise,* and *astute* flashed across the screen just long enough to register subconsciously. The other group had negative words like *senile, dependent,* and *diseased* flashed across their screens. The participants then walked down the same hallway again. This time, the positively influenced group walked 9 percent faster and had much more "swing time" and much less shuffling. The negatively influenced group didn't get any worse, perhaps because they, like most of us, had already been saturated by society's negative aging stereotypes.[54]

This study is clearly a wake-up call for becoming conscious of our own beliefs about aging and the physical effects of those beliefs. I've seen far too many women talk themselves into physical deterioration starting as young as thirty! And who hasn't witnessed the black balloons and jokes about being "over the hill" at birthday parties for friends turning forty?

Dr. Ellen Langer, a Harvard psychologist who wrote the classic book *Mindfulness,* observed: "The regular and 'irreversible' cycles of aging that we witness in the later stages of human life may be a product of certain assumptions about how one is supposed to grow old. If we didn't feel compelled to carry out these limiting mindsets, we might have a greater chance of replacing years of decline with years of growth and purpose."[55]

Amen.

11

From Rosebud to Rose Hip: Cultivating Midlife Beauty

I'll never forget the last time my former harp teacher, Miss Alice Chalifoux, came to borrow my harp for her students to use at the summer harp colony in Camden, Maine, where she taught for more than sixty years, and where I myself first took lessons when I was fourteen.

Though she never paid much attention to diet, exercise, or supplements, her skin was pink, fresh, and smooth, her eyes were bright, she was never sick, and her irreverent and earthy sense of humor was utterly delightful. With a twinkle in her eye, Miss Chalifoux told me that she had cut her schedule way back that summer. She only taught thirty-six hours a week—about half time by her standards. She was a perfect example of a woman who was beautifully attuned to the power of what I call the late rose hip stage of life, sowing her seeds of wisdom and inspiring others wherever she went. Her impish soul shone out through every pore, its youthful effects written all over her face. Miss Chalifoux was ninety-two years old.

No one would deny that every season of the year is imbued with its own special beauty and wisdom. The same is true of the seasons of our lives. Most of us know or have seen at least one woman like Miss Alice Chalifoux, who is living proof that beauty is possible at every season of our lives, depending upon how we live them.

Perimenopausal women can be likened to the full-blown rose of late summer and fall, as it begins to transform itself into a bright, juicy rose hip—the part of the rose that contains the seeds from which hundreds of other potential roses can grow. Until recently, our culture has worshipped only the rosebud stage of development, thereby rendering relatively invisible the beauty of the other stages. In fact, not so long ago, the dewy rosebud was often used as a prominent symbol for ads selling conventional hormone replacement drugs to women. The subliminal message was clear: if you used hormone replacement, you could stay at the rosebud stage of beauty for the rest of your life and never have to go through the process of maturing and ripening into the resilient and potent rose hip. But it's not true.

Once you're on the way to becoming a rose hip, you can't go backward to being a rosebud, though our culture certainly entices us to try. Learning how to maximize the strength and resilience of the juicy rose hip stage is absolutely necessary if you are to look and feel your very best as a woman in the full bloom of midlife! Just remember that when you're becoming a rose hip, any attempt to remain in the rosebud stage tends to look desperate and ridiculous. It's like trying to reglue the autumn leaves back onto the tree and then paint them all green to simulate the spring. It simply doesn't work. Instead, our task is to come to appreciate the beauty and power of the season we are in, instead of longing for what can no longer be.

This may be a particularly difficult task if, before menopause, you were the type of woman accustomed to using the power of your looks and body to attract the attention of men whenever you so much as walked into a room. If this has been true for you, then you're viscerally familiar with the power of external feminine beauty and have, perhaps, capitalized on it since adolescence. If your looks have charmed people for years, it is quite likely that you will have a harder time with becoming a rose hip than someone who didn't have this experience and therefore had to turn inward at an earlier age to find her sense of worth and beauty. I had an acquaintance like this once. When she turned forty-five, she bemoaned the fact that men no longer turned to look at her when she walked into a room. Since all of her influence and money had always come to her by virtue of her appearance and its effect on powerful men, becoming a rose hip was truly a harsh wake-up call, letting her know that her former wiles would no longer serve her in the second half of life. Those of you who've never had that experience in the first place will probably have a much easier time settling into the rose hip stage. In fact, if you're anything like me—and I know many of you are—you may happily find yourself becoming interested in clothing, skin care, and makeup perhaps for the first time in your life. What's more, you'll also find that the self-confidence and self-esteem from all you've done in the first half of your life have built a solid foundation of self-acceptance that leaves you feeling more empowered than ever before.

But whether or not we were ever raving beauties, all of us want to look our best at every age. During perimenopause, as we heed the call to truly come home to ourselves, we find ourselves lit from within by an inner glow. We find that we may never be rosebuds again, but we can still remain as attractive as possible by paying attention to good skin and body care. And we may even want to avail ourselves of plastic surgery or other cosmetic procedures. More choices are available to budding rose hips than ever before.

MAKING PEACE WITH YOUR CHANGING SKIN

One of the most distressing parts of midlife for many women is watching our skin begin to sag and get "crepey." I began to notice changes in my skin—a tendency toward more dryness and some fine wrinkles around my eyes—starting in my late thirties. When these first became noticeable, I decided to like them, since they reminded me of my father's eyes, which were always surrounded by the crinkles of lots of laughter and smiles. But I also wanted to do everything possible to keep those lines from getting deeper and more unattractive as time went on.

One of my newsletter subscribers eloquently shared the common dilemma of midlife skin changes and their potential emotional impact:

> I am forty-eight years old, at my ideal weight, and extremely fit. I work out on a regular basis and lift weights as part of my exercise program. I hike whenever I get the chance. However, it seems like almost overnight, the skin on my legs has become extremely slack. As I look down when I walk, I can see the skin on my thighs shake with each step. I'm sure it's the result of cumulative sun damage along with many years of gaining and losing those stubborn ten pounds. Is there anything that can be done? I now use sunscreen whenever I am outdoors, never bake in the sun, and try to keep my weight stable. Must I resign myself to wearing long dresses? Are there any supplements I can take? Is there anything that would rebuild the collagen? Any surgery

that would help? I'm in the process of a divorce after twenty-seven years of marriage and am, naturally, concerned about my appearance. I'd be very grateful for any suggestions.

Fortunately there's a great deal that we can do to both preserve the health of our midlife skin and even heal some of the damage that has already been done. While we're doing this, however, we still have to go through midlife with the courage to live our lives joyfully and fully, despite such things as aging skin and changing bodies. I know both from my practice and from my own life experience that this feels much harder when you're going through a divorce or loss of a life partner.

Nevertheless, it's important to remember that many women find love and happiness at midlife and beyond, regardless of a little sun damage or sagging here and there. This point was brought home to me rather dramatically recently during an event at which I spent time talking to two different women. One, a stunning woman in her late thirties with flawless skin and an almost perfect figure who was also a very successful businesswoman, was bemoaning the fact that there simply weren't any good men around with whom she could find happiness.

About half an hour later I met another woman. About fifty-five years old, she had a plain but lively face, unadorned by any makeup, and she was at least thirty or forty pounds overweight. Since we were discussing medical topics, she told me about a mastectomy she'd had years before that had left her chest quite disfigured. In the course of the conversation, she said, "I think we underestimate men, don't you? They can be so sweet." It turned out that she was dating three different men, one of whom she felt was the one she was destined to marry! This woman's inner beauty and sense of humor made me feel happy just being around her. When I compared her energy and attitude to that of the show-stoppingly beautiful woman I'd met earlier, I realized how transient the impression of mere physical beauty can be when it's not lit from within by a beautiful soul.

I'm very comforted by what I learned that day from those women and their experiences, and I return to it whenever I begin to succumb to the cultural and media-driven notion that after thirty-five it's all downhill for women, our best years are behind us, and no one will ever love us again because we are no longer twenty-five. I've come to see that nothing could be further from the truth. In fact, many men have told me that it's a woman's enthusiasm for her life, her self-acceptance, and her sense of fun that they find most attractive.

A Primer on Skin: Our External Nervous System

To prevent unnecessary aging of the skin—which manifests as dullness, sallowness, uneven pigmentation, dryness, and wrinkles—you first need to understand what your skin does for you and how it does it.

The skin is derived from the embryonic layer known as the neuroectoderm, the same tissue layer that becomes the brain and the peripheral nervous system. It functions as a kind of external brain, gathering information about our outer environment through its ability to sense pressure, temperature, pleasure, and pain. The skin is also the largest and most important part of the immune system.

The research of Tiffany Field, Ph.D., on the striking immune-system-enhancing benefits of massage is compelling evidence of just how intimately our skin is connected with and affected by every aspect of our health, from our emotions to our nutrient intake. Our skin is, quite literally, the boundary between us and our environment. As our first line of defense against the vagaries of that environment, including bacteria, viruses, excessive ultraviolet radiation from the sun, wind, air pollution, and secondhand smoke, it is not only vulnerable to what's going on outside of us, it's also affected by our internal environment, both emotional and nutritional.

The condition of your skin says a great deal about how well you're fitting into and feeling supported by your current environment. There's an unmistakable glow emanating from women who are happy and satisfied with their lives that no amount of cosmetic surgery can create. It comes only from connecting with Source energy. If, for any reason, you feel as though you cannot be safe or true to yourself in your environment, and you are not particularly aware of this, then your skin may react for you. That's why it is well known in dermatology that patients may need simultaneous treatment of their skin and their mind and emotions for best results. Dermatitis and hives, for example, are two of the conditions known to be caused by a mixture of psychological and physical factors, while disorders such as psoriasis, hair loss, and eczema may also be affected by psychological factors. Almost everyone has had the experience of developing a large pimple in a prominent area of her face just when she was most concerned about looking her best for some big social event, or breaking out in oral herpes (cold sores) just before going out on a date, or getting itchy hives on taking a new job or moving to a new city. Sooner or later all of who we are and have been shows up on our faces.

The Anatomy of the Skin

The skin consists of three layers: the outer epidermis, the middle dermis, and a fat layer underlying both of those. The paper-thin epidermis is a protective layer of dead skin cells that holds in moisture and oil. It is constantly being shed and replaced as fresh cells push their way up to the surface, get flattened, and then die. As we age, the sloughing process tends to slow down, which is one of the reasons why skin tends to lose its "freshness."

At the base of the epidermis are the basal cells, which contain the melanin-generating cells known as melanocytes. The amount and type of melanin determines the tone of your skin—a trait that is inherited from your parents.

The dermis layer, which makes up about 90 percent of the skin, is where the nerve receptors and blood vessels are located. It also contains sweat glands and sebaceous glands; the latter produce oil and are attached to hair follicles. Blackheads and pimples inevitably arise from clogged sebaceous ducts at the root of hair follicles. The sweat and oil secretions from the dermal layer help protect the skin from infection by creating a protective acid mantle, but this mantle is easily disrupted by using harsh detergent and non-pH-balanced soaps.

FIGURE 14: THE ANATOMY OF THE SKIN

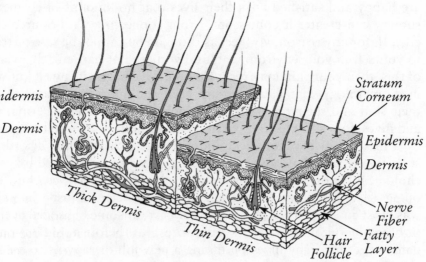

Two proteins known as collagen and elastin, which give skin its elasticity and flexibility, are also located in the dermis layer. On average, collagen production starts to diminish at a rate of 1 percent per year starting in our twenties. By midlife we may have lost up to 20 percent of our collagen layer, though there is enormous variation among different individuals and this is not inevitable. The darker your skin tone, however, the more collagen and elastin it has—which is why the skin and bones of dark-skinned women tend to be more resistant to the wear and tear of aging compared to those of Caucasian descent, and also why black- and brown-skinned women are less apt to have wrinkled skin compared to white-skinned women. The television personality Starr Jones Reynolds put it this way: "Black don't crack." Those with yellow skin tend to fall somewhere in between.

In addition to the thinning of the collagen layer of our skin with age, our oil glands tend to decrease their secretions, resulting in a greater tendency toward dryness. By about age fifty, the capacity of the skin to repair itself tends to slow down, for reasons that aren't entirely clear but may be related to free-radical damage. (See the next section.)

Free Radicals and Skin Aging

If you take a look at the skin on your buttocks and lower back, you'll notice something important: skin that has been protected from environmental pollutants and excessive sunlight is smoother and more wrinkle-free than elsewhere on our bodies. That means that skin aging is related to more than simply chronological age. It's also related to our environment—both inside and outside our bodies.

Premature aging of the skin—and of every other cell in our body—is related to the production of what are known as free radicals, oxygen molecules that have become unstable because they have lost an electron in the course of interacting with other molecules in our body during such basic metabolic processes as breathing and digestion. Free radicals are also produced when sunlight hits the skin, by repeated bouts of high blood sugar and insulin (glycemic stress), and by toxins of all kinds, including cigarette smoke and air pollutants. Emotional stress also results in free-radical damage secondary to the effects of cortisol and adrenaline. In the body, these unstable free radicals bounce around, attaching themselves to the cell membranes of virtually any tissue that is available in order to stabilize themselves with an electron from that tissue. If they take an extra electron from collagen in our skin, for example, this can damage the collagen. Over time the skin becomes stiff and discolored and loses its elasticity. It's much like the process by which iron rusts when left out in the open air.

Wrinkles result from the breakdown of elastin and collagen fibers in the deeper layers of the skin. Collagen and elastin are responsible for the resilience of the skin, allowing it to stretch and contract. When collagen gets broken down, skin tends to sag and wrinkle.

Free-radical damage can also harm and break down the fats within our cells and cell membranes, and the DNA of the cells, where the genetic code resides. Over time, cell membranes become stiff instead of fluid and flexible. There's no doubt that free-radical damage is one of the primary causes of aging, including skin wrinkling, and age-related diseases such as heart disease, Alzheimer's, arthritis, and so on. Glycemic stress from eating too many refined foods also contributes to premature aging.

Since some free radicals are produced as an unavoidable part of daily living, it's not surprising that our bodies have developed defense systems for dealing with them. This defense system is based on the effects of molecules known as antioxidants. These include vitamins C and E found in foods, and others produced in the body, such as glutathione, catalase, and superoxidedismutase. Antioxidants work by donating electrons to the unstable free radicals, thus rendering them harmless by preventing them from combining with other molecules and damaging our tissues.

Given this defense system, one might wonder why we age at all. As with all things, it's a question of balance. Though our bodies manufacture antioxidants and we ingest them in foods and as supplements, sometimes our antioxidant systems become overwhelmed by the sheer number of free radicals produced by such things as cigarette smoke, air pollution, sun exposure, diets that are heavy in trans fats or other suboptimal ingredients, high blood sugar, and emotional stress of all kinds. The resulting free-radical damage in our bodies is known as oxidative stress. Hundreds of research studies have now documented that we can keep the oxidative stress in our bodies to a minimum by ingesting antioxidants, applying products that contain them, avoiding environmental toxins, eating a low-glycemic diet, and maintaining emotional equilibrium.

How Smoking Damages the Skin

Midlife is the time when the ill effects of smoking become as plain as the nose on your face. Women who smoke heavily have a paler skin tone and more lines and wrinkles than nonsmokers. Some of this effect is from the decrease in circulation to the skin caused by nicotine. Decreased skin circulation results in fewer nutrients getting to the skin and a decreased ability of the skin to release the toxic waste products of cell metabolism. This results in a slowing of skin growth and rejuvenation.

In addition to this, smoking directly poisons the ovaries, leading to decreased levels of estrogen, which is necessary to help maintain elastin and collagen fibers.

How Excessive Ultraviolet Radiation Damages the Skin

It is estimated that about 70 percent of the change we see in our skin as we age is the result of damage done to collagen fibers in the dermis. Sun damage, in particular, causes the skin to lose its resiliency and elasticity.[1] Skin that is chronically overexposed to the sun is in a constant state of mild inflammation. Though we've all been brought up to feel that a tan makes us look more youthful in appearance, this is an illusion: the mild inflammation and swelling of tanned skin plumps the skin up, temporarily minimizing wrinkles, and gives the appearance of a more youthful look. But once the tan goes away, the wrinkles reappear, and what you're left with is skin that has lost its normal architecture.

Excessive exposure to ultraviolet radiation results in tissue inflammation that begins with free-radical damage to skin cell membranes followed by the release of harmful inflammatory chemicals that ultimately damage collagen and elastin fibers. Eventually collagen and elastin fibers that were originally flexible and fluid become stiff and hard. The aging process that your skin collagen goes through is much the same as what happens to a flexible and clear egg white when you drop it on a hot griddle: the fluid protein in the egg white is transformed into denatured protein, a dense, hard, inflexible type of protein. Ultraviolet radiation also damages the blood vessels in the skin, thus decreasing the flow of blood and other nutrients to this organ. This is in part the reason for those pesky dilated blood vessels on the cheeks and nose. Uneven pigmentation, roughness, and thickening of the skin result from disruption of both immune and cellular replication processes as we age. They are not inevitable but are brought about by DNA damage and oxidative stress from stresses of all kind, most importantly, UVR damage from the sun.

How Excess Blood Sugar and Nutrient-Poor Diet Damage the Skin

No one doubts the health benefits of nutrient-rich fruits, vegetables, lean proteins, healthy fats, and enough fiber. What most don't realize is that exactly the same diet that prevents diabetes and heart disease also provides you with a radiant complexion. A diet too high in refined carbohydrates raises blood sugar too quickly. And too much sugar in the blood results in a process known as glycosylation (or glycation), in which the sugar actually combines with proteins in the blood and the body. This is the basis for the blood test known as hemoglobin Alc, which is used to determine how well the blood sugar of a diabetic is being controlled. Hemoglobin Alc measures the amount of hemoglobin that has been adversely affected by blood sugar over a period of time. Too many refined carbohydrates and not enough nutrients also results in cellular inflammation and glycosylation in the collagen of the skin. When this happens, the collagen becomes stiff and inflexible—like the cooked egg white I mentioned earlier.

New healthy skin starts with healthy blood vessels. But when your fibroblasts (the cells that make collagen) don't get the nutrients they need, and your collagen is damaged from glycosalation, your skin simply doesn't look its best. You also need the right kinds of omega-3 fats to replenish your skin. The effect of a low-glycemic, nutrient-rich diet on the skin is the basis for *The Wrinkle Cure* (Rodale, 2000), by Nicholas Perricone, M.D., which provides the sound dietary advice that will also help prevent cancer and heart disease. (See chapter 7.)

PREVENTING OR TREATING WRINKLES

The key to younger-looking skin at perimenopause is to avoid smoking and overexposure to the sun (the earlier the better), follow a low-glycemic diet, and use antioxidants, both topically and internally. Uneven pigmentation, roughness, and hyperkeratinosis are the direct consequences of disruption of the cellular replication and immunological processes. As discussed above, these are brought about by DNA damage and oxidative stress resulting from absorption of UVR photons. Some women, by virtue of their genes, simply seem to have wrinkle-free youthful skin for a lifetime, regardless of how much sun exposure they get. But most of us have to give our skin a helping hand when it comes to midlife preservation or improvement.

Over the past decade or so, a huge amount of research has been done on the role of antioxidants in both preventing and even reversing the free-radical damage and tissue inflammation that are the root cause of skin aging. Excess sun exposure combined with the effects of a nutrient-poor diet and too much stress are what cause the kind of skin deterioration that we begin to notice during perimenopause. But these same factors can be addressed so that a great deal of the damage that has already been done can be stopped and even reversed.

Midlife Skin Care Regimen

~ CLEANSE YOUR SKIN REGULARLY. The skin has been called a "third kidney" because it removes almost as much waste material from the body each day as the kidneys themselves. If your skin is dry, you need to cleanse it thoroughly once per day. If it's oily, then twice per day may be better. Remove all makeup every night. When you care for your face, don't forget your neck—it's the first place you notice the effects of aging. Cleansing your skin thoroughly will clean out your pores and allow your skin to remove waste products efficiently from your body as you sleep, a time when your body is rejuvenating itself.

Use a cleansing lotion or soap that preserves the acid mantle of the skin, because it's one of your body's natural defenses against infection and breakouts. Look for the term "pH balanced" when shopping for a soap or cleanser. Many good brands are available.

If your skin is oily, be sure to avoid overuse of astringents, which usually contain alcohol. They can actually make an oil problem worse and also damage your skin over time.

~ CLOSE PORES AFTER CLEANING. Use a toner to close the pores after cleansing, especially if your skin is oily. Or simply use cool water to close the pores—it works well for all skin types.

~ RENEW SKIN WITH EXFOLIANTS AND TOPICAL ANTIOXIDANTS. One of the reasons that skin starts to look dull and old at midlife is that the rate of skin growth and cell turnover slows down. As a result, the plumper new skin cells that give your complexion a glowing appearance tend to stay below the surface. In order to help remove old dead skin from the surface, open your pores, and speed up new skin growth, you'll need regular exfoliation. This can be done either mechanically, with a washcloth, or with products that contain fruit acids, which include alpha hydroxy, beta hydroxy, or glycolic acids. (See below.)

Avoid using abrasive cleansers such as those made from the hulls of nuts, which is like cleaning your skin with sandpaper. This can lead to breakage of capillaries and microabrasions of the skin that raise the risk of infection and even acne.

If your skin is oily, apply a mild cleanser to a washcloth, and use that to exfoliate each night. Use a clean washcloth each time to decrease the amount of germs that your skin comes into contact with. Follow this with an application of a mild alpha hydroxy, beta hydroxy, or glycolic acid product and/or one of the antioxidant products I recommend below. Many products on the market today contain both antioxidants and fruit acids. If your skin is dry or sensitive, skip the washcloth and simply use an alpha hydroxy acid (AHA) or antioxidant preparation to do your exfoliating for you.

~ USE A SUNSCREEN EVERY DAY ON YOUR FACE, NECK, AND HANDS. Make a habit of putting sunscreen with an SPF of 15 or higher on your face, neck, and hands every morning except during the brief early-morning or late-afternoon "sun bath" that I advocate for optimal vitamin D levels. (See chapter 12.)

~ MOISTURIZE. If your AHA, antioxidant, or sunscreen formula is not in a moisturizing base, then finish off your daily skin care regimen with a light moisturizer for day and a richer formula for the evening. This helps much-needed moisture remain in your skin cells, keeping them plumped up.

Exfoliants and Antioxidants

FRUIT ACIDS: Alpha hydroxy acids (AHAs) and other fruit acids do double duty as exfoliants and antioxidants, boosting the effectiveness of the other antioxidants in your skin care preparation. As exfoliants, they work in three ways: (1) they help dissolve the "glue" that holds dead skin cells together, thus resulting in easier removal, so new and plumper cells can rise to the surface; (2) they increase the hydration of the skin through increasing the production of gly-cosaminoglycans (GAGs), which are present in the interstices of the collagen matrix,[2] thus boosting the amount of moisture in skin and reducing fine lines and wrinkles; and (3) they encourage the repair of elastin and collagen in the skin and even help thicken it a bit.

Commercial products usually contain from 5 to 10 percent fruit acids, concentrations that are low enough and safe enough for all skin types and tones. It's always best, however, to test any product first, either on the inner part of your elbow or just under your jaw-line. If your skin is sensitive, start with a 5 percent product. If you can tolerate that, gradually work up to a 10–12 percent product. You may experience a slight stinging with some products until you get used to them. Higher-strength AHAs (up to 70 percent) are used to lighten the skin or cause a deeper peel and should be used only by professional estheticians or doctors.

Fruit acids help normalize your skin whether it's dry or oily. If it's oily, they remove the top dead layer of cells, thus allowing oil to flow out of the follicle more easily so that it can be removed without strip-ping away essential moisture. If your skin is dry, fruit acids remove the dry dead layer and stimulate cell renewal.

It usually takes about two weeks before you'll notice a difference in your skin with regular use of a fruit acid. They can reduce wrinkles and improve roughness, sallowness, and hyperpigmentation at con-centrations as low as 5–8 percent.[3] Most people start by using AHAs only at night, but once you know they work for you, you can apply them twice per day.

As antioxidants, fruit acids can also alleviate some of the free-radical damage that results from exposure to sunlight and pollutants in the air.

ANTIOXIDANT VITAMINS AND HERBS: An ever-growing number of natural plants, vitamins, and herbs have been found to help the skin resist free-radical damage and inflammation when applied directly. Many can also help reverse the aging process. The effect of antioxi-dants is synergistic and they work best when used in combinations.[4] For example, vitamin C and vitamin E suppress the skin's sunburn re-action well when used together.[5]

Differing types of antioxidants exert their antioxidant effects through different pathways. Those that are known as nonenzymatic antioxidants (e.g., vitamins C and E) get depleted as they scavenge free radicals. Therefore they must be replenished regularly, especially under conditions where the free-radical burden is high, such as being under heavy emotional stress, or outdoors in the wind and sun. This is why it's best to apply at least one product in the morning for protection during the day, and another at night that is designed to replenish moisture as well as fight free-radical damage. A good antioxidant skin care regimen will improve skin circulation, decrease edema and puffiness (including under the eyes), decrease fine lines and wrinkles, possibly help shrink large pores, and also decrease ruddiness and restore a healthy, natural glow to the skin.

The following is a list of some of the best-studied antioxidants, though there are certainly more.

VITAMIN C: Research has shown that in the proper form, vitamin C, a powerful and ubiquitous antioxidant, can restore a smooth surface and youthful glow to aging skin. This is but one aspect of the very well-documented role it plays in protecting virtually every organ in our bodies from the effects of aging. In the skin, vitamin C is essential for the production and repair of collagen. It also helps heal inflammation because it blocks the production of some of the inflammatory chemicals.

The problem with using natural vitamin C topically is that it's very acidic, which is irritating to the skin. It is also water soluble and breaks down rapidly, losing its potency within twenty-four hours. That's why most products containing conventional vitamin C aren't effective. But when vitamin C is combined with substances that render it more bioavailable, it becomes nonacidic while maintaining its antioxidant and collagen-enhancing properties. Vitamin C that is rendered absorbable by the cells can penetrate the thin membrane that encases a cell, and it offers maximum protection against free radicals in the place they do the most damage—the outer membrane of the cell. Studies have shown that vitamin C in fat-soluble form is absorbed much more quickly and achieves levels in the skin that are ten times higher than natural vitamin C (ascorbic acid). Vitamin C in the form of such substances as tetrahexyl decyl ascorbate is stable and can be added to creams and lotions, where it will keep its potency for months.

Vitamin C creams help heal sunburn. And because fat-soluble vitamin C compounds help stimulate the growth of fibroblasts, the cells that help produce collagen and elastin in human skin, it has been shown to help reduce fine lines and wrinkles, firm skin that is sagging because of damaged collagen, and heal inflamed or irritated skin. It also gives skin a healthy glow. (See Resources.)

TOCOTRIENOLS AND VITAMIN E: Up until very recently, scientists felt that the tocopherols, particularly d-alpha tocopherol, were the most potent part of the vitamin E complex, and the alpha toco-pherols have been widely used in cosmetics and other products for over thirty years. Alpha tocopherol is often used in cosmetics in its ester form on the assumption that a process known as enzymatic hy-drolysis in the skin will restore it to an active form. But this isn't the case because, in the stratum corneum of the skin, where vitamin E's antioxidant defenses are most needed, there is only very limited enzy-matic activity necessary to change the ester into the right form. The result is that many "vitamin E" products remain largely inactive.

The ideal form of topical vitamin E is a natural blend of the toco-pherols and the tocotrienols (another part of the vitamin E complex). The tocotrienols inhibit peroxide formation—a measure of free-radical damage—much more efficiently than alpha tocopherol, and they're better at increasing the levels of the various skin enzymes that help protect the skin from ultraviolet damage. In fact, research sug-gests that the tocotrienols are forty to fifty times more powerful than other forms of vitamin E.[6] This relatively new type of high-potency vitamin E is made using a special extraction process on rice bran oil or palm fruit oil. The resulting liquid can easily be mixed into creams, lotions, shampoos, or other cosmetics. Topical tocotrienols can help dry, damaged hair, severely dry skin, and brittle fingernails. Look for the words *high-potency E* or *HPE* on the label to be sure you're get-ting the right products.

When applied topically, both tocotrienols and tocopherols rap-idly penetrate the skin and become most concentrated in the superfi-cial stratum corneum layer, right where the threat of UV damage is the greatest.[7] Vitamin E, like vitamin C, has also been found to in-hibit collagenase enzymes, which break down collagen following UVR exposure. (For more information about tocotrienols and skin care, visit the website of dermatologist Randall Wilkinson, M.D., creator of the Trienelle skin care line, at www.trienelle.com.)

COENZYME Q_{10}, OR UBIQUINONE: This powerful antioxidant is essential for the health of the entire cardiovascular system because of its ability to help cellular mitochondria produce energy. But it also functions as an antioxidant and helps inhibit collagenase.[8] In one German study there was a 23 percent reduction in fine lines on the face when a cream containing coenzyme Q_{10} was used topically.[9] Creams with coenzyme Q_{10} are readily available in natural food and other stores.

MELATONIN: Melatonin is best known for its effect on sleep and diurnal cycles, but it's also a potent antioxidant. Topical application of melatonin has been demonstrated to inhibit UV-induced redness, thus having a powerful anti-inflammatory effect.[10]

PROANTHOCYANADINS (OR PROCYANADINS) AND CATECHINS: Polyphenolic compounds are found in a variety of plants and have many beneficial effects in humans. For example, the polyphenols in green tea are what give it its beneficial effect on the lining of blood vessels. Procyanadins and catechins found in grape seeds, grape pips, green tea, green apples, and other sources, have substantial antioxidant activity.[11]

Other Skin-Enhancing Substances

MICROCOLLAGEN PENTAPEPTIDES: Fibroblasts are the cells that produce collagen in skin. These cells produce less collagen with age for reasons that aren't clear. We do know that they haven't lost the ability because when aging fibroblasts are placed in cell culture and stimulated by growth factors, they can produce significant quantities of collagen.[12]

One of the factors that stimulates fibroblasts to produce collagen is a small segment of the collagen molecule itself, known as a pentapeptide fragment.[13] Researchers have found that it is an effective stimulator of both collagen and fibronectin synthesis—both of which are important components of the interstitial matrix around skin cells.[14]

Testing of this pentapeptide (3 percent concentration) on a panel of thirty-five subjects for a period of six months demonstrated significant to highly significant changes over a placebo cream as well as a commercial 5 percent vitamin C product.[15]

LIPOSOMES: Liposomes are small, membrane-covered sacs approximately three hundred times smaller than the human cell that are very useful for penetrating the effective barrier that the skin provides for protection. They consist of a lecithin-based lipid membrane surrounding specific contents that the cells need. When applied to the skin, the structural similarity of the liposome to the cells, as well as its small size, allows it to penetrate readily into the various levels of the skin.

When it hits skin cells, the membrane of the liposome fuses into the cell membrane, discharging its contents into the cytoplasm of the cell over the course of six to eight hours. Lipsomal delivery systems thus dramatically increase the effectiveness of any active ingredient in a skin care formulation, making it approximately ten times more effective than when applied without the liposomal delivery system.[16]

How to Evaluate a Skin Care Formulation

The newest skin care ingredients are so effective that they belong to an entirely new category that has been dubbed "cosmeceuticals," given the fact that they have pharmacologic effects on the structure and function of skin. The FDA regards these products as cosmetics and they are regulated as such.

There are two things to consider about this as a result. The first one is that cosmetics manufacturers aren't allowed to make any claims (whether or not they are true) about a product or ingredient's ability to make permanent changes in the skin. This very much limits the ability of a manufacturer to provide consumers with independent referenced material about the action of a product or its ingredients.

Secondly, the labeling requirements for cosmetics do not require the manufacturer to disclose the amounts or percentages of ingredients, although all ingredients must be listed on the label. What that means is that the consumer doesn't know whether a product actually contains an ingredient in any meaningful quantity (i.e., the quantity and percentage that clinical studies have shown to be effective!). Labeling regulations require that ingredients be listed in descending order, from the greatest to the least, for those ingredients constituting 1 percent or more of the total weight. Ingredients making up less than 1 percent of the total may be listed in any order. The label, therefore, is of limited usefulness in determining the concentration of ingredients that may be highly effective at low concentrations. A product containing 1 percent of melatonin, for example, would be indistinguishable from a product containing .001 percent. A product might only contain a few molecules of an effective ingredient that will maximize marketing but minimize effectiveness! Therefore the consumer is forced to rely upon independent reviews of the scientific literature or independent reviews of individual products. In the resource section, I have endeavored to steer you to some products that I know are effective, both from personal experience and from my review of the science supporting them.

The Preservative Dilemma

The law requires that skin care products be preserved in order to prevent bacterial or fungal overgrowth, which is known to be dangerous. (There have been cases of blindness from mascara that was contaminated with pseudomonas bacteria.) Most companies accomplish this by adding traditional chemical preservatives known as parabens and also other formaldehyde-releasing chemicals. (Check product labels for the following: DMDM Hydantoin, Diazolidinyl Urea, Quaternium-15, benzalkonium chloride, benzalkonium bromide, chlorhexidine, cetylpyridinium chloride, or thimerosal.) Though preservatives are effective and give products a long shelf life, they themselves aren't entirely safe—especially when used on the skin over many years.

Some are found in very low levels in nature. Generally more than one paraben preservative is used to give broader germ-killing power. Parabens can cause skin irritation and contact sensitization over time. They may also act as environmental toxins that accumulate in tissue, including the breast. Further studies are necessary to evaluate how much risk is associated with longtime use of parabens and formaldehyde-releasing preservatives.

You may also see claims made for "natural preservatives." These products often use essential oils such as tea tree oil or grapefruit seed oil. These "natural preservatives" do not lend themselves to variations in formulas needed to produce an entire line of products; in other words, they have limited use and at times their effectiveness as a preservative or antimicrobial agent is questionable. It's prudent to consider using products that don't contain potentially harmful preservatives whenever possible to decrease one's total lifetime exposure to these common chemicals. (See Resources.)

Skin Care by Prescription Only

If you follow the insulin-normalizing diet I recommend in chapter 7 and institute the skin care regimen I've outlined above, including a good antioxidant product with at least two or three of the antioxidants listed, then you probably won't need anything else for your skin. Nevertheless, it's worth knowing about the popular prescription skin care medications that are available. There are two basic kinds: retinoic acid derivatives and hormone-containing products.

RETINOIC ACID DERIVATIVES: Retin-A, Retin-A Micro, and Renova are all prescription medications derived from retinoic acid, a form of vitamin A that helps prevent or reduce fine lines and wrinkles, reverse sun damage, and heal acne.

These substances are powerful antioxidants, and regular use of retinoic acid as prescribed by a physician can result in reduction of fine lines and wrinkles, stimulate blood flow to the skin, even out pigmentation, and help prevent wrinkles and lines from forming in the first place.

But retinoic acid is not for everyone. Side effects include redness, dryness, itchiness, and increased sun sensitivity. It takes anywhere from two to six months to notice a real difference if you're not taking any other steps to improve your complexion, and you must be absolutely committed to rigorous sunscreen use.

I personally used a form of Retin-A prescribed for many women before I discovered other more effective skin care products. Though the Retin-A worked and was nonirritating, it resulted in excessive flakiness of my skin, which I'd sometimes notice on my cheeks and jawline at the worst possible time—usually looking into the mirror just before leaving for a speaking engagement! Not all women have this effect, but I find I get much better results with the topical and systemic antioxidant program I now use.

TOPICAL APPLICATION OF HORMONE REPLACEMENT THERAPY: Skin contains receptor sites for hormones, and it is well documented that estrogen, which also has antioxidant effects, helps preserve the collagen layer of the skin. Declining hormone levels are one of the reasons for the thinning of the collagen layer during the perimenopausal years. Many women who've undergone surgical or medical menopause notice skin changes within a few months of the loss of their hormonal support unless they take steps to replace those hormones or take phytohormones.

Research has shown that topical application of estrogen can increase collagen thickness, decrease pore size, and help the skin hold moisture. In Europe, estrogen is often prescribed to help beautify the skin. You can get these same benefits by using hormones topically.

If you are already on bioidentical hormone replacement (see pages 142–149), ask your doctor to prescribe your hormones via a formulary pharmacist so that they can be put into skin lotion. In my experience, most women are delighted with this method of using hormone replacement. It improves the skin, enhances moisture, and provides the benefits of hormone replacement, all at the same time. As with any type of hormone replacement, it's always best to use the lowest dose that does the job. Levels that are too high can result in excessive oil secretion, acne, and even excessive growth of facial hair.

TOPICAL ESTROGEN: If you are not on hormone replacement already but want to try estrogen for its skin benefits, ask your health care provider to prescribe a small amount of estrogen just for this purpose. A formulary pharmacist can put a small amount of estradiol or estriol in an ointment or cream. Use of the cream is safe and effective, without the adverse side effects of too much estrogen. A 1996 study found that the use of dilute topical estrogen produced marked improvement of elasticity and firmness of the skin along with increased skin moisture, decreased pore size, and decreased wrinkle depth. The dose used in the study was 1 g of an ointment containing 0.01 percent estradiol and 0.3 percent estriol, applied daily to neck and face. Monthly determinations of blood hormone levels of estradiol, follicle-stimulating hormone (FSH), and prolactin failed to show any significant systemic hormonal changes using these dilute amounts on the skin.[17]

TOPICAL PROGESTERONE: Many of my patients have seen skin improvement, including decreased midlife acne, greater moisture, and fading of age spots, by using a 2 percent natural progesterone cream on their skin. This may be all you need without resorting to a prescription for estrogen cream.

Beautiful Skin from the Inside Out:
The Right Foods and Supplements

Good skin isn't just an "outside" job. The skin is a mirror for the health of your insides as well as your outsides. Take antioxidant vitamins (more about that below) and eat at least five servings of fruits and vegetables daily. Many of the hundreds of substances present in these foods, such as lycopene in tomatoes, lutein in dark green and yellow vegetables, and the antioxidants in berries, have been clinically proven to help prevent and heal sun damage to the skin. Since antioxidants work in concert with one another, the greater the variety of fruits and vegetables you eat, the better.

The insulin-normalizing diet I recommend for balancing hormones at midlife also helps keep your skin in good shape. Limit caffeine, and cut down as much as possible on high-glycemic-index foods such as cookies, candies, pies, cakes, and non-whole-grain breads, all of which can cause fluid retention from excess insulin secretion. They are devoid of skin-nourishing vitamins and minerals, and quickly break down into sugar, which, as I explained above, causes collagen to lose its flexibility. (This is one of the reasons why diabetic individuals whose blood sugar is not tightly controlled often develop cataracts in the collagen-rich lenses of their eyes and have difficulty with wound healing. It is also why oral supplementation with antioxidants has been shown to alleviate some of the side effects of diabetes.)

FIBER: Make sure that you're getting enough fiber. Nothing shows up on the skin faster than chronic constipation! I've seen many cases of acne clear beautifully once bowel function is normalized. One of the most effective ways to do this is simply by eating ¼ cup of ground golden flaxseed each day. In addition to the 11-plus grams of fiber you'll get, flaxseeds are also loaded with skin-beautifying omega-3 fatty acids and phytoestrogens. Fruits and vegetables are also rich in fiber in addition to their antioxidants.

WATER: You may also see a dramatic improvement in your skin if you drink eight 8-oz glasses of water per day.

FISH: Fish, especially salmon, sardines, and swordfish, is rich in both the omega-3 fats, which are important for building healthy cell membranes everywhere in the body.

SOY: One of the most common benefits women notice after several months of supplementing their diets with significant amounts of soy protein (100–160 mg of soy isoflavones per day) is improvement in their skin tone, hair, and nails. In a recent study of forty postmenopausal women taking Revival soy, 93 percent showed significant improvements in skin (namely, skin flaking and discoloration were reduced after three months, and wrinkling was reduced after six months). The women also reported significant improvements in hair roughness, dullness, manageability, and overall assessment as well as in nail roughness, ridging, flaking, splitting, and overall appearance.[18] One woman who takes the soy supplement Revival wrote, "Within two months of beginning this soy drink, my nails became stronger and more resilient than ever, my hair has taken on more body, and my skin has never looked more radiant. I'm thrilled." Soy's phytoestrogen content helps strengthen collagen everywhere in the body, whether in facial skin, vaginal tissue, or bone, while soy isoflavones may act as antioxidants to protect skin from free-radical damage.[19] Soy also provides high-quality protein needed for building and maintenance.

SKIN-AIDING SUPPLEMENTS: Though all of the various supplements that I recommend at midlife help the skin (see chapter 7), the antioxidants, such as coenzyme Q_{10}, vitamin C, vitamin E and tocotrienols, and proanthocyanidins are particularly important.

Research has shown, for example, that proanthocyanidins from pine bark or grape pips help protect skin from the damaging effects of too much ultraviolet radiation. In one study, this powerful antioxidant was shown to prevent ultraviolet activation of a certain area in the nucleus of skin cells, reducing the inflammation that occurs after a sunburn.[20] Many individuals have reported healthy changes in their skin, nails, and hair as a result. The usual dose is 40–120 mg per day; I personally take 60–80 mg per day and even more when traveling or under stress.

Coenzyme Q_{10}, which is found in every cell of the body, is fat soluble and concentrates in the plasma membrane of cells, where it protects against free-radical damage. This antioxidant is used up when skin is exposed to ultraviolet radiation and other environmental insults, so it makes sense to supplement your diet with it or apply it topically. It is also found in red meat, salmon, and nuts. Coenzyme Q_{10} assists in cellular metabolism. The usual dose in supplement form is 30–100 mg per day.

Vitamins E and C taken as supplements have also been shown to help protect against the UV-generated free-radical damage that can lead to skin changes. The dose of vitamin C used was only 200 mg; for vitamin E, it was 1,000 IU.[21] The results are apt to be even more impressive with the newer, more potent forms of vitamin E—the tocotrienols. The supplement regimen recommended in chapter 7 will give you all the skin-nourishing nutrients you need.

SKIN CARE FROM YOUR REFRIGERATOR

Once or twice per week, if you have the time, you can give your face a healthy dose of antioxidants, fruit acids, and plant hormones by using ingredients that you can find right in your refrigerator. Choose the food that most appeals to your sense of smell; you'll be getting aromatherapy benefits as well as direct benefit to your skin. Plain yogurt applied to your face makes a nourishing mask that gives your skin the benefits of lactic acid and also the hydrating effects of milk proteins. You can add pureed fresh fruit to it. (Don't use sweetened yogurt. The sugar is harmful to the skin.)

I love thinly sliced cucumber applied to my eyelids and cheeks to help me relax and get ready for evening. Green tea bags, moistened and applied to the eyelids, also give your eyes a soothing antioxidant life. And mashed-up fresh fruits such as peaches, strawberries, or apples can all be mixed with finely ground oatmeal to form a nourishing facial mask. You can also use parsley or even fresh basil, rosemary, or thyme. Remember, the skin will absorb the nutrients from these foods in about fifteen minutes, so you don't need to lie down any longer than that to benefit from a rejuvenating facial mask.

MIDLIFE ACNE

Anything that compromises the immune system, whether emotional stress or nutritional deficiency, will tend to exacerbate the underlying conditions that lead to acne. So will hormonal imbalances in which the body produces too much androgen. Anytime you are under stress, your cortisol and insulin balance is likely to be upset; this, too, can affect your skin—and the rest of you as well. At perimenopause, the same stormy emotions that were present at adolescence often arise again, along with the hormonal swings that exacerbate the situation. It's no wonder that skin breakouts are so common during this life stage.

Are You Thin-Skinned and in Need of Individuation?

Both adolescence and midlife are key developmental periods of our lives when we go through the process of individuating and defining who we are in relationship to others. The skin is the first contact surface between the mother and the infant, and for our entire lives it represents a boundary between us and other people. Some researchers believe that skin disease may be thought of as an attempt to define who we are in relationship to other people and what a healthy boundary between us should be.[22] I agree.

When I was in my early thirties, a time in life when hormones are relatively stable and skin is usually at its best, I developed a very troubling case of acne. It took me a while to understand what was going on. I'd never had much in the way of skin problems in my teenage years, and since I was exercising regularly, taking vitamins, and eating a whole-food diet, it seemed strange to me that I should suddenly be experiencing acne at my age. However, I was working at the time in an office where my ideas on nutrition, emotions, and the mind/body connection were not well accepted, a fact I dealt with by way of a lot of self-deprecating humor, hoping this would enable me to stay safe and fit in as best I could. I desperately wanted the approval of my colleagues and was so thin-skinned that I was constantly trying to forestall any criticism of my ideas and beliefs. Finally, at the age of thirty-five, I realized that I couldn't continue using so much of my energy to try to blend in, and so after a good deal of soul-searching, I took a leap of faith and left to cofound Women to Women. My four-year-long skin problem cleared up within three months and has never returned, even though I'm now smack in the middle of midlife hormonal changes!

THE ANATOMY OF ACNE

1. Androgenic hormones such as DHEA and testosterone increase production of sebum by the sebaceous glands.

2. Sebum makes the hardened outer layer of skin (the keratin-rich cells known as the horny layer) turn over faster. This results in pores and hair follicles that are clogged with dead skin cells and oil.

3. Skin bacteria of the type known as *Propionibacterium acnes* feed off the sebum and break it down into free fatty acids.

4. Free fatty acids attract white blood cells and other inflammatory molecules (eicosanoids) from the immune system.

5. An acne pimple or blackhead is the result.

Hormones and Midlife Acne

There are numerous studies showing that sebaceous gland activity is heightened by androgens such as DHEA and testosterone and reduced by estrogen or removal of the ovaries, which reduces androgen levels.[23] This is the reason why birth control pills often help clear up acne. But whether or not higher levels of hormones result in acne is an individual matter. Women with the most severe forms of acne generally have a genetic predisposition to androgen sensitivity in their skin, even at hormone levels that are normal.

When sebaceous glands are small, as in children and the elderly, acne does not occur. It is usually first seen in adolescence, when sebaceous gland development begins to take place. It occurs primarily on the face, back, and chest. Endocrinologists have long theorized that acne is an endocrine disease resulting from abnormal androgen production. Hair follicles and attached sebaceous glands contain a specific enzyme known as 5-alpha-reductase, which can convert estrogen into the androgen testosterone. That's why some women experience an increase in acne when their estrogen levels rise, due either to perimenopause or to being put on overly high levels of hormone replacement therapy. But two women who are on identical hormone replacement regimens, eat exactly the same diet, and have the same amount of stress in their lives may have skin reactions that are entirely different. That's why all treatments, including prescription medications, have their place and can be useful.

Natural Treatments for Acne

If your acne is mild to moderate, I'd recommend that you use the natural treatment program I outline below. If your acne is severe, you may also want to add one of the medications I discuss below, or follow the advice of a skin care specialist.

~ EAT A GOOD DIET. Follow the high-fiber, insulin-lowering diet outlined in chapter 7, because a diet too high in high-glycemic-index carbohydrates, as I've already stated, is associated with excessively high levels of insulin, which in turn can cause higher-than-normal production of androgens. For many women, this is all that is necessary to completely clear up acne.

~ TAKE SUPPLEMENTS. Take a comprehensive vitamin and mineral supplement daily. (See chapter 7.) It is well documented that zinc, vitamin C, and the B vitamins are essential for healthy skin functioning. Many women notice that their hair and skin improve dramatically when they start on a good supplementation regimen.

~ LOSE EXCESS BODY FAT. Get your body fat percentage into the healthy range. Excess body fat is associated with higher-than-normal androgen levels. Even a small fat loss of five to ten pounds can make a significant difference in insulin and androgen as it affects the sebaceous glands.

~ FOLLOW THE SKIN CARE REGIMEN FOR THE GENERAL CARE OF MIDLIFE SKIN (PAGES 355–356). Remember that the fruit acids alone often work very well for acne. A good antioxidant skin care program usually helps reduce or completely eliminate acne scars. Intense Pulsed Light (IPL) treatments can work wonders for old acne scars.

~ TRY HOME REMEDIES FOR PIMPLES. When you notice a pimple that hasn't come to a head yet, apply tea tree oil at night. The antibacterial properties in the oil will often result in significant regression of the pimple by morning. Some women use tea tree oil daily.

Another effective treatment is to make a paste of baking soda and lemon juice and apply it to the pimple. Baking soda also makes an excellent exfoliating agent unless your skin is sensitive.

~ REMOVE BLACKHEADS. For blackheads, get a professional facial with blackhead removal about once per month until your skin has cleared. After that, you can use one of the readily available blackhead removal strips, such as Bioré. Limit use to once per week to avoid overdrying the skin.

Acne Medications

VITAMIN A DERIVATIVES: Tretinoin (in Retin-A, Retin-A Micro, and Renova, applied topically) and Isotretinoin (Accutane, taken systemically) are prescription medications that increase skin cell turnover and allow sebum to be released more easily so that it doesn't get trapped. Accutane is an oral vitamin A derivative that powerfully inhibits both sebum production and growth of acne-causing bacteria. It is the single most effective treatment for severe acne that doesn't respond to other measures. However, it is very irritating and should never be used by anyone who is pregnant or trying to get pregnant, because it can cause birth defects.[24]

BENZOYL PEROXIDE AND SULFUR-CONTAINING PRODUCTS: Various lotions, creams, or gels containing benzoyl peroxide or sulfur are often used for their antibacterial and drying properties. Benzoyl peroxide penetrates the hair follicle and produces oxygen, thus suppressing the growth of acne-causing bacteria, which thrive in an anaerobic (oxygen-free) environment. Although often effective, these treatments can be very irritating for the skin. I recommend the Acne Recovery System Kit from Trienelle (www.trienelle.com), which allows users to adjust their dose of benzoyl peroxide and other effective anti-acne preparations to minimize irritation and maximize effectiveness.

ANTIBIOTICS: Tetracycline or erythromycin work by preventing the acne bacteria from breaking down the sebum into the free fatty acids that result in pimples. I do not recommend the use of antibiotics because they kill off the healthy bacteria in the bowel, which can lead to suboptimal absorption of nutrients, diarrhea, and repeated yeast infections. It can also lead to antibiotic resistance.

BIRTH CONTROL PILLS: Oral contraceptives are often used to reduce sebum production. They do this by decreasing the brain's signal to make hormones from the ovaries. I'd avoid these synthetic hormones unless you feel you have no other choice and are unable or unwilling to follow a healthier diet or use one or more of the topical treatments recommended above.

ROSACEA

Rosacea is a common condition at midlife (forties and fifties) and occurs equally in women and in men. Rosacea is, in essence, a neurological disorder of the facial blood vessels, which makes them hyper-responsive. This results in dilated blood vessels in the blush area of the face and upper chest. It is accompanied by facial flushing, a burning sensation in the face, and also papules and pustules. Rosacea clearly demonstrates the seamless connection between emotions and skin, for it always gets worse when women are under significant emotional stress. Psychological studies have linked rosacea with a disordered blushing reaction. Though blushing is a normal response to the emotions of excitement, shame, or embarrassment, in those with rosacea the body's normal response goes too far because the emotion is held too frequently or too long. Studies have shown, for instance, that people prone to this disorder are likely to be perfectionistic and have a strong need to please others. They also have a predisposition to excessive feelings of guilt and shame.[25] Rosacea "triggers" are numerous and include changes in temperature, certain foods, stress, changes in emotions, exercise, and several skin care products. Rosacea generally begins between the ages of thirty and sixty, though it can start as early as the teenage years and, although rare, in childhood.

CHERYL: *Rosacea and Shame*

Cheryl first came to see me when she was forty-two and having problems with irregular periods. She also had persistent reddening of the skin around her nose and cheeks, which her dermatologist had diagnosed as rosacea. Though she was on various topical antibiotics for the problem, they didn't help much. Her problem always seemed to be exacerbated premenstrually, but with such irregular periods, which sometimes came every two weeks, she never knew when her skin would look good and when it would flare up.

As I worked with Cheryl over the next year, we both noticed what a barometer her skin reddening was for emotional turmoil. And Cheryl had plenty. During the year that her rosacea first appeared, she was in the middle of an affair with a married professional—an affair that took place in his office. Over time she discovered that she wasn't the only woman with whom this man was sexually involved. When she discovered this, she felt deeply ashamed. Her childhood history revealed that she had been the victim of incest by her father, something she had also kept secret for years. But Cheryl had a great deal of courage. She began to go to groups for incest survivors and also started individual therapy. At the same time she committed to improving her diet and lifestyle on all levels. Over the next several years Cheryl became stronger and more independent. Eventually she even had the courage to forgive herself for becoming involved with an unscrupulous man in the first place. As Cheryl connected with her inner wisdom and supported herself physically through diet and exercise, her rosacea cleared up, slowly but surely. She now notices flare-ups only occasionally, and only when she reverts to old emotional patterns of shame and neediness, feelings that she now has the skills and self-esteem to work through effectively.

Treatment Options

The standard treatment for rosacea includes both oral and topical medications that are anti-inflammatory (antibiotics or accutane) and a topical anti-inflammatory (such as a metronidazole-based product). The treatment protocol is generally followed for four to six months until the rosacea is under control. (Often, antibiotics don't help—there's no evidence that rosacea is caused by abnormal skin bacteria.) After that, just topical treatment is continued. The obvious problem with oral antibiotics is that taking them over so many months can result in an imbalance of normal bowel flora. That's why I always recommend taking a probiotic (for example, acidophilus) if you're on an antibiotic. Cellular inflammation aggravates rosacea (and just about every other disease as well), so it's also helpful to follow a diet that keeps insulin levels normal. This means eating minimal amounts or eliminating "white" foods, including white bread, white potatoes, products containing sugar, and soda. It's best to include lots of fresh fruits and vegetables, which are also loaded with antioxidants to help fight inflammation. It's also helpful to use skin care products that are self-preserving and do not contain parabens and other irritants. (See Resources.) Be sure to avoid products with alpha-hydroxy acids, as they can be irritating. Hydrocortisone, benzoyl peroxide, and topical retinoids should also be avoided.

Some women report that supplementing their diets with betaine hydrochloride, which increases stomach acidity, helps rosacea, for reasons that aren't entirely clear. If you decide to take this supplement, which is available in natural food stores, make sure you take it with food. Otherwise it creates a sensation like heartburn. The usual dose is 500–1,000 mg with meals. IPL (Intense Pulsed Light) can also be very effective.

MIND/BODY APPROACH TO SKIN PROBLEMS

Did my description of the psychological profile of a rosacea patient or someone suffering from midlife acne strike home? If it did, then next time you feel yourself becoming overwhelmed by emotions of shame, anxiety, or anger, try the following.

1. Take a full, deep breath—all the way down into your belly. (We often stop breathing when we feel a strong emotion, as a way to stop feeling it.) Exhale and continue to breathe fully.

2. Close your eyes.

3. Identify where in your body you are feeling the emotion.

4. Describe what you are feeling. Does it have a shape or a color or a sound?

5. Don't try to change your feeling. Allow yourself to feel it fully, exactly as it is. Love yourself for it.

6. Keep breathing and moving around while doing this— breathing and moving will help you move the emotion right on through.

Here's what you're apt to notice: the minute you give your emotion a chance to be felt fully, it goes away. You can use this technique anytime you feel any difficult emotion. And guess what? You'll find that you have the ability to deal with it without outside help.

HAIR IN THE WRONG PLACES

Many women notice an increase in coarse or dark hair on their chins and upper lips starting at midlife. Although this can be quite distressing, it is perfectly natural and is the result of the higher androgen-to-estrogen ratio that prevails beginning in perimenopause. Androgen can transform fine peach-fuzz-type hair (known as vellus hair) into coarser hair (known as terminal hair). Sometimes, however, excessive facial hair can be a sign of an underlying hormonal imbalance, such as in the condition known as polycystic ovary disease. Coarse facial hair is also common in women whose diets are too high in refined carbohydrates, which shifts the hormones in the direction of androgens. But usually the growth of facial hair at midlife is not a sign of hormonal or nutritional problems, but simply the normal result of proportionally higher levels of androgens.

The same androgenic hormones that are associated with thickening and darkening of hair on your upper lip and your chin may cause hair loss on other areas, like the head. Androgenic hormones affect the hair follicles of the scalp by shortening what is known as anagen (the growth phase of the hair growth cycle), which causes the hair to regress to a finer, thinner texture. But how androgen affects the hair depends in part on where the hair is located. The androgen receptors in the hair follicles of other areas of the body vary in terms of numbers and sensitivity. That's the reason why excessive androgen can thin out the hair on your head while increasing the amount and thickness of the hair on your face. Of course, not only are there differences in androgen sensitivity in different bodily sites within the individual, but there are differences between individuals. Thus a relatively low level of androgen may result in facial hair growth in some women and not in others. Amount of body and facial hair also varies among different racial groups. Dark-haired, darkly pigmented Caucasians of either sex tend to be hairier than blonds or fair-skinned individuals.

Hair Removal Techniques

As normal as it may be, excess facial (or body) hair may be something you wish to deal with cosmetically. In general, I don't recommend plucking, waxing, or shaving, because over time this can distort the hair follicle, making permanent hair removal more difficult if you decide on that later. But before opting for permanent removal, you may want to try the insulin-balancing diet suggested in chapter 7. As an interim cosmetic intervention, it's best to simply cut the hair as close to the skin as possible or bleach it. If you do decide on permanent hair removal, keep in mind that fine, non-androgenized hair (the peach-fuzz type of hair that is present everywhere on the body) may undergo androgenization at any time during perimenopause or beyond. So even though you may have had your existing coarse hair removed, you may be producing new hair regularly, especially during times of stress, when androgenic hormone levels increase. Sometimes hair growth will also be encouraged by the hormones you're using or your diet and stress levels.

ELECTROLYSIS: Electrolysis is a procedure done by a trained professional that involves sending an electric current into the hair follicle via a carefully placed needle. It can take several treatments per hair follicle to truly destroy that hair follicle and prevent the hair from regrowing. Electrolysis is uncomfortable, so you may want your doctor to give you a prescription for a topical anesthetic known as EMLA (lidocaine and prilocaine), which must be put on the skin an hour before the treatment. Over time—usually a few weeks to a few months—regular electrolysis sessions will result in far fewer dark hairs. But you'll probably have to continue to go for treatments every month or so, as new vellus hairs are transformed into terminal hairs. Make sure that your electrolysis professional is well trained and certified.

LASER HAIR REMOVAL: Laser technology for hair removal is improving all the time and can be very effective. Like electrolysis, it is painful, so a topical anesthetic (EMLA) is used before the procedure. Make sure you go to a physician who is well trained in laser technology, because it is a rapidly evolving field.

PRESCRIPTION MEDICATIONS: The medications mentioned on page 379 for the treatment of hair loss on the head may also, ironically, be effective for treating hair growth on the face, since both may be a result of the hormonal shifts that occur at menopause. Spironolactone in particular is a potent anti-androgen that is sometimes effective when used topically.

Alopecia Androgenica: Midlife Hair Loss from Hormonal Imbalance

Though some women begin to experience some hair loss at menopause secondary to hormonal shifts in the body, most do not. Saying that significant hair loss is secondary to menopause would be like saying that dementia is a normal part of aging. Nevertheless, hair loss at perimenopause is a relatively common problem that erodes self-confidence and self-esteem and makes it difficult to enjoy yourself fully in a social situation.

Alopecia androgenica, which results in what we call male pattern baldness, is by far the most common cause of hair thinning and loss in women at midlife. Typically, the hair becomes finer and thinner and may eventually recede, though in women usually the front hairline is preserved. Up to 13 percent of premenopausal women and 37 percent of postmenopausal women suffer from hormone-associated hair loss to some degree.

I recently received the following illustrative letter from Evelyn, one of my newsletter subscribers.

> I am writing in an attempt to get some clarification on natural hormone replacement. I had a complete hysterectomy last July at the age of forty-four—fibroids. My doctor started me out on Premarin, and I had no problems that I was aware of. However, I had read many books on natural hormone replacements and decided to go with a formula my doctor prescribed for me. I have been using four drops of the hormone lotion to control hot flashes. I noticed after a while that my skin became oily and I am having problems with acne. Also, and what concerns me the most, is that my hair is thinning quite rapidly.
>
> I have had a blood test for hormones and thyroid—everything was within normal limits. The test showed that my hormone levels were higher than in a young, healthy female. I am trying to lower my dose to see if it will have an effect on my hair. I understand that too much estrogen can cause hair loss. My doctor encourages me to go back on the pharmaceutical alternatives, which he tells me he has used successfully for more than twenty years. At this time I am very confused and would do almost anything to keep my hair from falling out. Please, give me some advice on how to pursue this problem.

Clearly Evelyn is converting estrogen to androgen, and the androgens are having an effect at the level of her hair follicles. That's why her skin is getting oily, she's getting acne, and her hair is thinning.

Although the hormone regimen she is on works well for many women, transdermal hormones go right into the bloodstream and as such can give higher levels with lower doses than when the hormone is given orally. I suggested that Evelyn either switch to an oral estrogen-progesterone preparation or cut way back on her topical estrogen and progesterone. For reasons that aren't entirely clear, some women simply do better with oral hormones. I also suggested to Evelyn that she make sure she is following an insulin-lowering diet so that excess insulin from refined carbohydrates isn't pushing her body toward higher androgen production. She could also use a high-dose soy supplement to help her hot flashes and to keep her bones healthy. This infusion of phytohormones might allow her to cut her dose of estrogen, so there would be less of it around for her body to convert into androgen.

If you have hair follicles that are particularly sensitive to androgen, like Evelyn, any hormone replacement regimen that has too much androgen for your body can result in hair loss. The problem goes away once you stop the drug. Most hormonally associated hair loss is not caused by hormone replacement regimens, however; it is the result of an imbalance in your own body's hormonal production.

Androgen-associated hair loss can be likened to the canary in the mine. It is a symptom that often signals a much more pervasive hormone imbalance that affects many women to one degree or another. Though, as I mentioned, up to 37 percent of menopausal women will have some hair thinning from increased androgen production at menopause, about 10 to 15 percent of women have full-blown androgen-excess syndrome, characterized by facial acne, male pattern hair loss, upper-body obesity (apple-shaped figure), insulin resistance, increased facial hair, and adverse changes in lipid profile.

This syndrome, which overlaps with insulin resistance, which I've outlined in chapter 7, is associated with polycystic ovary syndrome, adrenal hypersecretion, genetic factors, excessive body fat, or unknown causes. Because all of these factors set the scene for early-onset cardiovascular disease and diabetes, your hormone-associated hair loss needs to be seen as only one aspect of a much larger systemic imbalance that you can do a great deal to help alleviate.

How to Get Your Hair Back—and Improve
Your Health at the Same Time

First, have your health care provider test you to see if there is a systemic cause for your hair loss. Diagnosing the type of hair loss you have will help clarify which options are most likely to work.

Make sure your hormone levels are normal. Even though the vast majority of women with hair loss will be found to have normal androgen levels, it's important to rule out the occasional rare abnormality, and also to remember that it's usually not your body's absolute level of androgen that's the problem, but your hair follicles' heightened sensitivity to androgen. Have your doctor check your thyroid, DHEA, free testosterone, and androstenedione levels. If you do fit the description of someone with full-blown androgen-excess syndrome, have your lipid profile, blood pressure, and blood sugar checked as well.

Even if your hormone levels check out as normal, do the following.

~ Follow the hormone-balancing diet outlined in chapter 7.

~ Lose any excess body fat. If your body fat percentage is above 30 percent, as measured in your doctor's office or fitness center, the excess fat is a factory for androgen and could drive your insulin levels, blood pressure, and blood lipids into unhealthy ranges. Excess body fat caused by a sedentary lifestyle and a diet too high in refined carbohydrates and trans fats is probably the key issue in combating not only androgen-associated hair loss, but also the health problems often associated with it.

~ Take a good vitamin and mineral supplement (see chapter 7) to help your new hair grow in fully.

~ Try Chinese herbs. Shou Wu Pian is a Chinese herbal medicine that often works very well to help restore hair growth. My acupuncturist has used it for years, and I have seen wonderful results, including a reduction in gray hair. (See Resources.)

TREATING THE SURFACE—MINOXIDIL AND TRETINOIN SPRAY: Minoxidil is currently the only drug approved by the FDA for its beneficial effect on hair growth. Minoxidil is a potent antihypertensive medication that when taken by mouth lowers blood pressure by dilating blood vessels. It was discovered by accident that it increases hair growth. Though it is not clear how it enhances hair growth when applied topically, it may increase the size of the hair follicle, prolong the growth phase of a hair follicle, increase blood flow to the skin, or enhance DNA synthesis. Side effects are rare but may include skin irritation and a short-lived increase in heart rate. In one study, a 2 percent solution of minoxidil increased the total weight of hair by over 40 percent over a forty-week period of use.[26] When researchers combined a 2 percent solution of minoxidil with 0.025 percent tretinoin (Retin-A) and used it four times per day as a scalp spray, 90 percent of the women in the study showed visible and cosmetically significant improvement in hair quality after six months.[27]

PRESCRIPTION MEDICATIONS FOR HORMONAL HAIR LOSS: The drugs doctors prescribe to rebalance systemic hormonal imbalances work well for some, though not all, women with hormone-associated hair loss. However, too often they help the symptoms without really addressing the underlying cause—too much body fat, unhealthy diet, sedentary lifestyle, and so on—or helping you learn how to heal yourself by using the body's own internal wisdom. If you use any of the following medications, complement them with appropriate diet and lifestyle changes.

~ *Birth control pills* with ethinyl estradiol, 30–40 mcg, for twenty days of the cycle: birth control pills sometimes work to stop androgenic hair loss for the same reason they help acne—they reduce the body's susceptibility to the effects of androgen on the hair follicle and its attached sebaceous gland.

~ *Dexamethasone*, 0.125–0.375 mg at bedtime. Dexamethasone is a powerful steroid that suppresses the production of androgens, thereby increasing the amount of hair on the head. It also treats the acne that accompanies male pattern hair loss in many women. Unfortunately, it has all the potential side effects of too much cortisol, such as an increase in insulin, thinning of the skin and bones, and an increased susceptibility to infection.

~ *Spironolactone* is an anti-androgen that can be taken orally or applied topically. Taken orally, it decreases total and free testosterone. Applied topically, it reduces the amount of androgen that directly affects the hair follicle.

In some women, an individualized hormone replacement prescription, such as the ones described in chapter 5 and above for skin, can help balance hormone levels and help alleviate androgen excess.

Making the Most of the Hair You've Got

While you're working from the inside out—or the outside in—you'll still want to look your best. Make the most of what you've got . . . and enhance it.

Consult a professional who specializes in hairpieces, hair extensions, weaves, and body perms. You might even want to inquire about hair transplantation for women by a dermatologist or plastic surgeon.[28]

Here are some more tips for making thin hair appear its best.

- Use gentle shampoos, and don't shampoo more than every other day.

- Don't brush your hair when it's wet—this stretches out the hair.

- Avoid teasing—it can break your hair.

- Chlorine damages hair. Shower with pure water. If your water is chlorinated, use a shower filter that removes it.

- Ask your hairdresser to recommend professional products for fine hair that will give you extra volume.

WHEN GOOD SKIN CARE ISN'T ENOUGH: DECIDING ON COSMETIC PROCEDURES

Sometimes the results you're looking for will be unattainable with diet and good skin care alone. If you have a "fixable" aspect of your face that bothers you every time you look in the mirror, it may be time to consider getting outside help. Whether you want to enhance your smile with cosmetic dentistry or get rid of the bags under your eyes that always make you look tired even when you're not, there's no doubt that fixing an energy-draining "ding" in your appearance can improve the quality of life. That's why so many women get braces at midlife, or have skin peels to give them a fresher look that simply can't be achieved any other way. Cosmetic surgery of all kinds is growing by leaps and bounds because of vast improvements in technology and increasing demand.

It seems to me that it is almost impossible to go through the normal process of facial aging in this culture and not wish that something could be done about certain parts of your face, especially the eyelids and jawline. If you're one of the lucky ones who really aren't at all bothered by sagging eyelids or jowls, bless you. If, however, you want an appearance-enhancing face-lift, eyelid surgery, skin peel, liposuction, laser surgery, or other cosmetic polishing of your exterior, then bless you, too. Through the years I've referred many patients for various plastic surgery or dermatological procedures. Just about 100 percent of them have been thrilled with the results.

In addition to giving referrals for plastic surgery, while I was still at Women to Women I even took a course in how to do deep facial skin peels. We did the procedure at the office and then cared for the women at a private home for four days thereafter. I always thought of this service as a kind of "cocoon" experience in which the newly peeled and vulnerable women were kept safe, warm, and healthy while they shed their old skins and prepared to face the world with a renewed countenance. I must admit that the results were spectacular for the women (and one man) who went through with the procedure. I was always thrilled on the last day to witness the "unveiling" as we helped our patients remove their masks of powder and apply makeup to cover their renewed but very red skin. This was especially true for those whose difficult and painful past histories had lined their faces with expressions of anger and depression they had since worked through. Virtually all of the women I treated had done lots of inner work. Now they simply wanted their outsides to match their insides.

One of my patients had her eyes done at the age of forty-one, about one year after a mastectomy. With the bags under her eyes surgically corrected, she looked brighter and fresher than she had in years. And her new look helped her outlook and possibly her immune system as well.

Particularly Effective Cosmetic Procedures

Led by the desires of baby boomers to look as young as possible for as long as possible, a whole new range of cosmetic and skin care solutions is now available to rejuvenate aging skin and keep it looking good for years. These include intermittent laser (called Intense Pulsed Light, or IPL) treatments, which are very effective at reducing wrinkles, evening out skin tone, thickening the collagen layer, and removing spider veins. IPL is generally done as a series of five or so treatments followed by maintenance of once every six months. IPL treatments can be alternated with glycolic peels so that you are having a mini-rejuvenation procedure every three months or so. Other acid and laser peels are available that can help remove the effects of sun damage and give you a clean slate that is easier to maintain with a good skin care regimen.

If you decide to consult a plastic surgeon or dermatologist or if you already have a procedure scheduled, I'd recommend the following.

~ Be sure that you're having a cosmetic procedure because it makes you feel better. Don't do it for your husband, boyfriend, or mother.

Over the years I've seen that the results of surgeries are always much better when our motivation for having them is clear.

~ Choose the right doctor. When it comes to cosmetic surgery, especially laser techniques, there is a great deal of crossover between the profession of dermatology and plastic surgery. For example, laser skin peels that include the eyelid area (usually done in a doctor's office) give a result that is often as good as a face-lift obtained with a surgeon's knife. Look for a board-certified plastic surgeon or, in the case of laser procedures, a dermatologist or other practitioner with extensive training in laser technology.

~ Don't choose a doctor just because he or she offers the lowest prices. All surgical and laser procedures carry a certain amount of risk. This risk increases if doctors cut corners on care and safety to keep prices low.

~ Make sure you go to someone with whom you feel completely comfortable. (This same criterion goes for body workers or anyone else who will be working with your body in any way—including a dentist.) Ask yourself: "Does this person have the kind of clinical, objective, and healing touch that will allow me to feel comfortable even if I have to stand in my underwear and have him or her look at my body and take pictures as part of my care?" A good doctor will put you at ease even in this kind of situation. If there's any feeling of discomfort, go elsewhere. That's what happened with a friend of mine who went to see a plastic surgeon in order to have both her nose and her deviated septum fixed. (She had had a broken nose since childhood.) The surgeon kept staring at her breasts, which are relatively small, while she kept trying to get his attention back on her nose. She had no desire to have breast implants. Though this man had all the right credentials, had trained at the best places in the United States, and is perfectly competent technically, he also had what I've come to call the sleaze factor. His attitude made her uncomfortable. So she chose someone else to do her surgery. Her feeling of unease was confirmed when she later heard via the grapevine that he had told his wife, also a physician, about some of the surgeries he had done and upon whom. This information had made its way around the community. Such a breach of confidentiality is completely unacceptable, but it happens. You can avoid this kind of situation by trusting your gut as well as a surgeon's credentials.

~ Keep your surgery decision to yourself as much as possible. You'd be amazed at the number of judgments your friends may have concerning cosmetic surgery, depending upon where you live. (The Southeast is currently the leader in plastic surgeries.)[29] Some of your friends won't think you're very spiritually evolved, for instance, if you want to remove the bags under your eyes. Frankly, how you look is none of their business.

~ If at all possible, go away to have your procedure done. Too many of my patients have had the experience of being home with a bruised face after plastic surgery, looking like battered women, and then having to answer the door for the plumber, the mail carrier, and everyone else who comes along.

~ Give yourself enough time. Recovery from eyelid or facial surgery usually takes a minimum of two weeks before you look presentable. So use this time for reading or taking a much-deserved retreat from your usual routine. It will speed your healing process and help the inside of you as much as the outside.

~ Make arrangements to be waited on for at least the first three days post-op. Though you may feel fine, you're apt to be more tired than usual and perhaps a bit weepy and emotional during this vulnerable time. Give yourself the space you deserve.

~ Stock up on the Chinese patent herb Yannan Pei Yan and begin taking it, one tablet four times a day, as soon as you possibly can after surgery. This herb speeds healing and cuts way down on postoperative bruising. I also recommend taking at least 2,000 mg of vitamin C for two weeks pre-op and four weeks post-op to help build up collagen in your skin. You can also use skin cream containing vitamin C ester to speed up healing.

~ Use guided-imagery tapes before and during surgery, and ask your surgeon and anesthesiologist to work with you. (See Resources.)

~ Be realistic. Cosmetic surgery won't change your life, despite what our culture would lead you to believe. If you are beautiful on the outside but ugly, depressed, or unhappy on the inside, your appeal will begin to fade within thirty seconds of walking into a room. I'm sure you've all had the experience of meeting people who become more and more attractive right in front of your eyes as you begin to know and appreciate the humor, joy, or fun they bring to every situation.

VARICOSE VEINS

Chances are you don't like the look of prominent blue varicose veins and want to do whatever you can to prevent them or, if you already have a few, minimize them. Appearance isn't the only problem with varicose veins, however. If they get bad enough, they are often associated with a painful, heavy feeling in the legs, especially at the end of the day. Happily, there are a number of strategies to help you prevent varicose veins in the first place, or keep them from getting worse if you already have a few.

Let's start by going over what varicose veins are and why they develop. The term *varicose* refers to a vein that is dilated, tortuous, and located just beneath the skin. Quite often the valves of these veins, which are designed to keep the blood from flowing backward, no longer work as they should. When a surface vein stretches and loses its elasticity, and the valves don't shut properly, blood flows backward, pooling in the affected vein, which then enlarges into a mass of blue tissue beneath the skin. Varicose veins can be large, having the appearance of blue worms, or they can be very small and purplish blue in color. These small "spider" veins often occur in a fanlike pattern in the thigh area. Varicose veins, whether large or small, are the end result of poor circulation.

Diet and Varicose Veins

It is very clear that the fundamental cause of varicose veins is a diet high in refined carbohydrates and low in fiber—the same kind that is also associated with heart disease, breast cancer, and bad skin. Such a diet often results in subtle nutritional deficiencies, excess weight, and constipation, all of which increase intra-abdominal pressure, which over the years puts too much pressure on the veins in our legs.[30] Chronic coughing does the same thing—and so does excess fat in the abdomen.

Varicose veins are virtually nonexistent in rural Africa, where the diet tends to be high in fiber-rich whole foods and very low in refined foods. But thanks to our own very different diet, almost all of us in this country are at an increased risk for developing at least a few dilated veins in our legs. Varicose veins can also be aggravated by the hormonal changes that women experience during three specific times in our lives: at the onset of our menstrual periods, during pregnancy, and at the beginning of menopause. These are the times when we are most susceptible to subtle changes in our blood flow that put us at increased risk for damage to our vein walls. Because of these hormonal changes, varicose veins can show up as early as age twenty. In men, by contrast, varicose veins develop evenly throughout the life span up until the age of seventy and don't appear to be hormonally related.

Program for Preventing or Treating Varicose Veins

Now that you know what you're dealing with, let's get down to the business of keeping your veins in top shape.

- GIVE YOUR LEGS THE SUPPORT THEY DESERVE. If you already have varicose veins or if you have a family history of varicose veins, make sure that you wear compression or support stockings of some kind whenever you know you will be on your feet for a long time. And elevate your legs as much as possible. I have a family history of varicose veins, so when I was a resident in training, I always wore compression stockings when I was on call at night. Putting those stockings on always gave me a new lease on life. Though I was only in my twenties at the time, I found that when I didn't wear them, my legs ached and my ankles got swollen after being on my feet all night. (I used Jobst brand stockings; another good brand is T.E.D.'s. These are available at your pharmacy. The cost is sometimes reimbursable from your insurance if you have a doctor's prescription.) Avoid standard knee-highs and thigh-high stockings if you have varicose veins, because the elastic at the tops of these impedes venous blood flow and increases the pooling of blood in the veins that is the cause of the problem in the first place.

- IF YOU TAKE ESTROGEN, MAKE SURE YOU'RE TAKING THE RIGHT DOSE. Low-dose estrogen replacement therapy does not appear to cause varicose veins in women, but occasionally a woman will notice that her legs ache and seem to swell more when she is on estrogen replacement, and existing varicose veins may seem to get worse. If you've noticed that your veins seem to be worse on estrogen replacement, consider lowering your dose.

- AVOID CONSTIPATION BY FOLLOWING A DIET THAT HAS ADEQUATE FIBER, PLENTY OF WATER, AND VERY FEW REFINED CARBOHYDRATES.

⁓ USE YOUR MUSCLES TO KEEP YOUR BLOOD MOVING. Rhythmic exercise such as walking, biking, running, or swimming keeps your blood moving and uses the mechanical action of your muscles to get the blood out of your veins and back to your heart. I've seen many women cure their symptomatic varicose veins and improve the cosmetic appearance of their legs by starting and staying with a regular exercise program.

⁓ NOURISH AND PROTECT YOUR VEIN LININGS. The herb bilberry (*Vaccinium myrtillus*) contains flavonoid compounds known as anthocyanosides, which are potent antioxidants that improve microcirculation and protect vein linings. Blueberries and currants do the same thing. These same substances also increase blood levels of a hormone known as prostacyclin (an eicosanoid), which prevents platelet aggregation, so blood flows more smoothly through the vessels. This herb has been successfully used to help prevent and treat varicose veins in pregnancy.[31] The usual dose is 160 mg per day for general prevention of varicose veins, and up to 480 mg per day to treat varicose veins that already exist. The flavonoid compounds in berries, particularly blueberries, blackberries, and raspberries, are also very helpful for keeping veins healthy.

⁓ KEEP YOUR VEIN WALLS SLIPPERY. Research has shown that individuals with varicose veins have a decreased ability to break down fibrin in their vein walls. Fibrin is a protein in blood that is involved in clotting. When it isn't metabolized properly by an enzyme known as plasminogen activator, it coats the inside of the vein, causing it and the surrounding skin to become hard and lumpy. Normally veins have enough plasminogen activator already in their walls to keep fibrin from building up. But when they become varicose, the levels of plasminogen activator decrease.[32] So you have to import your own.

A substance known as bromelain, found in pineapple, has been shown to act in a manner similar to plasminogen activator to cause fibrin breakdown.[33] In supplement form, it can be used to improve varicose veins that already exist or, in smaller amounts, to prevent them.

The usual dose of bromelain is 125–450 mg three times per day on an empty stomach. Use the smallest amount as general prevention, and the larger amount to treat veins that are already present. Bromelain is readily available at health food stores. You can also get bromelain by eating pineapple.

~ MAKE SURE YOU'RE GETTING ADEQUATE AMOUNTS OF VITAMIN E.
Since vitamin E deficiency has been associated with the exacerbation of varicose veins, you'll want to be sure to get enough of
this vitamin every day. An adequate dosage is 100–400 IU per
day, the amount I've already recommended for your daily multi-
vitamin/mineral combination.

When to Consider Treatment—Either EVLT or Sclerotherapy

If your varicose veins are causing you pain of any kind that
doesn't respond to the measures I've outlined (and pain includes feeling too embarrassed to wear shorts or a bathing suit), I'd recommend
that you look into a relatively quick, simple, and effective new treatment called Endovenous Laser Therapy (EVLT), performed by interventional radiologists (specialists who use ultrasound technology to
help diagnose and treat).

EVLT has a 98 percent success rate and typically requires only
one procedure (although you will need an initial consultation so the
specialist can evaluate your veins using ultrasound). Here's how it
works: After administering a local anesthetic (usually to the ankle or
knee), the doctor makes a very tiny cut and inserts a thin catheter
into the damaged vein. A laser fiber is threaded through the catheter
and is guided to the end of the problem vein. Additional anesthetic
then numbs the whole leg and causes the blood to leave the vein.
When the doctor fires the laser, it heats the inside of the vein wall,
causing it to collapse and seal shut. The laser is then withdrawn back
down the length of the vein to treat the entire problem area.

The doctor checks the vein with ultrasound to make sure it is
completely closed, after which the catheter is removed and the leg
is bandaged. The patient leaves wearing a waist-high compression
stocking to be left in place for seven to ten days. The whole procedure usually takes only ninety minutes, and the patient can resume
most activities right away—although lifting anything more than five
pounds is discouraged for the first week or so.

The most common side effects are mild swelling and bruising
or minor pain, which may worsen during the first week after treatment. Over-the-counter medications such as Motrin or Tylenol easily
take care of such problems, and some patients even report that their
post-op pain is less than the pain they experienced before surgery!
The incision site also occasionally becomes infected, which is treated

with antibiotics. Patients typically return for a follow-up exam after two weeks and again after two or three months to make sure that the vein remains closed.

Richard Baum, M.D., an interventional radiologist at Brigham and Women's Hospital in Boston, told me that of all the procedures he does, which include life-saving hemorrhage control, the patients who are the most grateful are those who have this procedure! (For more information, visit www.evlt.com or www.veins.nu. Also, if you are thinking about having this therapy, consider the Comprehensive Vein Care Center at Brigham and Women's Hospital, one of the best clinics in the country; for more information, visit www.bostonveins.com.)

On the other hand, if your problem is unsightly but painless spider veins, chances are all you need is a simple office procedure known as sclerotherapy—which has been safely used in Europe for the last fifty years and is finally catching on in the U.S. After an ultrasound evaluation, the physician (typically a dermatologist) injects the veins with a solution designed to irritate the wall of the vein, causing it to swell and cut off the blood supply. No anesthesia is necessary, although several procedures may be required.

Should you decide to go through with a vein procedure, I recommend that you follow all my suggestions for maintaining healthy veins before and after your treatment. Doing so will lower your chances of having any recurrent problems.

Despite our best efforts to appear youthful, life is full of challenges that sooner or later etch themselves on our faces and bodies. Happily, at midlife most of us are far better equipped to handle this than we were at twenty and still believed that our lives would be perfect if we could just lose that final five to ten pounds or if our noses looked different. We can still be beautiful—especially since the crucible of perimenopause removes some of our self-consciousness. We've had enough life experience to be happy that our legs still work, even if they don't look perfect, happy that there are amusing things to laugh at, even if doing so creates crinkles around our eyes. What a relief!

12

Standing Tall for Life:
Building Healthy Bones

During the summer before I wrote this book, I had the privilege of seeing rock-and-roll legend Tina Turner live in concert. At an age (sixty plus) when the majority of women have resigned themselves to slowing down and taking it easy, Tina tore up the stage in her towering heels (an athletic feat in itself), belting out her signature high-energy music for two solid hours while outshining dancers less than half her age. Her awe-inspiring performance laid to rest any notion about the inherent limitations in physical stamina that are supposed to come with growing older. I was thrilled that my two then teenage daughters were with me, so that they, too, could internalize this icon of female power and health. Watching Tina Turner that night, I was reminded anew that we midlife women can hone our physical strength and skills for years to come if we are willing to continue to move, to work our muscles regularly—and, of course, to unload any Ikes who are holding us back.

Tina Turner—and thousands of other older women who stand tall in their lives—offer a clear alternative to the realities of osteoporosis. You don't have to look very far to see women who are bent over or otherwise crippled by this devastating disease. Osteoporosis begins in earnest at perimenopause in susceptible women, but its effects may not appear until twenty or more years later, often when it is too late to do much about it. When it comes to bone health, prevention is absolutely essential. And that prevention needs to start as soon as possible. Perimenopause is an ideal time to shore up your bones—the part of you that is your foundation for moving forward in your life.

OSTEOPOROSIS: THE SCOPE OF THE PROBLEM

Bone loss starts silently, asymptomatically. In the early stages it is called osteopenia. As it progresses to osteoporosis, the bones become increasingly porous, brittle, and subject to fracture. The National Institutes of Health Consensus Conference defined osteoporosis as a disease of increased skeletal fragility, accompanied by low bone density (a T-score for bone mineral density below -2.5) and microarchitecture deterioration.[1] Make no mistake: this is a potentially fatal disease. It is estimated that by the year 2020, forty million American women will be over the age of sixty-five and that anywhere between 18 and 33 percent of all these women will suffer from a hip fracture by the time they reach the age of ninety. Of those who sustain hip fractures, 12–20 percent will die of related complications. (The lifetime risk of death from a hip fracture for a fifty-year-old woman is equal to the lifetime risk of death due to breast cancer.) Of those who don't die from complications, 50 percent will never regain their ability to walk and therefore will not be able to return to independent living.

Osteoporosis also increases the risk for wrist and vertebral crush fractures, which can result in pain, disability, and disfigurement. It is the vertebral crush fractures, in which the bone in the spine collapses, that result in the shrunken, hunched-over posture—complete with dowager's hump and pot belly—that is often seen in elderly women. If your mother or grandmother looks like this, you may be seeing your future—unless you act now.

By the age of eighty-five the majority of Caucasian women in the United States will have at least one partial deformity in their spine.[2] The risk for African-American women is less, while the risk for Asian-American women falls somewhere in between. This difference is related, in part, to the fact that women with more pigment in their skin also have a thicker collagen matrix upon which their bones are built. Men also have thicker, stronger bones than women, partly for genetic reasons and partly because of their higher levels of bone-building testosterone. Though men, too, may get osteoporosis, it's

FIGURE 15: FEMALE VERTEBRAE

(Bone cross sections)

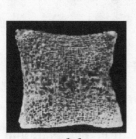 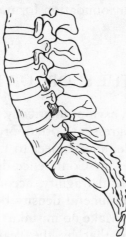 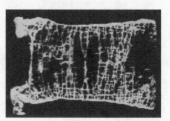

Healthy   *Osteoporotic*

often related to alcohol intake or steroid use and shows up at a later age than in women. Osteoporosis currently costs the health care system some $18 billion per year. Hip fractures represent 80 percent of the total expense, averaging $35,000 per patient.[3]

Given these discouraging statistics, it is little wonder that so many doctors are quick to prescribe drugs such as alendronate (Fosamax). Please remember, however, that statistics are derived from entire populations and may not have anything to do with you personally. In my practice I have seen eighty-year-old women with the bone density measurements of an average twenty-five-year-old. I have also seen twenty-five-year-olds with the bones of an average eighty-year-old. And today there are many safe and natural options available to help you either maintain the bone you have or build it to new, healthier levels.

WE'RE DESIGNED FOR LIFETIME STURDINESS

There is nothing inherent in the human condition in general, or the postmenopausal woman in particular, that causes our bones to weaken and break as we age. We were designed to live on this planet well supported by sturdy bones from youth to old age. Like other degenerative diseases so common in Western civilization, such as coronary artery disease, hypertension, and obesity, osteoporosis is either unknown or very rare among indigenous peoples living time-honored lifestyles characterized by a strong connection with the wisdom of the earth. A deep sense of connection to the earth shores up the health of our first emotional center—the part of our emotional anatomy that is associated with a sense of belonging, and with our basic sense of safety and security in the world. This sense of safety affects our bones, blood, and immune systems.

When an entire culture teaches us to regard our bodies as uncontrollable and unreliable, it is not surprising that so many women have lost their sense of connection and support—with resulting first-emotional-center disease such as osteoporosis. It is also not surprising that so many are beginning to lose bone at earlier and earlier ages, a side effect of a refined food diet, poor nutrient intake, and a sedentary lifestyle.

The gravity of the earth itself (weight-bearing exercise) and sunlight are two of the keys to bone health, as we will see in this chapter.

HOW HEALTHY BONE IS MADE

If you want to keep your bones strong and healthy, you need to understand the dynamic and effortless way in which your body is designed to build and remodel bone throughout your life. The process that results in osteoporosis is actually a survival mechanism created over millions of years of evolution to help your body maintain biochemical balance. Once you begin to work with that essential body wisdom, even bones that have already weakened can regain strength.

Bone metabolism is a complex process in which construction and demolition crews work side by side. Each of our 206 bones harbors cells that continually deposit a protein framework made from collagen. Minerals from the blood then attach to this matrix and harden into bone. Those same bones also contain cells that can break down that structure. In childhood, as we grow, the bone builders keep ahead of the bone destroyers. But the balance can shift as we get older. A wide variety of conditions—including depression, deficiencies of vitamin D and bone-building minerals, and steroid use—can allow the osteoblasts, the cells that make bone, to be outpaced by the osteoclasts, the cells that break down bone. The result is weakened bones.

Bones Are Storehouses for Essential Minerals

Bones are the major storehouses for calcium, phosphorous, and magnesium, as well as other minerals, all of which are necessary for the healthy functioning of every cell in the body. Calcium, for example, regulates processes ranging from the beating of the heart and the clotting of blood to the firing of nerve cells. When blood calcium levels become low, a series of complex and interrelated biological reactions is activated.

~ The parathyroid gland (in the neck) releases parathyroid hormone (PTH).

~ PTH stimulates the kidneys to convert the body's stores of vitamin D into an active form and release calcium from the surface of the bone. It also slows down the mineralization of bone, which uses calcium.

~ Activated vitamin D acts on the intestine to increase the absorption of calcium from food, encourages the kidneys to retain calcium that would otherwise be lost in the urine, and facilitates the release of more calcium from the bone.

As soon as calcium levels in the blood are restored to an acceptable level, all of these feedback mechanisms are reversed. Similarly, complex feedback loops are involved in the metabolism of the other essential minerals.[4]

It is the job of the osteoclasts to break down microscipic bits of bone, thus releasing minerals into the blood. Each day over 300 mg of calcium is dissolved from our bones. Over a year's time 20 percent of our adult bone mass is recycled and replaced as our bones continually undergo breakdown and renewal in response to the overall needs of our bodies. If more minerals are taken out than are replaced, the end result is low bone mass.

Bones Constantly Remodel Themselves to Adapt to Physical Stress and Strain

Among the amazing properties of the basic bone cell, the osteocyte, is its ability to act like a strain sensor, evaluating the amount of stress placed on a bone. Though the exact mechanism by which this happens isn't entirely understood, stress on a bone sets up a tiny electrical current that attracts calcium and other minerals to the site. This is known as a piezoelectric effect and is similar to the mechanism by which quartz crystals operate in electronics and clocks.

What is fascinating about this process is that it takes into account precisely where bone is needed and where it needs to be reduced. The old song about how "the hip bone's connected to the thigh bone" is about more than mere anatomical proximity. All of our bones, like every other cell in our bodies, are functionally connected to one another. A strain on a bone in our leg not only helps build that bone, but also helps determine the bone density in our spine and shoulders.[5] Regular stress on bones is absolutely essential to maintain strong bone. It's a case of use it or lose it. It's well documented, for example, that the weightlessness experienced by astronauts results in significant bone loss, as does prolonged bed rest.

One more piece of the puzzle falls into place when you know that osteoblasts and osteoclasts, the builders and the destroyers, communicate via proteins known as osteoprotegerine (OPG) and OPG-ligand. As one researcher explains it, "OPG-ligand is like the accelerator of your car. If you step on OPG-ligand, you lose bone. OPG is the brake of the system. If you step on OPG, then you have more bone. The balance between the two determines how much bone we have."[6] Scientists are now finding that almost all of the substances that stimulate bone loss do so by slashing production of OPG, boosting creation of OPG-ligand, or both. For example, the drug prednisone can set off quick and dramatic bone loss. In the lab, treating osteoblasts (bone builders) with prednisone inhibits their ability to make OPG but heightens their OPG-ligand production. In contrast, estrogen stimulates osteoblasts to produce OPG.

Immune status and bone health are also closely connected— which is not surprising, given that both are under the influence of the first chakra. Osteoclasts (the bone destroyers) are derived from the same bone marrow cells that make white blood cells. This helps explain why individuals with such seemingly unrelated diseases as rheumatoid arthritis, lupus, diabetes, multiple sclerosis, hepatitis, depression, and lymphoma have osteoporosis in addition to their other symptoms. Scientists have found that anything that stirs quiescent T cells, a ubiquitous part of our immune systems, into action also triggers them to make OPG-ligand. And anytime you turn on T cells (as in chronic infections and autoimmune disorders), you get bone loss.

The function of both osteoclasts and osteoblasts is influenced by many other factors as well, including levels of estrogen, testosterone, thyroid hormone, and insulin, nutritional status, and hormones (such

FIGURE 16: BONE REMODELING

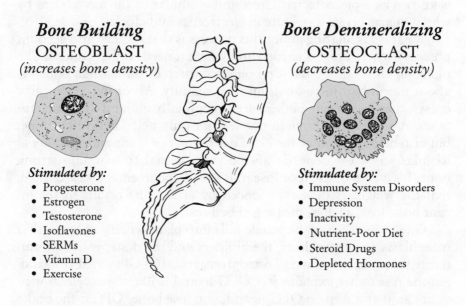

Bone Building
OSTEOBLAST
(increases bone density)

Stimulated by:
- Progesterone
- Estrogen
- Testosterone
- Isoflavones
- SERMs
- Vitamin D
- Exercise

Bone Demineralizing
OSTEOCLAST
(decreases bone density)

Stimulated by:
- Immune System Disorders
- Depression
- Inactivity
- Nutrient-Poor Diet
- Steroid Drugs
- Depleted Hormones

as norepinephrine and cortisol) produced by emotional stress.[7] There is also some evidence to suggest that OPG-ligand may stimulate osteoclasts or other substances, such as cytokines (one of the inflammatory chemicals), to degrade cartilage. This translates over time into joint destruction and arthritis. Clinical trials are now under way using a type of synthetic long-acting OPG to turn off osteoclasts and thus halt bone loss.

The Ups and Downs of Bone over the Life Cycle

We begin developing our skeleton in utero, and it rapidly increases in size throughout childhood, adolescence, and young adulthood. It reaches its maximum size and density (known as peak bone mass) somewhere between the ages of twenty-five and thirty. Over her lifetime a woman may lose 38 percent of her peak bone mass, while a man may lose only 23 percent of his.[8] But some individuals are resistant to bone loss.[9] One study, for example, showed that 38 percent of men and 2 percent of women age fifty-five to sixty-four lost almost no bone over a period of eleven years.[10] Nevertheless, many women begin to lose bone in their late thirties, long before estrogen levels begin to fall. This loss tends to accelerate perimenopausally. The average Caucasian woman loses 2–4 percent of her bone mass per year in the first five years after menopause. After that, loss slows down markedly or disappears.[11] In men, accelerated bone loss is more apt to begin in the late sixties.

It's important to remember that healthy women can lose some bone during menopause and not be at risk for fracture. Thousands of people walk around daily with very low bone density—yet only a small percentage of them experience fractures. It has been shown, for example, that in Japan hip bone density is markedly lower than it is in the United States, and yet the incidence of hip fractures is two and a half times less than it is here. And the Japanese consume less calcium than we do.[12]

What is the difference between bones that fracture and those that don't? The difference concerns two factors: basic bone architecture and the repair capability of bone. It appears that even those with osteoporosis still have enough bone mass to withstand the stresses and strains of daily life. Research has shown, for example, that a vertebra that has lost 50 percent of its bone mass is still strong enough to withstand five times the strain load that it would normally be subjected to. If the bone were otherwise normal, in other words, it shouldn't fracture. This means that many women who are diagnosed with low bone density will never go on to get fractures.

Still, we all know that bone fractures do occur in women with osteoporosis, even at very low strain levels—in fact, it has been documented that some women spontaneously fracture their hips and then fall as a result, not the other way around. So osteoporotic fractures must involve more than decreased bone mineral density. There must be something else wrong with the *quality* of the bone and its self-repair process.[13] Poor bone quality results from factors such as nutritional deficiencies, lack of exercise, too little vitamin D, and too much insulin.[14]

The Anatomy of Bone

Bone comes in two types: trabecular and cortical bone. Cortical bone is the tough, protective outer layer of bone. It is more calcified than inner trabecular bone, which is spongy and includes the marrow, where blood cells are made. About 80 percent of all bone in our bodies is cortical and 20 percent is trabecular. The arms and legs are mostly cortical bone; hips are a mixture of half and half; while the spine, ribs, jaw, and lower two-thirds of the wrist are mainly trabecular bone. Because trabecular bone is more loosely packed and porous and has more surface area than cortical bone, it is more susceptible to bone loss, which is one reason why fractures from osteoporosis tend to occur earlier in the spine and wrist, while hip fractures occur later.

Bones have to be strong enough to withstand hundreds of pounds of pressure, but flexible enough to withstand twisting and turning without breaking. This flexibility is provided by the living protein collagen, which makes up about 23 percent of all bone. (This is the same substance that gives skin its elasticity and thickness. Thin skin is also associated with thin bones.) The minerals attached to the collagen matrix are arranged in a crystalline structure that gives bone its rigidity and strength.

We were designed to maintain strong, heavy bones throughout our lives, as do all animals. If we have reached peak bone mass in our twenties, then we can stand a certain amount of bone loss as we age without being at risk for fractures. But because of the vagaries of our modern lifestyle, including lack of exercise or overexercise, smoking, poor diet, lack of vitamin D, or anorexia and bulimia, many women never reach their peak bone mass by age thirty. And it appears that the matrix of the bone that *is* present may not be normal. So many women begin perimenopause with a deficit in their bone banks.

Medical anthropologist Susan Brown, Ph.D., director of the Osteoporosis Education Project and author of the groundbreaking book *Better Bones, Better Body: Beyond Estrogen and Calcium* (Keats Publishing, 2000), points out that the bones of people who are living in Westernized countries are growing ever weaker, and that we now face a virtual epidemic of poor bone health.[15] Research shows that women living several centuries ago had stronger bones than modern women and that Near Eastern populations of some twelve thousand years ago had a bone mass that was nearly 20 percent higher than it is today.[16] (And they didn't consume lots of cow's milk!)

ARE YOU AT RISK FOR OSTEOPOROSIS?

To determine your personal risk for thinning, poor-quality bones, review the following list. If none of the risk factors applies to you, chances are good that your bones are just fine. You can simply continue the healthy lifestyle you are following. If, on the other hand, you can identify with several of them, you need to take steps right now to ensure that you'll be able to literally take steps in the future! Note that some of the risk factors for osteoporosis overlap those for heart disease.[17] As you get a handle on your bone health, you'll also be helping your heart.

~ Your mother has been diagnosed with osteoporosis or has had a hip or other osteoporotic fracture. Osteoporosis tends to run in families, but there's still a lot you can do to prevent it.

~ You are fair-skinned and blue-eyed. Because of genetic factors, blue-eyed blondes and those with red hair have less collagen in both their bones and skin than do those with brown, black, red, or yellow skin tones. This gives them less bony matrix on which to lay down minerals. Black women have the least risk for osteoporosis because they tend to have thicker bones and more robust collagen stores than Caucasian women.

~ You are quite thin or tall, or have a slight build and/or less than 18 percent body fat. Tall women, especially those with small bones, may be at risk for purely mathematical reasons: they enter menopause with less bone to lose. In addition, body fat is where much of a woman's natural estrogen during and after perimenopause is manufactured. The less fat she has, the less estrogen her body will produce to support her bones.

~ You smoke. Chemicals in cigarette smoke poison the ovaries and decrease your hormone levels prematurely. Estrogen, testosterone, and progesterone all have bone-protective effects.

~ You spend most of your time indoors. Women who are exposed to very little natural sunlight may be deficient in the natural vitamin D normally produced in sun-drenched skin. Vitamin D is necessary for healthy bone mineralization. Increasingly, we're finding that women who get osteoporotic fractures are the ones with serum vitamin D levels of 20 or lower. The sunlight–bone health link is so important that I've devoted an entire section to it later in this chapter.

~ You are sedentary and spend less than four hours per day on your feet. Bones stay healthy only when they have vertical vectors of force placed on them regularly. A sedentary lifestyle provides insufficient weight-bearing exercise to stimulate bone growth. Many studies have shown that bed rest is associated with osteoporosis. In contrast, weight training has been shown to build bone density even in postmenopausal women who aren't on estrogen.

~ You are (or were) a "fitness fanatic," that is, you become irritable and unreasonable if you are unable to get in your daily run or other exercise. The lifestyle of the fitness fanatic includes dieting for weight loss and/or engaging regularly in strenuous exercise such as marathon training. Dietary restrictions and the chronic stress of overtraining can impair mineral intake and absorption. It also messes up what is known as the hypothalamic-pituitary axis— the exquisite feedback loop between the brain, the body, and our hormone levels. Chronic overexercise without adequate caloric or mineral intake results in stress fractures in ballet dancers, gymnasts, soccer players, and competitive runners, among others. Such fractures are currently on the rise in young athletes and can set the stage for later osteoporosis.

~ You have a history of amenorrhea (no periods) associated with excessive exercise and/or anorexia nervosa.[18] Amenorrhea results in a derangement of the hypothalamic-pituitary axis similar to that seen in depression. The end result is lower estrogen, androgen, and progesterone, and an eicosanoid profile that favors osteoporosis and other diseases.[19]

~ You drink more than 25 g of alcohol per day. (The following servings each contain about 10 g of alcohol: 12 oz of beer, 4 oz of wine, and 1.5 oz of 80 proof beverage.)[20] Alcohol interferes with the function of both osteoblasts and osteoclasts, thus inhibiting your body's ability to lay down new bone and to remodel old bone.[21]

~ Your liver is overstressed. The liver's ability to produce and metabolize estrogen is essential for the growth and maintenance of strong bones at any age. Drinking more than two alcoholic drinks per day, taking medication known to be hard on the liver (such as certain cholesterol-lowering drugs), and infection with viral hepatitis are among the significant liver stressors that can harm bone health.

~ You drink more than two units of caffeine per day (8 oz of coffee = 1 unit; 12 oz of cola = 0.4 units). Caffeine results in increased urinary excretion of calcium; the more you consume, the more calcium you lose. If your calcium intake is relatively low to begin with, regular caffeine consumption could result in significant loss of bone over time. If, on the other hand, your calcium and mineral intake is high, a couple of cups of coffee a day probably won't matter much. *Note:* Even though tea contains caffeine, both green and black tea have been shown to build bone mass—probably because of their phytoestrogen content.

~ You are or have been clinically depressed for a significant period of time. Numerous studies have shown that depression is an independent risk factor for osteoporosis. Depressed people have high levels of the immune system chemical known as IL-6, which overstimulates the osteoclasts (cells responsible for breaking down bone). Depression is also associated with abnormalities in the hypothalamic-pituitary-adrenal axis and with elevated cortisol secretion, which predispose one to bone loss.[22]

~ Your diet is poor—little fresh food, few leafy green vegetables, and lots of junk food. Such a diet doesn't provide minerals and other nutrients necessary to support the growth and maintenance of a solid bone foundation.[23]

~ You went through premature menopause (before age forty), have had your ovaries removed surgically, went through menopause as a result of radiation or chemotherapy, and/or have prematurely gray hair. A woman who enters menopause prematurely for any reason is at increased risk for osteoporosis unless she gets adequate hormone replacement during the years when her body would normally have been producing higher levels of hormones. Nonsurgical premature menopause, and the premature graying of the hair that often accompanies it, are the result of an autoimmune reaction affecting the ovaries and hair follicles. The cause of these reactions isn't clear.

~ You take steroid drugs regularly for conditions such as asthma or lupus. Steroid drugs result in accelerated breakdown of tissue in the body—including the collagen matrix for both skin and bone.[24] Steroids also diminish the sensitivity of the bowel to vitamin D, which in turn reduces calcium absorption.[25] Prolonged steroid use may also significantly decrease estrogen and androgen levels.[26]

~ You use anticonvulsant medication regularly or benzodiazepines such as diazepam (Valium), chlordiazepoxide (Librium), or lorazepam (Ativan).[27] These drugs have also been found to interfere with bone metabolism.

~ You've had at least two consecutive bone density tests at least six months apart, done on the same machine, that reported scores more than 2.5 standard deviations below normal for your age.

~ You have a thyroid disorder. Women who suffer from hyperthyroidism are at risk because the excess thyroid hormone (thyroxine) that their bodies make stimulates the osteoclasts to break down bone. Those with hypothyroidism may also be at risk if their dose of thyroid medication is too high. If you have thyroid disease, make sure you are on the lowest dose of thyroid replacement possible for your situation, and follow a sound program for maintaining bone health.[28] (For a holistic approach to thyroid disease, see *The Thyroid Solution: A Mind-Body Program for Beating Depression and Regaining Your Emotional and Physical Health* [Ballantine Books, 1999], by Ridha Arem, M.D.)

Whether or not you are at high risk for osteoporosis, understand that, like the rest of your body, bone is a living work in progress. That means that there is always something you can do—ranging from drugs to dietary change—to help yourself build bone.

MEASURING BONE DENSITY

Women with no risk factors for osteoporosis do *not* need bone density screening. Those that do should get a baseline bone density screening either before or during perimenopause. Though bone density screenings cannot measure the quality of bone, they can measure quantity. And low bone mineral density is statistically associated with an increased fracture risk. Although fractures aren't likely to show up until a woman is in her seventies and eighties, now is the best time to do something about any potential problems. Unfortunately, many insurance plans won't pay for bone density screening unless you've already had documented osteoporotic fractures. This is typical of the Western crisis approach to medicine, which too often neglects prevention. However, I urge you to make this investment in your health.

Heel Bone Density

Heel bone density testing, with a machine such as an Osteo-Analyzer, is an accurate and cheap method of screening for women of all ages. For example, it is being used to do baseline screening on teenage girls who are at risk for not achieving maximum bone density because of dieting. Heel density tests do not require a doctor's prescription and may even be offered at your local drugstore. They are not as accurate as a full-scale DEXA test (see below) because they measure only one area of your body. But they are a valuable early warning system.

DEXA Testing

Dual energy bone densitometry (DEXA) is the current gold standard. It uses a very low dose of X-rays to measure bone density both in the spine and in the hips. A woman's bone density is then charted on a graph to see how it stacks up against normal bone densities for a given age. The National Osteoporosis Foundation (NOF) and World Health Organization (WHO) both rate bone density according to a standard curve on which 0 equals the norm. Severity of bone loss is then determined by how far a given measurement falls below that mean. As you can see from the chart below, WHO and NOF differ slightly in their classifications of osteopenia and osteoporosis.

Like heel bone density, DEXA is a static test—a snapshot in time. One reading won't tell you whether your bone density is increasing, decreasing, or remaining the same. You need at least two successive tests at least six months apart to determine what the trend is and whether or not you need to make adjustments in your bone health routine. For example, small-boned women may register on the low end of a DEXA test even if their bones are not at risk.

DEXA testing is available at all major medical centers and in many doctors' offices. It requires a doctor's prescription. Because readings vary from machine to machine, try to have your consecutive measurements taken on the same machine.

BONE DENSITY CLASSIFICATION		
	WHO	**NOF**
NORMAL	0 to −1.0	0 to −1.0
OSTEOPENIA	−1.0 to −2.5	−1.0 to −2.0
OSTEOPOROSIS	Less than −2.5	Less than −2.0

Source: World Health Organization, *Assessment of Fracture Risk and Its Applications to Screening for Postmenopausal Osteoporosis,* Technical Report, Series 843 (Geneva: WHO, 1994).

Skin Thickness Testing

A number of studies have shown that ultrasound measurement of skin thickness (which is dependent upon healthy collagen) predicts fracture risk as accurately as conventional bone density testing.[29] The accuracy increases when both skin thickness and bone density are combined. Unfortunately, this test has not caught on widely in the United States. But it's worth asking your doctor about it; you may be near one of the medical centers that perform it.

Urine Test for Bone Breakdown Products

As bone breaks down, it releases minute collagen fragments into the urine that can be measured. Because a certain amount of bone breakdown is normal, everyone's urine contains some collagen fragments. But when the breakdown products in the urine skyrocket, you may well be losing bone faster than is healthy.[30] Several different types of urine tests, such as Pyrilinks and Osteomark, are available. Unlike the static measurement of the scans, these tests can give you a day-by-day reading of the metabolic state of your bones long before a bone density test will register a problem. They also give you a way to monitor your progress once treatment is initiated. Test kits are available without a prescription, and results can be mailed directly to your home. (See Resources.)

The Bottom Line

Bone density screening and urine testing are a marriage made in heaven. A simple bone density (either heel density or full-fledged DEXA test) will give you a baseline if you are at risk. Normally you have to wait six months to a year to know if you are gaining bone, losing bone, or staying the same. But sometimes the subsequent tests continue to read on the low side, even though you have stemmed the bone loss or begun building new bone.[31] That's where the urine test comes in. It can tell you immediately whether or not you are losing bone, and if you are, you can repeat it every month or so to make sure that the bone-building program you're on is working. Your test will show you when you are no longer peeing out your bones! Once your tests indicate that your bones are stable, I suggest that you retest your urine for bone loss every year or two.

These tests can let midlife women know how they're doing in time to prevent further bone loss and even increase bone density years before osteoporosis becomes evident. They allow you to create health daily, not wait until symptoms start!

HELGA: *Exercise Daily, Bone Loss Daily*

Helga first consulted me when she was fifty-seven, five years after her periods had stopped. Active and healthy, she rode horses nearly every day, spent long periods of time outside, and did much of the heavy stable work herself. She had never smoked, and drank only an occasional glass of wine. She wanted to avoid estrogen and wasn't really having any symptoms that bothered her. She simply wanted to be sure that her overall health was good and that her bones were in good shape.

Helga was blond, blue-eyed, and fair-skinned and had always been trim and small-boned, weighing only 105 pounds at her 5'4" height. When her initial bone density test showed that her bones were a bit more than two standard deviations below the mean, I wasn't too concerned, given that her slight build, not significant bone loss, was apt to be the reason for this low reading. I put her on a good supplement regimen (see below) and suggested that we repeat her screening test in six months. When that result came back, it was a bit lower than the first time but not significantly so. To be on the safe side, however, I suggested a Pyrilinks urine test. I was very surprised when this test showed that she was losing bone rather quickly.

Given her reluctance to take estrogen or other bone-building medications, I suggested a whole-soy product that delivers 180 mg of soy isoflavones per day, a dose that has definitely been shown to help preserve and build bone density. I also recommended 30 mg of natural progesterone per day in the form of a skin cream.

I wondered if Helga's ongoing bone loss in the face of a healthy lifestyle could be related to depression or some other loss. Helga had emigrated to this country from Sweden when she was thirty years old and married an American with whom she had three children. She and her family had always enjoyed regular visits to Sweden to visit her mother. But her mother had recently died, leaving Helga without any remaining family in Sweden. Her youngest child had also recently left home. I told Helga that our bone health is often at risk during times when the very foundations of our lives undergo dramatic and irrevocable change. Though emotionally stoic by nature, Helga acknowledged that she had been feeling a great deal of grief in the past year.

Though we can never replace our families or go back to "the way it was," it is possible for all of us to re-create sustaining relationships in our lives. So in addition to adding the soy estrogens and progesterone cream to her regular exercise and supplement program, I suggested to Helga that she seek out some new social ties with other friends of Swedish descent in order to reconnect with her heritage. Within two months, her Pyrilinks tests returned to normal and she stopped losing bone.

LOUISE: *Never Too Late*

Louise was eighty-six when her son first brought her in for a consultation for osteoporosis. A very slight white woman who weighed no more than 100 pounds, Louise had broken her hip the year before and had twice dislocated the hip replacement that had been inserted. She had been told that she had very severe osteoporosis and her doctors weren't sure there was much they could do for her. One even suggested putting her in a body cast for six months, which alarmed her (and rightly so—immobilization always causes further deterioration of bone).

Louise was mentally very sharp and, up until the hip fracture, had maintained a very active social life, managed a large stock portfolio, lived alone, and took care of herself. She told me the following: "Back in the early 1990s, I was part of the Women's Health Initiative study to determine whether or not calcium was necessary for building bone. I recently found out that during all those years I was on placebo, not calcium or vitamin D. I am furious." Indeed, Louise is the kind of "at risk" woman who really needed minerals, an exercise program, and vitamin D. She was afraid it was now too late. I told her that nothing could be further from the truth. I put her on a good supplementation program (see chapter 7), as well as 1,200 mg calcium, 1,000 IU of vitamin D, and also 600 mg of magnesium. I also helped Louise find an orthopedic surgeon who would repair her hip properly and not relegate her to life in a wheelchair just because of her age. Louise had the correct surgical procedure and recovered beautifully. Refusing pain medication, she entered a vigorous physical therapy program. Two months after her surgery, a doctor friend came up to her at church and said, "Louise, you might as well give that walker to me because I need it more than you." The fact is, Louise had been walking around actually carrying her walker in front of her instead of using it. She is now building bone, growing healthy fingernails for the first time in years, and is back to her former full social life—as well as driving!

BONE-BUILDING PROGRAM

No matter how many risk factors you identified, it's never too late (nor too early) to build your bones—even if you are ninety or already have significant bone loss. As long as you're alive, your bones are dynamic, living organs that respond daily to every aspect of your life—from your emotions to your diet. First, address the risk factors that are under your control.

⁓ CUT BACK ON OR ELIMINATE ALCOHOL AND CAFFEINE.

⁓ QUIT SMOKING. Acupuncture can help you a great deal with this.

⁓ FOLLOW THE PERIMENOPAUSAL DIET PLAN OUTLINED IN CHAPTER 7. Eat five servings of low-sugar fruits and vegetables per day. These are all high in potassium and boron, which help protect your bones by reversing urinary calcium loss.[32]

⁓ EAT PHYTOESTROGENS. Soy and ground flaxseed are particularly potent in this regard. Several studies have suggested that regular intake of soy protein has a bone-protective effect that is equivalent to that provided by estrogen. A six-month double-blind study at the University of Illinois found that postmenopausal women on a diet that was high in soy isoflavones were protected from spinal bone loss.[33] In the fall of 2005, findings of a study of more than 24,000 Chinese women were reported in the *Archives of Internal Medicine*. Researchers noted that women consuming 13 gm or more of soy protein every day were half as likely to incur a bone fracture as those eating 5 gm or less per day.[34] This is pretty exciting, especially when you consider that you can get this amount of soy protein simply by drinking two glasses of soy milk.

In a Danish study, half of the participants were given two glasses of soy milk with isoflavones; the other half drank the same quantity without the isoflavones. Bone loss was measured after two years, and then four years. The first group of postmenopausal women had virtually no bone loss at either interval! The second group saw a decrease in bone mass by a little more than 4 percent, which is still lower than what many postmenopausal women experience. Researchers concluded that although the soy milk they drank didn't have isoflavones, the daily intake of soy protein still provided some protective benefits for these women's bones.[35]

Yet another study followed fifty postmenopausal women who consumed three servings a day of soy milk (about 7.5 oz each) or three handfuls of roasted soy nuts, for a total daily dose of 60–70 mg of isoflavones. In twelve weeks the study noted a 13 percent increase in osteocalcin, a marker of bone formation, and a 14.5 percent decrease in markers for osteoclasts, cells that cause bone loss. The benefits of soy were not compared side by side with hormone replacement therapy, but soy protein revealed a bone-forming benefit that estrogen does not provide.[36]

~ GET YOUR VITAMIN D LEVEL CHECKED AND MAKE SURE YOU TAKE 800–5,000 IU PER DAY—AND ALSO GET SOME NATURAL SUNLIGHT! I recommend up to fifteen minutes of exposure during early morning or late afternoon, three to four times per week—but never enough to burn the skin. In the winter, you can use a tanning booth for eight to ten minutes once per week.

~ DRINK GREEN TEA. Green tea is especially rich in phytohormones and antioxidants. Research has shown that women who drink either green or black tea regularly have stronger bones than those in a control group.[37] I keep a pitcher of naturally decaffeinated green tea in my refrigerator and drink it regularly throughout the day.

~ DO REGULAR WEIGHT-BEARING EXERCISE. You need three exercise sessions per week, minimum. If you are lifting weights, two sessions per week are sufficient—but activities such as walking and yoga, can help, too.

~ IF YOU ARE DEPRESSED, GET PROPER TREATMENT. Regular exercise and exposure to natural light are sometimes all that is necessary. If you work under fluorescent fixtures, replace them with full-spectrum lightbulbs. Though most full-spectrum lights don't provide the UVB light necessary to stimulate vitamin D and calcium uptake, they definitely can help relieve depression and seasonal affective disorder. Interestingly, the nutritional supplement Saint-John's-wort, which has proven antidepressant effects, also lowers a cytokine known as IL-6, which is one of the chemicals that causes cellular inflammation and is involved with immune system activation. When its levels are normalized, bone density may be positively affected. It is unclear whether standard antidepressant medications also have this effect.

⁓ GET YOUR HORMONE LEVELS CHECKED. Many postmenopausal women have testosterone levels that are normal even for a pre-menopausal woman, making them much more resistant to osteo-porosis without additional hormones. Some women also have estrogen levels that remain in the low-normal premenopausal range long after menopause. If this is the case, you won't need to worry about taking a drug to support your bone mass.

Hormones That Help Build Bone

Supplementing with estrogen (which is far more common than supplementing with DHEA or testosterone) has been shown to help prevent bone loss, but given some of the risks of HRT, I recommend vitamin D, minerals, exercise, and—when nothing else works—antiresorptive drugs such as Fosamax as the first line of treatment. But if you're on HRT for other reasons, it's helping protect your bones as long as you're on it. In fact, the first FDA-approved indica-tion for estrogen replacement was the prevention of osteoporosis. Some studies have demonstrated a nearly 50 percent decrease in risk of fractures with conventional HRT.[38] The 2002 WHI study corrobo-rated this data. But that doesn't mean women need estrogen therapy to maintain healthy bone mass. Those women whose bodies continue to make even a small amount of estradiol or testosterone naturally have been found to have a significantly decreased risk of osteoporosis compared to those whose bodies are no longer able to make these hormones.[39]

Keep in mind, however, that bone mass is affected by far more than just hormones. For example, it has been demonstrated that one-half of the total vertebral bone loss that a woman in the United States will experience during her lifetime occurs before she goes through menopause.[40] In addition, some studies have failed to find any signif-icant differences between the spine and hip bone densities between pre- and perimenopausal women and their postmenopausal counter-parts. For example, research at the USDA Human Nutrition Research Center on Aging failed to show any accelerated rate of bone loss in the hip or wrist among women close to menopause. Nor did they find any significant change in bone mineral density in the group of women as a whole, a finding that has been duplicated in a Swedish study.[41] Some authorities even hypothesize that only 10–15 percent of a woman's skeletal mass is affected by estrogen.[42] And some women on estrogen replacement still lose bone mass over time.[43] While it is clear that hormones play an important role in bone health, they are just one factor. If you do take estrogen, for example, I recommend taking the lowest dose possible, since bone protection has been demonstrated even at very low doses.

Consider hormone replacement or other bone-building drugs if you've had any of the following conditions associated with decreased hormone levels:

~ History of amenorrhea lasting a year or more
~ Premature, surgical, or medical menopause
~ History of steroid use
~ Strong family history of osteoporosis (mother or grandmother with obvious osteoporosis)
~ A diagnosis of osteopenia or osteoporosis

Remember, hormone replacement or bone-building drugs help preserve bone density only as long as you take them. Once you stop, you begin losing bone. The same is true for the effect of exercise on bone.

If you can't use estrogen or androgen, consider natural progesterone, as either a 2 percent transdermal cream, a prescription pill (Prometrium), or from a formulary pharmacy. Synthetic progestin (medroxyprogesterone, or MPA) has been shown to stimulate osteoblasts (bone builders), and natural progesterone may have the same positive effect on bone density.[44] Double-blind, randomized, placebo-controlled studies show that low-dose MPA with estrogen prevents hip and other fractures.[45] Further controlled studies show low-dose MPA with lower-than-normal doses of estrogen significantly increases spinal bone density.[46]

Endocrinologist Jerilynn Prior, M.D., founder and scientific director of the Centre for Menstrual Cycle and Ovulation Research (CeMCOR) in Vancouver, B.C., believes progesterone therapy is just as effective as the bisphosphonates, the strongest bone medicines available. (See "What About Bone-Building Drugs?" later in this chapter.) Dr. Prior recommends dosages of either 10 mg per day of synthetic progestin or 300 mg a day of natural progesterone (taken at bedtime because it promotes sleepiness)—enough to get blood levels up at least 18 or ideally 45 nmol/L.[47]

Bone-Building Nutrients

Currently only 11 percent of women in the United States get adequate calcium every day—not to mention all the other nutrients that are needed to build healthy bone. Even if your diet is good, make sure your daily supplement program includes the following:

Magnesium	600–800 mg (because of farming practices, many foods are low in this key mineral, so it must be supplemented)[48]
Calcium	600–1,200 mg[49]
Vitamin D	800–5,000 IU
Vitamin C	1,000–3,000 mg
Boron	4–12 mg[50]
Zinc	15 mg
Manganese	2–5 mg
Copper	2–3 mg
Vitamin K	70–140 mcg

Calcium and Magnesium Supplements

Studies have clearly demonstrated that calcium supplementation helps build bone mass and prevent fractures.[51] It also helps to make other modalities such as exercise, vitamin D supplementation, and hormone replacement more effective in those who are already being treated for osteoporosis.

I prefer mineral supplements that are chelated with amino acids for maximum absorption—calcium citrate, calcium citrate-malate, or a mixture of any of the following: calcium ascorbate, calcium fumarate, calcium succinate, or calcium tartrate. Microcrystalline hydroxyapatite is also a good source of bone-building calcium. Make sure that you take magnesium along with the calcium. A 1:1 ratio of calcium to magnesium is ideal, but 2:1 is also acceptable. (See Resources.)

Although Tums are now being promoted as calcium supplements, I do not consider them a good choice. For one thing, Tums is an antacid that decreases hydrochloric acid levels in the stomach—and hydrochloric acid is necessary for optimal absorption of cal-

FIGURE 17: SOURCES OF CALCIUM

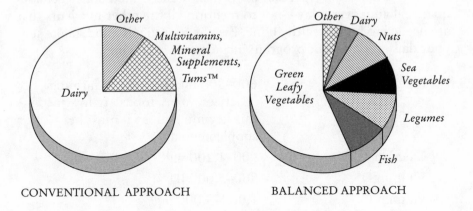

CONVENTIONAL APPROACH   BALANCED APPROACH

cium. Many people already have inadequate levels of hydrochloric acid as they age, which can lead to digestive problems. Why make that worse? For another, Tums contains no magnesium or any of the other nutrients needed for bone building. Magnesium deficiency is as much a problem in bone health as inadequate calcium, and because calcium and magnesium work in critical balance, they should be supplemented together. In fact, too much unbalanced calcium can actually decrease the body's ability to absorb magnesium from food. Dietary surveys have shown that 80–85 percent of American women consume less than the RDA for magnesium already. High, unbalanced calcium intake can also block the uptake of manganese, decrease iron absorption, interfere with vitamin K synthesis, and increase fecal phosphorous excretion. Finally, very high doses of calcium carbonate (4–5 g per day), which is the type of calcium in antacids, can cause a serious, kidney-damaging disorder known as milk alkali syndrome.[52]

The Protein-Calcium Connection

Rachel, one of my newsletter subscribers, had a query about protein that I've heard from many women.

I am fifty years old and perimenopausal. I have recently been diagnosed with osteoporosis from a DEXA scan, although my gynecologist would not yet classify me there, since I score -2.0 in my spine and -2.4 in my hips. The point remains [that I feel] I am in dangerous territory and I am not yet in menopause. My risk factors are that I recently stopped smoking (in fact, this news is what finally did it), my father has osteoporosis, and I have a small frame.

I am determined to try to reverse this through nutrition, supplements, and exercise, rather than take HRT or Fosamax.

Here's my program so far: I work out at least five times a week doing fast walking, free weights, and tai chi. I am having a difficult time finding a nutritionist who has expertise with osteoporosis. All the research I've read has said that a high-protein diet leaches calcium out of the body through urine. However, I recently read in *Women's Bodies, Women's Wisdom* that some recent research disputes this. Can you give me more information on your findings? How much protein should I be taking in daily? Does it matter if it's animal protein or not?

Many nutritionists blame too much protein for osteoporosis and kidney disease, and there is some research that supports this view.[53] However, Larrian Gillespie, M.D., a urological surgeon and the author of *The Menopause Diet* (Healthy Life Publications, 2003), points out that much of the relevant research has been conducted in hospitals on patients with insulin-dependent diabetes or otherwise compromised health.[54] Though some research has shown that even in healthy people, excess protein, especially in the form of red meat, may cause calcium loss in the urine, this effect is minuscule in comparison to the adverse bone effects of the imbalanced inflammatory chemicals produced by too much stress, alcohol, and refined carbohydrates.

The fact is that for the vast majority of time that humans have been on this planet—about one million years—our main source of food has been nuts, seeds, and fruits foraged in season, plus animal protein. Agriculture, and the grain- and dairy-rich diets that it made possible, has existed for a mere ten thousand years. And recent research into Paleolithic nutrition has found that hunter-gatherer societies—even those in existence today—are healthier on all levels than those whose food sources are primarily grain-based. Plus they don't have osteoporosis.[55]

Here's the bottom line: the same amount of protein that supports overall health supports healthy bones. For a 5'4", 140 lb female (the average woman in the United States), that means about 27 g of protein at each of three meals per day (about 81 g per day total). One ounce of meat or fish contains about 7 g of protein; a serving of 4 oz meets the requirement. Eggs contain 6 g of protein each. An egg white has 4 g. Hard cheese contains 6–7 g per ounce. Soft cheese has 3–4 g per ounce. Curd cheese such as cottage cheese or cheese curd has 7 g per ¼ cup, and tofu has 10 g per ¼ cup. Check the nutrition labels at the grocery store; they almost always include this information.

People who are physically active need more protein than those who are sedentary. Larger women also need more. The fact is that because of dieting and misinformation, far too many women don't get enough protein.

HIGH-CALCIUM FOODS[56]

There are many good sources of dietary minerals. Yogurt is one of the most easily digestible. One cup of yogurt contains about 300 mg of calcium. However, Americans have been culturally conditioned to focus on dairy as the key to healthy bones. Consider that a 3.5 oz can of sardines also contains 300 mg of calcium and is loaded with health-enhancing omega-3 fats.

Food	Amount	Calcium (mg)
Green Leafy Vegetables (cooked, unless specified)		
collard greens	1 cup	300
wild greens (lamb's-quarters, wild onions)	1 cup	350
broccoli	1 cup	150
kale	1 cup	179
spinach	1 cup	278
turnip greens	1 cup	229
beet greens	1 cup	165
bok choy	1 cup	200
mustard greens	1 cup	150

Food	Amount	Calcium (mg)
rhubarb	1 cup	348
watercress (raw)	1 cup	53
parsley (raw)	1 cup	122
dandelion greens	1 cup	147
Sea vegetables (cooked, unless specified)		
hijiki	1 cup	610
wakame	1 cup	520
kombu (kelp)	1 cup	305
agar-agar (Kanten flakes) used as a thickener for sauces, etc.	1 cup (dry flakes) (16 tbsp)	400
dulse	1 cup (dry)	567
Fish (bones: the major source of calcium in fish)		
sardines (with bones)	3½ oz can (drained)	300
salmon (canned)	1 cup	431
oysters, raw	1 cup	226
Beans and Legumes		
tofu, firm	4 oz	80–150
tempeh	4 oz	172
garbanzo beans (chickpeas)	1 cup (cooked)	135
black beans	1 cup (cooked)	135
pinto beans	1 cup (cooked)	128
tortillas, corn	2	120
Nuts and Seeds		
sesame seeds (must be ground for absorption)	3 tbsp	300

Food	Amount	Calcium (mg)
almonds	1 cup	300
sunflower seeds	1 cup	174
Brazil nuts	1 cup	260
hazelnuts	1 cup	282

Other Sources

blackstrap molasses	1 tbsp	137
orange juice calcium fortified (Minute Maid)	1 cup	210

Mineral Waters

Perrier	1 liter	140
Mendocino	1 liter	380
San Pellegrino	1 liter	200
Apollinaris	1 liter	91
Contexeville	1 liter	451

Dairy

milk		
skim	1 cup	300
whole	1 cup	288
cheese (American, Swiss, cheddar)	1½ oz	300
ice milk	1 cup	204
nonfat yogurt	1 cup	294
cottage cheese (low fat)	1 cup	150

Foods High in Magnesium

In mg per 100 grams (3½ oz) servings

- Kelp 760
- Wheat bran 490
- Wheat germ 336

~ Molasses 258

~ Almonds 270

~ Dulse 220

~ Peanuts 175

~ Millet 162

~ Tofu 111

~ Collard greens 57

~ Cooked beans 37

WHAT ABOUT BONE-BUILDING DRUGS?

Far too many doctors prescribe one of the newer bone-building drugs as the first line of treatment for any woman who shows any sign of decreased bone mass—even those who are very far from having actual osteoporosis or even significant osteopenia. However there are many safe and effective alternatives that work more naturally with the wisdom of the body.

Here's a brief rundown of the most commonly available bone-building prescription drugs. Like hormone replacement, these work only as long as a woman is on them.

BISPHOSPHONATES: The bisphosphonates are the most widely prescribed antiresorptive agents and are currently considered the first-line treatment for postmenopausal osteoporosis. These drugs interfere with osteoclast function, thus preventing bone breakdown. They have been shown to increase spine and hip bone mass and to reduce the risk of spinal fractures about as well as estrogen replacement.[57] Trials have shown that in women with osteoporosis, alendronate (Fosamax), risedronate (Actonel), and ibandronate (Boniva) reduced the incidence of hip, vertebral, and nonvertebral fracture by almost 50 percent, particularly in the first year of treatment.[58] However, these drugs may cause side effects. Fosamax, for example, may cause nausea, constipation, and heartburn. In some studies, up to a third of the participants had stomach-acid-related complaints, and one in eight required treatment. Some even developed severe esophageal ulcers.[59] About 50 percent of women stop treatment within a year. However, bisphosphonates may be appropriate for women at risk for osteoporosis who cannot or will not take other medications or other measures to build bone mass. Some of the more common side effects of Actonel include back pain, joint pain, stomach pain, nausea, and vomiting. I'm very concerned about untoward long-term side effects from these drugs. For example, they've been shown to cause severe jaw bone loss in some women.

EVISTA (RALOXIFENE): This selective estrogen receptor modulator (SERM), like the related drug tamoxifen, has an estrogenic effect on bone but anti-estrogenic effects on breast tissue. Though Evista has been shown to help build bone, and though it decreases spinal fractures by 40 percent, it has not resulted in a decrease in the incidence of hip fractures, for reasons that aren't yet clear.[60] Side effects include hot flashes. I'm also very concerned about the possibility of dementia risk with this drug because, like tamoxifen, it blocks the well-known beneficial effects of estrogen (including the estrogen our bodies make on their own) on brain cells.

CALCITONIN: Calcitonin is a naturally occurring peptide that partially blocks osteoclast activity and regulates calcium loss in the urine. This is an injectable or nasal synthetic form of the parathyroid hormone. It reduces the risk of spinal but not hip fractures and also reduces pain from new spinal fractures. Side effects include nausea and flushing. Most experts agree that the bisphosphonates work better.[61]

Bottom line: everyone with low bone density needs to have enough vitamin D, calcium, and magnesium. Many might also benefit from alendronate or risedronate once weekly (or ibandronate once monthly)—but I'd prefer all women try natural methods first.

GET STRONG

Regardless of your diet, supplements, or any drugs you may be on, the big news is that weight-bearing exercise in general and strength training in particular play a crucial role in creating and maintaining healthy bones. If you don't currently exercise regularly, you're not alone. Sixty percent of the U.S. population is sedentary, which is one of the main reasons why osteoporosis has reached such epidemic proportions. Remember, it is not the aging process per se that causes bones to thin—it's the fact that too many women slow down and stop using their muscles.

Weight-bearing exercise helps build bone by stimulating the mineralization and remodeling process. Every major muscle in our bodies is attached to underlying bone by tendons. Every time a muscle contracts, it exerts a force on the bone to which it is anchored. Any activity that builds up muscle also puts stress on bone and helps build bone mass. We know, for example, that in tennis players the bone density in the racket arm is significantly greater than in the other arm. Yoga and tai chi can also help build bone mass. But the most studied method of strengthening bone is weight lifting.

Miriam Nelson, Ph.D., of Tufts University, has done groundbreaking research that shows how weight training can slow down and even reverse bone loss. Dr. Nelson studied two groups of postmenopausal women, none of whom were on estrogen replacement, bone-building drugs, or any special supplements. Both groups were sedentary but healthy at the start of the program. One group remained sedentary while the other began a simple exercise program. At the end of one year the women who lifted weights for forty minutes twice per week had turned back the clock in several ways. Their scores on strength tests increased to match those of women in their late thirties or early forties. Without dieting, they trimmed down; muscle is less bulky than fat. Their balance improved greatly, warding off falls. The biggest payoff: while the sedentary control group lost about 2 percent of their bone density during the year, the women who strength-trained gained 1 percent.[62]

But stronger bones aren't the only benefit of getting strong. Nelson noted an unexpected but very exciting change in the women who did weight training—a change that I've also seen repeatedly in my own practice. Within a few weeks the weight-lifting women felt happier, more energetic, and more self-confident. As their muscles began to get stronger, they became more active and daring. In order to control the study, they had agreed not to join other fitness programs. But these former couch potatoes were now going canoeing or inline skating or dancing because they wanted to. Nelson also confirmed that weight training, like aerobic exercise, lifts depression and helps arthritis.[63]

The joys and benefits of fitness are so numerous that I want to do everything in my power to motivate you to get strong. Of all the ways to stay vital, healthy, and attractive, exercise probably gives the most return for the time spent. Whatever your age and condition right now, physical exercise can improve it and give you a new lease on life—guaranteed. In 1994 researchers proved this by instituting a strength-training program in frail nursing-home patients with an average age of eighty-seven. The exercise group did forty-five-minute strength-training sessions for the hips and knees three days per week. Within ten weeks, their strength increased by over 100 percent. In a non-exercising control group, strength declined by about 1 percent. The improved muscle strength after exercise was unrelated to the age, sex, medical diagnosis, or functional level of the participant. After the strength-training program some of the participants who had previously used walkers required only a cane. Exercise also improved stair-climbing ability, speed of walking, and overall level of physical activity.[64]

If these kinds of results are possible in frail octogenarians in nursing homes, think what could happen for a fifty-year-old couch potato. The average midlife woman of today is expected to live until at least age eighty-five, if not a hundred. You cannot afford to let your muscles and bones slip into decline at midlife. There are too many potentially high-quality years ahead. And there's not a single drug, technological breakthrough, or genetic development on the horizon that can or ever will come close to providing you with the benefits you can derive yourself from getting and staying strong. Besides, women who exercise regularly live six years longer than non-exercisers. If you think you don't have time to exercise, I suggest that you rethink this belief. Slowly shuffling along with a walker instead of striding confidently takes up a lot of time. And dying six years prematurely is truly a colossal waste of time.

Almost every woman I know is too busy to exercise. There are always more things to get done in a day than you have time for. If you wait to exercise until you get everything else done, you are waiting for a miracle. Like muscles that won't get stronger until you reach down and pick up a heavy weight, exercise won't happen in your life unless you make it as much a priority as brushing your teeth or taking a shower. The first thing that must change if you are to exercise regularly is your mind. No excuses.

What Would It Take to Get You Moving?

~ Do you enjoy moving your body? Recall a moment in your life in which you were captivated by the sheer joy of dancing, running, swimming, or jumping. When was the last time you felt this way?

~ When was the last time that you felt that pleasurable sense of complete relaxation that comes from spending a day immersed in the pleasures of some activity—skiing, hiking, sailing, dancing, or inline skating?

~ What types of activities did you enjoy as a child? As a teenager?

~ If you do not exercise now, why not?

~ If you don't exercise now, when did you stop? Why?

~ Do you feel that you don't have time to exercise? Why not?

HEALING YOUR FITNESS PAST

My mother turned eighty this year, and in celebration the whole extended family gathered in my hometown for a big party and other activities that included downhill and cross-country skiing, as well as snowshoeing. My mom kept right up with her grandchildren and still skis beautifully. Every summer, she leads a group of forty-somethings on a hiking exedition in the Adirondacks that they call Camp Edna. These women love benefiting from my mother's experience and expertise. So at an age when many women have relegated themselves to the sidelines, my mother is not only coaching the game, she is also actively playing it. She often gets up at six, mows the huge lawn on the farm where I grew up, waters all the flowers, then plays two sets of tennis with her friends. Sometimes she plays eighteen holes of golf, too.

My mother's physical activity level is way out there, and I don't see it as a standard to which I or anyone else should aspire unless they find it as satisfying as she does. But my mother's physical condition and prowess have helped me (and my daughters) understand that physical decline and weakness need not be part of growing older. In fact, it's a legacy I received before birth: my mother skied and hiked through all her pregnancies and later carried each of us children in a backpack during these same activities.

Despite this legacy, I had to work through some unfinished business around sports and fitness. In contrast to my mother and siblings, I was not interested in spending every free moment on the ski slopes or hiking up mountains carrying a heavy backpack. I liked to read books—by the fire in winter and sitting up in a tree in summer. As an adolescent, I longed for a Christmas morning in which we could all sit around, relax, talk, and drink cocoa, like they did in the movies. But invariably, as soon as the presents had been opened, everyone rushed out the door to get in a couple of runs at the local ski area before our relatives arrived for dinner. My only chance for having the loving family connection that I longed for was to haul out my gear and join them. So I did. And I learned how to ski pretty well. (This year, I went home for the holidays for the first time in thirty years and finally experienced the Christmas of my dreams—sitting around the fire and visiting with my mother and siblings. No one went skiing!)

But my overall sports skills lagged behind those of my mother and siblings no matter how hard I tried. During the summer of my thirteenth year, for example, I practiced my tennis strokes daily against the barn door for six solid weeks. My father's only comment was "You're swinging that racket as if it were a broom." This left me with considerable baggage around sports. So at midlife I decided to release this baggage and pick up some barbells—and some insight— instead. When I was forty-five I took tennis lessons, more as therapy to recover from my past than from a desire to play regularly. By the end of the season I realized that I was perfectly capable of playing and enjoying a game of tennis. Later that summer I even played doubles with my mother and brother. What a healing!

John Douillard, D.C., Ph.D., a fitness expert and the author of *Body, Mind, and Sport* (Three Rivers Press, 2001), points out that 50 percent of women experience their first personal failure around organized physical activity in school gym class, and that this sense of being a physical "loser" can stay with you the rest of your life. At perimenopause you have to ask yourself, "Do I really want to continue limiting my health and happiness because of something that happened to me in eighth-grade gym class, or with my parents when I was six?"

Get out your journal and write down everything you remember about physical activity and sports from when you were eleven to thirteen years old. What did you love to do? What activities felt good? What are your memories from gym class? What is your family legacy around fitness? What do you honestly believe about the physical capabilities of a woman your age? Age seventy-five? Age ninety? What was the fitness level of your mother? Your grandmother? What happens to you when you walk into a gym?

My colleague Mona Lisa Schulz has been able to transform her fitness legacy several times, finally reaching balance. When she was growing up, her family's idea of a vacation was to drive to the base of a mountain in New England, eat a sandwich, and then drive back home. She desperately longed to get out of the car and actually climb a peak. But her mother always had a bad back, and her father always had a headache and chest pain. Once, when she was sixteen, she wanted to go skiing. Her mother said, "Don't go or I'll disown you. You've put your father and me through enough already." (By then Mona Lisa had already had major surgery for scoliosis.) She went skiing anyway, and eventually a large part of her individuation from her family of origin involved proving herself by becoming a competitive athlete in both running and bike racing—which she tended to do excessively as a way to cope with the stress of her family. Though continuing spinal problems eventually halted these activities, she has worked around her physical challenges and still remains strong and fit through walking, biking, and daily workouts on a variety of fitness equipment. She, too, has reached balance.

Exercise for Vibrant Health on All Levels

At midlife I finally figured out what type of exercise was right for my body and temperament by realizing that my sports skills, strength, and fitness levels were all about me and my body, not a way to win family approval or measure up to a cultural standard. Regardless of your own fitness past or legacy, you need to know that vigorous regular exercise is an absolute necessity if you intend to live well beyond midlife. Vigorous exercise sends positive signals to your entire body that increase your levels of human growth hormone. Exercise tells your body to stay vigorous, vibrant, healthy, and growing. Sitting on the couch and eating junk food and drinking too much alcohol gives your body the opposite message: get old, deteriorate, and go into decline. It's that simple.

Ask yourself what activities you want to be able to participate in for as long as you live. I tried for years to enjoy running—it was very "in" in the 1970s and 1980s. But it never felt good. Though I ran regularly throughout medical school and residency, I never felt that elusive runner's high, no matter how long or hard I ran. In fact, I hated it. I finally gave myself permission to stop.

I now go only for those activities that feel right. I love Pilates, the mind/body fitness approach developed by Joseph Pilates that engages the mind, the muscles, breathing, and stretching all at once. I also love seeing how far I've come since I started in 1998. I'm now stronger, leaner, and more flexible than I was eight years ago! Pilates, like any discipline that uses the mind as fully as the body, ends up transforming both. I also enjoy yoga occasionally, and I do regular weight training. I like being able to lift heavy objects—I know I could easily remove the window from an airplane exit row if necessary! Strong muscles help you move confidently through the world.

RUTH: *Couch Potato No More*

Ruth, fifty-five, came to see me complaining of aches and pains and not being able to sleep well at night. She told me she had raised five children and was now looking forward to retirement from her job as a government secretary. She had never done any regular exercise. Her initial bone density test showed a slight bone loss despite the fact that she had been on estrogen for seven years following a hysterectomy with ovary removal for heavy bleeding. In addition to recommending dietary improvement and a supplement program, I stressed to Ruth that she needed to begin an exercise program: her couch-potato status was putting her at risk for significantly tarnishing her dreams for her golden years.

Ruth decided to start a walking program every morning with some of her friends. Within three months she had lost ten pounds without changing her diet at all, her aches and pains were gone, and she was sleeping better than she had in years. Later that year she and her husband both took up skiing and hiking. Though I'm still trying to convince Ruth to begin a weight-training program, her bone density has stayed steady even without it. Fitness and outdoor exercise have become a regular part of her life.

Start Somewhere—Anywhere

If you simply can't see yourself doing something like weight training just yet, commit to doing some kind of physical activity for just ten minutes daily for thirty days. Here's what I recommend: put on some music you love and dance around your house. Even if you're in a wheelchair, you can sit and move your upper body. No kidding. No excuses. I guarantee that by the end of thirty days or much sooner, you'll be looking forward to your daily dance. Just this simple exercise will wake up the inherent, irresistible desire to move that lies within each of us—albeit more deeply buried in some than others!

Movement is contagious. Today's dancing around your living room will eventually wake up enough of your muscles that you'll want to do more. You can always pick up your cat and dance around with him or her. (This is weight training, after all!) Start very slowly and breathe in and out through your nose—this will expand your lower lungs optimally. It can take a while to create flexibility in your rib cage, so don't get discouraged if nose breathing makes you feel out of breath at first. Don't ever push beyond what is comfortable for your breathing and heart rate. But every day ask your body to move a little faster or bend a little deeper. Simply moving your body begins the bone-building process.

Get Support

After you've done your one month of dancing, you'll have created the movement habit in your life. Now's the time to begin adding some weight training. I suggest that you go to a Y, an adult education class at your local high school, or a gym and have one of the staff members guide you through a personal strength-training program. This way you'll be learning proper technique, which you can later adapt for home use.

Whether you work out at home or in a gym will depend upon your lifestyle and temperament. I've done both and find advantages and disadvantages to each approach. The beauty of the gym is that the phone doesn't ring and no one interrupts you. And the entire environment is dedicated to fitness, so you're more apt to get into the spirit of it. But sometimes taking the extra time to go to the gym is too much. My current personal fitness regimen combines one-hour Pilates sessions in a studio with a teacher, thirty-minute Pilates mat sessions on my own at home, and one hour of aerobic weight training with videos, each done twice per week. I also take regular forty-five-minute walks. I haven't always been able to get this amount of exercise in. One of the benefits of being perimenopausal is that my time is more my own than at any other time of my life. And I find that I like exercise more now than I ever have.

Build Strength into Your Day

Here are a few tips for adding some strength training to your day-to-day activities. Try these exercises when you're on the phone or have a few spare moments. They cover all the major muscle groups.

~ TOE STANDS. Face a wall and stand twelve inches away from it with your feet shoulder-width apart. Rest your fingertips lightly against the wall for balance. (As you improve you can use the wall less and less.) Now raise yourself as high up as you can; remain on your toes for a count of three, breathing normally, then lower yourself slowly. Breathe. Repeat a total of eight times. Gradually hold each toe stand for thirty seconds as you become stronger.

~ HEEL STANDS. Stand facing a wall so that you can put your hands against it if necessary. Slowly raise the toes and balls of your feet until you are balanced on your heels. Remain on your heels for a count of three. Slowly lower. Breathe. Repeat. Try for a total of eight repetitions, and gradually increase the amount of time you balance on your heels so that eventually you're holding each heel stand for a count of thirty.

Both heel and toe stands use your own body weight to strengthen your legs and to improve balance and flexibility.

~ PUSH-UPS. Although many women hate them, nothing beats a push-up for strengthening the upper body. You can ease into this exercise with wall push-ups. Stand with your feet about three feet from a wall. Lean forward with elbows bent and palms touching the wall. Now push off the wall, keeping your back perfectly aligned with your legs, making sure that your head is aligned with your back and not pitching forward. Repeat this wall push-up eight times. Build up to three sets of eight repetitions.

After this becomes easy, you'll be ready for push-ups on the floor. Start on your hands and knees with arms straight. Now bend your elbows and dip your chest to the floor. Go slowly and keep breathing. Try for four knee push-ups. Gradually build up to two sets of eight.

When you get strong enough, you'll be ready for full-blown regulation push-ups. Start on your hands and knees. Then straighten your legs out behind you so that you are supported by your toes and your arms. Your body should form a perfectly straight line with your head in alignment with your spine. Don't allow your hips to jackknife up in the center. Now dip down so that your chest almost touches the floor. Push back up. Hold. Repeat. Do four, working up to eight. Eventually you'll be aiming for two sets of eight push-ups.

~ WEIGHTS. Place a set of graduated dumbbells (5–20 lb, depending upon your strength level) in front of your TV. During commercial breaks or even during your favorite shows you can easily do a few sets of biceps curls, overhead presses, bent rows, flat rows, or triceps kickbacks. The point is to keep the weights out where you'll run into them regularly.

Take your time. Your body is very forgiving and very responsive if you approach it with respect and love. Each time you lift weights, ask your body if it is willing to breathe a little deeper and lift a bit more weight. Don't push it. On the days when you feel wonderful, do more. When you feel lousy, cut back. Exercise is a discipline, it is true. But once you've made the commitment to do it regularly, get that abusive coach out of your head. The best motivator is the pleasure, joy, and awareness that come from being in your body.

Preventing Hip, Shoulder, and Back Pain

Many women begin to experience joint problems during perimenopause, including decreased range of motion in one shoulder or in the hip joints. When I started Pilates, I personally had a chronic right hip problem that responded well to exercises directed at loosening the hip joints. I knew intuitively that this approach was going to prevent me from needing a hip replacement someday. (Right hip problems run in my family. My father needed one when he died but had refused to get it.) I also developed severe right shoulder pain and decreased range of motion in my early fifties. Once again, gentle exercises and the stretching that is part of Pilates helped me work through it. Now my range of motion is better than it was when I was thirty!

You must maintain your range of motion and also keep your spine well-aligned and stretched in order to keep the spinal nerves free from impingement, which can lead to back, hip, and other pain. Pilates does this beautifully, and so does yoga. There's also an ingenious at-home program that anyone can do called The Core Program, developed by physical therapist Peggy Brill. The Core Program is a series of exercises that can be done in a small space with only a mat and some ankle weights. Thousands of women have had their bodies transformed by doing The Core Program, including my mother, who does the program regularly. (For more information, read *The Core Program: Fifteen Minutes a Day That Can Change Your Life* [Bantam Books, 2001], by Peggy W. Brill, or visit her website at www.brillpt.com.)

Supplements for Joint Health

Because the cartilage in your joints tends to undergo wear and tear over the years, it's very important to supply your joints with the nourishment they require. NSAIDs such as Advil and Motrin have been implicated in the destruction of cartilage over time. Though these popular OTC drugs definitely decrease joint pain, they do more harm than good over the long haul. Alternatively, many women get significant relief from joint pain and arthritis with the following supplements, taken in addition to a good multivitamin:

~ Glucosamine sulfate: 1,000 mg twice per day

~ Turmeric: 250 mg twice per day

~ Omega-3 fats: 1,000–4,000 mg per day

~ Proanthocyanadins (OPCs), made from grape seed or pine bark: Start with a loading dose of 1 mg per pound of body weight. Take it in divided doses for 10–14 days. After that, you can decrease to a maintenance dose of 60–200 mg per day. (See Resources.)

THE SUNLIGHT–BONE HEALTH CONNECTION

Everywhere we turn, we are warned about the dangers of exposure to the sun, from premature skin aging to fatal skin cancer. Though these risks are well documented, they are overstated, especially for those of us who live in northern climates, where sunlight isn't a glaring issue for most of the year. Women past menopause lose up to 3–4 percent of their bone mass every winter if they live in northern latitudes, above a line approximately from Boston through Chicago to the California-Oregon border.[65] Even on a bright sunny day in December in northern Maine, you cannot get enough ultraviolet exposure to produce vitamin D unless you expose a great deal of your skin to the sun at midday for thirty to fifty minutes or so, a level of exposure that is uncommon. The problem is compounded if your diet is already low in calcium and vitamin D. Forty percent of individuals with hip fractures in northern latitudes are vitamin D deficient. In women whose diets are adequate in calcium and other nutrients, however, bone mass can be regained in the summer months with regular sunlight exposure.

The truth is that sunlight can help you become healthier and can literally save your life. That's because ultraviolet rays from the sun help your body manufacture necessary vitamin D. As with just about everything else, the key is moderation.

Vitamin D is a hormone that helps your bones absorb calcium. If you don't have enough vitamin D circulating in your blood, you won't be able to use the calcium from your diet or from supplements. Therefore, it is an important factor in preventing osteoporosis. Right now the RDA for vitamin D is based on the amount you need to prevent rickets. Rickets is a disease where vitamin D levels are too low, resulting in the body's decreased ability to produce new bone. In adults, this is called osteomalacia, a gradual softening or bending of bones secondary to failure of bones to calcify.

To prevent rickets, you need just a minimal level of vitamin D (200–400 IU per day). But prevention of rickets isn't the only benefit of optimal vitamin D levels. For example, adequate vitamin D can decrease hypertension, so people with higher vitamin D levels enjoy lower blood pressure.[66] It can slow the progression of osteoarthritis and also decrease the prevalence of multiple sclerosis.[67] Vitamin D also helps prevent some cancers, such as breast, ovarian, prostate, and colorectal cancer. In fact, suboptimal levels of vitamin D may be one of the reasons why breast cancer incidence is higher in the northern latitudes than in the South.

But in order to lower your risk for these diseases, especially breast, ovarian, and colorectal cancer, you need much higher serum levels than you can get with a teaspoon of cod liver oil or the usual vitamin D supplement. Your safest and most effective route for this is routine sun exposure.

Sunlight Versus Vitamin D Supplementation

Our bodies were designed to get vitamin D from the sun. Our ancestors ran around the plains of Africa for millennia with large surfaces of their bodies exposed to sunlight. Exposure to outdoor sunlight is a much more reliable predictor of vitamin D levels in your body than your dietary intake. In fact, vitamin D intake in your diet correlates poorly with the amount of vitamin D in your blood. This is partly because oral vitamin D requirements have been found to vary tremendously between individuals. And while it is possible to take in toxic levels of vitamin D from supplements, it is impossible for sun exposure to result in too much vitamin D. That's because our bodily wisdom contains a built-in mechanism whereby we manufacture exactly what we need from the sun—no more and no less. The vitamin D that your body makes on its own from exposure to the sun's ultraviolet rays (specifically ultraviolet B, or UVB) is superior to oral supplementation for helping your body absorb calcium.[68]

Sunlight alone can bring your vitamin D levels into the healthy range. If you expose your face and hands to sunlight without sunscreen for about twenty minutes three to five times per week for four to five months per year (between April and October in northern latitudes—above the fortieth parallel), you probably will get enough UVB rays to keep your bone mass intact, because your body has the ability to stockpile vitamin D for use during low-sunlight times. This is nature's wisdom at work, because not all regions of the country are equal when it comes to ultraviolet exposure. If you have very dark skin, you need to be in the sun longer—even an hour or two hours to get the same result.

The more skin you expose, the quicker you make vitamin D, which is why some experts recommend full-body exposure regularly. In fact, full-body exposure for fifteen minutes is the equivalent of an oral dose of 10,000 IU vitamin D. (But UV exposure beyond this does not give you higher vitamin D levels.) However, as we age, our bodies become less efficient at making their own vitamin D. So if you are older than sixty-five, you may need more time in the sun to get the same benefit. Here's a general rule: if there's enough sunlight to cause a reddening of your skin when you're outside for any length of time, then there are enough UVB rays to assist your body in making vitamin D.

How to Have Your Sun and Be Safe, Too

Everyone can get the amount of sunlight she needs safely by getting outdoors regularly. The benefits of small amounts of UVB light are so striking that endocrinologist Michael Holick, M.D., and his colleagues at Boston University Medical Center are studying the effects of providing artificial UVB light to seniors. NASA has also contracted Dr. Holick to put this special light into spaceships for long missions to counteract the effects of weightlessness on bone.[69]

Early-morning or late-afternoon sun exposure is the safest. I personally take a forty-five-minute walk about four mornings per week during the warm months, wearing shorts and a tank top to ensure adequate sun exposure. When I can't get out in the morning, I try for late afternoon or early evening, when there is still some sunlight available but when the risk of overexposure is minimal. Other than these "vitamin D–enhancing times" I wear sunscreen.

Avoid midday sun and sunburn. Almost all skin cancers are associated with the harmful effects of sun overexposure without adequate antioxidant protection. In fact, UV exposure beyond pre-erythema levels (reddening of the skin) doesn't enhance your vitamin D levels. In other words, vitamin D reaches maximum levels in light skin twenty minutes after exposure.

Other easy ways to get a little vitamin D enhancement are rolling down the window in your car as you drive, riding in a convertible, or even opening the windows in your house. Why not create a sunroom or sun corner—a place where you can easily open a window and expose yourself to warm sunlight without even having to go outside? This is a good option for city dwellers.

What to Do When You Can't Get Enough Sunlight

Vitamin D is an essential hormone. In the absence of sunlight, you must get it in your diet. While it is nearly impossible to get the high levels of vitamin D you need in your blood without adequate sun exposure, vitamin D supplementation has definitely been shown to help women build or maintain bone mass.[70]

People under sixty-five should take 800–1,000 IU per day. People sixty-five and older should take 800–2,000 IU per day unless they have a known sensitivity to it. (You may need more or less. The point is that sunlight is more reliable than any supplement.) Good food sources of vitamin D are liver, cod liver oil, and egg yolks.

Why Fortified Milk Isn't the Vitamin D Answer

Though all of us have been taught that it's possible to get all the vitamin D we need from fortified dairy foods, that's not always the case. When Dr. Michael Holick studied the vitamin D content of fortified milk, he found that there's often not enough vitamin D present because of processing problems. In fact, up to 50 percent of the milk tested had less vitamin D than noted on the label. Fifteen percent of the milk had no vitamin D at all! And in skim milk there is a problem getting vitamin D into the solution because vitamin D is fat soluble and requires some fat to blend with the product. That's why skim milk products may have little or no vitamin D whatsoever.[71]

When in Doubt, Measure

If you have any evidence of osteoporosis from either bone density screening or a urine test, then I'd recommend getting a serum vitamin D level as well. This is a simple blood test. A blood level of vitamin D of 20–25 nmol/l or lower indicates a severe deficiency. We're now finding that women with osteoporosis have vitamin D levels of 20 mg/dl or lower! You want to shoot for a level that is in the upper range of normal, about 45–250 nmol/l. Levels greater than 100 nmol/l have been shown to decrease hypertension.[72] Levels of 75 nmol/l and above slow the progression of osteoarthritis. Studies of lifeguards and farmers—people who are out in the sun all the time—show that they have vitamin D levels of around 100 nmol/l. You may also want to have your serum levels checked if you're healthy but you are in doubt about how much vitamin D you're getting or manufacturing from sun exposure. If your levels are low, get more sun exposure to prevent later problems, even if your bones seem healthy now.

I once did a consult for a woman in her mid-forties who summered in Maine and ran regularly for exercise while covered in sunscreen and clothing. Though she lived most of the year in the Southwest, an area with abundant sunshine all year around, she avoided the sun at all costs because she was worried about skin cancer. When I ordered a serum vitamin D level, it came back at 25 nmol/l, indicating severe deficiency. Since then, she has been taking daily fifteen-minute early-morning sun baths in her backyard. Within two months her serum vitamin D level had increased to a very healthy range, and both her mood and her immune system improved dramatically. Within six months her bone density had also improved. She discovered some other benefits as well: She completely recovered from a tendency to catch colds and have aches and pains.

Should You Use a Tanning Salon?

Though dermatologists cringe at tanning salons because of the danger of overexposure, I recommend them for those who are at high risk for osteoporosis, depression, or certain cancers and who have no other way of getting UVB radiation.

A short five- to ten-minute sun bath in a facility once or twice per week in the winter months can boost your brain serotonin levels, lift depression, help build bone, help calm arthritis, and maybe also help prevent some cancers. The key, as with natural sun exposure, is to be sure you never burn or get red skin, and also that your body is fortified with antioxidants.

Take Antioxidants

Increasing numbers of studies have shown that antioxidants such as vitamin E, vitamin C, proanthocyanidins, and beta-carotene help protect the skin from sun damage, and also help it heal more quickly. (See chapter 11 for further information.)

Beware Drug-Induced Sun Sensitivity

Remember that many very common drugs actually increase sun sensitivity and will therefore increase your chances for getting a sunburn if you stay out too long. These include the following: antibiotics such as azithromycin (Zithromax), minocycline (Minocin), tetracycline, and sulfa; diabetic medications of the sulfonylurea family; skin treatments such as Retin-A and Renova; and diuretics of the thiazide family. It's always best to check with your pharmacist.

SHORE UP YOUR EARTH CONNECTION WITH PLANT MEDICINE

Traditional herbalists teach that when we consume plants regularly, our bodies take in their energetic qualities as well as their vitamins and minerals—a perfect way to help us connect with nature and shore up our first emotional centers. Oats (*Avena sativa*) and oat straw (the grass, leaf, and flower of the oat), for example, thrive in chilly, wet climates characterized by harsh winds and sudden storms. These hardy plants are rich in calcium, iron, phosphorous, B complex, potassium, magnesium, and vitamins A and C.[73]

The noted herbalist Susun Weed has found that regular consumption of herbal infusions with their highly bioavailable nutrients helps increase bone density as well as providing other benefits. One of my nutritionist colleagues also recommends them. Using infusions regularly is a very inexpensive and effective way to increase mineral intake.

How to Make an Herbal Infusion

Infusions are stronger than herbal teas. Use 1 oz (30 g) of dried leaves (two handfuls of cut-up leaves, or three handfuls of whole leaves). Put in a quart or liter jar. Fill jar with boiling water, put the lid on, and steep for four hours at room temperature. This can be kept in the refrigerator.[74] Use 2 cups daily.

When using oat straw or other plant medicines, open yourself to the wisdom of the earth and nature as they have manifested in the plant you are taking into your body. Be patient and persistent. Feel your bones becoming as strong and sturdy as the mountains and rocks that form the backbone of the planet.

13
Creating Breast Health

I remember the many evenings I sat in the labor-and-delivery area of the hospital with one of my midwife colleagues. Though her own children were nearly grown, this woman would sometimes clutch her chest when she heard a baby cry or saw a particularly adorable newborn. "My breasts are tingling so much, I feel as though I could nurse this child myself," she would say at such moments.

Breasts are both literally and symbolically a source of nurturance and pleasurable bonding. Their dual role is in part the result of a brain hormone known as prolactin. This chemical, which is activated during birth, keeps the breasts full of milk and also enhances the process of bonding, so that when a mother breast-feeds, prolactin facilitates the flow of both milk and love to the child. The mother in turn is rewarded not only with pleasurable physical sensations, but with the emotional fulfillment that comes from providing for a being she deeply loves. Prolactin has such a powerful effect that many women experience the letdown reflex, which fills the breasts with milk, even when they're not actually nursing. Merely thinking about their child or hearing the child's cries can set the reflex in motion.

But prolactin secretion doesn't occur only during breast-feeding. Prolactin levels have been found to increase in both men and women when they are involved in pleasurable, mutually beneficial relationships. Not surprisingly, the emotions of love and compassion, which nourish our very souls, are often accompanied by the same tingling sensation in the breasts that nursing mothers feel—and that my midwife colleague described so eloquently.

I like to think of that tingling as proof that the "milk of human kindness" is more than a mere metaphor. Love is hardwired into our biology. That's why nurturing and supporting others feels so good to most women, and why we so often find ourselves "mothering" others. When the emotion of love can flow freely, our bodies are filled with the same hormone that sustains all human bonds, and our breasts are bathed in the energy of health.

OUR CULTURAL INHERITANCE: NURTURING AND SELF-SACRIFICE

Love has a healing, life-enhancing effect if our relationships are truly reciprocal, allowing us to receive as much as we give. But this ideal is not so common. Most women have been brought up to nurture others in ways that often require us to put our own well-being at risk. Throughout history, we women have been revered for our ability to sacrifice ourselves for the good of those around us. It is no wonder that Tammy Wynette's song "Stand by Your Man" is the best-selling country song of all time. But as it turns out, the man Tammy was standing by for much of her married life was beating her, which brings home very powerfully the degree to which our nurturing tendencies can tip the balance toward dangerous self-sacrifice.

Our breasts are the part of our anatomy most identified with nurturing. And they are also perhaps the most highly charged area of our bodies, flagrantly exploited by the culture we live in as our most potent weapon in the battle to win the love and approval of a man. Powerful symbols, these breasts. In the movie *Erin Brockovich* the sassy legal-assistant heroine is asked by her astounded boss how she has managed, without any experience or training, to accumulate so much sensitive, damning information concerning a large utility company's environmental pollution practices. Looking resplendently voluptuous in her overflowing bustier, actress Julia Roberts replies, "They're called boobs, Ed."

No wonder one of my friends, when she heard I was getting a divorce, asked if I was going to get breast implants. Our culture leads us to believe that without a stunning new set of breasts, it would be impossible for a woman at midlife to attract a new man. What more vivid proof could we find of our need for love—and the lengths to which we are willing to go to get it?

The Midlife Breast Challenge

Midlife is when we hear the wake-up call that demands that we start honoring our own needs. Our children are leaving home or long gone, the time for the kind of self-sacrifice demanded by raising a family is coming to an end, and we now have the opportunity to re-examine our lives. If we are involved in relationships that are getting in the way of self-realization, we need to think about how we can change them. Perimenopause challenges us to get real, to create relationships that are true partnerships with people who will love us for who we really are.

Learning to form such mutually nurturing relationships, as part of a commitment to love and nurture ourselves on every level, will improve the health of every organ in the body. But the breasts are particularly likely to be affected, because the breasts are located in the fourth emotional center, which is associated with the ability to express joy, love, grief, and forgiveness, as well as anger and hostility. If those emotions are blocked, then the health of all the organs in the fourth emotional center, which include the lungs and heart as well as the breasts, may suffer.

Forming loving relationships that nurture us, and nurturing our-selves directly through the choices we make about how we live our lives, can help us to create breast health. Such nurturing is not selfish; in fact, it allows us to have within us something that is worth giving to others. Here again we can look to breast-feeding for the wisdom inherent in our bodies. Both the quality and quantity of a mother's milk are improved when the mother herself is well rested, well nour-ished, and happy. We need to remember this lesson at midlife, when the opportunity for transformation is boundless and the costs of turning our backs on it may be very high.

Midlife Breast Pain

Because of the hormonal changes associated with perimenopause, many women experience breast pain, especially during the second half of the menstrual cycle, from ovulation through the onset of menses. Often because of skipped ovulations and overstimulation by estrogen, breast pain comes and goes seemingly at random. This problem often subsides on its own and is not a sign of cancer. Dietary improvement and taking a good multivitamin often quell the inflammation that causes the pain. (See chapter 6, "Foods and Supplements to Support the Change.") Also, eating foods such as soy and flax can help. Breast expert Dixie Mills, M.D., finds that a sonogram is often very reassuring for women who are really worried.

Many times breast pain is a sign that a woman needs to do some emotional updating. The following story is a wonderful example of the power of mind/body breast healing at midlife.

CATHERINE'S STORY

Catherine had fibrocystic breasts that had hurt premenstrually for as long as she could remember. Around the time she turned forty, the pain and lumpiness increased to the point where she had only one pain-free week a month. She quit drinking caffeine, took every supplement she had heard might help, used castor oil packs, and regularly went for acupuncture treatments. She also saw an herbalist who created an herbal remedy just for Catherine. "My breasts were taking over my life!" she told me. Her doctor was sympathetic but said he wasn't sure what else she could do that she wasn't already doing and, trying to be reassuring, told her that as fibrocystic breasts go, hers weren't all that bad.

Then she went to visit her family for two weeks over Christmas. She was in such a rush taking care of last-minute shopping and errands before she left that she forgot to pack her supplements. "Without having to focus on pill-popping, rushing around to practitioners, or figuring out how to tactfully ask my friends about their breasts, I found that mine started hurting less," she discovered. "But I knew that the fact that I wasn't taking any supplements and was spending less time worrying about my breast pain was not causing the pain to go away. What I realized was that I needed to pay more attention to this problem on a different level." She decided to take an inventory. In so doing, she realized that the pain had first come on strong during another family visit about four years ago. The trigger was a comment her uncle made in jest about her grandmother complaining about her breasts hurting all the time. "I was very close to my grandmother," Catherine told me, "and my uncle and mother regularly made comments I perceived as negative about her, many of them in the context of she and I having a special relationship—the subtext being that those negative comments they made about her were also meant to apply to me."

Catherine realized that while she had recognized her emotions on an intellectual level, she hadn't really allowed herself to feel them completely. Remembering that one of her yoga instructors used to say, "In order to heal, you have to feel," Catherine decided to dedicate her yoga and meditation practices to those emotional elements that might be contributing to her breast pain. "I literally dedicated my practices to my breasts!" she told me, and also to the practice of forgiveness, which is a wonderful tonic for all fourth-emotional-center manifestations (including breasts, lungs, heart, and shoulders). For the next several months, she let go of a lot of unspoken anger toward her family, much of it anger she had held in her whole life. And it worked. "While my family needs a lot more support from me lately due to my uncle going through the last stages of lung cancer and an incredible amount of drama surrounding this," she reports, "my breasts are fine—no matter what I put into my body, caffeine included. Since I started letting go of the emotional baggage through forgiveness, my breasts have, in effect, forgiven me. It is truly a miracle."

BREAST CANCER RISK FACTORS

Midlife is also the time when, statistically speaking, your chances of getting breast cancer are on the rise. In fact, for women living in industrialized societies, age is first on the list of established risk factors for breast cancer,[1] but that's only because age is generally associated with the cumulative risk of unhealthy lifestyle patterns. Remember—the vast majority of women *don't* get breast cancer.

~ Age (over fifty years old; risk increases with age until eighty years old)

~ Early onset of menstruation (before age twelve)

~ Family history of breast cancer, in either a first-degree relative (mother, sister, daughter) or a second-degree relative (maternal or paternal aunt, grandmother)

~ Late menopause (after age fifty-five)

~ Giving birth to a first child after age thirty

~ No full-term pregnancies

~ Long-term hormone replacement therapy (greater than five years)

~ Benign breast disease with biopsy showing atypical hyperplasia

~ Significant weight gain after menopause

~ Regular alcohol consumption

~ Low levels of vitamin D

~ History of high-dose radiation to the chest

~ Not getting enough sleep at night

Note: Early or surgically induced menopause decreases the risk for breast cancer.

THE EMOTIONAL ANATOMY OF BREAST CANCER

Like all diseases, cancer has an emotional component as well as a physical one. Many women with breast cancer have a tendency to hide their emotions behind a stoic face and to stay in relationships where they give much more than they receive. The core belief at the heart of this behavior is that we're not worthy of anything better.

The refusal to honor and express our own emotions can sometimes reach pathological extremes. A woman once came to see me because she said she was having trouble breathing. She arrived alone and unsupported, and the tests I had done on her soon confirmed my fear that her breast cancer, which had been diagnosed a year before, had spread to her lungs. She had never sought treatment for her condition because she had not wanted to "inconvenience" her husband or her children. In fact, she had not even let them know about her condition. I told her as gently as possible that her choices, though made in the spirit of generosity and self-sacrifice, were not really helping anyone, least of all herself. She needed support and nurturance, and her family needed to be included in what was happening to her.

In my experience, many women have been denying their needs for so long that they do not even know they have them. One of my friends recalled growing up with a mother whose automatic response to any desire she ever expressed was "Don't ask, don't even think about it." Imagine what that does to a person's ability to ask for what she needs, to express her feelings honestly or to even know what they are! No wonder so many women will do almost anything to avoid appearing self-centered—to the point of putting themselves at risk of dying of terminal illness.

There are now many scientific studies confirming the idea that our emotional style may influence both the incidence of breast cancer and our ability to recover from it. One study, for example, involving 119 women between the ages of twenty and seventy who were referred for breast biopsy because of suspicious breast lumps, looked into the impact of adverse life events on the likelihood of the breast lump being cancerous. Severe crises such as divorce, death of a loved one, or loss of a job in the five years preceding the breast lump did indeed increase the chance of its being cancerous. But interestingly, the way in which a woman dealt with adversity was also a significant factor in whether she developed cancer. Those who had allowed themselves to experience their grief fully when they confronted devastating losses were three times *less* likely to suffer from breast cancer than those who hid their emotions behind a brave face or submerged their grief in various forms of activity.[2]

Clinical psychologist Lydia Temoshok, Ph.D., shares similar ideas in the book *The Type C Connection* (Random House, 1992), which she coauthored with Henry Dreher. Drawing on hundreds of case histories, she identifies what she calls the Type C behavior pattern: those who are unfailingly pleasant, self-sacrificing, compliant, and appeasing—and also unable to express their emotions, especially anger. This behavior pattern, Dr. Temoshok discovered, is associated with various cancers, including breast cancer.

"The most common comment of this kind of cancer patient with breast or gynecological cancer is, 'I'm not worried about me, I'm only worried about my family,' " notes Dreher. "Those patients with thicker and far more aggressive and life-threatening cancers were more severely self-sacrificing and nonexpressive of their needs and feelings."[3]

Not allowing ourselves to grieve uses up vital energy, depriving us of the resources we need to heal. At times of loss we must go through the painful and difficult process that I refer to as radical surrender: we must surrender to a power and order that is bigger than we are. Call it what you will—God, the universe, whatever—we must allow this power to heal our lives, and this can happen only through the full experiencing of our grief.

442   THE WISDOM OF MENOPAUSE

Another study showed that a woman's feelings about the communication between her and her family, and about the availability of help from her family, affected the function of her immune system and therefore her ability to recover. Women with breast cancer who perceived a lack of social support were found to have immune system depression and a poorer prognosis.[4] On the other hand, social support doesn't have to be from your family to have a positive impact on survival. Studies have shown that breast cancer or other support groups characterized by open and honest sharing of experience are associated with increased longevity and decreased rate of tumor recurrence.[5]

MARY: *The Ten-Year Plan*

Mary was forty-one when she called my colleague Mona Lisa Schulz, M.D., Ph.D., for an intuitive reading. Married to a fiercely competitive businessman who spent more time on the road than he did at home, Mary longed for the day when her husband's business would finally be self-sustaining enough to allow him to stop traveling so much. She herself had once been a high-powered executive in the computer industry but was now a stay-at-home mom with two children, ages six and nine. As part of the ten-year plan for work, finances, and family that she and her husband had developed, she had left her career in order to devote herself full-time to rearing the two children they had and the two they were planning to have in the time remaining on that plan.

The problem was, only five years into the plan, Mary was exhausted. As she told Dr. Schulz, she was putting off having a third child until she could get a handle on why she felt so terrible all the time. She wanted to know what her body was trying to tell her through her fatigue. That was why she had scheduled a reading with Mona Lisa.

The reading Dr. Schulz did on Mary revealed an energy pattern that was like that of "a widow pacing back and forth on a widow's walk, forever looking out to sea, waiting and pining for her husband to return." On the basis of what she had read energetically, she told Mary that she, like other women with this pattern of behavior, could have a tendency to form hormonally sensitive densities in her breasts. (Since Dr. Schulz does not make diagnoses during readings, she would never use the term "breast cancer" or even "benign breast lump," both of which are diagnostic terms.)

At this point, Mary revealed that she had, in fact, been diagnosed with breast cancer four years earlier. The surgery, chemotherapy, and radiation seemed to have successfully eradicated the cancer, but she still felt completely drained by the experience.

Dr. Schulz asked Mary what she thought was going on in her life. Mary knew that something was painfully out of balance, but she didn't know exactly what. She missed her old job and was aware that staying home didn't suit her temperament, but she felt that she should just learn to make the best of it in the interest of the plan she had agreed to. She was also aware of how much she longed for her husband to share in the raising of their children, but felt she couldn't voice this longing because it would interfere with his ability to complete his part of the ten-year plan.

Dr. Schulz explained to Mary that all illness is a hologram that contains genetic, environmental, physical, nutritional, emotional, spiritual, and behavioral aspects simultaneously. For Mary, the understanding of that hologram would require her to question the validity of the plan that had locked her and her husband into a way of life that was in fact unsatisfactory to both of them. Her breast cancer had been a signal to her, and the fatigue that had enveloped her ever since then was another signal. Her task was to awaken to the message that her body was trying to give her. She needed to accept the fact that she was not temperamentally suited to be a stay-at-home mother. Some women would, of course, thrive in such circumstances if, like Mary, they had the economic wherewithal to support that lifestyle. Mary just didn't happen to be one of them.

But Mary hadn't allowed herself to own her dissatisfaction consciously because she and her husband were both wedded not just to their plan, but to an outdated view of gender roles: the woman is to be the full-time nurturer, the man the good provider. Mary's unhappiness seemed to her to be her own fault, a sign that she was not a good mother—so it was something she thought she needed to fight against, not act on.

Program for Creating Breast Health
Through Full Emotional Expression

The following is the program Dr. Schulz and I put together for Mary and other midlife women who are ready to create breast health more fully.

⌐ BE HONEST ABOUT WHAT YOU'RE FEELING. Dr. Schulz noted that Mary was too sweet and nice, despite being in a very difficult situation. She'd say things like "It's not that bad. It's okay, I can handle it." And then two seconds later she'd tell Dr. Schulz how frustrated she actually was with her situation. Her response reminded me of an episode of the old TV sitcom *Golden Girls,* in which Blanche was trying to come to grips with her son's decision to marry a much older woman who was pregnant with his child. When a friend of hers asked her what she planned to do, she replied, "Do what mothers always do. Tell my son I love him and that anything he does is fine with me, then complain like hell to anyone else who will listen." This pattern, though funny in a sitcom, is exactly what creates disruption in the energy of our fourth emotional center.

Creating health instead of havoc in your emotional centers requires you to extinguish those "I'm really fine" phrases from your vocabulary when they are covering up real and painful emotions that need to be expressed. You may need to work with a therapist to help you learn how to be honest first with yourself, and then with your mate or other family members.

You also need the courage to be honest with yourself about any aspect of your life that you aren't ready to change. Given our cultural inheritance about our breasts, it is little wonder that women's fear of breast cancer far overshadows our risk for those things that are more likely to kill us either directly or indirectly, such as heart disease or being battered by a husband or boyfriend. *I've come to believe that the fear of breast cancer serves to numb us to what we're really afraid of—being abandoned and left alone while continuing to pine for true love and the improvement of the relationship we're in.* (Note: When my colleague, breast expert Dixie Mills, M.D., read this, she said, "This sentence is so important, I wish there were a way to make it stand out.") One of my patients, a woman with breast cancer who was also supporting her husband financially and had the means to change her life, finally admitted to me that she continued to stay in her loveless marriage because it felt so much easier for her to die than to risk being the one to be abandoned or left alone first.

⌐ CREATE A LIFE PLAN. You have the power to improve your relationships and love life right now! This process begins with improving your relationship with yourself. Draw up a one- or two-year life plan just for yourself (not for your mate or family members).

Spend at least thirty minutes dreaming about how you'd like to fill your time, where you'd like to go, whom you'd like to be with, and so on. When we went over the life plan concept with Mary, she admitted that even the thought of having a third child exhausted her. Gradually she began to come to terms with the fact that the two additional children called for in their infamous ten-year plan might not be right for her. Clearly Mary's body in general, and her breasts in particular, had been trying to tell her this for a long time.

⁓ CREATE AN ENERGY BUDGET. Draw up a balance sheet with one column listing the activities that rejuvenate you and the other listing the activities that drain you. Then make a daily expenditure plan that tips the balance in favor of rejuvenation. (If you have young children, for example, I'd suggest that you trade off child care with other mothers or grandmothers in your neighborhood.) Commit to engaging in at least one activity per week that is pleasurable to you—regardless of what your family members think of it. Understand that this is a process, not a destination. It took me four years to tell my husband that I was getting massages every month. Until then, even though I had made them part of my regular schedule, I didn't have the courage to admit to him that I was actually spending time and money on something so nurturing and pleasurable that didn't have an immediate, tangible payoff.

⁓ MAINTAIN A RELATIONSHIP WITH YOUR OWN CREATIVITY AND PLEASURE. Keep your mind engaged. Mary felt hers was rotting away. She was clearly someone who needed the stimulation of a job. Don't allow your mind and your creative pleasure to wither or permit your true self to get lost in the daily grind of living. If you're not working a regular job, consider taking a class or engaging in some other stimulating activity on a regular basis. I've found time and again that the very act of having a schedule tends to help us conserve and direct our energies. (I always practiced my harp with much greater focus when I knew I had a performance coming up.) There is no substitute for having some order, discipline, and structure in your daily life. Just be sure that you are creating the structure, not the other way around.

⁓ PERIODICALLY REEVALUATE YOUR GOALS AND PLANS. I do this each year around my birthday, and also during the solstices and equinoxes of the year—times when the creative energies of the earth are maximally available to us. Let go of anything that is clearly obsolete and incompatible with your emerging inner wisdom. Mary told us later that when she asked her husband how *his* body was responding to their ten-year plan, he told her that his old ulcer had been acting up lately. But he hadn't wanted to share that with her, because he felt that he needed to show his love and support for his family by remaining a "good provider." This is an example of how a basically good marriage can change and grow when people are honest with each other—and themselves—about their needs.

LIFESTYLE AND BREAST HEALTH

Though I'm convinced that the most important part of creating daily breast health is achieved through the energetic influence of self-nurturance, releasing resentments, and mutually reinforcing relationships, the health of our breasts, like that of every other bodily organ, is also affected by what we eat and by other lifestyle choices.

The Diet Connection

A substantial body of research has linked the consumption of dietary fat with various breast symptoms and breast cancer. That's why for many years I advised my patients, particularly those at high risk for breast cancer, to follow a low-fat, high-fiber diet—the one that I felt was the most likely to keep breast tissue healthy. Because this type of diet was so often nutritionally superior to the ones my patients had been on previously, they often experienced improvement in symptoms such as breast pain and the lumpiness of fibrocystic breasts. (Though often termed a "disease," this is simply an anatomical variation in which the glandular areas are more prominently palpable to the touch.) A low-fat, high-fiber diet also increases the excretion of excess estrogen, thus lowering potential overstimulation of estrogen-sensitive breast tissue.

However, recent research suggests that the breast cancer–fat connection is not as straightforward as previously thought. It comes from an analysis of the diets of 88,795 women, ages thirty to fifty-five, from the famous Nurses' Health Study, who had completed detailed questionnaires about their eating habits every four years from 1980 to 1994. This phase of the study focused on fat because it was known that Asian women, who eat a diet much lower in fat than ours, also have a much lower rate of breast cancer. However, breast cancer was found to be no more common among the women in the

Nurses' Health Study who ate a lot of fat than among those who consumed less than 20 percent of their calories in the form of fat. Furthermore, there appeared to be no difference in breast cancer incidence among those who ate saturated fats, or even the infamous trans fats, versus those whose fats were derived mainly from vegetable sources or from fish!

In response to these surprising results, the study's lead author, Michelle Holmes, M.D., an instructor of medicine at Harvard, said, "Our research indicates it's highly unlikely that women who consume a low-fat diet are protected against breast cancer. Equally, it appears that a high-fat diet also poses no increased risk for the disease."[6]

Though I would have been surprised by this study back in the 1980s, I'm not surprised now. Breast cancer is multifactorial, with nutritional, emotional, and genetic aspects. Nutritionally, it's becoming clear that sugar and refined carbohydrates are a far bigger risk factor for breast cancer than dietary fat content, but unfortunately they weren't taken into account in this study. Nor were other factors that may help account for the low rate of breast cancer in Asian women. The different micronutrient intake, the high intake of plant hormones such as the isoflavones found in soy, and a lower amount of refined carbohydrates in their diet may all turn out to be factors that lower breast cancer risk.[7]

The dietary fat–cancer link is still worth considering, however, given that there's so much data that links excess fat consumption with heart disease and other serious medical conditions. I recommend avoiding excess dietary fat, especially saturated and trans fats. In fact, recent findings from a large prospective study of postmenopausal women with breast cancer found that women who reduced their fat intact also reduced their risk of reoccurrence of their cancer from 12 percent to 8 percent in five years. They also lost at least four pounds.[8]

The Sugar-Insulin Connection

Breast cancer is definitely associated with a substance known as insulin-like growth factor (IGF-1). This substance affects the growth of breast cells in utero, during puberty, and during adult life. Abnormal IGF-1 activity is caused by insulin levels that are too high—a direct result of a diet too high in refined carbohydrates. High insulin levels trigger a metabolic cascade that results in cellular inflammation.

And inflammation is a precursor for cancer. (See chapter 7.) High insulin levels also suppress sex hormone–binding globulin (SHBG), which ordinarily circulates through the body binding estrogen and lowering its activity. With less SHBG in the bloodstream, more biologically active estradiol reaches the breast tissue and stimulates its growth. Over the course of many years, this relative excess of estrogen may increase the risk of breast cancer.[9] A new study conducted in Italy found a direct association between breast cancer risk and consumption of sweet foods with high glycemic index and load (including biscuits, brioches, cakes, puffs, ice cream, sugar, honey, jam, marmalade, and chocolate), which increase insulin and insulin growth factors.[10]

Alcohol Consumption

Many studies have linked the consumption of alcohol with increased risk for breast cancer. The risk increases with the amount of alcohol consumed. In the Nurses' Health Study, for example, researchers found that the risk of breast cancer in women who had one or more drinks per day was 60 percent higher than the risk in women who did not drink.[11] Part of this is due to alcohol's effect on the liver's ability to process estrogen effectively.

For women who are taking oral estrogen replacement therapy, the risk of drinking alcohol may be even higher. In one study, women on oral estrogen and synthetic progestin replacement who drank the equivalent of half a glass of wine experienced increases in estradiol levels in their blood of 327 percent, a rise that didn't happen in women not on oral hormone replacement. Significant rises in estradiol were noted within ten minutes after drinking the alcohol.[12] In the Nurses' Health Study participants this was prevented in those women whose average intake of folic acid was at least 600 mcg per day. (I recommend 800 mcg per day for everyone!) Alcohol is a known inhibitor of folic acid, and folic acid is required for DNA repair mechanisms. High folic acid intake may therefore prevent some of the gene mutations that lead to cancer.[13]

Another part of the alcohol–breast cancer link is that women too often use alcohol as a way to stay out of touch with the painful feelings of sorrow, anger, and pining for love and relationship that may be associated with increased risk for disease in the fourth chakra organs.

Smoking

A study published in the *Journal of the American Medical Association* in 1996 noted that a flawed enzyme present in millions of Americans (in half of all white women and in an even larger number of those of Middle Eastern descent) may raise the risk of breast cancer in women who smoke. Of those with the flawed enzyme, heavy smokers who had reached menopause had about four times the risk of breast cancer as nonsmokers. Postmenopausal women who had the flaw and who had smoked any amount at or before age sixteen also ran a similar risk, which supports the theory that exposure to certain toxic substances adversely changes the way DNA gets expressed during the stages of life when breast tissue is developing.[14]

Smoking, like alcohol consumption, also tends to shut down the energy of the fourth emotional center, rendering us numb to the situations we're in and less capable of doing anything to change them for the better.

Exercise

As many studies have shown, regular exercise decreases the risk of breast cancer considerably, along with all its other well-documented benefits.[15]

That's because regular exercise normalizes insulin and blood sugar levels and also tends to decrease excess body fat, all of which keep estrogen levels normal. Women who exercise for about one hour four times per week reduce their breast cancer risk by at least 37 percent.[16] You don't need to do strenuous exercise to get this benefit. Walking, gardening, and dancing will all do fine.

Sleep

Women who consistently sleep nine hours or more a night have less than one-third the risk of breast tumors compared with those who get seven or eight hours of sleep nightly, according to a 2005 Finnish study of more than twelve thousand women.[17] Several recent studies have shown that exposure to light late at night may increase the risk of breast cancer. The reason is that nighttime light (if it's bright) interrupts the production of the hormone melatonin.[18] Harvard researcher Eva Schernhammer, M.D., Dr.P.H., showed that women with above-average melatonin concentrations are less likely to develop breast cancer.[19] (Dr. Schernhammer's previous research found that female night-shift workers have about a 50 percent greater risk of developing breast cancer than other working women.)[20] So be sure to get plenty of sleep in a dark room every night. (Using a nightlight, if it is dim, is not associated with higher risk.)

EATING FOR BREAST HEALTH

Based on current evidence, I'd suggest that you follow the insulin-balancing diet I've already outlined in chapter 7. Above all, I urge you to nurture yourself fully every day by eating food that is delicious as well as healthy. Eat well, because doing so is a way of reaching your full potential.[21]

I have a fundamental problem with any approach, dietary or otherwise, that promises to "prevent" anything. Although there is an extensive body of evidence supporting the hormone-balancing and health-enhancing effects of the nutrient-dense, insulin-balancing diet I've suggested, here's the problem: even women who eat perfectly sometimes get breast cancer. If you make food choices only out of the desire to "prevent" something, then by the law of attraction, you'll actually be carrying the energy of the disease you're afraid of right into your body along with the healthy food!

In the study mentioned above, for example, the nurses who ate the lowest amount of fat (less than 20 percent of their daily calories) actually had the highest rate of breast cancer in the group. Though surprising at first glance, these data support a link between breast cancer and self-sacrifice, an association that has been scientifically documented. If you are afraid of breast cancer, it will not be helpful for you to become a dietary martyr, always depriving yourself of the foods you love and find nurturing. Imagine eating a small green salad, all the while craving something more substantial, and thinking, "Well, I'll deprive myself because I'm preventing breast cancer." Does this feel nurturing or healthy to you? It doesn't to me. (Personally, I can't imagine living well without some high-quality chocolate!)

That said, let me review the basics.

~ EAT LOTS OF FRUITS, VEGETABLES, AND FLAXSEED. Research has shown that women who excrete the highest amount of lignans—which are formed in the intestinal tract from plant materials—

have the lowest risk for getting breast cancer.[22] The food source with the highest known concentration of health-promoting lignans is flaxseed. I suggest that you consume ¼ cup of freshly ground flaxseed daily. Diets high in plant materials also tend to be higher in fiber, which has been shown to help the body excrete excess estrogen in the stool.[23] Start with one tablespoon per day and work up. (I have a small coffee grinder that I use only for flax seeds.)

Numerous studies have also demonstrated that fruits, vegetables, and seasonings, such as broccoli, kale, collards, cabbage (the cruciferous vegetables), tomatoes, turmeric, garlic, and onions, contain antioxidants and other phytochemicals that protect against cell damage and mutation caused by free radicals. They may also block carcinogens from reaching or reacting with critical target sites throughout the body.[24] Indole-3-carbinol, the active estrogen-modulatory ingredient in the cruciferous vegetables is also available in supplement form.

~ KEEP REFINED CARBOHYDRATES TO A MINIMUM. Breast tissue is sensitive to excess androgens as well as excess estrogen, both of which are normalized with a diet that keeps insulin and blood sugar normal. Over time this will become your favorite way of eating.

~ EAT SOY. Whole soy foods often help women with breast tenderness and pain, and they may even offer protection for women with breast cancer, or with high risk for it, thanks to soy isoflavones, which protect estrogen-sensitive tissue against overstimulation by estrogen.[25] It is best to get your isoflavones from whole foods, rather than from the purified extracts of soy found in isoflavone tablets or capsules. The more soy you eat, the greater your protection.

Some women have expressed concern about the phytoestrogens in soy and in some herbs recommended in menopause. None of the breast cancer risks associated with estrogen replacement apply to the consumption of these plant hormones. The plant hormones found in whole soy food, dong quai, chasteberry, and black cohosh have never been associated with the promotion of breast cancer in any study. In fact, many studies have shown that they are protective because of their adaptogenic qualities, meaning their ability to modulate the activity of estrogen in our bodies in a healthy, balanced way.

Why Soy Is Safe for Breast Tissue

A study in mice that showed increased mammary tumors when the mice were exposed to Prevastein, an isolated soy isoflavone, received a great deal of media attention in the fall of 2005.[26] Obviously many women were concerned, particularly those who eat soy. Here's what you need to know.

Prevastein is a chemically extracted form of purified isoflavones. Soy products made from whole soy do not contain this kind of ingredient. Purified extracts from broccoli, carrots, potatoes, brussel sprouts, tomatoes, etc. have been shown to be toxic and I don't recommend consumption of chemically purified plant chemicals.

Mouse models are considered by most experts to be irrelevant to human studies because they metabolize soy differently from humans (just like dogs can't eat chocolate). Mice and rats make thousands of times more soy metabolites than humans do. The mouse model used in this study spontaneously develops breast cancer on any diet (they are bred for this very reason) and the amount of isoflavones administered (130 mg/kg of body weight) in this study would be impossible for a human to consume who is using a product made from whole soy (e.g., the average 140 pound woman would have to consume thirty soy shakes of a product such as Revival that already contains 180 mg soy isoflavones per serving). Mouse studies using soy germ (the whole soybean) have not been shown to increase breast cells[27]—only the highly purified extracts do this in mice. Recent monkey and human studies have administered soy at 200 mg to 1,000 mg per day and have not found breast stimulation. In fact, these new studies note that soy decreases estrogen levels, improves estrogen metabolism to healthier metabolites, and decreases mammogram density.[28]

One year-long study involving Revival (one shake per day) and breast cancer patients found that it actually decreased tissue inflammation.[29] In fact, soy shakes made from whole soybeans are currently being used in three new breast cancer studies at Johns Hopkins University, where these shake samples (Revival brand) are available in the lobby of the breast cancer center for the breast cancer patients! In another three-year monkey study (using a model that is the standard for humans—not mice or rats), the monkeys were given 400 mg per day of soy isoflavones from whole soy. At the end of three years, no breast or endometrial stimulation occurred and the hormone profile was favorably improved to reduce breast cancer risk.[30]

~ EAT OMEGA-3 FATS. Studies have shown that women whose diet is high in omega-3 fats have a lower risk for developing breast cancer. Research has also shown that supplementing the diet with omega-3 fats can create a healthier ratio of omega-3 to omega-6 fats in breast tissue within three months.[31] I've had several patients who have had significant softening of firm scar tissue around their breast implants when they've supplemented their diets with omega-3 fats daily. A diet that contains adequate amounts of omega-3 fats also helps prevent inflammation and tumor growth throughout the body. You can get enough omega-3 fats by eating salmon, sardines, or swordfish two or three times per week. Or you can take 100–400 mg per day of DHA or fish oil supplements (1,000–5,000 mg of omega-3 per day). Another convenient source of omega-3 fats is ground flaxseed. As mentioned above, I consider flaxseed a true perimenopausal superfood and recommend ¼ cup per day to all women.

~ GET ENOUGH VITAMIN D. Clinicians are increasingly finding low serum levels of vitamin D in women with breast cancer (and other cancers as well). Those with the lowest levels (less than 25 mg/dl in blood) have the highest risk. We've been brainwashed into avoiding the sun, and women don't get nearly enough vitamin D in food or supplements. There are vitamin D receptors on all the immune system cells and optimal amounts of this hormone/vitamin are essential for proper immunity. In addition to moderate sunlight exposure (about ten minutes or so per day), I also recommend taking at least 1,000 IU of vitamin D_3 per day. This will also help to increase bone density. (See chapter 12.)

~ TAKE COENZYME Q_{10}. Coenzyme Q_{10} (also known as ubiquinone) is present naturally in the body and in organ meats. It has been shown to improve immune system functioning. Hundreds of studies have also demonstrated its ability to help those with congestive heart disease. Several studies have demonstrated that women with breast cancer have deficiencies in coenzyme Q_{10}.

Taking coenzyme Q_{10} in relatively high doses, 90–350 mg per day, has been associated with partial or complete remission of breast cancer.[32] In chapter 7 I recommended that all perimenopausal women take 10–100 mg per day. If you are at high risk for breast cancer, I'd increase the dose to 70–100 mg per day. Since statin drugs (prescribed to lower cholesterol) decrease levels of coenzyme Q_{10}, all women on these drugs should take this supplement.

BREAST CANCER SCREENING

Most women have been taught that regular mammograms and breast self-exams are the key to breast health. And there is indeed heartening evidence that the mortality rate for breast cancer is decreasing as a result. What isn't clear, however, is whether this decrease in mortality is simply because we're now diagnosing more pre-cancers that would never have resulted in death in the first place. Recently sonograms have also been found helpful in the early diagnosis of breast cancer.

Though screening may be an important part of early detection, keep in mind that it cannot actually *prevent* breast cancer. At best, it diagnoses it at an earlier and presumably more treatable stage. I'm also concerned that the massive national campaigns aimed at getting women to have regular mammograms have taught an entire generation that breast cancer screening is synonymous with creating breast health. Participating in disease screening is no substitute for learning and practicing the preventive, health-building thoughts and behaviors that can transform us.

Depending on individual circumstances, I recommend mammograms, breast self-exams, and all the other screening technologies. But every perimenopausal woman needs to know about the limitations of screening and take responsibility for creating healthy breast cells daily by nurturing herself with healthy food and supplements, avoiding excessive alcohol, stopping smoking, and engaging in mutually satisfying relationships.

The Pros and Cons of Early Detection

The idea that breast cancer can be cured by early detection and prompt treatment rests on the belief that all breast cancers grow at the same rate. They don't. Some cancers grow rapidly and others slowly, which is one of the reasons why just about every one of us has heard about or knows a woman whose regular mammogram screening was normal but who was diagnosed with breast cancer several months later. One possible explanation for this is that mammography screening is far more likely to detect slow-growing, nonaggressive tumors than the kinds of cancers those women had. A study conducted at Yale–New Haven Hospital of all the women who received their first treatment for breast cancer in 1988, for example, showed that those women whose cancers were detected via mammography screening alone had an excellent prognosis, not just because of early detection, but because the cancers so detected were relatively slow-growing or even dormant, thus requiring minimal therapy. Many of the women, for example, had a condition known as ductal carcinoma in situ (DCIS), a type of breast pathology that can often remain completely dormant for a woman's entire life.

In fact, autopsy studies of women who died of other causes, such as accidents, have shown that 40 percent have some degree of DCIS in their breasts.[33] Other studies have confirmed that the incidence of DCIS has increased more than fourfold since 1980; this type of cancer now accounts for a quarter of all cancers detected by mammogram. The main reason for this dramatic increase is the widespread use of mammographic screening. Dr. Gilbert Welch, a researcher at Dartmouth-Hitchcock Medical Center, puts the dilemma well when he writes, "Our ability to detect subtle forms of breast cancer is a two-edged sword. On the one hand, it offers the hope of preventing some cases of advanced breast cancer through early detection and treatment. On the other hand, it fosters increased worry and labels more women as having disease, many of whom would never develop invasive cancer.[34]

The DCIS Dilemma

DCIS, or Stage 0, breast cancer presents a real dilemma for women and doctors alike. Although our increasingly sensitive technology keeps improving our ability to detect early forms of breast cancer, our understanding of what to do with this knowledge is lagging behind. What is clear is that in the majority of women DCIS may or may not go on to become invasive cancer. But fully 98 percent of the time it doesn't spread—and women don't die from it, which means that only minimal treatment (if any) is necessary. Yet many women with DCIS are subjected to very aggressive treatment: surgery (often mastectomy), sometimes followed by radiation or tamoxifen or both. Because we are unable to identify which types of DCIS or which women are likely to progress, we treat everyone. And many women understandably want to be treated because of fear. The Yale investigators noted, for example, that of the thirty-one women with DCIS in their study, all of whom survived without recurrence, fully 48 percent underwent mastectomies. The authors noted, "Since none of these patients had cancer death or recurrence, regardless of the extensiveness of treatment, the need for aggressive forms of therapy might be reconsidered."[35] That's one of the understatements of the decade. The high rate of DCIS that is picked up on mammograms may also be a factor in the much-celebrated reduction in breast cancer mortality that we've seen over the past twenty years; the women so diagnosed would not have died in any case. They'd die "with" their so-called disease, not from it.

Breast-Screening Concerns

Several years ago I gave a lecture in California to a group that included physicians, allied health care professionals, and others interested in a more holistic approach to health. I presented the data on mammograms and DCIS and suggested that women may want this information when making decisions about if, when, and how often to have mammograms. I was dismayed by the reaction.

In the ladies' room during a break, women from the audience were confused and upset. They deeply believed in mammograms and felt safe when they had them. I had introduced doubt. I couldn't help wondering if, by telling the truth about the diagnosis and treatment questions raised by our improved technology, I had inadvertently broken my Hippocratic oath: "First, do no harm." But I decided that confusion is often the first step on the road to clarity and personal power. If a period of uncertainty and questioning was required for these women to rely more on their inner wisdom, then I figured that over the long haul I'd done more good than harm. After all, there is nothing benign about surgery, radiation, and drug therapy, with all their well-known side effects, when they aren't absolutely necessary.

When I came back from the ladies' room I was met onstage by an infuriated radiologist who ran a breast-screening center. "You're dangerous. Do you know that?" he spat at me. "I cannot believe that you're telling women this stuff. I am so disappointed in you. You're putting women's lives at risk." He wasn't interested in the scientific reasons for my statements, and it was clear to me that we weren't about to have a balanced discussion about the mammogram issue. His mind was made up. Then and there I learned directly and painfully that when it comes to breasts and mammograms, emotions run very high, and this has nothing to do with science.

In January 1997, the National Institutes of Health convened a panel of prestigious experts who spent six weeks reviewing more than a hundred scientific papers and hearing thirty-two oral presentations on this issue. When they concluded that there wasn't enough evidence to recommend routine mammography screening for all women ages forty to fifty,[36] they, too, were met with vicious attacks. In an editorial on the subject, which also included a reply to one radiologist's particularly vehement objections, Kenneth Prager, M.D., the chair of the Ethics Committee at Columbia-Presbyterian Medical Center in New York, wrote, "Could it be that the radiologist who vilified the panel's conclusion has not only the welfare of women in mind but radiologists' own wallets, in view of the millions that would be spent in the wake of an official recommendation for all women in their forties to undergo mammography?"[37]

And the debate is still raging. Case in point: a study reported in the July 2005 edition of the *Journal of the National Cancer Institute* found mammography screening performed in the community setting yielded no benefit in terms of lives saved.[38] But later in the same year, a study in the *New England Journal of Medicine* showed that half the decrease in mortality from breast cancer was attributed to mammography.[39]

The argument isn't just over whether or not annual mammograms are cost efficient or even whether they save lives. The debate is also bringing to light the fact that routine annual screening may actually cause harm. First of all, the procedure itself isn't always benign. A 1994 study in *The Lancet* showed that the breast compression required by mammograms may cause small, in-situ tumors to rupture, spreading cancer cells into surrounding tissues and possibly resulting in more invasive cancers and metastases.[40]

But the most frequent harm done by routine screening involves the incidence of false positives (saying that there's something abnormal when there isn't), which occur in about 10 percent of mammograms. And this risk increases over time. In 2000, the *Journal of the National Cancer Institute* pointed out that the cumulative risk of having false positive mammograms is quite significant in many women. By the ninth mammogram, the study reported, the false-positive risk can be as high as 100 percent in women with multiple high-risk factors.[41] Another study estimated that after ten mammograms, about half of all women (49 percent) will have had a false positive result, which will have led to a needle biopsy or an open biopsy in 19 percent.[42]

In two reviews published in *The Lancet*, Danish researchers Ole Olsen and Peter Gotzsche examined seven randomized controlled mammography studies and found that the screening tool not only didn't save lives but also often led to needless treatments and were linked to a 20 percent increase in mastectomies—many of them unnecessary.[43]

A 2000 study from the *Journal of the National Cancer Institute* followed nearly forty thousand Canadian women between the ages of fifty and fifty-nine, concluding that annual mammograms were no more effective than standard breast exams in reducing breast cancer mortality. Mammography didn't increase the survival rate of those who were diagnosed with breast cancer.[44] And still another study published in the *Journal of the American Medical Association* found that women age seventy and older benefited very little from mammography.[45] The cancers detected at this age would never have killed them.

Despite the evidence against routine screening, nineteen medical organizations (including the American College of Obstetricians and Gynecologists) currently recommend that women get annual mammograms. Yet I agree with Cornelia Baines, professor emerita at the University of Toronto and former deputy director of the Canadian National Breast Screening Study, who recently said, "I remain convinced that the current enthusiasm for screening is based more on fear, false hope, and 'greed' than on evidence."[46]

My Breast-Screening Suggestions

~ HAVE REGULAR BREAST EXAMS FROM A HEALTH CARE PROFESSIONAL AT AN INTERVAL THAT YOU FEEL COMFORTABLE WITH. For some women, that's yearly. For others who really know their breasts, it may be far less frequently. The next time you have a physical, ask your health care provider to go over your breast anatomy with you so that you can know exactly what normal feels like. (Far too many women think that their breasts are lumpy when they're simply feeling normal glandular tissue.) Once you know what normal feels like, get to know your breasts at different times during your menstrual cycle, because they feel different depending upon hormone levels. Breasts are usually easiest to examine during the first half of the menstrual cycle, when hormonal stimulation is at a minimum. During perimenopause, however, when menstrual periods are erratic and irregular, there's no way to tell for sure what part of the cycle you are in. Breasts may feel swollen and "premenstrual" for weeks at a time. This is generally because progesterone levels are low, not because something is wrong. It's important to appreciate this variation.

~ TRANSFORM THE REGULAR BREAST SELF-EXAM. For decades, women have been encouraged to examine their breasts regularly as a way to find breast cancer at the earliest possible stage, get it treated early, and thus save their lives. This has led to a "search-and-destroy" approach to breast exams that encourages you to make your hands into mine sweepers in search of something that may kill you. No wonder so many women skip this routine but end up feeling guilty as a result. As Dr. Francis Moore of Harvard Medical School wrote, "What man would enjoy lowering his trousers in front of a mirror once a month and examining his testicles carefully, by rigorous palpation, looking for testicular tumors?"[47] Still, no one seriously questioned the advisability of doing regular breast self-exams (BSE) until recently, when the results of a large randomized trial of BSE were released, which found that the practice didn't change breast cancer mortality.

The study involved over 260,000 women in Shanghai who were divided into two groups and followed for five years. Half of the group was trained in BSE and had that training reinforced at the workplace, while the other half, the control group, had no training in BSE nor were they encouraged to perform BSE of any kind. At the end of five years, the study found that those women in the BSE group found more benign breast lumps than the control group, but their breast cancer mortality was not reduced at all. The death rate from breast cancer was the same in both groups. The study authors concluded that "women who choose to practice BSE should be informed that its efficacy is unproven and that it may increase their chances of having a benign breast biopsy."[48]

This doesn't mean that you shouldn't get to know your breasts. It simply means that a paradigm shift is called for. When a woman attends to her breasts with loving care and a loving consciousness on a regular basis, it is entirely possible that she will be influencing her breast cells in a positive, health-enhancing way. That's why I recommend a monthly breast self-massage as a healthy and viable alternative to the outmoded BSE. (Do not do this if you have been recently diagnosed with breast cancer, because it may increase tumor spread; it's fine once treatment is finished.) Many women never touch their breasts with love or tenderness, having been led to believe that their breasts are the property of their mates and not really part of their own bodies. Invite your breasts into your life by getting to know them and touching them regularly. Then your regular breast self-exam becomes an opportunity for healing. Breast massage activates lymph drainage, increases blood flow, and oxygenates tissue—all good ways to help create breast health. After all, for millions of years of human evolution, women nursed babies for most of their reproductive years, a process that provides a great deal of breast stimulation. This massage can also be done by your partner in a nonsexual, supportive way.

Here's a technique developed by Dana Wyrick, who practices lymphedema therapy at Mesa Physical Therapy/San Diego Virtual Lymphedema Clinic in San Diego, California.[49]

Self-Massage of Chest and Breast

I recommend doing this massage in the most pleasurable environment possible, e.g., in a rosewater-scented bath with your favorite music playing. Do each side of your chest independently. Instructions below are for the left side; simply reverse "hand" instruction to do your right side. Use a light touch. Your object is to *move the skin,* not to massage the muscles. The following routine, when done properly, will assist the lymphatic capillaries in removing toxins and impurities from the body tissue. The stroking will also accelerate transport of impurities to the lymph nodes, where they will be processed and rendered harmless. Finally, cleansed lymph will be returned to the bloodstream, where the now harmless impurities may be carried to the lungs, kidneys, and colon for elimination.

1. With the first three fingers of your right hand, locate the hollow above your left collarbone. Stroking from your shoulders toward your neck, lightly stretch the skin in the hollow. Repeat this movement five to ten times.

2. Now cover the hairy part of your left armpit with the fingers of your right hand held very flat. Stretch the skin of your armpit upward five to ten times.

3. Next, again using a flat right hand, lightly stroke ("pet") the skin from the breastbone to the armpit. Do this above the breast,

FIGURE 18: THE LYMPH SYSTEM

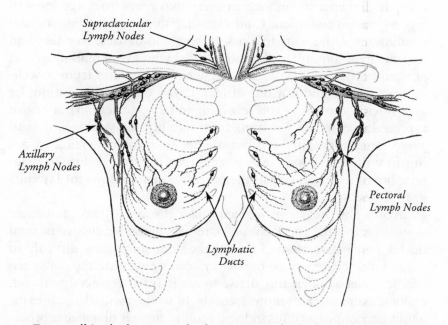

Supraclavicular Lymph Nodes

Axillary Lymph Nodes

Pectoral Lymph Nodes

Lymphatic Ducts

Every cell in the breasts and other organs is bathed in lymph. Lymph carries nutrients and immune cells throughout the body and filters waste products through the lymph nodes, where they can be detoxified. Stimulating lymph circulation through regular massage of the breast and chest wall area can help maintain healthy breast tissue.

over the breast, and below the breast, repeating each path five to ten times.

4. Finally, using a flat right hand, lightly stroke from your waist up to your armpit on your left side, repeating five to ten times.

Now change hands and massage the right side of your chest.

~ MAMMOGRAMS FOR WOMEN AGES THIRTY-FIVE TO FIFTY. Get annual or biennial mammograms and/or sonograms or other screening if you have a positive family history for breast cancer or if you find that getting this screening puts your mind at ease. (Peace of mind produces very positive biochemical changes in the body.) If you have a first-degree relative who got breast cancer before menopause, consider annual screening mammograms starting five years before the age your relative was diagnosed.

Many practitioners recommend a baseline mammogram at age thirty-five, then a mammogram every two years from age forty to fifty in low-risk women. I individualize this recommendation depending upon the woman's risk factors and desires. I've also had patients (and a number of good friends) who avoid mammograms altogether. I respect this decision when it is made from a well-informed place and not out of fear. If you choose this option, let your doctor know that you're willing to be a partner in your health care and release her (or him) from liability for your decision to avoid mammography. Tell him or her that you're willing to put this in writing and sign it as a legal release form. Failure to diagnose breast cancer is one of the most frequent reasons for lawsuits against doctors!

Note: The breasts of women under the age of fifty (and some who are fifty and older) can be extremely dense because of normal ductal connective tissue. This makes mammograms difficult to read and interpret, since the X-rays can't penetrate the dense tissue. In older women this dense tissue is often replaced with fat, making mammograms more accurate. In women with dense breasts, about fifty out of a thousand will require further diagnostic procedures, such as additional mammograms, sonograms, and even biopsies, to determine whether or not they have breast cancer. Of these, it is estimated that only two will have breast cancer.[50] The others will often go through a great deal of anxiety, which I wish could be avoided! Dr. Dixie Mills says, "I often recommend a woman get a baseline mammogram and see how dense her tissue is (a factor that cannot be determined by feel) and add this information into her choice of manner of screening. Women should not be made to feel that they are to blame for their breasts being dense; it is a factor of mammogram pictures being limited to shades of black and gray and white on a flat photo."

~ MAMMOGRAMS FOR WOMEN AGE FIFTY AND OVER. All major medical associations agree that after the age of fifty, annual mammograms result in early detection and decreased mortality from breast cancer. Ideally, mammograms should be done at a multidisciplinary breast center, where your film can be read immediately and where you can also get additional diagnostic procedures or treatment if necessary. Most major medical centers now have these centers. However, I continue to be concerned about the cumulative effect of yearly radiation on breast tissue health.

If You Find a Breast Lump

⁓ IF YOU FIND A LUMP, GET A DIAGNOSIS. It's important to see a practitioner who can help you through the process of finding out whether your breast lump is benign or cancerous. The waiting and imagining the worse is obviously not healthy. Dr. Dixie Mills says, "Many women who come to see me have already reviewed their wills."

⁓ ALWAYS TAKE SOMEONE WITH YOU. Many women who have found a breast lump are too frightened and overwhelmed to ask questions and explore all their options with their doctor or other medical professional. Having a companion can help you focus; if he or she takes notes, you can review them together later.

⁓ DON'T LET ANYONE RUSH YOUR DECISION. Many options are available for the diagnosis and treatment of breast lumps, ranging from breast cyst aspiration to needle biopsy to open biopsy. Most breast lumps or thickenings actually turn out to be benign. Many are simply fluid-filled cysts, which can be aspirated right in the office. If the fluid is clear, you have both your diagnosis and treatment at the same time. Nothing further needs to be done. Oftentimes breast lumps or thickenings are the result of hormonal stimulation and will go away after you get your period. This is particularly true during perimenopause, when estrogen overstimulation of breasts is so common. One of my patients developed large, painful lumps in both of her breasts throughout her perimenopause. This really scared her and also made it difficult to tell what was really going on in her breasts. After she finally had her last period, however, her breasts returned to their normal consistency, and her lumps went away for good.

⁓ GET A SECOND OPINION IF YOU'RE NOT COMPLETELY COMFORTABLE WITH THE FIRST. Even if you do have cancer, in the vast majority of cases your treatment will not be compromised if you take a couple of weeks or even months to find a doctor you trust and feel comfortable with.

IF YOU HAVE BEEN DIAGONOSED WITH BREAST CANCER

Join a breast cancer or other support group in your area. Studies have shown that support groups characterized by open and honest sharing are associated with increased longevity and decreased rate of recurrence of tumor. Besides, a support group is a very safe place to learn how to ask for what you need—or even discover those needs in the first place.

The following books and other resources provide powerful support for your inner wisdom during this time, as well as a wealth of practical information.

> *Sacred Choices: The Gentle Art of Disarming a Disease and Reclaiming Your Joy,* by Judie Chiappone (Holistic Reflections, 2000).
>
> *My Healing from Breast Cancer,* by Dr. Barbara Joseph (Keats Publishing, 1996).
>
> *Breast Cancer Survivor's Club,* by Lillie Shockney, R.N. (Windsor House Publishing Group, 1996).
>
> *The Cancer Report: The Latest Research in Psychoneuro-immunology (How Thousands Are Achieving Permanent Recoveries),* by John Voell and Cynthia Chatfield (Change Your World Press, 2005). (For more information on this research, visit www.cancer-report.com.)

The Moss Reports by Ralph W. Moss, Ph.D. (at www.cancerdecisions.com).

Dixie Mills, M.D., maintains an excellent breast health website (www.drdixiemills.com).

PUTTING BREAST CANCER RISK IN PERSPECTIVE

Most women grossly overestimate their risk for breast cancer. Recent surveys of women between the ages of forty-five and sixty-four show that 61 percent feared cancer (predominantly breast cancer) more than any other disease. Only 9 percent feared heart disease the most, despite the fact that it is the leading cause of death in women, claiming more women's lives each year than the next four-teen causes combined.[51] Breast cancer isn't even the leading cause of death from cancer in women. That distinction goes to lung cancer.

Though every one of us probably knows a woman with breast cancer, and though breast cancer is the most common cancer among North American women, the lifetime risk for breast cancer—the widely touted one-in-eight women (or one-in-seven for Caucasian women) figure[52]—applies only if you live beyond the age of eighty-five.[53] The one woman in eight who does develop breast cancer has a 50 percent chance of receiving the diagnosis after the age of sixty-five and a 60 percent chance of dying from another cause.

Kelly-Anne Phillips and her colleagues at Princess Margaret Hospital in Toronto, Ontario, Canada, have constructed a very help-ful chart based on the 1995 incidence and mortality rates in the Ontario Cancer Registry. Here's what it shows.

Out of 1,000 females born healthy and alive:

~ Ages 35–39: 986 will be alive. Of these, 1 will get breast cancer, 0 will die from it, and 2 will die of other causes.

~ Ages 40–44: 983 will be alive. Of these, 5 will get breast cancer, 1 will die from it, and 4 will die of other causes.

~ Ages 45–49: 977 will be alive. Of these, 8 will get breast cancer, 2 will die from it, and 6 will die of other causes.

~ Ages 50–54: 968 will be alive. Of these, 11 will get breast cancer, 3 will die from it, and 11 will die of other causes.[54]

The irrational fear of breast cancer creates a great deal of suf-fering for women and prevents many from enjoying the benefits of perimenopausal treatments—such as high-dose soy, bioidentical pro-gesterone, low-dose bioidentical estrogen, and testosterone—that can relieve symptoms and help prevent diseases that are far more apt to be a threat to longevity or quality of life.

THE BREAST CANCER GENE: SHOULD YOU BE TESTED?

Fully 95 percent of all breast cancers have little or nothing to do with genetics. The rest is attributable to inherited mutations in two different genes: BRCA1 and BRCA2. Women who inherit a BRCA1 mutation have a higher risk than those with a BRCA2 mutation.

They have a 56 percent lifetime risk of breast cancer and also an estimated 15 percent risk of developing ovarian cancer by the age of seventy. Though less is known about the BRCA2 mutation, it is estimated that it will account for an additional 40 percent of hereditary breast cancers.[55]

The true frequency and implications of breast cancer gene mutations are still uncertain, in part because the BRCA1 gene is very large and many different mutations have been found within it. One particular BRCA1 mutation has now been detected in approximately 1 percent of Jews of Eastern European descent. Different mutations have been found in other populations. In addition, there are other gene pathways besides those governed by BRCA1 and BRCA2 mutations that may lead to breast cancer. When you add to this the technical problems of sequencing an entire gene, it is clear that genetic testing for breast cancer risk is an incomplete science. A negative test for the gene may have little meaning in a setting of a strong family history of breast and ovarian cancer.[56] On the other hand, if there is only one individual in the family with breast or ovarian cancer, the chances of this cancer occurring due to a mutation in either BRCA1 or BRCA2 is quite small.

Dr. Francis Collins of the National Center for Human Genome Research in Bethesda, Maryland, summarized the current dilemma associated with testing positive for the breast cancer gene.

> We are still profoundly uncertain about the appropriate medical care of women with these mutations. Despite the general usefulness of mammograms for the early detection of breast cancer in women over the age of 50, there are no data to instill confidence that regular mammography at a younger age, in concert with self-examination and examination by doctors or nurses, will reduce the risk of death from metastatic breast cancer among very-high-risk women with BRCA1 mutations. We do not yet know the appropriate use of more drastic measures, such as prophylactic mastectomy, especially given the anecdotal evidence that cancer can still occasionally arise in the small amount of epithelial tissues remaining after surgery. . . . Clinical research is urgently needed to address all these uncertainties.[57]

Though federal legislation is in progress to protect those who test positive, testing also raises the potential for health insurance discrimination, life and disability insurance discrimination, and discrimination in employment.[58]

Here's the bottom line: though a negative test for the breast cancer gene can be a great relief for an individual with a positive family history for breast cancer, it's not a guarantee against getting breast cancer. I do not recommend being tested unless you have at least two or more close family members who've had breast or ovarian cancer.

Proactive women between the ages of thirty-five and seventy-four who have never been diagnosed with breast cancer but have a blood-relation sister who has been can participate in the Sister Study. This national study conducted by a branch of the National Institutes of Health plans to follow fifty thousand women for at least ten years to learn how environment and genes may affect the risk of getting breast cancer. (For more information, visit www.sisterstudy.org.)

You should also undergo thorough genetic counseling from a professional with extensive knowledge and training in the field, both before and after getting your test results. If your test is positive, seek medical care from a professional who is actively engaged in research protocols to further our knowledge of these troubling disorders. The National Cancer Institute Cancer Information Service (1–800–4–CANCER) can supply information about genetic services at cancer centers supported by the institute.

A third option: genomic testing done by a physician skilled in nutritional and functional medicine may help you decrease your risks further through targeted lifestyle changes. (See www.functionalmedicine.org.) It's also crucial to remember that many, many women have healed their lives—and their cancers—through lifestyle changes which include updating old, outmoded, self-destructive childhood programming!

THE EFFECT OF HRT ON BREAST HEALTH

Despite the fact that most women, with or without supplemental hormones, will not get breast cancer, the documented link between hormones and breast cancer is worrisome for everyone concerned. Nearly every woman asks, "What is the effect of hormones on my risk for breast cancer?" The answer depends on which hormones she is taking, what her dosage is, and what her inherent risk factors are to begin with. These issues were raised by a letter I received from a man concerned about his wife's hormone supplementation program.

My wife has recently switched from taking Premarin, which she originally took to quell hot flashes, to taking natural progesterone in the form of a skin cream. As a result, her breast pain and tenderness have gone away and so have her headaches. What's more, my wife has had almost complete relief from her hot flashes, too. But, as a result of some things I have read about the possible connection between progesterone and breast cancer, I want to be reassured that my wife is on the right track—and that no unscheduled trains will be coming down that track which could cause her harm in the future.

The experience of the woman described in this letter beautifully illustrates the side effects that often result from taking Premarin, until recently the most commonly prescribed estrogen drug for perimenopausal symptoms. Breast pain is one of the most common adverse reactions to estrogen replacement of all kinds, with anywhere from 20 to 35 percent of women complaining of it when given standard, non-individualized doses.[59] This is especially frightening for women who have a personal or family history of benign breast disease (also known as fibrocystic breast disease), which, in the past, was felt to be associated with an increased risk for breast cancer. Newer research, however, has failed to show any consistent association between benign breast disease and increased risk of breast cancer.[60]

Headaches are also a common side effect, since estrogen can be metabolized into a substance that is similar to adrenaline and can result in pounding temporal headaches. Bioidentical progesterone, on the other hand, has been shown to stop hot flashes and has none of these side effects.

Many people, however, are uncertain about potential long-term health problems resulting from progesterone, because of recent studies from the National Cancer Institute and the Women's Health Initiative, both of which documented an increased breast cancer risk for those women on long-term estrogen/progestin hormone replacement. What most people (including doctors) do not understand is the difference between the synthetic hormones at non-individualized doses used in the NCI and WHI studies and bioidentical estrogen and progesterone used at low, individualized doses.

Here are the facts: the National Cancer Institute study was a large epidemiological study involving 48,355 women who were on both estrogen and progestin for varying periods of time between the years 1980 and 1995. Women of normal weight who took this hormone combination for five years had a 40 percent increased risk for breast cancer compared to those who were not on hormone replacement. (Intriguingly, women who were overweight did not have this increased risk, although overweight women are at higher risk in any case because body fat makes estrogen.) They also had a greater risk for developing breast cancer than those on estrogen alone.[61] The 2002 WHI study showed that out of 10,000 women on Prempro, there would be an additional 8 cases of breast cancer compared to placebo.

Though the 40 percent increased-risk figure sounds very scary, here's what it really means: If you take 100,000 normal-weight women, ages sixty to sixty-four, who are not on hormone replacement, you could expect 350 cases of breast cancer to develop over a five-year period. If all these women took a combination hormone replacement consisting of conventional estrogen with progestin, then the number of cases would increase to 560. As you can quickly see, the vast majority of women would not get breast cancer, with or without hormones.

Here's another way of saying this: Statistically speaking, out of 1,000 women who have never taken conventionally prescribed hormones, 77 will get breast cancer by age seventy-five. For women who have taken hormones for five years, that figure climbs to 79; after ten years, it is 83; and after fifteen years, it is 89. Again, the vast majority of women who take hormone replacement (even what I consider a suboptimal form) do not get breast cancer.

The other key point to keep in mind is that virtually all the women in the NCI study—and in most of the other studies that link hormone replacement with breast cancer—were using non-individualized doses of conjugated estrogens (most likely Premarin) in combination with the synthetic progestin Provera. Premarin has been the most-prescribed estrogen in this country for decades, and it is almost always given together with a synthetic progestin such as Provera, often in the combined preparation known as Prempro. In the WHI study, *all* the women were taking Prempro. Each of these non-bioidentical hormones has its own risks.

Studies have shown that when Premarin is metabolized in the body, its breakdown products are biologically stronger, and therefore potentially more apt to promote cancer, than the breakdown products of bioidentical estrogens.[62] It has also been demonstrated that there can be a greater than tenfold variance in blood levels of estrogen among women on the *same* standard dose of Premarin—usually 0.625 mg.[63] What is even more disturbing is that many of the women in these studies are on even higher doses, 1.25 mg per day.

Synthetic progestins present their own set of problems. They can bind to both estrogen and androgen receptors in cells and thus stimulate unhealthy tissue growth. They can also *increase* the biological activity of estrogen. This may explain why women in the National Cancer Institute study who were on both estrogen and synthetic progestin had an even greater risk for developing breast cancer than those women who were on estrogen only.[64] This same association has been found in the Million Women Study in the U.K.[65] and also in the Women's Health Initiative study. If you are on hormone replacement, you may want to check to see whether or not you are taking anything containing the following synthetic progestins: medroxyprogesterone acetate—MPA (brand names Provera, Amen, Prempro); norethindrone (brand names Femhrt, Activella); or norgestimate (brand name Levlite). If you are, I suggest a change to bioidentical hormones.

A new study from Australia that analyzed several studies on HRT and breast cancer risk suggests that breast cancer risk linked to estrogen is not as high as assumed. They estimate that the use of HRT for about five years starting at age fifty hardly affects the cumulated breast cancer risk up to age seventy-nine. Extended use for ten years increases risk by 0.5 percent and for fifteen years by 0.9 percent. Upon stopping HRT, the relative risk quickly declines to zero.[66] The same researchers found the same thing with HRT use in California.[67]

What it boils down to is this: HRT appears to slightly increase the risk for breast cancer, but not as much as previously thought. It's probably safer to use bioidentical hormones at individualized doses if you're going to use HRT.

BIOIDENTICAL HORMONES AND CANCER RISK

There is good reason to believe that the long-term use of bioidentical low-dose estrogen, balanced with bioidentical progesterone, would result in a very limited increase in breast cancer risk, if any.[68] Here's what every woman should know.

Estrogen

The breasts are glandular organs that are exquisitely sensitive to cyclical hormonal changes in the body. In the first half of the menstrual cycle estrogen tends to increase breast tissue growth; in the second half progesterone stabilizes and refines this growth. During our menstrual periods our breasts are at their smallest, with both hormones at their lowest levels. During perimenopause, which is characterized by estrogen dominance and a relative lack of progesterone, a woman's breasts may become larger and more tender with no cyclical waxing and waning to keep breast tissue more stable.

For decades numerous studies have demonstrated that, with the exception of phytoestrogens in whole foods, estrogen of all kinds, even that produced by our own bodies, can promote breast tissue growth. In susceptible individuals, this may be associated with an increased risk for breast cancer.[69] It is this sensitivity to long-term, uninterrupted estrogen exposure that explains breast cancer risk factors such as early menarche, late menopause, no children, and obesity. Eating a diet that increases insulin also increases hormonal stimulation of breast tissue. Therefore, to preserve breast health, use the least amount of bioidentical estrogen that gives you the results you seek. And get your hormone levels tested when necessary to make sure you're not getting overdosed.

If you have a family history of breast cancer (grandmother, mother, sister, or maternal aunt) or have the gene for breast cancer, you will probably want to avoid estrogen replacement despite its known benefits.

Opting not to use estrogen doesn't mean you have to suffer in silence. Many alternatives can relieve your symptoms, improve your health, and also protect your breasts: exercise, dietary improvement, whole soy, herbs, and natural progesterone. These alternatives are very effective.

ESTRIOL: Preliminary studies have shown that women who excrete the highest levels of estriol in their urine appear to have a lower risk of breast cancer. One study from Hebrew University of Jerusalem showed that estriol actually has an anti-estrogen effect when given in sufficient dosages, preventing estradiol from binding to estrogen-sensitive tissue, including the breast and endometrium, so tumors don't form.[70] In a recent study from Berkeley, rats receiving a three-week treatment of estriol along with progesterone had a significantly reduced incidence of breast cancer.[71] Because of such evidence, many physicians have sometimes used estriol, a non-patentable bioidentical estrogen, in their patients' hormone replacement regimes. Estriol is biologically weaker than estradiol and estrone, the two other estrogens produced naturally in the body; as already discussed in chapter 9, it works very well when applied locally to estrogen-sensitive tissue such as the vagina. Estriol is widely used in Europe and gives good relief of menopausal symptoms. It is important to note that estriol has been linked with otosclerosis in some women, a genetically linked condition in which three small bones in the middle ear fuse together and thus fail to transmit sound to the brain. Exercise caution with estriol if you have a family history of otosclerosis. *Note:* The studies on estriol have not been replicated—most likely for financial reasons. Therefore, despite its promise, estriol requires more study.

Progesterone

Though the widely publicized NCI and WHI studies mentioned previously proved synthetic progestin is not protective against breast cancer and may even promote it, their conclusions cannot be applied to the natural, bioidentical progesterone found in such preparations as Emerita cream or Prometrium capsules. In fact, it makes biological sense that adding bioidentical progesterone (which has no androgenic or estrogenic activity) to estrogen replacement regimens may actually help protect the breasts against overstimulation from estrogen and thus further decrease the risk of breast cancer as long as the dose is low. Bioidentical progesterone has been shown to reduce estrogen-receptor production on breast cells and also to decrease the production of estrogen within breast cells. Some women experience transient breast tenderness in the first week or so of bioidentical progesterone use, since it initially increases estrogen receptors in the breasts. However, this effect is very short-lived and goes away after several days. There is no convincing evidence that low-dose bioidentical progesterone causes continued growth of breast tissue. In fact, it appears to do just the opposite.

We simply do not have enough data on women using bioidentical estrogens and progesterone. We urgently need studies that compare bioidentical, individualized hormone replacement with standard synthetic regimens. The Women's Health Initiative study results have at least created a dialogue about the need to study other forms of HRT. Unfortunately, these studies have also produced a backlash against HRT in general.

Genes, Hormones, and Breast Cancer: The Cell Growth–Cell Death Cycle

If we were to do a very large, long-term study on natural progesterone, we would probably find that it offers some protection to the breast, especially when used without estrogen during perimenopause, when estrogen dominance is so common. The reasons for this have to do with the fact that progesterone plays a role in cell death. Let me explain why this turns out to be a good thing.

Nature in all her wisdom has created a balance between breast tissue cell growth and breast tissue cell death. Breast cancer is one of the health problems that arises when there's an imbalance between these two processes. Breast cancer—like all cancers, actually—is characterized by two processes: (1) excessive and uncontrolled cell division, and (2) a lack of normal, healthy programmed cell death.[72] The signals that direct cell growth, cell development, and programmed cell death (called *apoptosis*) are directed by the interaction between our genes and our environment. Though this process is extraordinarily complex, we are beginning to understand it, thanks to advances in molecular biology. For instance, we now know that a gene known as the BCL2 gene blocks cell death. This function is appropriate for the times when breast cell tissue needs to grow (such as at puberty and at the ovulatory stage of the menstrual cycle).[73] However, when the BCL2 function is not modulated by other factors, it can cause inappropriate cell longevity and possible uncontrolled growth, which can lead to an increased risk of breast cancer. BCL2 is known as a proto-oncogene, which means that it promotes cancer if its expression goes unchecked. (And that depends on its environment.)

Another gene that influences breast tissue is p53. The p53 gene, in contrast to BCL2, is a tumor suppression gene; it halts uncontrolled cell division by increasing apoptosis (cell death). Activation of this gene helps to prevent cell overgrowth and subsequent cancer.

As it turns out, the p53 and BCL2 genes are influenced by sex hormones in ways that either favor cancer or protect against it. Estrogen increases the expression of the BCL2 gene and thus promotes breast cell growth. As I already mentioned, this isn't necessarily a bad thing. But unabated expression of the BCL2 gene due to excessive amounts of estrogen can result in increased growth of estrogen-sensitive tissue in the breasts, uterus, and ovaries. It is well known that the risk of cancers in these organs is associated with excessive estrogen stimulation.[74]

In contrast, progesterone decreases the expression of the BCL2 gene while increasing the expression of the p53 gene, leading to an increase in programmed cell death at an appropriate time and thus to a decreased risk of cancer in estrogen-sensitive tissues.[75]

Estrogen and progesterone also differ in the *kinds* of breast tissue they stimulate. Estrogen causes breast cells known as ductal tissue to divide and grow. Unopposed estrogen has the capacity to create uncontrolled growth of breast tissue—including cancerous growth. Progesterone, on the other hand, causes the breast cells to differentiate into lobular cells—nature's preparation for milk production if pregnancy were to happen. If a woman does not get pregnant, these lobular cells simply undergo programmed cell death, dying off naturally at the end of their life cycle. In other words, a well-differentiated lobular cell is not capable of growing into a cancer.

A very helpful analogy was given to me by David Zava, Ph.D., a researcher with years of experience studying the effects of hormones on breast tissue.[76] Dr. Zava likens the different parts of breast tissue to the different parts of a tree. The ductal tissue, whose growth is promoted by estrogen, is like the trunk and branches of the tree. The lobular cells, whose growth is promoted by progesterone, are comparable to the leaves that grow from the ends of the branches. Once a tree cell becomes a leaf, it can never go back to being a trunk or a branch. It simply grows up, matures, and eventually dies at the end of its programmed life cycle. This is not true with the trunk or branches, however. Their cells can grow at any time and make an infinite number of branches or growths on the branches or trunk itself—just like the infinite cell proliferation of a breast cancer.

Given the processes I've just outlined, it makes sense that women subject to excessive estrogen stimulation—whether the estrogen is produced in their own bodies (e.g., during periods of estrogen dominance, so common during perimenopause, or from excessive production of estrogen in body fat cells) or is taken in from the outside (through estrogen replacement or through environmental agents with estrogen-like activity)—would be at increased risk for getting breast cancer. But if they take enough progesterone to balance this estrogen, the risk would diminish. And that is precisely what the scientific literature suggests.[77]

Research by endocrinologist Jerilynn Prior, M.D., founder and scientific director of the Centre for Menstrual Cycle and Ovulation Research (CeMCOR) in Vancouver, B.C., shows that women's estrogen levels are significantly higher than normal during perimenopause. In an effort to counterbalance this, Dr. Prior, also the author of *Estrogen's Storm Season: Stories of Perimenopause* (Centre for Menstrual Cycle and Ovulation Research, 2005), successfully prescribes progesterone to her patients with menopausal symptoms. Quelling any concerns that the progesterone will increase risk for breast cancer, Dr.

Prior points to studies showing progesterone opposes the effects of estrogen and so may decrease the risk of breast cancer.

For example, a study of women with progesterone *deficiency* from anovulation, who were being followed at an infertility clinic, has shown those women to have a risk for premenopausal breast cancer 5.4 times greater than those in a control group. And in a 1995 study in which transdermal bioidentical progesterone was placed directly on the skin of the breast, researchers found that the progesterone was able to inhibit breast cell proliferation. The dosages used were approximately the same as when a woman is using a transdermal cream such as Emerita or Phytogest—in other words, a 2 percent progesterone cream twice per day at recommended dosages. These levels are about equal to those found at ovulation in most women.[78]

Another study showed that those women who had physiologically adequate levels of progesterone at the time of breast cancer surgery had a decreased risk for recurrence, compared to women whose progesterone levels were low.[79] This study has been repeated with the same results, which has led some breast cancer surgeons to suggest that women use 2 percent progesterone cream on their skin for a week or so before breast biopsy or surgery. It appears that bioidentical progesterone can enhance immune response. It also seems to make any tumor cells that may be released during surgery less apt to attach to other sites and grow. This may be why women with breast cancer who are operated on during the luteal phase of their menstrual cycles—when progesterone levels are the highest—have a significantly decreased rate of recurrence.[80]

A 1996 review of the evidence on progesterone and breast health concluded that bioidentical progesterone not only reduced the rate of spread of breast cancer, but may even be responsible for reducing the incidence of new cases.[81]

Though no one has done a definitive long-term clinical trial of bioidentical progesterone, my clinical experience and that of many of my colleagues, including the late Dr. John Lee, a pioneer in bioidentical hormone research, has led me to believe that bioidentical progesterone can benefit many women, especially if used during perimenopause, and will very likely be found to decrease the risk for breast and other estrogen-responsive cancers that may well get their start during this time of life.

Progesterone Preparations and Progesterone Receptor–Positive Breast Cancer

One of the questions I'm frequently asked is whether a woman whose breast cancer has tested positive for progesterone receptors can safely take progesterone. There is a great deal of confusion about what it means to have a breast biopsy that shows that the tumor is positive for progesterone receptors, especially in those women who have been using bioidentical progesterone at the time of their diagnosis.

Here are the facts. All breast cancers that are positive for progesterone receptors are also estrogen receptor–positive. Because estrogen is known to stimulate growth of these types of cancer cells, many people automatically assume that progesterone must do the same. Just the opposite is true. Positive progesterone receptors indicate that a cancer is receptive to the balancing and anti-cancer effects of progesterone.

To understand this apparent paradox, remember that hormones in the bloodstream and the fluid surrounding cells work by uniting with receptors on the surface of the cell. The hormone fits the receptor like a key in a lock. If the right receptor is there, the hormone message makes its way to the chromosomes and turns on the appropriate gene to produce a specific cellular effect. Progesterone signals the cell to stop multiplying, while estrogen signals the opposite. For that reason, bioidentical progesterone is probably beneficial for women with progesterone receptor–positive breast cancer.

In general, women with estrogen- and progesterone-positive breast tumors have the best prognosis, since the presence of both these receptors means that the tumor is well differentiated and slower growing than more poorly differentiated tumors.

Though I'm convinced that bioidentical progesterone is safe and even beneficial for women with estrogen- and progesterone-positive breast cancers, this is a controversial area. Use your inner guidance and consult with your doctor.

My Advice About Progesterone

~ If you are currently perimenopausal and using a progesterone cream or another form of bioidentical progesterone such as Prometrium or Crinone, you are helping your body create hormonal balance that may well protect your breasts from overstimulation by estrogen and androgen. I recommend that you continue to use it until after menopause, unless your inner guidance tells you otherwise.

~ If you are at risk for estrogen or androgen dominance, consider adding bioidentical progesterone. Conditions associated with estrogen dominance are the following: irregular periods, body fat percentage greater than 28 percent, sedentary lifestyle, polycystic ovary syndrome, fibroid tumors of the uterus, breast tenderness, a low-fiber diet high in refined carbohydrates, heavy menstrual periods, and hormone replacement with estrogen only. Androgen dominance is associated with acne, polycystic ovarian disease, and male pattern baldness.

~ Though not all women's health experts agree on the progesterone question, I personally would recommend that every woman who is concerned about her breast health avail herself of the substantial benefits of bioidentical progesterone, especially during the perimenopausal period, when it is well known that she is likely to start skipping ovulations and therefore to have low progesterone levels. Substantial doses of soy protein would be a reasonable alternative to progesterone. Use progesterone for two to three weeks out of the month and then take a week off. This is the most beneficial and physiological way to use it. If you are postmenopausal, get a blood or saliva test done to be sure you're not converting progesterone to estrogen.

What About Testosterone?

Androgens such as testosterone and even DHEA can be converted into estrogen in the body, which means that taking testosterone could theoretically increase your risk for breast cancer. Use the lowest dose that gives you the results you need, or try alternatives first.

Here's the bottom line: it is in our best interest to make the wisest choices we can if we opt for hormone replacement—which means using bioidentical, individualized hormone replacement regimens when needed at the lowest doses that give us the results we want. Once we've done that, we simply have to let go of our illusion of control and realize that there are no perfect solutions. We all do the best we can with the information we have at the time. But that information, like us, keeps evolving and changing. This year's best solution may differ from next year's. Nevertheless, most of the time our bodies and our cells maintain their health—which is why the vast majority of women, either on or off hormone replacement, do not get breast cancer.

THE TAMOXIFEN DILEMMA

Tamoxifen (trade name Nolvadex) is commonly prescribed to women with certain types of breast cancer and also to prevent breast cancer in high-risk women. It is one of a class of drugs called selective estrogen receptor modulators (SERMs). Other SERMs include raloxifene (Evista), which is used to prevent and treat osteoporosis and is also now recommended as an alternative to tamoxifen in postmenopausal women. Tamoxifen's anti-estrogenic effect on breast tissue has been shown to prolong the disease-free interval and overall survival rate in women with estrogen receptor–positive breast cancer. It has been prescribed for hundreds of thousands of women, making it the most commonly used anti-cancer drug in the United States. Tamoxifen became a generic drug in the early part of this century, thus reducing its cost and the profits made from it. As a result, attention has turned to newer, more expensive drugs.

Tamoxifen has significant risks, sometimes due to its estrogenic properties, other times due to its anti-estrogenic effects. Some researchers are concerned that its anti-estrogenic effects on brain tissue may put women at increased risk for dementia or depression.[82] It has been my experience that many women who are taking tamoxifen suffer from depression but don't tell their doctors because they don't want to bother them. This is particularly true for women who no longer have periods. In its estrogenic mode, tamoxifen results in changes in the endometrial lining of the uterus, ranging from atypical hyperplasia (abnormal thickening) and polyps to invasive cancer. The longer you're on it, the greater the risk.[83] This means that any woman on tamoxifen needs to have regular uterine screenings by ultrasound or other means to make sure she doesn't develop uterine cancer. Another problem with tamoxifen is that if a woman continues to take it beyond five years, it may stop acting like an anti-estrogen in her breasts and start to act more like an estrogen.[84] In other words, a woman may develop resistance to it, and, if she does get breast cancer again, it may even increase the chance of the cancer being resistant to treatment.[85] Tamoxifen is also associated with increased risk for stroke, cataracts, and blood clots.

Tamoxifen for Breast Cancer Prevention

Although placebo-controlled, randomized clinical trials have never been done, tamoxifen is currently approved for and marketed to healthy women considered at increased risk for breast cancer. In a highly publicized study done by the National Cancer Institute, the drug reduced the rate of expected breast cancers in a group of 13,000 women in the United States and Canada from 1 in 130 women to 1 in 236 women. Statistically, this represented a 50 percent reduction in the risk of breast cancer in those women who took tamoxifen prophylactically—a figure that certainly got everyone's attention. Though two other studies, done in Europe, did not show any breast-cancer-decreasing benefits, the drug was approved for prevention of breast cancer in women at high risk for the disease.[86]

After its approval for prevention in 1998, many ads for Nolvadex appeared in mainstream magazines. One read, "If you care about breast cancer, care more about being a 1.7 than a 36B. Know your breast cancer risk assessment number. You can call 1–800–898–8423 to learn more about Nolvadex and the Breast Cancer Risk Assessment test."

The NCI tamoxifen prevention trial included women with a 1.7 percent risk. This "risk number" is based on what is known as the Gail model, which was developed by a group of statisticians at the National Cancer Institute in the late 1980s. Its purpose was to try to assess the theoretical risk of breast cancer using data developed on only 28,000 white women. Those who came up with this assessment tool admitted that it represented only a "best guess," not the last word in scientific proof.[87] The updated Gail risk assessment that was developed to promote tamoxifen has been controversial from the start, with critics contending that it tended to overstate risk. Even the original creators of Gail cited "three major sources of uncertainty" about their risk model. However, these uncertainties, as well as the risks of the drug itself, tended to be underplayed.

For example, women taking tamoxifen for prevention are two to three times more likely to develop uterine cancer or blood clots in the lung and legs than controls. Stroke, cataracts, and cataract surgery are more common with the drug, too. Most postmenopausal women also experienced hot flashes and bothersome vaginal discharge. Quite a few healthy women knew intuitively that the risks outweighed the benefits and decided to take their chances without tamoxifen. And it turns out that their inner wisdom was correct.

In 2006, a new study reported in the journal *Cancer* showed that women at the lower end of the risk range did not, in fact, live longer as a result of taking tamoxifen. The study, which was based on a hypothetical population model of a group of 50-year-old women considered at high risk (1.7 percent or higher) took into account the calculated incidence of breast and endometrial cancers, end-result statistics, and non-cancer outcomes of those on tamoxifen. Researchers found that tamoxifen actually *increased* mortality in women with a uterus whose risk was under 2.1 percent. For those with a very high risk number, 3 percent or more, however, there was a potential benefit in terms of decreased mortality. This beneficial effect was especially strong in women who'd had hysterectomies.[88]

The pendulum has now swung back to center when it comes to SERMs and breast cancer prevention. In an article on *Medscape* news, V. Craig Jordan, Ph.D., (dubbed "the father of tamoxifen" by the media), the scientific director for the medical science division at Fox Chase Cancer Center in Philadelphia, said, "This drug has got to be used very specifically. It is not one that should be added to the water supply, and it calls for a huge amount of physician discretion."[89] I couldn't agree more.

My Advice on Tamoxifen and Other SERMs

~ If you are already on tamoxifen, feel good about it, and are having no side effects, then I'd recommend that you stick with it for up to five years.

~ If taking tamoxifen reduces your fear of breast cancer significantly and brings you peace, then by all means take it. This is especially true if you've watched your sister or mother die of breast cancer. In this case, the overall benefits of tamoxifen—including the sense that you are doing something to protect yourself—may well outweigh the risks.

~ If you're offered raloxifene, remember that it is a "same doll, different dress" drug. Though it is touted as having a lower incidence of serious side effects than tamoxifen, they are still significant. Remember, too, that it is recommended only for postmenopausal women.

~ If you've had breast cancer, discuss with your doctor whether your type of cancer has shown a response to tamoxifen, and, if so, how long you should take it. Remember that neither tamoxifen nor raloxifene decreases your risk for breast cancer that is estrogen receptor–negative—the type of breast cancer that tends to be more aggressive.

~ If you are at increased risk for breast cancer, decrease that risk by following the suggestions I've given earlier in this chapter. Discuss taking a SERM with your doctor if your risk is 3 percent or greater, but let your inner guidance have a voice in your decision.

~ If you opt to take tamoxifen or raloxifene, get regular medical care, including screening for endometrial abnormalities and cataracts.

~ You can decrease some of the side effects of tamoxifen by taking soy, using supplements, and following the dietary guidelines given on pages 450–454.

~ Don't take tamoxifen for longer than five years unless you and your doctor feel strongly that your individual situation warrants it.

THE NEWEST DRUGS FOR FIGHTING BREAST CANCER: HERCEPTIN (TRASTUZUMAB) AND ARIMIDEX (AROMATASE INHIBITORS)

Two extremely promising new drug treatments for breast cancer are helping us to make great strides against this disease. One, the antibody trastuzumab (the generic name for the drug Herceptin), specifically targets a protein called HER-2/ neu that is present in 15 to 25 percent of breast cancer patients. Although traditionally reserved for treating women with advanced breast cancer, trastuzumab has recently been proven to delay the growth and spread of tumors in women who are in the early stages of the disease as well. Evidence presented at the May 2005 meeting of the American Society of Clinical Oncology showed that trastuzumab reduced the risk of breast cancer recurrence in this group by about 50 percent and the risk of death by about 33 percent. Yet this drug is not a silver bullet—it was also associated with a small but real increase in the risk of developing weakening of the heart muscle. It is the first of what researchers hope will be other more targeted drugs. If you have breast cancer, your tumor should have been tested for this HER-2/neu gene.

Aromatase Inhibitors

The aromatase inhibitors are another class of drug (including anastrozole, the generic name for Arimidex; letrozol, the generic name for Femara; and exemestane, the generic name for Aromasin). These drugs inhibit the adrenal glands, fat stores, and breast and other tissues from converting precursor steriods into estrogen, thereby lowering estrogen levels in the body. When given to postmenopausal women in early-stage breast cancer, these drugs reduce the rate of cancer recurrence and lengthen the time between bouts for those who do have recurrences. In one of the early trials, Arimidex delayed tumor progression for an average of 11.1 months (while Tamoxifen delayed tumor progression for only 5.6 months). Aromatase inhibitors also cause fewer side effects than tamoxifen, although those taking them did report more joint pain and broken bones, as well as osteoporosis. Women have complained to me about the severity of their joint pain. Clinical trials are now being conducted for prevention using this class of drugs for DCIS.

In conclusion, please realize that the problem of breast cancer can't be solved only at the physical level. Don't be fooled into believing that you must always take a drug to help your body stay well. To create healthy breast tissue, each of us needs to be willing to participate in creating a life that is healthy in mind and spirit as well as body. Sometimes we may need drugs or surgery; at other times we need only the natural strategies I've emphasized in this chapter and throughout this book—eating healthfully, getting exercise, stopping smoking, cutting down on or eliminating alcohol, expressing your feelings, loving, and being loved.

14

Living with Heart, Passion, and Joy: How to Listen to and Love Your Midlife Heart

T he years around menopause are the time when women's risk for heart disease, hypertension, and stroke rise significantly as our hearts and the network of blood vessels that carries nourishment to every cell in our bodies call out to us more loudly than ever, demanding that we listen well and allow ourselves to feel the exquisite joy of life more fully than ever. Because heart disease in all its guises claims more lives than any other illness, midlife is a time when a change of heart may save your life.

Despite the fact that eleven times more women die of heart disease than breast cancer, failure to diagnose heart disease in a timely manner is rarely the subject of lawsuits, whereas suits for failure to diagnose breast cancer are very common. Statistics (which need not apply to you) show that one in two women will eventually die of some kind of heart disease—either coronary artery disease causing a heart attack or a stroke (a stroke is just a "heart attack" of the brain)! In contrast, one woman in twenty-five will die of breast cancer.

Many women never realize that they have a heart problem until the disease is well established. Breast cancer, on the other hand, is seen as an invader from outside ourselves, so we tend to take a fighting stance toward it, for better or for worse.

When it comes to your heart, however, you can't fight it—you must instead follow its dictates if you are to achieve the vibrant cardiovascular health that will nourish and rejuvenate every organ in your body for the rest of your life. The heart teaches us directly and persistently. And it is quite forgiving if we will simply heed its messages.

THE HEART HAS ITS SAY AT MENOPAUSE: MY PERSONAL STORY

In chapter 3 I wrote about my first experience of the "empty nest": how I had picked up my younger daughter at camp, taken her to Dartmouth for a college tour, driven the three long hours home with her sound asleep in the car—and then found myself face-to-face with the realization that her physical presence wouldn't heal my emptiness. There is a sequel to that story. The next morning I went for a walk. About halfway through I began to experience an ache in my throat that radiated up into my jaw. No matter what I did, I couldn't make the pain go away. It felt as though a fist were squeezing my esophagus. I kept walking, wondering what this symptom was all about. When I got home the pain was still there and impossible to ignore. So I called my physician friend Mona Lisa Schulz and asked her to come over and help me through the situation.

The throat is in the fifth emotional center, which has to do with communication, so I wondered if there was something I needed to say. Mona Lisa reminded me, however, that I've never had any trouble expressing myself. Instead, my family legacy of stoicism and heart disease pointed to challenges in the fourth emotional center.

Together we sat down and took out the Motherpeace tarot cards to try to get some clarity. My intuition, which was reflected in the cards, suggested that my throat and jaw pain had in fact originated in my heart. I was also reminded that the classic symptoms of heart attack in women are often located in the neck, jaw, and upper chest. As I reviewed the events of the prior twenty-four hours, I came to see that my literal "heartache" stemmed from my disappointment and grief over my reunion with my daughter—a reunion in which my own needs for partnership and companionship had not materialized at all. (*Note:* Both my physician friend and I knew that my pain didn't require a visit to the E.R.!)

Setting Myself Up for Heartache

Looking back, I see now how I had set myself up for heartache. For several days before going to pick up my daughter, I had fantasized about how loving and warm our reunion would be. I anticipated her every emotional and physical need as I prepared for the trip. I thought that her return would help me heal from the heartache of my divorce. In retrospect, I see that by trying to truly be there for her, I was actually treating her the way I wished someone would treat me. In addition to the drive together, I had hoped that she'd want to spend some time shopping and having a meal with me. I didn't ask for this outright. I've never wanted to be the kind of mother who manipulates her children into taking care of her needs by staging after-all-I've-done-for-you-at-least-you-could-have-dinner-with-me kinds of scenes. Knowing that this approach confuses love with guilt and obligation, I went to the opposite extreme. It never occurred to me, for instance, that it was okay to ask my daughters to spend an evening or a day with me now and then. Instead, I had led my daughters—and myself—to believe that I didn't have any needs that I couldn't fulfill on my own. No wonder my heart was forced to speak up!

The Stoic Heart: My Legacy

By asking for so little, I was unconsciously carrying on a legacy I had inherited from my stoic maternal line, a legacy that is a setup for heart disease: If you don't ask for much, you won't be disappointed. Instead, you can earn love by providing service. And if you become strong enough and capable enough to meet your needs for yourself, you'll never have to feel vulnerable, never have to face possible rejection.

My frenzied redecorating in the three weeks prior to my younger daughter's return was not motivated purely by the desire to create a living space that was pleasing to me, though that was part of it. It was also meant to please and delight my daughters. I had envisioned the newly decorated family room as a space in which they could stay up late and watch movies with friends with no fear of keeping me awake. I wanted their approval.

After my daughter and I arrived home, I eagerly showed her the new rooms, anticipating oohs, ahhs, and praise. She looked around briefly, said she liked it, wondered why I had chosen those particular couch cushions, and then settled into phoning the six friends who had left messages for her.

As I unpacked the car to the background of her enthusiastic conversations, I felt as though I had just provided a very nurturing taxi service. When my children were little, providing a warm, safe place for them to grow up was enough. Now I wanted more. But I didn't know that yet. I was simply aware of vague discontent within me. After all, my daughter's behavior was completely normal for a healthy sixteen-year-old with a burgeoning social life.

Why was I so heartsick? Why did I get chest pain the next morning? My daughter certainly wasn't responsible for that. What was my heart trying to tell me? Over the next few days I began to unearth and to let go of a big heartache-inducing legacy that was now obsolete.

Keeping the Peace at Any Price
Is a Big Pain in the Heart

Like my mother before me, I had been brought up to believe that it was my job to keep the peace in the family and make a comfortable home for my husband and children. I did this—mostly single-handedly—for most of my marriage. After my husband and I separated, I characteristically plowed ahead, believing that my good-natured efforts would make it okay for the children. The truth is that I was heartsick about putting them through the pain of my divorce and also about stepping down from my position as cheerful emotional buffer for the family. In all this I had neglected the fact that I, too, had emotional needs and that I, too, was hurting and grieving over the loss of my marriage.

In trying to protect my children from their own inevitable pain, I had been doing everything in my power to maintain the illusion that our lives hadn't changed. I shielded them from the reality of bills to be paid and a household to be maintained, and never asked for their help. But my heart was giving me the painful message that this coping style wasn't working.

Intellectually I knew that staying healthy on all levels was far and away the biggest help and support I could provide for my daughters during this difficult time. My chest pain was a sign that I needed to tend to the needs and desires of my own heart if I was going to accomplish this. As soon as I began this process my upper chest and neck pain went away completely and have not returned.

At midlife I came face-to-face with an unconscious, deeply buried sense of unworthiness that had, for as long as I could remember, motivated me to prove myself to others through service. In the case of my family, this giving was laced with unconscious guilt for having and loving my career while simultaneously thinking that maybe I really should be spending more time as a stay-at-home mom. I made up for the time I spent on the job—or at least I told myself I did—by becoming as efficient and cheerful as possible, my nurturing providing steady background music in the lives of those closest to me. It was simply expected.

Part of my legacy of stoicism and unworthiness was that I had almost no "receptor sites" in my own body and psyche for the experience of someone actually anticipating and making space for my personal emotional needs. In other words, even if someone had wanted to be there for me in the way I was there for my children and husband, I would not have been open to attracting or even recognizing it. The music may have been playing, but my personal radio dial was always set on another station.

My divorce awakened me to the presence of those friends who had always been there for me—and who always would be. But I first had to open my heart and feel vulnerable and needy enough to allow myself to ask for help and then accept it when it was offered. This didn't come naturally or easily. But it was preferable to the old pattern.

Over the years I've observed that many women use pleasing behaviors to make themselves acceptable to others. One of my friends told me that whenever she feels that she doesn't belong or fit in, she does what she did in her family of origin to relieve the tension: she cooks, she cleans, she buys food, and she makes meals for others.

When we first recognize the patterns within us that shut down the energy of our hearts, our tendency is to beat ourselves up for them—which simply closes our hearts further. The first step we each must take is to acknowledge that the patterns that are causing us heartache in adulthood began as successful adaptations to difficult childhood circumstances. They worked for us then, and they have allowed us to become who we are. So the first thing we want to do when we recognize these patterns is to congratulate ourselves. Now, in retrospect, I can't imagine living a life in which I put my desires on the back burner. Now I know that my desires are an important part of my inner guidance and that ignoring them is a health risk.

Yearning for Connection: Needing to Be Free

I'm not suggesting that at midlife we need to give up serving others. Participating in true service—where you're not in it for love and approval—is good for the heart. Most women, however, don't get to true service until we learn to balance our need for connection with our need to be free. Like the parasympathetic and sympathetic aspects of our autonomic nervous system, which so exquisitely control the minute-to-minute caliber of our blood vessels, we need both freedom and connection. Nanna Aida Svendsen, a writer and teacher originally from Denmark, eloquently articulates this balance.

> The heart, it seems, yearns for connection. A great grief arises when connection to others seems to come at the cost of connection to ourselves. I notice how dead I become inside, even if only subtly, when I try to conform to other people's idea of who and how I should be and forgo my own feelings—my connection to myself. When the natural generosity, compassion, and caring of the heart becomes distorted or usurped, then all sense of aliveness, generosity, creativity, and true self-expression seems to go and I am left feeling empty and drained. It takes a great deal of energy to shape oneself to fit someone else's needs and expectations, to conform to their demands, to be codependent. And no matter how tempting it is in the hope of gaining love, or of being kept safe, it always costs. Just as it always costs to demand conformity to our needs by others—to be in a hierarchy when the heart is yearning for partnership. You can see that cost in the faces of so many couples. You can see the suppressed anger or the deadness that resides there. Though the heart may long for connection and love, it also, it appears, longs to be free.[1]

CARDIOVASCULAR DISEASE: WHEN THE FLOW OF LIFE IS BLOCKED

Cardiovascular disease results, in part, from an accumulation of oxidized fat in blood vessels that calcifies and eventually causes blood vessel and heart damage. Strokes, which kill ninety thousand women per year, can be likened to a heart attack in the head. Both heart attacks and strokes are caused by clogged vessels; what differs is their location. In addition to arteriosclerotic plaque deposits, emotions such as depression, anxiety, panic, and grief have been shown to cause constriction in blood vessels, thereby impeding the free flow of blood.[2]

Your heart beats a hundred thousand times per day and thirty-six million times per year. Anything that causes constriction in your blood vessels makes your heart and your vessels have to work harder to do their job. Clearly both emotional and physical factors are involved in creating or maintaining heart health. Over my years in practice I've seen happy, joyful women with high cholesterol counts live healthy lives into their eighties and even nineties, while much younger women whose lives were characterized by depression, anxiety, or hostility might have their first heart disease symptoms in their early fifties despite normal cholesterol levels.

Cardiovascular disease in any one area means that it is also present throughout your entire body. Though most of us wait until midlife to take steps to prevent or treat it, heart disease actually begins in childhood—the minute we learn to start shutting down our hearts to avoid feeling disappointment and loss.

At midlife our hearts ask us to wake up and live our personal truth so that there is a seamless connection between what we say we believe and how we actually live our day-to-day lives. As astrologer Barbara Hand Clow writes: "The heart does not open if one is lying to oneself or others, is manipulating or controlling others, or is separated from other people." She goes on to explain, "The heart chakra is experienced very physically, and it is possible to actually feel the heart opening at mid-life as the kundalini energy flows in: Many of my clients, for example, report a burning in their heart areas." If we don't follow our body's lead and fuel our hearts and lives with the energy of full emotional expression, full partnership, and heeding our desire for more pleasure in our lives, then heart attack, hypertension, stroke, and dementia are more likely to result.

When we have the courage to open our hearts at midlife, however, we are opening ourselves up to the possibility of living more fully and joyfully than we have since we were young children—only now we have the skills and power of an adult with which to direct our openhearted energy. Clow writes, "The heart chakra opening is the signal of 'radical embodiment'—the soul totally in the body—which is the most exquisite experience available on Earth. The integrity of a person with an open heart is always astounding."[3]

HEART DISEASE FACTS

~ Heart disease actually begins in childhood but often doesn't manifest until around menopause.

~ Heart disease (including hypertension and stroke) is the most frequent case of death in women over the age of fifty.[4]

~ Heart attack, though usually occurring later in life, is twice as deadly in women as in men.[5]

~ One in two women will eventually die of coronary artery disease or stroke.

~ Only one woman in twenty-five will die of breast cancer.[6]

PALPITATIONS: YOUR HEART'S WAKE-UP CALL

There's no question that heart palpitations at menopause are related to changing hormones. However, my experience has been that in many midlife women heart palpitations are primarily from increasing heart energy trying to get in and be embodied in a woman's life. At midlife our hearts and bodies often become increasingly sensitive to those things that don't serve us, like caffeine, refined carbohydrates, aspartame, alcohol, or monosodium glutamate, all of which may overstimulate our hearts. You also might need to avoid scary, violent, or emotionally draining news, movies, books, or individuals.

The following letter from Terri, one of my newsletter subscribers, is typical of how midlife heart palpitations often present.

I am a forty-eight-year-old female with no major health problems. I do not take any prescription medicine. I walk five times a week and go to the gym about twice a week to do some light weight lifting. My periods are still fairly regular. I have a fairly healthy diet, although it could be better. I drink about a cup of coffee a day but usually don't drink soft drinks. About a month ago, after a fatty fast-food meal and a large cup of coffee in the early evening, I started experiencing heart irregularities. I felt like my heart was skipping a beat and was going to beat out of my chest! This went on for a couple of days and I went to see my doctor. She did an EKG, which was slightly abnormal, and scheduled me for a stress echocardiogram and Holter monitor. Of course, by the time I had these tests, the palpitations had stopped and they were normal. Then about a week later, they started again. I have cut out drinking coffee and started doing more yoga. I have also started taking more magnesium in addition to my multivitamins. I have monitored what is going on with my life and I can't seem to find any pattern to when these occur. Most nights when I lie down in bed they usually start up, especially when I lie on my left side. My doctor wants to start me on a low dose of a beta-blocker. I told her I would like to start using natural progesterone cream routinely for a couple of months because I feel these palpitations may be related to hormonal changes. I would really like to avoid taking heart medications. However, these palpitations can interrupt my sleep and are very uncomfortable. Are these palpitations hormonally related?

My suggestion to Terri was that she go through the program for creating heart health I outline in this chapter. Her midlife heart is obviously becoming very sensitive, alerting her to the need to balance freedom and connection and also to nourish her heart fully. I concur with her intuitive desire to start on some natural progesterone as a way to balance potential estrogen dominance. Besides, progesterone is known to be very calming to the nervous system. It may well help her with sleeping. In addition, her heart is telling her to stop caffeine. The caffeine in one cup of coffee can take up to ten hours to be metabolized in women, so it exerts a stimulatory effect on the central nervous system and the nerves of the heart for quite some time.

For many women, heart palpitations stop as soon as they begin to take progesterone cream or estrogen, stop caffeine, and also normalize blood sugar and insulin levels through dietary change. (See chapter 7.) But it's also important to find out what your heart is yearning for. One of my patients with heart palpitations found that they stopped soon after she asked for a promotion at work, something she hadn't had the courage to do before. She got the promotion and finds her work more fulfilling than ever. Her heart no longer has to speak so loudly.

The Brain-Heart Connection

Recall that the emotional and psychological changes of the perimenopausal years are to the entire life cycle as the week before one's
period is to the monthly cycle. All the issues that have been occurring
premenstrually and which perhaps had been avoided until now—
"Should I quit my job?" "Should I stay in this relationship?"—now
come up and hit us between the eyes rather relentlessly, demanding
that they be dealt with at this time. Though women with palpitations
often tell me that they have examined their lives and there don't appear to be any personal issues bothering them, my experience has
been that our bodies speak to us only when we can't seem to "hear"
them any other way. When issues of love, issues of the soul, or issues
of a woman's unmet passions cry out for attention, they often take
the form of heart palpitations. If we are willing to be open to their
meaning, we will be giving our hearts a chance to be heard. If we act
on what we hear, the symptom often goes away.

FIGURE 19: THE HEART-EMOTION CONNECTION

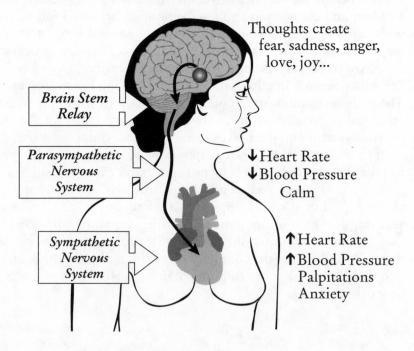

Emotions have direct physical effects on the heart and cardiovascular
system, via the sympathetic and parasympathetic nervous systems.

In his foreword to the book *The HeartMath Solution*, Stephan Rechtschaffen, M.D., writes that "the heart is a physical object, a rhythmic organ, and love itself."[7] We need to think of our hearts as all of these things simultaneously and care for them with this perspective in mind. Because of the intricate connections between our brains and our hearts, our thoughts and emotions can and do have a powerful effect on the heart's rhythm.

Let's take the dramatic example of sudden, unexpected cardiac death. This condition claims more than 450,000 lives per year in the United States, and research, which focuses on the physical condition of the heart itself, has made relatively little headway in decreasing these numbers. Sudden cardiac death is caused by a fatal arrhythmia known as ventricular fibrillation (VF), a disorganized, self-perpetuating electrical instability of the heart muscle that results in a failure of the heart to pump blood.

VF can occur spontaneously in a completely normal heart and is usually seen when there is some pathological hindrance to the flow of blood in the heart vessels, a condition that often happens in humans in association with some psychosocial stress, such as bereavement, job insecurity, or marital strife. Whether or not a stressor affects the heart physically is dependent on the meaning that stress has for a given individual.[8]

GENDER BIAS AND HEART DISEASE: OUR CULTURAL INHERITANCE

For thousands of years our culture has valued male hearts more than female hearts. The heart-strengthening dreams, desires, and aspirations of women, as well as the vulnerable and tender hearts of men, have all suffered as a result. Here are the facts.

~ The vast majority of research on both heart disease and its treatment has been done on men, even though the female's cardiovascular system is different from the male's.

~ Women's brain connections to the heart are different from men's. Men's brains are more lateralized than women's, which means that in general most men use only one hemisphere at a time, usually the left, which is associated with linear, logical thinking. Women, on the other hand, use both hemispheres simultaneously, and they have more frequent access to their right hemispheres. The right hemisphere is associated with music, emotions, intuition, and a deep experience of oneself. Here's where things get interesting. There are more neuronal connections between the heart and the right hemisphere of the brain than between the heart and the left hemisphere. So in any given moment a woman has a greater neurological and emotional connection to her heart than do most men.

~ Given the difference in their brain-heart connections, women with heart problems have different symptoms than men.[9] Men who are having a heart attack typically present with chest pain that begins under the breastbone and spreads to the jaw and the left arm. Women with heart attacks may not have chest pain at all. Instead, they may experience primarily jaw pain and indigestion. Or the first sign of a heart attack in women may be congestive heart failure, with no evidence of the heart attack preceding it except for telltale changes on an electrocardiogram. They may die from this "silent" heart attack.[10] Women who do have chest pain often experience more functional limitation than men, but fewer women are referred to cardiologists for a complete workup.

~ Until very recently, most doctors have not appreciated this difference. Consequently, serious heart problems go underdiagnosed and undertreated in women. In fact, women are only half as likely as men to undergo acute catheterization, angioplasty, thrombolysis, or coronary bypass surgery. The risk of dying of heart disease in a hospital is two times as great for a woman as it is for a man.

~ When a woman with chest pain or a racing heart shows up at a doctor's office or emergency room, she may appear anxious and depressed, and an affective disorder rather than heart disease may be the first diagnosis considered. While it is true that affective disorders, including depression, phobias, and panic and anxiety, are twice as common in women as in men, they aren't "just in women's heads"—they affect the body as well. One of my most vivid memories of my maternal grandmother is how she often wrung her hands at night. Though she always maintained a wonderfully friendly and cheery demeanor, her hands belied her outward peacefulness. She died of a sudden heart attack at age sixty-eight.

~ If a man shows up who appears to be under stress, his symptoms are more apt to be correctly associated with heart attack—even if he acts hostile.

~ Women's blood vessels are smaller and have a different organization from men's. This is one of the reasons why coronary bypass surgeries and angioplasties don't work as well in women as they do in men and also why more women die after these procedures. More women than men with so-called normal coronary arteries also have heart attacks, angina, and myocardial ischemia. As a result, a normal angiogram (blood vessel study) in a woman with symptoms doesn't necessarily mean that she doesn't have heart disease.

~ The rate of early death after heart attack is higher for women than men, even if the women receive treatment. Researchers don't know if this difference is caused by older average age at diagnosis, narrower vessels, greater frequency of coexisting illnesses, or inadequate or delayed medical care.

~ The thought patterns and behaviors that are associated with heart disease in women are different from the patterns associated with heart disease in men. In research on men, sudden death from heart attack is related to hostility—so-called type A behavior. This hasn't yet been demonstrated in women. This doesn't mean that men are inherently more hostile than women. In women, hostility just gets expressed differently. Recent studies have shown a correlation between hostility and hardening of the arteries in both men and women starting as young as age eighteen.[11] But men tend to act out their anger and frustration physically in the outer world, whereas women are taught that this is unacceptable and unladylike. Therefore women learn to hold these feelings inside, where they ultimately can set the stage for a great deal of heart trouble.[12]

Let's use the analogy of two pots of water on a stove. The pot on the right—the woman—is on simmer, with a lid on top. The pot on the left—the male—has no lid, and the heat is on high. The heat of the male's anger will cause the water in the pot to boil vigorously, with a lot of steam and noise. In a typical male heart attack, the pot boils over. The woman's pot will never boil over, but the heat is there nonetheless, and the next thing you know, the water has evaporated and the pot has cracked. But because there was no noise and steam, no one was alerted to the problem. The same thing happens with a woman's cardiovascular system.

In the past few years, health care providers have been warned about these differences and have been urged to do a full cardiac evaluation of women with symptoms such as anxiety and chest pain. As we move toward a partnership society, our awareness of gender bias in heart disease treatment is becoming stronger. It is encouraging to know that the National Institutes of Health and the FDA have called for the inclusion of women in cardiac-related clinical trials. And the government has also founded the Office of Women's Health Research, which sponsored the Women's Health Initiative.

ARTERIOSCLEROSIS: REDUCING YOUR RISK

Arteriosclerosis is a thickening or hardening of the arterial wall. It underlies all coronary artery disease and is responsible for the majority of deaths in the Western world. Medically speaking, it is now well documented that hardening of the arteries is caused by damage to the endothelial lining of blood vessels from free radicals. This is caused by glycemic stress, trans fats, emotional stress, and micronutrient deficiencies. I'll use a case from Dr. Mona Lisa Schulz's intuitive practice to show how emotional factors become entwined with family history and other risk factors.

KAREN: A Heart at Risk

When Karen called Mona Lisa, she provided nothing more than her age, fifty-three, with a request for a reading. Mona Lisa quickly intuited that she was burned out from meeting the demands of her family. She also saw that Karen hid her emotions behind a brave and stoic face, especially her feelings of frustration, exhaustion, and weariness. She never complained.

When Mona Lisa proceeded to a physical reading on Karen's head, she saw decreased flexibility in her blood vessels. These stiff blood vessels were also present in her heart. Mona Lisa perceived that she had symptoms of dizziness and an odd imbalanced feeling. She also sensed blurred vision and a change in her heart rhythm. In addition, she saw that Karen was profoundly fatigued.

After this initial reading, Karen told Mona Lisa that she had become the mother of a combined family when she remarried. She cared not only for her three children, but also for her husband's children from his first marriage. One of Karen's children suffered from multiple handicaps and cerebral palsy. His medical problems made his care very complicated. But Karen told Dr. Schulz that God had always been good to her and that although her family burden was great, she didn't feel she should complain. It seemed to Karen that others had it worse than she did. After all, she was a nurse and had seen this firsthand. She finally admitted that she allowed herself to be used by her children but didn't feel that she had the verbal skills to do anything about it. She had recently picked up her stethoscope and heard a blockage in the carotid artery in her neck. Frightened, she went to her doctor and was sent to a cardiologist, who told her the carotid artery was 75 percent blocked and that there were some blockages in her coronary (heart) arteries as well.

Illness has many different aspects. It is in part genetic, partly due to diet, and partly due to environmental toxins. The area that medical intuition focuses on is the emotional and behavioral aspects of health. Karen's history combined all of these factors. Her mother had died of a stroke and her father of a heart attack. Her father had always been very careful about his diet but had still had high cholesterol and hypertension despite good medical care. Her mother had always been overweight, no matter how hard she tried to lose the extra pounds. Both parents were stoic Minnesotans who cared for their kids on very little money and with little support from the extended family. Karen had never heard either of them complain, get mad, or even have a disagreement. Clearly Karen took after her parents, both genetically and emotionally. And her risk for blood vessel disease was the same as theirs.

Even if your family history looks like Karen's, you can break this chain of inheritance and lower your risk. The first step is a review of exactly what hardening of the arteries is, why it happens, and what to do about it.

The Anatomy of an Artery

Arteries carry blood away from the heart to all the organs and tissues of our body. They are lined with endothelial cells, which actually secrete anticoagulants (molecules that prevent blood clots, coronary occlusion, heart attacks, and embolic strokes) as well as pro-clotting proteins (which prevent bleeding or hemorrhagic strokes). If this endothelial lining is damaged or overproduces the pro-clotting factors associated with stress and subsequent cellular inflammation, the risk for heart attack or stroke rises.

Blood vessels undergo changes beginning in childhood, depending upon diet, genetic tendencies, and how we learn to handle emotional expression. In the famous Bogalusa Heart Study, for example, the beginnings of heart disease were discovered in children as young as age nine.[13]

The following describes the three stages of development of arteriosclerosis.

1. DEPOSITION OF FATTY STREAKS. These can be found in children. Immune cells called macrophages on the surface of the blood vessel endothelial cells swallow LDL cholesterol as it floats by. The fat droplets accumulate, causing fatty streaks to develop in the coronary arteries and the aorta. LDL cholesterol and other components of arterial plaques won't stick to the endothelial lining of vessel walls unless there is some kind of damage to these walls in the first place— usually the result of free-radical damage to cells from a refined-food diet, the wrong kind of dietary fat, environmental toxins (such as cigarette smoke), chemicals caused by stress, a nutrient-poor diet, or a combination of all of these.

2. FORMATION OF FIBROUS PLAQUES. Over time the fatty streaks enlarge, causing scarring in the underlying endothelial lining, and these scars can eventually grow into plaques, which are elevated areas of scarred or fibrous fatty tissue in the aorta, the coronary arteries, and the carotid arteries in the neck that bring blood to the brain and are often involved in strokes. (This is where Karen heard the disrupted flow of blood.) These domelike bulges have a central core of cholesterol crystals.

3. COMPLICATED LESION. The dome of the lipid plaque eventually grows large enough to significantly narrow blood vessels, which eventually results in decreased blood flow and thus decreased flow of nutrients and oxygen to tissue—in the same way that mineral buildup clogs plumbing. The calcified plaque may begin to ulcerate. When this happens, there is a much greater risk for blood vessel rupture and bleeding, resulting in a stroke or hemorrhage. Bits of calcified artery can also break off and be propelled by the flow of blood into distant areas where they lodge in a vessel and further cut off blood flow, thus resulting in stroke (dead brain tissue), heart attack (dead heart tissue), or dead tissue in other areas of the body.

Disorders that are characterized by arteriosclerosis include diabetes, insulin resistance, hypertension, a diet too high in refined carbohydrates and too low in antioxidants, decreased thyroid hormone, and a genetic tendency toward producing too much homocysteine.

How Do You Know If Your Vessels Are Healthy?

Only rarely will a doctor be able to diagnose arteriosclerosis from hearing an odd sound (known as a *bruit*) in the carotid artery, or from hearing a click or abnormal rhythm in the heart. If you have diabetes or high blood pressure, are significantly overweight, never exercise, follow a poor diet, or are a smoker, I can virtually guarantee that you already have arteriosclerosis.

Most of the time, arteriosclerosis is not diagnosed until an individual has a cardiac event of some kind, such as a stroke or heart attack. Individuals with chest pain or difficulty walking because of vascular insufficiency often undergo an X-ray test known as an angiogram, which visualizes blood vessels that are injected with dye. Sometimes an ultrasound technology known as a Doppler device will be used to diagnose vessels that are blocked.

The good news is that arteriosclerosis can be largely prevented or reversed by diet and lifestyle factors. In fact, the famous Nurses' Health Study, which has followed more than eighty-four thousand women for over fourteen years, has demonstrated that the risk of arteriosclerosis is very low in those women who exercise regularly, abstain from smoking, and follow the kind of diet I recommend in chapter 7.[14] I'll discuss selected risk factors in more detail below. It's important for every perimenopausal woman to get a complete checkup from a health care provider who is qualified to evaluate her cardiovascular status. This evaluation should include, as a minimum, a thorough history and physical exam, EKG, blood pressure check, and lipid profile.

FACTORS ASSOCIATED WITH AN INCREASED RISK FOR CARDIOVASCULAR DISEASE

- You are/were a habitual smoker.
- You have high LDL ("bad") cholesterol (greater than 130 mg/dl).
- Your HDL cholesterol ("good" cholesterol) is low (less than 46 mg/dl).
- You have high triglycerides (greater than 200 mg/dl).
- You have high blood pressure (greater than 130/85).

~ You have high levels of the amino acid homocysteine in your bloodstream.

~ You are overfat (body mass index greater than 25) with an apple-shaped figure (a preponderance of body fat above the level of the hips).

~ Your waist measures 34.5 inches or more.

~ You have periodontal disease.

~ You have diabetes.

~ You are sedentary and don't exercise.

~ You have a history of significant clinical depression.

Cholesterol

A lipid profile is a measure of your total cholesterol, LDL cholesterol, HDL cholesterol, and triglyceride levels. Here are the numbers to shoot for on the lipid profile.

TOTAL CHOLESTEROL: Below 200. (*Note:* If your cholesterol is slightly higher than 200, don't worry about it if your HDL is sufficiently high.)

HDL (HIGH-DENSITY LIPOPROTEIN): HDL—the "good" cholesterol—should be 45 or higher; 67 or above is ideal. Low HDL cholesterol has been shown to be a more potent risk factor in women than it is in men. Women with low levels of this cholesterol subtype (a reading of 35 or less) have a sevenfold increase in heart disease risk compared to those whose HDL levels are normal.[15] Low HDL is one of the first indicators of insulin resistance.

LDL (LOW-DENSITY LIPOPROTEIN): LDL—the "bad" cholesterol— should be 130 or below. LDL cholesterol rises after menopause in many women, a fact that was the basis for promoting estrogen replacement, which decreases LDL levels. If your LDL is greater than 150 mg/dl (some doctors use even lower numbers), you're considered at high risk for coronary artery disease. LDL cholesterol undergoes free-radical damage and forms plaques in the arteries.

TRIGLYCERIDES: This number should be 150 or lower. Triglycerides are an independent risk factor for women. An ideal triglyceride level for a woman is around 75. A woman with a triglyceride level of greater than 200 has a 14 percent risk of developing coronary artery disease. High triglycerides are associated with toxic abdominal fat and glycemic stress in part because the liver, as well as other areas of the body, stores excess blood sugar as triglycerides.

RELATIONSHIP OF TOTAL CHOLESTEROL TO HDL: Neither type of cholesterol is inherently bad or good. Both are necessary for good health. They need to be balanced in the body. Divide your total cholesterol by your HDL cholesterol. If the resulting number is 4 or less, you are at low risk, regardless what your total cholesterol number is. The ratio of total cholesterol to HDL is a much better predictor of risk than simply your total cholesterol number. Ask your doctor to give you a copy of your lipid profile so that you can get to know your numbers. It's very motivating to watch your lipid profile improve every year when you commit to becoming healthier than ever before at midlife.

Currently 40 percent of women older than fifty-five have elevated cholesterol levels.[16] Though interpretation of lipid profile results will vary from lab to lab, a total cholesterol level as high as 225 to 240 does not necessarily indicate that a woman is at increased risk for heart disease if her HDL cholesterol is also high (45 or above). Because most of the studies of heart disease and blood lipid levels have been done on men, we still don't know exactly what levels of blood lipids are optimal for women. What we do know is that women can have higher total cholesterol levels than men and not be at increased risk for heart disease.

Get the lipid profile repeated at least every five years if it's normal. If your blood sugar is high, get the test repeated more frequently.

If your cholesterol levels are high, know that dietary change and a good supplement program can lower cholesterol significantly and quickly. Though there are a number of ways to do this, I'm partial to the Reset Program from USANA. (See page 225.) Oftentimes these positive changes are so motivating that they spur permanent lifestyle changes that maintain healthy cholesterol levels and permanent fat loss. If you cannot or will not institute lifestyle improvements, at least take omega-3 supplements and consider taking garlic, which has antioxidant properties (either lightly cook it, or take a garlic supplement with the equivalent of 4,000 mg fresh garlic and a guaranteed amount of the active ingredient allicin).

What About Statins?

I am very concerned about the overuse of statin drugs, e.g., Lipitor, Crestor, Zocor, etc., which are being prescribed to millions of women in the belief that because they lower LDL cholesterol levels, they will prevent heart disease. This is the same line of reasoning that led doctors to prescribe Premarin to millions of women back in the '80s and '90s because it was shown to raise HDL (good cholesterol) levels. Unfortunately, this line of reasoning is seriously flawed. High LDL cholesterol is not a disease—at least half of all people who get heart disease don't even have high cholesterol! Simply lowering LDL cholesterol will not prevent heart disease. The cause of heart disease is cellular inflammation and arterial wall damage, which oxidizes LDL and causes it to stick to damaged blood vessel walls and build up plaque. This can be prevented (or ameliorated) through proper diet, exercise, stress reduction, and supplementation with the right nutrients. *Note:* The level of LDL cholesterol that is considered "normal" has been continually reduced over the years, largely because of the behind-the-scenes influence of the pharmaceutical industry, which supplies the majority of research grants to academic medicine. The American Heart Association's 2004 recommendations for "normal" LDL were lowered to 70, which I consider ridiculous.[17]

Here's what all women should know about statins: despite all the hype, many large studies involving statins have failed to show much benefit. Here's a partial list.

~ The ALLHAT clinical trial (announced in 2002) was the largest study in the world using Lipitor.[18] Ten thousand participants with high LDL cholesterol were treated either with statins or lifestyle changes. Though the subjects in the group that took Lipitor did, in fact, lower their LDL cholesterol significantly compared to the control group, there was no difference in death rate from heart attack between the two groups!

~ The Heart Protection study supposedly conferred "massive" benefits to participants who took Zocor for five years compared to controls who didn't take the drug.[19] After five years, those on the drug had an 87.1 percent survival rate compared to an 85.4 percent survival rate for those who didn't. But the survival rates were independent of the lowering of cholesterol, so there was no difference between the two groups in reduction of death from heart disease.

~ The Japanese Lipid Intervention Trial of 2002 was a six-year study of 47,294 patients treated with Zocor. The drug lowered LDL cholesterol dramatically in some participants and moderately or not at all in others. After five years, there was no correlation between LDL cholesterol levels and death rate.[20]

~ A 2003 meta-analysis of forty-four clinical trials involving 9,500 patients found that the death rate for those taking statins was identical to those taking no drugs. More worrisome is that 65 percent of those taking statins experienced adverse side effects that caused many to withdraw from the study. The bottom line: statin drugs showed no benefit in reducing the overall number of deaths.[21]

~ The 2003 ASCOT-LLA (Anglo-Scandinavian Cardiac Outcomes Trial—Lipid Lowering Arm) study compared the benefits of Lipitor versus placebo in patients with normal LDL cholesterol but with high blood pressure and other risk factors for heart disease.[22] After three years, Lipitor was credited with decreasing the risk of heart attack and stroke. But no reduction in deaths occurred. And there were actually more deaths in the women taking Lipitor than in those who didn't take it!

~ The 2003 University of British Columbia Therapeutics Initative Study found that statin drugs did not prevent heart disease in women.[23]

Statin Drugs Deplete Vital Nutrients

If statins were wildly effective in decreasing the mortality rate from cardiovascular disease, then their benefits might outweigh their risks. But this is clearly not the case. And the risks, though vastly underreported, are considerable. The serious side effects resulting from statins are the result of how they work. Statin drugs block cholesterol production in the body by inhibiting an enzyme called HMG-Co-A reductase. This is the same pathway that the body uses to create coenzyme Q_{10} and substances called dilochols, both of which are absolutely essential for proper cell health. By blocking cholesterol production, statins also block production of these vital nutrients.

Dilochols direct proteins to the areas of the cells that need repair. Without them, the cells can't carry out their genetic programming for cellular functioning and restoration. Statins therefore wreak potential havoc with cellular repair. Coenzyme Q_{10} (ubiquinone or CoQ_{10}), which is far better known than the dilochols, is a critical cellular nutrient that is necessary for producing energy in the form of ATP in the part of the cell known as the mitochondria. ATP is a molecule that carries energy for cellular function much like gasoline powers the engine of a car. Without it, nothing can run. The heart, in particular, requires an enormous amount of energy and CoQ_{10} to function efficiently. CoQ_{10} is also necessary for the vital role played by cell membranes (the actual "brain" of the cell) and also for the formation of collagen and elastin that make up the connective tissue in skin, muscles, and blood vessel walls. Because every cell in the body requires coenzyme Q_{10} to function properly, depletion of this enzyme from statin drugs causes problems throughout the entire body.

SIDE EFFECTS OF STATIN DRUGS

~ *Muscle weakness and fatigue.* This is the most common side effect of statins and it is the direct result of depletion of CoQ_{10} in the muscles and heart. Beatrice Golomb, M.D., Ph.D., has studied statin side effects and has reported that nearly all patients taking Lipitor and about one-third of patients taking Mevachor have experienced muscle problems.[24]

~ *Heart disease and heart failure.* CoQ_{10} levels fall naturally as we age, decreasing by about 50 percent between the ages of twenty and eighty. This is one of the reasons why heart attack, stroke, and cancer increase with age. Statin drugs deplete this nutrient even further, thus increasing the risk of cardiomyopathy and heart failure. The heart is the worst place in the body to deplete CoQ_{10} because it requires so much energy that must be constantly replenished. Cardiologist Peter Langsjoen, M.D., has reported on the adverse effects of Lipitor among twenty patients who started on the drug with completely normal hearts. After six months and a low dose of Lipitor (20 mg per day), two-thirds of the patients started to show signs of heart failure.[25] Dr. Langsjoen credits this effect to CoQ_{10} depletion. While heart attack rate has decreased somewhat over the last twenty years, cardiomyopathy and heart failure incidence have increased. I'm concerned that this problem will increase even more in those taking statins.

~ *Liver damage.* The liver constantly detoxifies the blood and carries out a huge number of enzymatic reactions. So it, too, requires a good supply of CoQ_{10}. Even a modest deficiency can cause liver problems, reflected in increased liver enzymes on a blood test. People on statins need to get liver enzymes checked regularly. Liver damage can begin the moment one begins taking statin drugs.

~ *Brain and nerve damage.* CoQ_{10} is essential for normal brain and nerve function. When it is depleted, dementia can result. This is why many people on statins have difficulty with memory, mood, and clear thinking. In a study in Denmark of 500,000 people, researchers found a significantly higher incidence of neuropathies, including peripheral neuropathy, in those taking statins.[26] Another study showed a fourteenfold increased risk of neuropathy after two or more years on statins compared to controls.[27]

~ *Depression.* It is well documented that low cholesterol is associated with depression and may even increase the risk of suicide. This makes sense. Cholesterol is an essential building block of brain and nerve tissue. It is like the "coating" on the wires that govern nerve conduction and function—including maintaining a stable mood. It is fairly common for women to begin experiencing anxiety and mood problems after beginning statin drugs. One study of 121 women aged eighteen to twenty-seven found that women with low cholesterol are twice as likely to have depression and anxiety.[28] Supplementing one's diet with the right type of omega-3-rich fats often helps this problem dramatically. So does getting off statins.

~ *Cancer.* Statin drugs have been found to suppress the immune system (which is why they are sometimes prescribed for those with inflammatory conditions such as arthritis). And that also explains why they've had some effect on decreasing cardiovascular events such as stroke, which results from inflammation in blood vessel walls. In fact, any benefit from statins may be from this anti-inflammatory effect. Unfortunately, it is well documented that drugs that suppress the immune system increase the risk of cancer. That is why statin drugs have been found to cause cancer in rodent studies.[29] The most likely reason that we haven't yet seen this effect in studies on humans is that clinical trials haven't lasted more than two to five years. It would take longer to see this effect. Not surprisingly, CoQ_{10} is effective at lowering the risk of many cancers, including colon, rectum, breast, lung, prostate, and pancreas.[30]

I'm also very concerned about the increased risk of breast cancer in women on statins.[31] In fact, the CARE (Cholesterol and Recurrent Events) trial at Brigham and Women's Hospital in Boston found twelve new cases of breast cancer in the 250 women taking Lipitor, while there was only one new case in the placebo group.[32] While not proving a cause and effect relationship, it's certainly worrisome. Though other studies have failed to show this effect, they have not been double-blind, placebo-controlled.[33]

A Word About the Pharmaceutical Industry

It's important to your health that you realize the degree to which the pharmaceutical industry influences medical research, medical reporting (in both medical and mainstream media), and medical prescribing. The overuse of statins is a stellar example of this influence. Marcia Angell, M.D., the former editor-in-chief of the prestigious *New England Journal of Medicine,* has documented the way in which drug companies influence medical research, prescribing, and reporting very strongly and effectively in her book *The Truth About the Drug Companies: How They Deceive Us and What to Do About It* (Random House, 2004). (For more information on the statin debate, read *Lipitor: Thief of Memory, Statin Drugs and the Misguided War on Cholesterol* [Infinity Publishing, 2004] by Duane Graveline, M.D., a former astronaut and aerospace medical research scientist who twice developed global amnesia after taking Lipitor on his doctor's recommendation.)

The current situation with the pharmaceutical industry can be likened to the influence of the tobacco industry on the medical profession back in the '40s and '50s when doctors and the AMA espoused the "benefits" of smoking to their patients and were paid handsomely by big tobacco. Eventually the truth won. And it will again.

High Blood Pressure

Blood pressure fluctuates all the time, hour by hour, and day by day, and there has been extensive overdiagnosis and unnecessary treatment of millions of people because of this. It's not uncommon for blood pressure to rise simply in response to a doctor's visit! This is called the "white coat syndrome" and I've seen it repeatedly. On the other hand, bona fide hypertension is a well-known risk factor for heart attack, kidney disease, and stroke. Blood pressure should be 130/85 or less. Twenty percent or more of North American women between the ages of forty-five and sixty-four have mild to severe high blood pressure, a condition that, in the famous Nurses' Health Study, has been found to increase the risk of coronary artery disease by 3.5 times.[34]

Blood pressure can be significantly lowered by any one of the following lifestyle changes: regular exercise (such as brisk walking), biofeedback, dietary improvement, or weight loss. Even in very overweight women, losing only ten to twenty pounds will often lower blood pressure significantly. If these measures fail, then it's advisable to use blood-pressure-lowering medication, even though these medications can have side effects such as dizziness, headaches, and fatigue.

Be sure to get your lipid profile and blood pressure checked again within three to six months. *Note:* If you follow the insulin-normalizing diet I recommend at perimenopause, you can expect substantial improvements in your lipid profile, your blood sugar, and your blood pressure within two to four weeks.

Homocysteine

Elevated blood levels of the amino acid homocysteine, which is found in high amounts in animal protein, constitutes a strong risk factor for cardiovascular disease. At least 10 percent or more of the population has a genetic tendency for elevated levels of homocysteine but there are other factors besides genetics that elevate it. When high homocysteine levels are reduced, the incidence of heart attack is cut by 20 percent, the risk of blood-clot-related strokes decreases by 40 percent, and the risk of venous blood clots elsewhere in the body plunges by an impressive 60 percent. Studies have shown that dietary intake of vitamins B_{12}, B_6, and folate can help combat an elevated homocysteine level, as can cutting back on the amount of animal-based protein in your diet. Ask your health care provider to determine your homocysteine level. (It should be below 7.) If it's too high, you need to add activated folic acid (L-methyl folate), vitamin B_{12}, and vitamin B_6 to your diet. L-methyl folate is the most biologically active and usable form of folic acid. It has been shown that conversion of folic acid is frequently disrupted by genetic factors, age-related factors, and metabolic problems. Taking activated folate bypasses these problems.[35] You may also need folate supplements of 1,000–2,000 mcg for three months or so, after which point you can decrease the supplements to a maintenance amount. (As one of those with a genetic tendency toward high homocysteine, I was able to lower my levels to normal by taking extra folic acid.)

Peridontal Disease and Cardiac Risk

Periodontal disease (inflammation and infection of the gums) is present in a significant percentage of adults in the United States. In recent years, a number of compelling studies have shown that gum disease is a risk factor for coronary artery disease and stroke. Although no one can say that periodontal disease directly causes cardiovascular disease, research has clearly shown that periodontal disease is more prevalent in patients with acute and chronic heart disease. This association may be due, in part, to the fact that inflammation plays a central role both in gum disease and in hardening of the arteries. It has also been shown that the inflammation seen in periodontal disease is associated with narrowing of the carotid arteries, a risk factor for stroke.[36]

Periodontal disease is easily preventable (and often treatable) from the outside through proper brushing, flossing, and regular visits to the dentist for professional evaluation and cleaning. Dietary improvement and supplementation help treat it from the inside. Caring for your teeth and gums is a practical and easy way to decrease at least one risk factor for cardiovascular disease or stroke.

Smoking

Smoking is responsible for 55 percent of the cardiovascular deaths in women less than sixty-five years old because smoking increases oxidative stress enormously in every cell of the body. The Nurses' Health Study followed more than 117,000 female nurses ages thirty to fifty-five. In that study the relative risk of total coronary artery disease among smokers was four times higher than that of women who never smoked. But in women who stopped smoking, the relative risk of coronary artery disease immediately decreased to 1.5. Two years after stopping smoking, the risk dropped to that of a woman who has never smoked. Smoking is also responsible for approximately 29 percent of all cancers. Since 1987 lung cancer has been the leading cause of cancer deaths among women.[37]

At least thirteen studies have shown that smokers cease menstruation one to two years earlier than nonsmokers. The effect is dose-dependent, and the difference persists after controlling for weight. Female smokers sixty years and older also have significantly reduced bone mineral density of the hip compared with nonsmokers.[38]

HOW TO QUIT

You have to want to quit to be successful. With each subsequent attempt, however, the chances for successfully staying off tobacco increase. The biggest problem women have with successfully quitting smoking is that they often have to change their friendships and behavior patterns and begin to think of themselves as nonsmokers.

Acupuncture can help people quit, because it's helpful for detoxing addictions. Some women also do well with Smokers Anonymous programs or with one of the nicotine patches.

I recommend calling your local hospital to see what is available. Or discuss stopping smoking with your doctor.

Age

The only reason that age is a risk factor for heart disease is that by the time you reach fifty or so, the processes that clog arteries are often well established. Coronary artery disease starts in many by the teenage years. It's the result of your day-to-day decisions on all levels: emotional, physical, and psychological. To treat it, reverse it, or prevent it, you need to change those day-to-day actions that led to it in the first place.

A large study of coronary risk factors in fifteen-year-olds and young adults, for example, showed that of 197 males and 197 females, 31 percent of the males and 10 percent of the females had calcification of their coronary arteries by age fifteen. We know that these calcifications are closely associated with heart attack, stroke, and aneurysm in later life. To further figure out which individuals were more likely to have these lesions, the investigators found that the following factors were most predictive of coronary artery pathology: high body mass index and low HDL ("good") cholesterol.[39] All roads lead back to glycemic stress!

Powerful Versus Powerless

If you perceive that you are valuable and powerful in the world and have choices, then your heart will be more apt to work optimally. The opposite is also true. At least two studies have shown a relationship between a woman's job and her health. One study found that women who are employed and married have the best health, with or without children. If their husbands are supportive, so much the better. Good health is also associated with more complex and challenging jobs characterized by autonomy.

But if you feel that you have no autonomy, the risk for heart disease goes up. Clerical workers whose supervisors are demanding and whose job situations do not allow them to express anger are at increased risk for developing heart disease. Time pressure is also a risk factor that has been associated with poor health.[40]

If a woman's heart isn't in her work, she cannot express her anger about this, and she perceives that she can't leave, this conflict hits her right in the heart, an organ that is exquisitely sensitive to the effects of excessive catecholamines over time. A woman in a stressful job in which she feels she doesn't have a say is also more likely to smoke, which results in higher blood pressure and cholesterol—both additional risk factors for heart disease.

Studies suggest that low educational standing is consistently associated with higher risk of coronary artery disease in women. This isn't necessarily related to formal education, however; rather, it is tied more to the fact that those who are better educated tend to take better care of themselves and to know that they have choices. Also, body mass index and cigarette smoking are inversely related to educational attainment. Vigorous leisure-time activity is also related to educational attainment. Fitness levels assessed by treadmill have been directly related to educational attainment in women but not in men.[41] The good news is that you don't need to go back to school for an advanced degree to change your perception and take charge of your lifestyle.

The number and diversity of your friends and associates also contributes to heart health or lack of it. Women with greater numbers of children and too many demands on their time combined with a lack of emotional support have been shown to be at greater risk for heart disease. But women who perceive that their families are supportive are at lower risk.

SHARON: Dying for Her Benefits

Sharon had been a patient of mine for years. Though she was about twenty pounds overweight, she walked regularly and was in a very happy, supportive relationship. Her blood pressure and cholesterol were normal, and she was in good health. She was also on Premarin and Provera—two hormones that had been prescribed for her at the beginning of her menopause for hot flashes. She had done well with this approach and there was no reason to change the prescription. (At the time, we didn't have the data on alternatives that are now available.) At the age of fifty-four Sharon developed chest pain, and a cardiac workup showed that she had narrowing of her coronary arteries. She underwent bypass surgery. When I asked Sharon if she was going through any unusual stresses around the time of her chest pain, she told me that she had been hoping she could take early retirement from her job as a university professor. She and her husband had bought a house in Florida, where they spent as much time as possible. But she discovered that if she took early retirement, she wouldn't be eligible for her full pension benefits. So she halfheartedly decided that she had no choice but to stay another ten years. It was shortly after she made this decision that she developed her chest pain. As I did her annual pelvic and breast exam, I asked her if she really felt it was worth it to stay another ten years in a job that was literally shutting off the joy to her heart. And I was reminded that people who stay in jobs they hate strictly for their benefits rarely get to use them.

Hidden Emotions Lead to Hypertension

There is no question that factors such as obesity, salt intake, and a sedentary lifestyle are associated with hypertension. And so is stress. But not in the way we've been led to believe. Samuel J. Mann, M.D., professor of clinical medicine at the Hypertension Center of The New York–Presbyterian Hospital Weill Cornell Medical Center in New York City has seen thousands of people with all varieties of high blood pressure. Over the years, he began to notice a pattern that didn't fit with the common view of hypertension. In his book *Healing Hypertension: A Revolutionary New Approach* (John Wiley, 1999), he notes, "Even patients with severe hypertension did not seem more emotionally distressed than others. If anything, they seemed less distressed. Their high blood pressure appeared to be more related to what they did *not* seem to be feeling than to what they *were* feeling."[42] He began to see that old, unhealed, repressed trauma seemed to be a major culprit in his patients. After all, anger and stress can elevate blood pressure, but they do this temporarily and aren't the root cause of hypertension. Instead, it is our hidden emotions, says Dr. Mann, the emotions we do not feel, that lead to hypertension and many other unexplained physical disorders. To deal with hypertension at its core (or anything else for that matter), it is necessary to bring those hidden emotions to the light, to consciousness, and to deal with them.

My friend and colleague Annemarie Colbin, Ph.D., the founder of the Natural Gourmet Institute for Health and Culinary Arts in Manhattan, shared her personal experience with hypertension after she herself was diagnosed with hypertension despite her very healthy lifestyle.

I can testify to the validity of this approach. In the summer of 2000, I read about Dr. Mann in a little free newspaper that covers my New York neighborhood. At the time this seemed a surprising synchronicity, as I had suddenly found myself grappling with some episodes of extremely high blood pressure—as high as 220/120. I was unable to sleep at night, or at most slept two to three hours, a completely new development for me. I also had trouble concentrating. Although I am very opposed to taking pharmaceutical drugs, I did consult a physician and took some anyway. I also went to my usual alternative medicine practitioners, such as my chiropractor, homeopath, and acupuncturist, which helped a little, but I knew it wasn't enough.

After reading the article about Dr. Mann, I bought his book and read more on his unique perspective. Then I went to see him, and with his encouragement started looking at what kind of hidden emotions I could be harboring. It didn't take long to figure out that the place to look would be in my repressed, or perhaps pre-verbal, memories of the three years I spent during World War II in Budapest, Hungary, when I was two to five years old. I was there with my mother (my father, I found out years later, was in a forced labor camp), and we spent many nights in cellars and basements with 30 to 40 strangers, hiding from the bombs and grenades. In terms of emotions, I knew there was something there, but I had no memory of it.

One day in August, after a weekend of sleeping one night out of three, I found myself again with high blood pressure, 200/100, and I went for a walk in the park, barefoot in the grass. (I had taken this up as a de-stressor.) Thinking about the war years, and also about how I felt the sleepless night before, I realized that my night wakefulness was quiet and watchful. I did not think, worry, toss, or turn. I was just on high alert. It felt as if I was just waiting. What, I wondered, was I waiting for?

Then I remembered my mother telling me about one time when we were staying in a basement, and she was summoned upstairs by the occupying soldiers for a party, together with another young woman there. Thus, she had to leave me alone in the dark cellar with all the strangers, none of whom cared about me. I suddenly got in touch with a profound terror that a three- or four-year-old would feel—the fear that my mother might not come back. I remembered knowing that I would die if she didn't return. I had no home, no family, no friends around, nothing—it was just the two of us, and without her I had no chance of survival. I think I must have stayed awake all that night waiting for my mother, and now, in my sleepless nights, I was reliving it. I lay in the grass, on the safe ground, and shook and cried, feeling and releasing that old terror.

After a while of shaking and crying, I calmed down, got up, and went home, feeling strangely relieved. Then I checked my blood pressure. It had gone down to 137/82—in one hour! I knew I was on the right track. Since then, it still has gone up and down, and I had to do quite a lot more spiritual work, but at the time of this writing, four months later, my blood pressure seems to be keeping itself normal with no medication. It's been a harrowing four months, and I'm not finished yet, but I am certainly on the path to cleaning out that old emotional baggage, thanks to Dr. Mann's revolutionary insights.

Depression

Depression is consistently related to a high risk for heart disease in both men and women. In a recent survey of my newsletter subscribers, 46 percent listed their biggest health concern as depression and anxiety. In contrast, only 18 percent indicated that heart disease was their greatest concern. What these and most other women don't realize is that the emotions associated with sadness or grief, anger or depression, and fear or anxiety are very much connected to heart disease (as well as bone health).

Women's blood vessels are smaller than men's and are extremely sensitive to the biochemical changes that occur in response to the emotions of daily life. These biochemical changes result in either constricted or dilated blood vessels. When your blood vessels constrict in response to emotions such as anger, grief, and fear, they do so because of an outpouring of chemicals from the sympathetic nervous system; blood flow is reduced, and tissue damage and high blood pressure are the result.

Because at least 25 percent of women suffer from depressive episodes at some point in their lives, and because women are more apt to suffer from depression than men, depression emerges as a very important and modifiable risk factor for women. Though it is well documented that both men and women often suffer from depression after a heart attack, newer data conclude that depression is an important independent risk factor for heart disease. A study from the Ohio State University College of Medicine and Public Health recently showed just how profoundly depression affects coronary artery disease in women. Even after adjusting for other factors such as smoking, obesity, and lack of exercise, the risk for non-fatal coronary artery disease was 73 percent higher in depressed women compared to a control group.[43] In their research, depressed women were also shown to be twice as likely to develop coronary artery disease as were normal, nondepressed women.

CARBOHYDRATES, SUGAR, AND HEART HEALTH: WHAT EVERY WOMAN SHOULD KNOW

By now you know that overconsumption of refined carbohydrates plays a role in developing type 2 or adult-onset diabetes, a disease whose incidence is rapidly increasing as our population grows fatter and fatter. But what most women don't know is that the same carbohydrate consumption pattern that results in obesity, poor skin, and hormone imbalance is also a potent risk factor for heart disease, hypertension, and stroke. The diet most commonly prescribed for treatment and prevention of heart disease in both men and women is a high-carbohydrate, low-fat approach. Unfortunately, this diet may have exactly the opposite effect. When compared to a higher-protein, higher-fat diet with exactly the same number of calories, the high-carbohydrate diet has been shown to increase risk factors for ischemic heart disease, such as high triglycerides and insulin, in healthy postmenopausal women. It also lowers HDL cholesterol.[44] Eating a high-carbohydrate meal has also been shown to trigger angina sooner and reduce exercise tolerance in patients with known heart disease. This is because high insulin levels can cause constriction of arteriosclerotic coronary arteries.[45]

The experience of many women whose husbands go on high-carbohydrate, low-fat diets following heart attacks is that the men lose weight and lower their total cholesterol while their wives gain weight and may lose some of their HDL ("good" cholesterol) on exactly the same food plan. To prevent this, women need to be sure to eat only those carbohydrates that don't raise insulin levels too high or too quickly.[46] (See chapter 7.)

To understand how excessive carbohydrate intake can contribute to heart disease, we have to return to the subject of insulin. When you eat carbohydrates that are converted into sugar rapidly, your body pours insulin into your blood from your pancreas. Insulin is necessary to move the sugar from your bloodstream into your cells, where it is used for energy. But insulin doesn't simply regulate your blood sugar; it also helps control the storage of fat in your body. And heart disease is basically a disease associated with too much fat in our arteries.

Here's how it happens. Insulin directs amino acids, fatty acids, and carbohydrate breakdown products into our body tissues. It also regulates the body's production of cholesterol. Insulin tells the liver to begin making LDL cholesterol ("bad" cholesterol), which at high enough levels—and under the right circumstances—actually sticks to blood vessel walls that have already been damaged by glycemic stress (blood sugar that's too high) and forms a plaque. And that is the essence of coronary artery disease and also cerebrovascular disease—the kind of arterial disease that affects brain function and enhances your risk for stroke and also dementia.

If you eat a lot of sugar or a lot of high-glycemic-index carbohydrates, such as pasta, bread, candy, cookies, and potatoes (and/or alcohol), and you are prone to high blood sugar or insulin resistance (as about 75 percent of us are), your liver may well increase its synthesis of LDL, which tends to stick to your inflamed blood vessels, forming plaques and subsequently causing arteriosclerosis, or hardening of the arteries.

Insulin also drives your kidneys to retain fluid, in a way that is similar to the kind of fluid overload that is seen in coronary artery disease and congestive heart failure. Excess insulin therefore poses a significant risk for hypertension, coronary artery disease, obesity, and high cholesterol levels, not just diabetes. Fluid retention from insulin is the reason why susceptible individuals can easily put on three or four pounds after a single large carbohydrate-rich meal. (I call these "liquid" pounds.)

Insulin and Blood Vessel Wall Thickening

In addition to all its other important roles, insulin is also a growth factor in the body: excess insulin and high blood sugar result in inflammation in the lining of blood vessels throughout the body. Over time, this process promotes smooth muscle growth in your blood vessel walls, which contributes to the formation of plaque, causing your artery walls to thicken and become rigid. Excess blood sugar from chronic carbohydrate consumption irreversibly attaches to the LDL cholesterol molecules that are already stuck to the blood vessel walls. This disease process in blood vessels also includes free-radical damage, a type of cellular damage that is akin to rust on a car.[47]

Here's the bottom line: if you eat too many high-glycemic-index carbohydrates and don't exercise, then your body will convert those carbs into excess blood sugar, fat, and LDL cholesterol. In addition, the higher your intake of refined carbohydrates, the more cellular inflammation, which is the final common pathway for heart disease.[48]

Follow a diet that keeps insulin levels low—the same diet that also prevents middle-age spread, balances your hormones, and improves your skin.

Some women are able to keep their weight and cholesterol levels normal by eating a lot of complex carbohydrates, including whole-grain breads, and others—like me and millions of others—are not. You can't go wrong, however, if your diet consists mostly of lean protein, healthy fats, and lots of fruits and vegetables. Choose the most colorful ones, such as blueberries, strawberries, collard greens, squash, and kale. These are the highest in antioxidants. Hundreds of studies have confirmed that foods rich in flavonoids, carotenoids, and other antioxidants can reduce your risk for cardiovascular disease. Women who routinely eat four to five servings of fruits and vegetables per day (particularly the green, leafy, cruciferous, and citrus varieties) have a 28–35 percent decreased risk of stroke—an estimated 7 percent decrease in risk for each serving.[49]

The isoflavones and other substances in soy have also been shown to have a beneficial effect on blood lipids. For example, an analysis of thirty-eight controlled clinical trials found that the consumption of soy protein rather than animal protein resulted in significantly decreased levels of total cholesterol, LDL cholesterol, and triglycerides.[50] Regular consumption of soy protein and ground flaxseed is also associated with lowered cholesterol and a decreased risk for arteriosclerosis.[51]

Last but not least, avoid trans fats.

CARDIOPROTECTIVE SUPPLEMENTS

The following is a list of some of the best-studied cardioprotective foods and supplements. You don't need to take all of them. Many will be present in a good comprehensive formulation for women. But others, like a higher dose of vitamin C, a cup of green tea daily, or a clove of garlic, are easy to add to your day.

Magnesium

Among its many roles in the body, magnesium helps stabilize electrical conduction in the cardiac muscle. It also helps relax the smooth muscle in blood vessels,[52] contributing to maintenance of normal blood pressure and vascular tone, and assists insulin in transporting glucose into cells, fighting glycemic stress. Because it helps all muscles (including coronary artery muscles) relax, it's very effective in helping prevent cardiac damage and even death after a heart attack. (In fact, up to 40 to 60 percent of sudden deaths from heart attack are caused by spasm in the arteries—not blockage from clots or arrhythmias!)[53]

Magnesium deficiency is relatively common; because commercial agriculture today relies heavily on inorganic fertilizers, our food supply tends to be poor in this mineral. Food processing results in decreased magnesium as well. Chronic emotional and mental stress is also associated with magnesium deficiency because the stress hormones cortisol and adrenaline release magnesium from the cells; eventually it is excreted in the urine.

Diuretics result in the loss of magnesium in the urine, too, which is why the chronic use of diuretics has been associated with sudden cardiac death. If you're on diuretics for high blood pressure or any other reason, make sure that you take additional magnesium, potassium, and zinc. Excessive use of the stomach acid inhibitors cimetidine (Tagamet) and ranitidine (Zantac) can result in magnesium deficiency as well. Take 400–1,000 mg per day in divided doses with meals.

In general, organically grown whole grains (including wheat germ and wheat bran) and vegetables are rich sources of magnesium, as are good quality sea salt and sea vegetables (such as kelp). Other good sources include almonds, peanuts, and tofu. You can even get magnesium by adding Epsom salts (which are magnesium sulfate) to your bath, which allows the magnesium to be absorbed through the skin.

Magnesium supplements come in several forms, including magnesium oxide, magnesium chloride, and chelated magnesium. (Magnesium is also sold in combination with calcium.) If you're healthy, start with 200 mg twice a day. If you have cardiovascular challenges, boost it to 500 mg twice a day. (You'll know you've reached your limit when you develop loose stools.) Transdermal magnesium formulated by Norm Shealy, M.D., Ph.D., is also available. (See Resources.) (For more information on magnesium, read *The Miracle of Magnesium* [Ballantine Books, 2003] by Carolyn Dean, M.D., N.D.)

Calcium

Calcium is needed by every cell in your body, including the electrical system of the heart. Adequate calcium intake also helps keep blood pressure normal. This mineral works in tandem with magnesium, and therefore it's important to make sure you get enough of both. In general you want to be sure that your calcium is balanced with magnesium in either a 1:1 or 2:1 ratio. Take 400–1,200 mg/day with meals, depending upon how much calcium is present in the diet.

Antioxidants

Thousands of studies have documented the ability of antioxidants to help your heart, blood vessels, and every other tissue in your body resist free-radical damage and thus stay healthy. Here's an overview of my favorites—though there are others.[54]

COENZYME Q_{10}: This nutrient is concentrated in organ foods such as liver, kidney, and heart. It helps produce ATP, the basic energy molecule in every cell of the body. It is also a powerful antioxidant. Numerous studies have documented its beneficial effects on the heart, both in maintaining health and in healing from disease. (High doses have even been found to reverse some types of cardiomyopathy.)[55]

Coenzyme Q_{10} improves the ability of the heart to pump effectively and has also been shown to help reduce high blood pressure and congestive heart failure in those who already have heart disease. Coenzyme Q_{10} is also very important for breast health. Coenzyme Q_{10} levels in heart muscles can be ten times greater than in other tissues because the heart functions continuously, without resting. That's why any condition that impairs the ability of the heart to do its work leaves this organ more susceptible to free-radical damage.

As already noted, coenzyme Q_{10} can be depleted in women who take statin drugs, including lovastatin (Mevacor), pravastatin (Pravachol), and atorvastatin (Lipitor), to lower their cholesterol.[56] Studies have shown that almost half of patients with hypertension have coenzyme Q_{10} deficiencies. Taking 50 mg twice a day for ten weeks has been shown to significantly lower blood pressure.[57] For those individuals already on medication for elevated blood pressure, the need for antihypertensive medication declined gradually in about four and a half months in half of the patients who took coenzyme Q_{10} (225 mg per day); some were able to stop taking blood pressure medication altogether.[58] A randomized, placebo-controlled study of people taking coenzyme Q_{10} supplements with or without statin drugs found that coenzyme Q_{10} supplementation reduced the risk of heart attack and death by 50 percent, whether the subjects were on the statin drug or not.[59]

The minimum dose of coenzyme Q_{10} I recommend is 30 mg/day. For anyone with any family history of heart disease, I'd recommend 60–90 mg/day to help prevent the disease from developing. The dose can go up to 300–400 mg per day for those with advanced heart disease.[60] (For more information, read *The Coenzyme Q_{10} Phenomenon*, by cardiologist Stephen Sinatra, M.D. [Keats Publishing, 1998].)

CAROTENOIDS: There are dozens of studies that show that individuals who consume high amounts of pigment-rich foods are at lower risk for heart disease. These foods are loaded with carotenoids such as beta-carotene, which has been shown to decrease risk of free-radical damage to the heart and blood vessels. In one study of individuals who had already had unstable angina and had undergone coronary artery bypass, the addition of beta-carotene to their diets decreased subsequent major cardiovascular events such as heart attack, stroke, need for additional bypass procedures, and cardiac death by 50 percent.[61] Beta-carotene prevents the lipoprotein LDL ("bad" cholesterol) from becoming oxidized. The usual dose of beta-carotene is 25,000 IU per day in supplement form.

However, a mix of the carotenoids is better than taking just one. For example, lutein is present in HDL ("good") cholesterol and may help prevent LDL cholesterol from oxidizing. The best way to get lutein is in fruits and vegetables, but it is also available in health food stores as a supplement; take 3–6 mg per day. Lycopene is another good antioxidant; eating tomatoes a couple of times a week will give you all the lycopene you need.

VITAMIN E: This antioxidant has been shown to keep blood platelets "slippery," thus decreasing the risk of blood clots. Vitamin E is an anti-inflammatory in the heart muscle. It may also inhibit arrhythmia and cardiomyopathy. In the Nurses' Health Study, participants taking 400–800 IU of vitamin E per day reduced their risk of heart attack by 30 percent.[62] The Cambridge Heart Study, which looked at the effects of vitamin E on two thousand patients with documented heart disease, found that those who took between 400 and 800 IU of vitamin E per day had a 77 percent decrease in cardiovascular disease over a year's time.[63]

A 2005 meta-analysis of previous studies by Edgar Miller III, M.D., Ph.D., created quite a stir when it suggested that high-dose vitamin E supplementation may increase mortality in adults.[64] Yet Dr.

Miller's analysis excluded many of the larger studies with thousands of subjects because the total mortality rates were low. None of those studies showed that vitamin E increased mortality. On the other hand, many of the studies Dr. Miller did include were smaller (with less than one thousand people), and it's only the smaller studies that showed significant adverse effects from taking vitamin E. Quite a few of those studies looked at abnormal populations, i.e., older adults who already had advanced chronic degenerative disease. Also telling is that the researchers' secondary analysis showed that differences in death rates were statistically insignificant; at the highest dose of vitamin E, the risk of death was actually lower! The bottom line: not only is there solid evidence like that from the Nurses' Health Study and the Cambridge Heart Study showing vitamin E boosts cardiovascular health, but other studies show that vitamin E is associated with a significant reduction in bowel cancer,[65] reduces the risk of dementia,[66] and even slows the development of cataracts.[67] Vitamin E should definitely be part of a comprehensive supplementation program.

Dosage is 200–800 IU per day of d-alpha-tocopherol (natural vitamin E; check the label) or mixed tocopherols.

TOCOTRIENOLS: Tocotrienols are part of the vitamin E family of compounds. But compared with regular vitamin E, they are 40 to 60 times more powerful as antioxidants. Tocotrienols have a positive effect on all three of the major physical risk factors for coronary artery disease: total cholesterol levels, oxidation of low-density lipoprotein (LDL, or "bad" cholesterol), and the clumping of red blood cells that makes stroke more likely.[68] Free-radical damage (oxidative stress from poor diet, psychological stress, smoking, etc.) that accompanies LDL oxidation is particularly dangerous because it can cause serious injury to artery and vein walls.

Tocotrienols lower cholesterol by promoting the natural degradation of an enzyme (HMG-CoA reductase) that controls your liver's breakdown of LDL cholesterol. This is the same enzyme that statin drugs affect, except that tocotrienols work through a different mechanism. For that reason, you can often lower your cholesterol with tocotrienols instead of statins.

Most multivitamins don't have significant amounts of tocotrienols, so you have to add them. If you plan to use tocotrienols to lower cholesterol, take about 50 mg per day daily for a month, and then lower the dose to about 30 mg (two capsules per day) thereafter. (If you're already on a statin drug, add tocotrienols, because they work synergistically with statin drugs, thus enhancing their effectiveness;

use about 30–55 mg per day.) Sometimes tocotrienols are included in a vitamin supplement and sometimes they are available separately. Fresh fruits, dark green leafy vegetables, almonds, peanuts, and wheat germ also contain tocotrienols and the other types of vitamin E.

SELENIUM: This antioxidant has been shown to decrease the risk of free-radical damage to blood vessel walls. The usual dose is 50–200 mcg per day.

OLIGOMERIC PROANTHOCYANIDINS (OPCs): The proanthocyanidins are in the class of foods known as the flavonoids. Cardiovascular disease risk is inversely proportional to flavonoid intake.[69] OPCs are derived from grape seeds or pine bark (one brand is Pycnogenol). This is a supplement I wouldn't live without because of its many benefits. OPCs are quickly absorbed into the bloodstream, help to regenerate the body's levels of vitamin E, and also prevent the oxidation of LDL cholesterol by free radicals. In addition, they improve blood vessel and skin elasticity by helping prevent free-radical damage to collagen, reduce or eliminate the discomfort of arthritis, help prevent circulation problems, and reduce excessive blood clotting. They also help prevent all the symptoms of allergy and hay fever. The usual dose is 40–120 mg/day.

ALPHA-LIPOIC ACID (ALA): Alpha-lipoic acid is a unique antioxidant in that it is both water- and fat-soluble. That means that it can stand guard against free-radical damage in every part of the cell. It has also been shown to help preserve intracellular levels of vitamins C and E and to help regenerate another antioxidant known as glutathione. Alpha-lipoic acid is also helpful for the metabolism of insulin, and in Germany it has been approved for the treatment of diabetic neuropathy (nerve damage). It has been shown to improve blood flow both to the nerves and to the skin. The usual dose is 50–200 mg/day.

VITAMIN C: This powerful antioxidant helps protect the endothelial lining of your blood vessels and has also been found to aid the absorption of calcium and magnesium, two key minerals for heart health. A dose of 1,000 mg per day has been shown to significantly reduce systolic blood pressure, though the mechanism is not clear. I recommend taking it in the form of plain old ascorbic acid. If you have a sensitive stomach, use the ascorbate form. I recommend at least 1,000–3,000 mg/day.

B Vitamins and Folic Acid

Over half of all women don't get the folic acid they need. This not only puts their babies at risk for neural tube defects such as spina bifida, but also increases their risk for arteriosclerosis and heart disease. It has been found that the individuals with the highest homocysteine levels also have the lowest levels of folic acid, B_{12}, and B_6. A higher dose of folic acid than the RDA is associated with a lower risk of heart attack (it may inhibit platelet aggregation and prolong clotting time) and is also the antidote for high homocysteine.[70] Women with adequate B vitamin and folate levels have a definite decreased risk for heart disease.[71]

The usual doses are: vitamin B_6, 40–80 mg per day; vitamin B_{12}, 20 mcg per day; folic acid, 400–1,000 mcg per day. It's always best to take these together with the entire B complex. (See chapter 7.)

FOODS FOR HEART HEALTH

FISH: Studies have shown that 3 g per day of fish oil containing both EPA and DHA is cardioprotective because it makes platelets more slippery and decreases cellular inflammation.[72] Alternatively, you can eat three servings of cold-water fish per week, such as salmon, mackerel, swordfish, or sardines. One 4-oz serving of salmon contains about 200 mg of DHA.

If you don't eat fish regularly, supplement your diet with omega-3 supplements, from either fish oil, flax oil, hemp oil, or algae-derived DHA (good for vegans). The usual dose of DHA is 100–200 mg per day; for other omega-3 fats it is 1,000–5,000 mg per day.

GREEN TEA: The flavonoids in green tea are known as polyphenols. These substances have powerful antioxidant effects that may be greater than or equal to that of vitamins C and E. As little as one cup of green tea per day will provide protection.[73]

GARLIC: Garlic has a long history of use in the treatment of hypertension. One pilot study showed that high doses of garlic (2,400 mg of deodorized garlic per day) significantly lowered both diastolic and systolic blood pressure. Like alpha-lipoic acid, garlic appears to increase the activity of the endothelial cells that produce nitric oxide, which is a blood vessel relaxant.

Numerous studies have also shown that regular consumption of garlic reduces cholesterol by 10 percent or more and lowers triglyceride levels by up to 13 percent. It may also inhibit platelet aggregation and blood clot formation.[74]

The German Commission E, which evaluates therapeutic claims for natural substances, recommends a dosage level equivalent to one to four cloves of fresh raw garlic a day. This is the amount estimated to provide 4,000 mcg of allicin, one of garlic's most beneficial compounds. Many good garlic supplements are on the market. Look for one with the active ingredient alliin, because this substance is relatively odorless until it is converted into allicin in the body. Products containing this substance supply all the benefits of fresh garlic but are more socially acceptable. A daily dose should be 10 mg of alliin, or a total allicin potential of 4,000 mcg. (See Resources.)

HAWTHORN: In her inspiring book *Herbal Rituals,* master herbalist Judith Berger points out that hawthorn leaf, blossom, or berry (*Crataegus oxycantha*) extracted into water or spirit-based preparations is a "fierce and protective ally for those seeking to prevent heart-related conditions which are passed on from generation to generation."[75] Hawthorn berry extract can calm palpitations, help restore blood vessel elasticity, ease fluid buildup in the heart, halt fatty degeneration of the heart, help dilate coronary arteries, and also reduce blood pressure. It can be used by those already on cardiac medication and may help you decrease your dosage. I take my hawthorn as a tea. You just buy a bag of organically grown hawthorn berries at a natural food store and steep them in hot water to taste. There is nothing standardized about this method, but I see myself as creating a healthy heart by drinking a little tea, not treating heart disease. Hawthorn has not been shown to have any adverse side effects.

If you prefer to take your hawthorn as a pill, look for a standardized extract, and use a product that contains 10 percent proanthocyanidins or 1.8 percent vitexin-4"-rhamnoside. The usual dose is 100–250 mg three times per day.

SOY: For years, studies have shown that soy lowers triglycerides and total cholesterol levels, including LDL ("bad") cholesterol, while raising HDL ("good") cholesterol.[76] Soy has further been shown to reduce blood levels of C-Reactive Protein (CRP)[77] and homocysteine,[78] both markers for cardiovascular problems. Some studies even document improvements in the width of the arteries.[79] This may be due to soy's antioxidant properties, which could prevent LDL cholesterol from clogging the arteries.[80] The data has been so overwhelming that on October 26, 1999, the FDA approved the health claim that consuming 25 gm of soy protein per day reduces the risk of coronary artery disease.[81]

Recently, a study was conducted using meal replacement shakes and nutrition bars, both soy- and milk-based. For those using the soy-based products, researchers noted a decrease of 15.2 percent in total cholesterol and 17.4 percent LDL cholesterol after six weeks, as well as a significant decrease in triglycerides. Stats for those using milk-based meal replacements were 7.9 percent and 7.7 percent, respectively, with no drop in triglyceride levels.[82]

Sodium-Potassium Balance

Decreasing sodium and increasing potassium in your diet can help control high blood pressure, which is an important risk factor for heart and circulatory problems.[83] For the 60 percent of individuals whose hypertension is related to sodium intake, the effect of sodium on blood pressure can be relieved by increasing one's intake of potassium. Dietary potassium deficiency is caused by a diet that is low in fresh fruits and vegetables and high in sodium. This is your basic fast-food diet! A diet rich in fruits, vegetables, and whole grains can supply you with 4,000–6,000 mg of potassium a day. Drugs such as diuretics, laxatives, aspirin, and others can also deplete your potassium. Prolonged exercise is associated with loss of potassium as well—up to 3,000 mg of potassium can be lost in one day by sweating. A diet high in potassium and low in sodium protects against high blood pressure, stroke, and heart disease. Potassium supplements have been shown to significantly lower both systolic and diastolic blood pressure, but these have side effects, including nausea, vomiting, diarrhea, and ulcers, when given in pill form at high dosage levels. This won't happen if you increase your levels through diet alone.

Most Americans have a potassium-to-sodium dietary ratio of 1:2, but researchers recommend a 5:1 ratio. One trip to a fried-chicken joint or pizza place will mess up this ratio. Because fruits and vegetables like potatoes, bananas, and apples are such rich sources of potassium, don't get too hung up on their high glycemic indexes. Because they are whole foods, they will not raise your insulin levels high enough to really cause damage unless they are highly processed into something like french fries. It is the simple carbohydrates in white-flour products that really mess things up as far as both insulin and potassium-to-sodium ratios are concerned. This is yet another reason why you want to try for five servings of fruits and vegetables per day in your diet.

Because magnesium and potassium work together at the level of the cell, they are often low at the same time.

FOODS TO IMPROVE YOUR POTASSIUM-SODIUM RATIO

Potatoes	110:1 (ratio of potassium to sodium)
Carrots	75:1
Apples	90:1
Bananas	440:1
Oranges	260:1

WHAT ABOUT ASPIRIN?

In 1982 John Vane, Ph.D., won the Nobel Prize by showing that aspirin can inhibit the clumping of platelets in blood vessels. This led to the widespread recommendation to take aspirin to decrease the risk of heart attack and stroke by preventing clots from forming in arteries that have been narrowed by arteriosclerosis. Studies strongly suggest that those who have evidence of ischemia of the heart muscles (decreased oxygenation of the heart) can definitely benefit from taking aspirin.[84]

A recent study of 40,000 female health workers over the age of forty-five, known as the Women's Health Study, found that women who took the equivalent of a baby aspirin every other day reduced their risk of stroke by 17 percent. There was no reduction in risk of heart attack, however. Aspirin use has its risks, though they are small at low doses. There were 127 hospitalizations for gastrointestinal bleeding among the aspirin users compared to 97 cases among the non-aspirin users.[85] (Excess alcohol intake is a well-known risk factor for gastrointestinal bleeding!)

Aspirin works by decreasing cellular inflammation and subsequent platelet "stickiness." But there are other far more effective and healthy ways to do this without any possible side effects.

Eat fruits and vegetables: Studies have shown that women who eat five to six servings of fruits and vegetables per day lower their risk of stroke by 31 percent. The strongest effect comes from the cruciferous vegetables, such as broccoli, cauliflower, Brussels sprouts, and cabbage, followed by green leafy vegetables and citrus fruit and juice.[86]

Eat carrots: JoAnn Manson, M.D., Dr.P.H., and her colleagues at Harvard Medical School tracked 87,000 nurses for eight years in the Nurses' Health Study and found that women who ate just five large carrots per week lowered their risk of stroke by 68 percent compared to those who ate only one carrot per week.[87]

Drink tea: Both black and green tea consumption have been shown to have beneficial effects on the endothelial lining of blood vessels, which helps decrease the risk of stroke.[88] The Zutphen Elderly Study in the Netherlands found that foods rich in an antioxidant known as quercetin (such as apples, tea, and onions) also decreased the risk of stroke. Black tea consumption (five or more cups per day) decreased the risk of stroke by 69 percent.[89]

Take tocotrienols: Tocotrienols do the same thing as aspirin without the risks of gastrointestinal bleeding. They decrease blood clotting or "stickiness" the same way aspirin does, by inhibiting the production of a potent coagulation factor known as thromboxane. As thinner, more freely-flowing blood is associated with the lower risk of stroke, heart attack, and transient ischemic attack, tocotrienols have also been shown to decrease platelet aggregation by as much as 15 to 30 percent, an effect equivalent to that of baby aspirin.[90] (If you're already on aspirin, you can still take tocotrienols because they don't enhance the effect of aspirin significantly, if at all.)

Eat fish: Eating fish or taking fish oil (or another source of omega-3 fats) has consistently been shown to decrease the risk of stroke.[91]

GET MOVING!

Exercise provides enormous cardiovascular benefits and has been shown repeatedly to significantly reduce the risk of heart disease, hypertension, and stroke.[92] Exercise training after diagnosed coronary artery disease has also been shown to improve blood flow to the heart by improving the ability of the blood vessel lining (endothelium) to keep vessels open and also by recruiting collateral vessels in the heart muscle that help bypass vessels that have been blocked.[93]

The benefits of exercise to help your heart even after a heart attack are evidence of just how forgiving the heart and blood vessels are when we care for them.

Your goal should be to exercise five or six days per week for at least thirty minutes. Walking is fine, but remember that true fitness includes strength, flexibility, and endurance so activities should promote all three. Weight training, for example, builds lean muscle mass that not only increases strength but also increases your metabolic rate. Yoga is great for flexibility. Aerobic activities increase endurance. Exercise also decreases insulin and blood sugar levels and will give you a much bigger "grace factor" in terms of your diet. In other words, when you exercise, you'll have a bit more leeway with your diet.

The Role of Lymph

One of the main reasons why exercise has such healing power is that it vastly increases the lymph circulation in your body. Lymph is the clear fluid that drains from around your body's cells into the lymphatic system, a network of thin-walled vessels found throughout every organ and tissue in your body. Lymph vessels contain small valves to keep the lymph from flowing backward. Bean-shaped structures known as lymph nodes are found at frequent intervals along lymph vessels, with major centers occurring in the groin, neck, and armpits and alongside the aorta and the inferior vena cava in the chest and the abdomen. The function of the lymph nodes is threefold: (1) to filter out and destroy foreign substances, such as bacteria and dust; (2) to produce some of the white cells called lymphocytes that help fight tumors and other invaders; and (3) to produce antibodies that help in the body's immune surveillance system. All lymph eventually gets emptied into a large central vessel in our chest cavities, known as the thoracic duct, which eventually empties into our hearts, so that the lymph and blood get mixed together once again after our lymph nodes have removed the waste, bacteria, and other flotsam and jetsam from it.

In addition to its role in helping keep bacteria and other invaders in check, the lymphatic system is essential to the mechanism by which fats are processed by the body. Lymph vessels that drain the small intestine collect the digested fat from the foods we eat and pass it directly into the main blood circulation, bypassing the liver. Once fats are in the blood, they may or may not get laid down in the blood vessels of the heart, forming fatty streaks that eventually lead to hardening of the arteries and the beginning of cardiovascular disease. Whether or not this happens depends upon our diet, our exercise habits, and our emotional and psychological state.

I interviewed Jerry Lemole, M.D., a leading cardiovascular surgeon from Philadelphia, many of whose patients suffer from end-stage heart disease. His research on the role of the lymph system is both intriguing and motivating.

The HDL-Lymph Connection

The lymphatic system in the heart is intimately involved with the process that leads to coronary artery disease. LDL, the so-called bad cholesterol, is a large, fluffy fat molecule that can get into blood vessel walls through breaks in the intimal tissue that forms the blood vessel lining. This is especially apt to happen when LDL cholesterol becomes oxidized. Once LDL gets stuck here, it tends to break down and leave cholesterol deposits behind.

HDL cholesterol, the "good" cholesterol, is a smooth football-shaped molecule that is small enough to actually get into the tissue around the blood vessel wall and vacuum up the cholesterol deposits left behind by the LDL.

In order for HDL to do its job of vacuuming up cholesterol deposits, it needs to get to where the cholesterol is located. It does this through lymph circulation. Dr. Lemole likens HDL molecules that pick up cholesterol in the artery walls to taxicabs in New York City. If you view Manhattan from a helicopter, you'll see a certain number of cabs. At any given time, because traffic in New York is so often backed up in the tunnels that lead to and from the city, you'll have many cabs unavailable to passengers in the street who need to be picked up. If you could speed up the passage of the cabs through the tunnels, there would be more cabs available on the streets.

The same is true with the cholesterol-carrying capacity of HDL. When lymph flow is sluggish, HDL molecules simply are not available to pick up excess cholesterol deposits. If you speed up the circulation time of lymph, you'll also improve the efficiency of HDL to scavenge excess fat from your arteries.[94]

How to Speed Up Lymph Flow

I. DON'T SIT FOR LONG PERIODS OF TIME. Women who sit for long periods of time at sedentary jobs are more likely to get heart disease because the lymphatic flow through their thoracic cavity is limited.

2. BREATHE DEEPLY AND REGULARLY. Breathing fully in through your nose and inhaling air down into the lower lobes of your lungs followed by a brisk exhalation massages the thoracic duct and all the lymph vessels and nodes in your chest cavity, which helps HDL get to the places it needs to go to do its work.

3. MOVE. Lymph flow depends upon the muscles in the body to move it along. Every time you walk, do yoga, breathe deeply, run, or move your muscles briskly, you are helping move the lymph along. Dr. Lemole reports that the average turnover time for proteins in lymph is once to twice per day. But when you exercise regularly, you can increase this figure to three to five times per day. So exercising gives your body three to five times more opportunity to get rid of excess cholesterol deposits in the blood vessels around your heart.

4. AVOID OVEREXERCISE. When we exercise, we actually increase the oxidative stress in our bodies, which results in the production of free radicals in our bodies. Over time this can do more damage than good. That's why so many endurance athletes have impaired immune function, which makes them more susceptible to infections and illness. This needn't be the case if you always breathe in and out fully through your nose as you exercise and never exert yourself beyond what is comfortable with this way of breathing. (For further information about this, read *Body, Mind, and Sport,* by John Douillard.)

Dr. Lemole recommends that you walk at a pace of about 3.6–4.0 miles per hour, which means that it should take you about thirty to forty minutes to cover two miles. Any faster than that and you will incur a lot of oxidative stress in your body that will require you to take additional antioxidant vitamins to cover the potential damage. Remember that if you exercise so that you're breathing comfortably in and out through your nose, your body will also be operating at a pace that decreases free-radical damage, because comfortable nose breathing results in a balance between your sympathetic and para-sympathetic nervous systems.

Exercise lowers many cardiovascular risks, including high blood pressure. In one study, those who did not engage in vigorous exercise regularly had a 35 percent greater risk of hypertension than those who did. Though it helps to have been active in high school and college, you will not be protected unless you continue regular vigorous exercise throughout your life.

THE HEART-ESTROGEN LINK: WHAT'S REALLY GOING ON?

Because the incidence of heart disease in women rises at about the age of fifty, the same time that estrogen levels start to decrease, scientists assumed that heart disease after menopause must be related to an estrogen deficiency. And because studies have demonstrated that estrogen lowers LDL cholesterol, raises HDL cholesterol, and helps support blood vessel walls, scientists naturally assumed that giving everyone estrogen would solve the problem of heart disease. But the original WHI study was halted when researchers found that Prempro (Premarin plus Provera) actually increased the risk of blood clots, heart attack, and stroke in healthy women. In addition, the Heart and Estrogen/Progestin Replacement Study (HERS), the Estrogen Replacement and Atherosclerosis (ERA) study, and the WHI study all showed that estrogen replacement did *not* decrease the incidence of heart attack in women who already have heart disease, and in fact even increased the risk for a while. These results certainly decreased the unbridled enthusiasm for prescribing Premarin that had characterized the medical profession during the 1990s.[95]

But now there's a new wrinkle in the estrogen-heart connection that scientists have long suspected. In 2006, an analysis of the data from the Nurses' Health Study cowritten by researcher JoAnn Manson, M.D., Dr.P.H., who was also one of the lead researchers in the WHI study, found that nurses who began taking hormone replacement therapy near menopause did indeed have about a 30 percent lower risk for heart disease than women who didn't use hormones.[96] In comparison, nurses who started HRT ten years or more after menopause showed no benefit. The study showed no difference between those who took estrogen alone and those who took it combined with synthetic progestin. The study also reanalyzed data from the WHI study and confirmed that the risk of heart problems increased in women who began taking HRT ten years or more after menopause. (There was a 22 percent increase in those who started HRT from ten to nineteen years after menopause.) But those who started it within a couple years after their last menstrual period experienced an 11 percent lower risk of heart disease. Even more striking, in the estrogen-only branch of the WHI, published in 2006, women who started HRT between ages fifty and fifty-nine had a 44 percent lower risk of heart disease.

This latest study makes sense given the large body of research showing that estrogen has a beneficial effect on the heart and blood vessels (at least in younger women). Here's a summary of the documented beneficial effects of estrogen on the heart and blood vessels.

- Estrogen exerts a cardioprotective effect on blood vessels and helps coronary arteries dilate (not constrict inappropriately).[97] It directly modifies and normalizes the function of the endothelium and vascular smooth muscle.

- It has a favorable impact on lipoproteins, cholesterol, and fibrinogen levels and reverses some adverse effects of lipid metabolism.

- It decreases endothelium retention of LDL by coronary arteries.[98]

- Estrogen has been used as an alternative to cholesterol-lowering drugs such as lovastatin and pravastatin. There may even be an additive effect on cholesterol and lipoproteins by combining ERT and pravastatin.[99]

The 2006 reanalysis of the WHI and Nurses' Health studies data is definitely intriguing and encouraging—and it certainly helps clear up some of the confusion created by earlier studies. Despite this new data, however, I still wouldn't prescribe HRT to everyone just to prevent heart disease. There are too many other factors to consider, including breast cancer and stroke risk. As always, women and their physicians need to make the HRT decision in partnership with their own intuition and body wisdom.

HOW TO LOVE AND RESPECT
YOUR MIDLIFE HEART

The energies of love, enthusiasm, joy, and passion actually enliven your heart. To promote a healthy heart, you must have a goal, a passion, a reason for living.

Many women get heart disease when, for any number of reasons, their heart is no longer in their work or their life. A very healthy eighty-five-year-old patient without any signs of heart disease recently told me that she didn't think she'd be around much longer. Her ninety-year-old husband had been hospitalized with heart disease and wasn't back to his usual state of health. She said, "We've been married for sixty years. I couldn't go on living without him." It is well known that elderly spouses often die within weeks of each other. Even in the medical profession this is known as "dying from a broken heart."

At midlife, more than ever, our hearts are calling us home. We must remember that for every behavior—whether health-enhancing or health-destroying—there are emotions that are processed by the heart and the entire cardiovascular system. And behind every emotion, there is a belief—a perception about reality. Thoughts and beliefs that support self-love and self-worth enhance health and well-being, and the lifestyle behaviors that support them. The more women truly care for themselves, the better their health is.

Emotions that we can't deal with directly and elegantly go into our bodies and drive our behaviors, pure and simple. The truth of this comes down the track like a freight train at midlife.

Though it has been said that "home is where the heart is," in my experience home is also where the heart most easily gets broken. One of the greatest challenges of midlife is to come home to ourselves. We can do this only when we allow ourselves to get to the heart of the matter—and our emotions will always lead us there. Too many women use addictions—to food, alcohol, smoking, too much or too little exercise, or recreational drugs—as a way to avoid the feelings that will lead them home. It is only through achieving emotional balance that we will truly reach the feeling of being at home within ourselves. And it is only through learning emotional balance that we will be willing to stick with the healthy diet, exercise, and supplement programs that will help our hearts. Though I suggest that you follow the dietary and exercise guidelines I've outlined, I believe that it is even more important to learn what it is to love and accept yourself. This journey home is always poignant and often painful, but inevitably always worth it, too.

One of my perimenopausal friends whose mother had been mentally ill, and who knew that she had always used food as a way to cope with the craziness of having to care for both her mother and her younger siblings, told me that when she turned forty-three she finally was able to allow herself to really feel the pain of all those childhood years and let it go. She said, "I remember the first time I sat in my therapist's office and actually allowed myself to feel the absolute panic and terror within that was the result of fear that I'd become just like my mother. And in that moment I knew why people with severe weight problems often don't lose weight—or why they put it right back on. They prefer overeating and obesity to allowing themselves to feel the depth of despair and pain within them." Luckily my friend has a very strong faith, and with the help of God she allowed herself to finally get all those old feelings out in the open, a process that took several months and a lot of tears.

She credits this to the fact that she sailed through menopause with nary a symptom. She no longer uses food to quell her emotions and has kept her weight stable for over ten years. The only way out was through!

Whether or not you have midlife heart symptoms such as palpitations, hypertension, high cholesterol, chest pain, jaw pain, arm pain, or any other evidence of heart disease, or if you simply want to prevent heart disease in the future, you owe it to yourself to learn the language of your heart.

THE HEART-OPENING EFFECT OF PETS

One of the first things I did after my husband moved out was to go down to the animal shelter and get two cats, something I'd wanted to do for a long time—my husband had been allergic to them. Few things have done me and my health as much good as my two cats, Buddy and Francine. One of my midlife friends from New York City, a professional woman with a high-powered job, recently got a dog. She told me, "It's really true that happiness is a warm puppy. What a wonderful thing to wake up each morning to such unconditional love! Everyone in my building loves him. And when I take him for a walk, I make all kinds of new friends!" Scientific literature on the health benefits of pets proves beyond the shadow of a doubt that our hearts are touched and healed, quite literally, by the unconditional love that animals can bring to our lives.

Though animals can't offer all the different types of support that we humans need, they still provide companionship, security, and a feeling of being needed. They also help connect us to the world around us and give us a focus outside ourselves—which is very helpful for those who suffer from depression. Larry Dossey, M.D., an internist who has extensively researched the healing power of prayer, refers to companion animals as "four-legged prayer."

The presence of a pet is associated with decreased cardiovascular reactivity—which means that the influence of a pet helps us stabilize our blood vessels and heart rhythm. People have been found to have lower heart rates and lower blood pressure when they are with their pets. This translates into thousands of fewer heartbeats over months and years, which can slow the development of arteriosclerosis. Research at Brooklyn College has shown that pets slow heart rate even among highly stressed, high-intensity type A personalities.[100]

Pets of all kinds lower blood pressure. Petting a dog has been shown to decrease the blood pressure of healthy college students, hospitalized elderly people, and adults with high blood pressure. When bird owners talk to their birds, their blood pressure drops an average of ten points. And watching fish in an aquarium has been shown to bring blood pressure below resting levels. Research has also shown that when children are sitting quietly and reading, their blood pressure is lower when a dog is in the room.[101]

Support from animal companions has been linked to increased survival in those with coronary artery disease. This survival was independent of marital status and living situation. University of Pennsylvania researchers Aaron Katcher, M.D., and Erika Friedmann, Ph.D., found that people with pets lived longer after experiencing heart attacks than those without pets.[102] Subsequent research has shown that among people who have heart attacks, pet owners have one-fifth the death rate of those who do not have pets.[103] If you can't own a pet yourself, volunteer at an animal shelter or visit other people's pets. They're a cardiac tonic with no side effects.

THE INTELLECT IS CERTAIN IT KNOWS, BUT THE HEART ALWAYS WINS

It has taken me half a lifetime to know one thing for sure: the intellect exists to serve the wisdom of the heart. Our intellect-driven society, however, leads us to believe that it's the other way around. And so we wait for the next drug or technological breakthrough, thinking it will save us. But in the end, the wisdom of the heart always wins.

All the drugs and technology in the world can't mend a broken heart or heal someone whose heart is no longer in the game of life. The EKG signal coming from the heart is sixty times stronger than the EEG signal from brain waves. So when there's a conflict between the intellect and the heart, the heart always wins. And the only way to heal the true discomforts of the heart is to feel them fully, have faith in a power greater than yourself, and then live your life robustly.

My Prescription for Preventing and Healing Heart Disease

~ Understand that each heart is self-healing if given the space and permission to feel what it needs to feel.

~ Be willing to bravely and compassionately enter the unhealed places in your heart. When you are on intimate terms with your own pain and suffering and have made a commitment to heal them, you will eventually come to the joy that is your natural state. And you will also find that you have far less difficulty keeping your heart open to others. Your very presence becomes part of the healing as everyone around you realizes that they are not alone and are also worthy of openhearted acceptance, too.

~ Know that it's part of the Great Mystery why some people open their hearts to themselves and do the work of healing and others do not. Still, maintain hope and compassion, no matter how dim they may seem.

~ Rather than take on the impossible burden of thinking it is our job to fix others, we must also remember that the biggest gift we can give to another is a healed, joyful, and compassionate heart. And that is, and always will be, an inside job.

Whether or not you get a new pet, a new job, or a new mate, midlife is a time of rebirth. The newly opening midlife heart is tender, green, and new. Don't allow it to be stepped on. Learn how to protect yourself; ask for help and allow yourself to receive it. Open your heart, care for your heart, and let it lead you home.

The Calm After the Storm

O ne day during the winter after my divorce, I awoke at six to go to my regular morning exercise class in Portland. Though the weather report said it was raining, I opened the door and walked out into a snowstorm that was dumping about two inches an hour all around me. Nevertheless, I set out. After all, I'm a veteran of snowbelt winters in western New York. As I headed south, however, I could scarcely see, and I briefly considered turning around. But in my characteristically stoic fashion I continued, certain that the weather would lighten up momentarily. Suddenly my car started fishtailing. I was spinning in a circle, wildly out of control and heading for the guardrails. I braced myself for the crash, wondering simultaneously whether I would survive being broadsided by the oncoming traffic. After my car slammed to a halt against guardrails cushioned by snow, I braced for further collisions. Miraculously, the cars behind me were able to stop in time. Not sure what to do next, I hesitantly put my car into gear. I was able to pull out onto the highway, and I slowly continued my drive into Portland. As I entered the city the weather did indeed clear, and I ended up going to my class. Though I was shaken, the damage to my car was mostly cosmetic—I had shattered my left rear bumper, nothing else. I felt very lucky. I knew that I could have been killed.

My accident seemed like a swift energetic reenactment of my perimenopause, complete with the shattering of my marriage and of the parts of my personality that now needed to die if I was to stay healthy and grow. The accident happened almost one year to the day from the time when my husband and I had separated and started divorce proceedings. For the past year my old life and personality had, like my vehicle on that icy road, been seized by a force beyond my control. Despite my worst fears, I had ended up able to move forward under my own power. And though at the time the impact of the breakup had felt as though it might destroy some essential part of me, the damage, like the damage to my car, turned out to be largely cosmetic. My life no longer looked as picture-perfect as it once had. Yet I discovered that the only thing of true significance that had been shattered was the closely guarded and comforting illusion that something or someone outside of myself could and should save me from living the life that I was destined to live. After twenty-four years of marriage, I had managed to spend a year without a man. I had survived a great deal of grief and pain, found that I was able to support my children and myself, and, though shaken, had emerged more fearless than ever before.

The morning after my accident I awakened to a beautiful sunny day, my two cats asleep on the foot of the bed. Yes, I was alone in the house. Yes, my nest was empty. But my heart was more full of love, joy, and anticipation for the future than it had been in over a year. I was free, and for the first time in my life I could create the rest of my life on my own terms instead of trying to please someone else—whether parents, teachers, husband, or children.

I also knew, right down in my bone marrow, that I needed to cherish my newfound moments of solitude in my own home, because they might not last forever. If I meet a man with whom I can be fully myself, sharing both my vulnerability and my competence and valuing the same mix of qualities in him, then I would love to have a life partner again. For now, though, I know that my primary relationship has to be the one with myself. I can no longer lose myself in a relationship with anyone else or put anyone else's welfare ahead of my own. So at this transitional time of my life I am savoring every sunset and every morning of awakening to new possibilities, new adventures.

Whether or not I ever find that life partner, I know I am not alone. And neither are you, whether or not you're married, have children, or live in community. You and I are part of a massive group of capable, healthy, and self-assured women who are redefining what it means to be a woman at midlife: physically, emotionally, financially, and spiritually. All of the things we were passionate about in our adolescence are now coming up for us again. But this time we have the skills, connections, and savvy to act on our passion and make it real. Once we truly become partners with our own spirits at midlife, we not only restore our faith in ourselves, but also become part of a force to be reckoned with.

In the first edition of this book, I wrote, "Every morning I look at myself in the mirror, and I like the woman I see. I like her physical and emotional strength and her compassionate heart, a heart that has been broken but has now become courageous enough to love again—if (and only if) I can find someone who can love me in return without asking me to compromise any part of myself." Now, six years after writing those words, I have finally found that special someone who can love me without compromise. It's me! It took a while, but after I finally learned to accept, celebrate, and really enjoy myself, I of course also found a wonderful man who is proud of me and can celebrate me, too. I had to change inside before that change was reflected on the outside in an actual relationship. This is always the case. No exceptions.

We're waking up together, you and I. Don't let anyone tell you that the passions that are now shaking you to the core are simply a hormonal storm. Don't let anyone tell you that you're asking too much or that you should be more "realistic." Your passions are real, and they are calling out to you to be acted upon. But don't panic if you feel some pain. Whenever we give birth to anything important, like the new relationship with our souls that is possible at midlife, there are going to be labor pains. You don't have to make this transition overnight. You have months, even years.

Never forget that the big wisdom of life comes at menopause. There is enormous power here. Though the mainstream media has tried to make midlife women all but invisible, we're at a turning point. There is a critical mass of us, and we're beginning to know our own power. No one yet suspects how much we can accomplish when we go into our businesses, churches, clubs, and families and, quietly and peacefully, like the stealth missiles we are, set about changing everything for the better.

What happens when each of us, in her own unique way, starts refusing to say the lines that have been handed to us, refuses to play the roles that we've inherited from the women before us—women who did the best they could but whose roles are now as obsolete as the role I chose to play in my marriage back in the 1970s?

It is estimated that by the year 2008 women between the ages of fifty and sixty-five will be the largest demographic group in the United States. And for the first time in human history, the money we will be using will be money we have earned ourselves. What happens when we wake up to the power that has always been there but that our mothers and grandmothers were talked out of? What happens when, because of our sheer numbers and the circumstances of our formative years, we wake up and realize that the people we've been waiting for are us? As we flex our economic, mental, and physical muscles and put our money and energy where our ideals are, the world will change in ways that reflect our inherent women's wisdom, wisdom that has the potential to benefit every woman, man, child, and living being on this planet.

Resources

Note: The phone numbers and addresses listed in this section were current as of the publication date of the book.

General Resources

Women's Health Resources from Christiane Northrup, M.D.

Christiane Northrup, M.D., F.A.C.O.G., P.O. Box 199, Yarmouth, ME 04096; www.drnorthrup.com.

Dr. Northrup's interactive website (www.drnorthrup.com) is the best place to find regularly updated information on her lectures and other resources. Dr. Northrup also welcomes your letters. Many of her readers' questions are answered in her monthly newsletter, *The Dr. Christiane Northrup Newsletter.* (See below.)

MEDICAL AND EDUCATIONAL LITERATURE FOR WOMEN
Women's Bodies, Women's Wisdom: Creating Physical and Emotional Health and Healing (Bantam, 2006)

This groundbreaking book is now completely revised, offering up-to-date information on the entire range of women's health problems.

With over 1.2 million copies now in print, and translated into eleven languages, Dr. Northrup's first book has been described as contemporary medicine at its best, combining new technologies with natural remedies and the miraculous healing powers within the body itself.

Mother-Daughter Wisdom: Understanding the Crucial Link Between Mothers, Daughters, and Health (Bantam, 2005)

Dr. Northrup's latest book explains how the mother-daughter relationship sets the stage for our state of health and well-being for our entire lives. Because our mothers are our first and most powerful female role models, our most deeply ingrained beliefs about ourselves as women come from them. And our behavior in relationships—with food, with our children, with our mates, and with ourselves—is a reflection of those beliefs. In this book, Dr. Northrup shows how once we understand our mother-daughter bonds, we can rebuild our own health, whatever our age, and create a lasting positive legacy for the next generation.

Women's Health Wisdom Monthly E-Letter

Through her monthly e-letter, Dr. Northrup provides a forum for discussing safe, effective, and natural solutions to women's health problems. With her characteristic compassion, she presents the most up-to-date information on topics from help for hot flashes to choosing the best foods for your body. She also answers readers' health questions, shares personal success stories from readers, and recommends further reading. E-letter subscribers also have access to a wide range of products and services designed to help women live their lives more fully and healthfully. Available at www.drnorthrup.com.

The Dr. Christiane Northrup Newsletter

Dr. Northrup's monthly newsletter covers topics ranging from sexuality and menopause to the link between financial and physical health. In each issue, Dr. Northrup includes articles, recommended reading, and helpful tips so you can get to know your body, nurture your soul, and discover that "true health comes from within." Dr. Northrup also answers readers' questions and offers guest columns by well-known authors, including Louise Hay, Terah Kathryn Collins, and Caroline Myss, Ph.D. Available at www. drnorthrup.com or through Hay House (800–654–5126 or 760–431–7695; www.hayhouse.com).

HEALING CARDS

Women's Bodies, Women's Wisdom Healing Cards, a Fifty-Card Deck and Guidebook

The Women's Bodies, Women's Wisdom Healing Cards were created by Christiane Northrup, M.D., to help women reach clarity, fulfillment, and success in each of five major life areas: fertility and creativity, partnership, nurturance and self-care, self-expression, and the development of an enlightened heart and mind. The deck comes with a seventy-two-page instruction booklet that offers a variety of practical ways to access intuitive, grounded information on a number of issues. Available from Hay House,

Inc. (800–654–5126 or 760–431–7695; www.hayhouse.com) or www.drnorthrup.com.

AUDIOTAPES

Dr. Northrup's audiotape programs are all available through www.drnorthrup.com or through Hay House (800–654–5126 or 760–431–7695; www.hayhouse.com).

Mother-Daughter Wisdom: Creating a Legacy of Physical and Emotional Health

Dr. Northrup narrates an abridged version of her latest book, *Mother-Daughter Wisdom,* discussing the bonds passed from generation to generation that shape our physical, mental, and spiritual well-being.

Intuitive Listening: How Intuition Talks Through Your Body

Six-CD audio program by Christiane Northrup, M.D., and Mona Lisa Schulz, M.D., Ph.D.

Drs. Northrup and Schulz help you tune in to your inner guidance by understanding the language your body talks. The program covers immune-system health, endocrine-system and hormonal health, digestive health, the structural system, and the brain and mind.

Igniting Intuition: Unearthing Body Genius—Six Ways to Create Health, Happiness, and Almost Everything Else in Your Life

Six-tape audio program by Christiane Northrup, M.D., and Mona Lisa Schulz, M.D., Ph.D.

Dr. Northrup and Dr. Schulz teach you powerful, energizing, and life-changing tools for personal growth—how to use your body's own unique intuitive language to help you heal body, mind, and soul. With over thirty years of combined medical practice between them, Drs. Northrup and Schulz describe the seven emotional centers that are associated with the major organ systems in the body, and show how both good health and illness communicate information you can use to change your life. With wit and wisdom, they teach you how to recognize the patterns associated with disease so that you can change the conditions of the cells themselves by changing your thoughts, your relationships, and your activities.

Igniting Intuition

Two-tape audio program by Christiane Northrup, M.D., and Mona Lisa Schulz, M.D., Ph.D.

Drs. Schulz and Northrup explore the basics of how intuition is wired in the body and brain.

Chapter 2: The Brain Catches Fire at Menopause

Toxic Emotions/Forgiveness

SUGGESTED READING

Hay, L. L. (1998). *Heal Your Body: The Mental Causes for Physical Illness and the Metaphysical Way to Overcome Them*. Carlsbad, CA: Hay House, Inc.

Levine, S. (1989). *Healing into Life and Death*. New York: Doubleday and Co., Inc.

Luskin, F. (2002). *Forgive for Good*. San Francisco: HarperSanFrancisco.

Northrup, C. (2006). *Women's Bodies, Women's Wisdom*. New York: Bantam Books.

Chapter 3: Coming Home to Yourself

Deliberate Creating

Esther and Jerry Hicks
(830–755–2299; www.abraham-hicks.com)

Jerry and Esther Hicks publish books and tapes containing spiritual messages on everything from how to create deliberate intent and how to discover your life purpose to the value of your relationships with others. I have enjoyed their material for many years.

Feng Shui

SUGGESTED READING

Collins, T. K. (1996). *The Western Guide to Feng Shui: Creating Balance, Harmony, and Prosperity in Your Environment*. Carlsbad, CA: Hay House.

Collins, T. K. (1999). *The Western Guide to Feng Shui: Room by Room*. Carlsbad, CA: Hay House.

Proprioceptive Writing

Proprioceptive Writing Center
(212–213–5402; www.pwriting.org)

Proprioceptive writing (PW) is a practice that uses writing to explore the psyche, using the intellect, intuition, and imagination simultaneously. PW was developed twenty years ago by Linda Trichter Metcalf, Ph.D., and Tobin Simon, Ph.D., after a decade of teaching writing to college students. I personally worked with them privately and in group settings for seven years. Workshops at the center in New York City and online courses (both private and group) are available.

Chapter 4: This Can't Be Menopause, Can It?

Holistically Oriented Physicians

American Holistic Medical Association
(505–292–7788; www.holisticmedicine.org)

The AHMA (founded in 1978) is an organization of licensed medical doctors (M.D.s), doctors of osteopathic medicine (D.O.s), and medical students studying for those degrees. Physicians from every specialty are represented. The AMHA website contains both an online physician referral directory as well as a guide to choosing a holistic practitioner.

Hormone Testing for Adrenal and Ovarian Function

Genova Diagnostics
(800–522–4762 or 828–253–0621; www.gdx.net)

Genova (formerly Great Smokies Diagnostic Laboratory) offers salivary hormone testing, as well as a wide range of other functional testing for bowel health, cardiovascular health, and more. Collection kits, articles, abstracts, and other publications regarding test methodology, clinical applications, and patient aids are available. I particularly recommend the Women's Hormonal Health Assessment (available at www.gdx.net/home/assessments/womenshealth).

Formulary Pharmacies

See chapter 5 Resources.

DHEA (dehydroepiandrosterone)

Pharmaceutical-grade DHEA is available from formulary pharmacies or Emerson Ecologics (800–654–4432 or 603–656–9778; www.emersonecologics.com).

I recommend 5-mg DHEA Sublingual manufactured by Douglas Laboratories. Suggested dose: one-half to one tablet daily, or as directed.

Migraines/Headaches

Bioidentical progesterone

A few drops of concentrated bioidentical progesterone (6,000 mg/30ml propylene glycol) applied to the skin can sometimes halt a migraine. This concentrated preparation can be obtained by prescription from any formulary pharmacy. (See also chapter 5 Resources.) Two percent progesterone cream is also effective if used daily one to two weeks prior to one's menstrual period.

Feverfew

Tanacetum parthenium works like aspirin to inhibit prostoglandins, preventing the blood vessel spasms that trigger migraines. Mygrafew, manufactured by Nature's Way, contains dried feverfew extract (leaf) 12 mg, delivering 600 mcg parthenolides (standardized to 5 percent parthenolide). Recommended dose is one tablet daily. Available from Emerson Ecologics (800–654–4432 or 603–656–9778; www.emersonecologics.com).

Chapter 5: Hormone Replacement

See chapter 4 Resources for information on hormone testing.

Individualized Hormone Therapy

Many physicians and formulary pharmacists work in partnership with their patients to provide individualized hormone-replacement solutions. Ask your physician about this kind of customized care; he or she can call a local formulary pharmacy to consult with a knowledgeable pharmacist. To locate a pharmacy that provides individualized prescriptions, contact:

International Academy of Compounding Pharmacists (IACP)
(800–927–4227 or 281–933–8400; www.iacprx.org)

IACP (formerly known as Professionals and Patients for Customized Care, or P2C2) is a nonprofit organization made up of more than 1,300 compounding pharmacists nationwide. The IACP website has a locator feature that can help you find a compounding pharmacy in your area.

American Hormones, Inc.
(888–801–5777 or 845–296–1973; www.americanhormones.com)

This compounding pharmacy was founded by Erika T. Schwartz, M.D., renowned expert in the field of natural hormones. American Hormones offers high-quality pharmaceutical-grade hormones shipped nationwide and internationally. The website has extensive information on bioidentical hormones.

For additional information on individualized hormone therapy, contact:

Natural Woman Institute
(www.naturalwoman.org)

The Natural Woman Institute was founded by Christine Conrad, author of *A Woman's Guide to Natural Hormones* (New York: Perigee, 2000). NWI maintains a database of physicians and health practitioners nationwide who prescribe natural, bioidentical hormones.

Progesterone Cream

Progesterone cream (2 percent strength) is available from a number of different sources. I have personally used the following preparations and find them comparable in quality and effectiveness.

Pro-Gest Cream, by Emerita. This is the first brand I ever used or recommended. Available from Emerson Ecologics (800–654–4432 or 603–656–9778; www.emersonecologics.com).

Bioidentical progesterone in capsule, suppository, or transdermal form is available through any formulary pharmacy. It is also available in regular pharmacies under the brand name Prometrium or Crinone vaginal gel.

Chapter 6: Foods and Supplements to Support the Change

Herbs

Many quality herbal supplements are available. Some of my favorite suppliers are listed here.

SUPPLIERS
Avena Botanicals
(866–282–8362 or 207–594–0694; www.avenabotanicals.com)
For dried organic herbs in 3-oz size.

Blessed Herbs
(800–489–4372; www.blessedherbs.com)
For bulk herb sales.

Emerson Ecologics
(800–654–4432 or 603–656–9778; www.emersonecologics.com)
Emerson Ecologics provides high-quality nutritional supplements, antioxidants, vitamins, minerals, herbs, standardized herbal extracts, green foods, and essential fatty acids from the world's leading manufacturers of professional supplements.

Specific Herbal Products

Phytoestrin. This all-natural botanical formulation contains phytoestrogens from five different sources. Ingredients include soy isoflavones, black cohosh, vitex (or chasteberry), licorice root, and dong quai. Available through USANA (888–950–9595 or 905–264–9863; www.usana.com).

Black cohosh. The rhizome of *Cimicifuga racemosa* has been used by Native Americans for centuries in much the same way as the Chinese have used dong quai. It is used for the treatment of menopausal ailments due to increasing ovarian insufficiency, mild postoperative functional deficits after ovariectomy or hysterectomy, PMS, and adolescent menstrual disorders. Many different preparations are available. I recommend Black Cohosh Standardized Extract from Nature's Way, 40 mg twice a day. Available from Emerson Ecologics (800–654–4432 or 603–656–9778; www.emersonecologics.com). Remifemin is another widely used brand available in many natural food stores and pharmacies, as well as from Emerson Ecologics. Start with one tablet (20 mg per tablet) twice per day, or take as directed.

Chasteberry. Femaprin is manufactured by Nature's Way from dried chasteberry. Best results are obtained with continuous use. Available from Emerson Ecologics (800–654–4432 or 603–656–9778; www.emersonecologics.com).

New Life Formula for Women is made by Sweet Annie Herbs from Siberian ginseng, black cohosh, angelica, blessed thistle, licorice, nettle, red clover, red raspberry, wild yam, sarsaparilla, dong quai, lemon balm, yellow dock, skullcap, and vitex. Available from Emerson Ecologics (800–654–4432 or 603–656–9778; www.emersonecologics.com).

Women's Phase II (Vitanica) is a combination of dong quai, licorice root, burdock, motherwort, and wild yam. This formula was developed by Dr. Tori Hudson, a naturopathic physician and professor at the Bastyr University of Natural Health Sciences. It has been tested clinically and found to help relieve many common menopausal symptoms. Available from Emerson Ecologics (800–654–4432 or 603–656–9778; www.emersonecologics.com).

Women's Menocaps (also known as Women's Hormone Balance/Menopause Formula). These capsules contain the highest-quality wild-crafted dong quai, burdock, *Vitex agnus-castus,* black cohosh, motherwort, and licorice. Wise Woman Herbals was founded by Dr. Sharol Tilgner, a naturopathic physician who formulates all of the company's products and is the former head of the pharmacy at the National College of Naturopathic Medicine. Available from Emerson Ecologics (800–654–4432 or 603–656–9778; www.emersonecologics.com).

Soy

Information regarding soy can be obtained at the website www.soyfoods.com. The intent of this site is to promote the consumption of soy foods throughout the world by providing reliable, scientifically based information about health benefits, taste-tested recipes that include nutritional information, and other resources for consumers, dietitians, journalists, scientists, and soy foods companies.

Revival Soy products.
Available from Physicians Laboratories (800–738–4825 or 336–722–2337; www.revivalsoy.com). The following soy products are available.

> **Revival Soy.** Of all the numerous soy products on the market, my favorite is Revival, a meal replacement drink that contains 20 g of protein and ~160 mg of soy isoflavones per serving, the equivalent of six servings of soy. Gram for gram, Revival Soy contains more isoflavones than soy milk, for example, simply because it is formulated from whole, genetically pure soybeans to be six times more concentrated than most other soy products. This healthy, protein-based meal replacement won't cause weight gain and has many benefits for both men and women.

> **Revival Digestive enzymes.**
> If you experience any flatulence (gas), constipation, or bloating with soy, this supplement has fifteen times the strength of the leading retail digestive enzyme.

> **Revival Soy Bars** are made from crunchy, puffed soy crisps blended with marshmallow, chocolate chips, or peanuts. Flavors include Smart-Carb Chocolate Peanut Paradise, Smart-Carb Chocolate Raspberry Zing, Smart-Carb Autumn Apple Frost, Peanut Chocolate Buddy, Peanut Pal, Chocolate Temptation, Apple Cinnamon Celebration, and Marshmallow Krunch. One serving equals six servings of regular soy foods, providing ~160 mg soy isoflavones (genistein, daidzein, glycitein), ~1,000 mg saponins, and 15–17 g medical-grade soy protein. All Revival Protein Bars are free of hydrogenated oils and meet the FDA's criteria for reducing cholesterol and risk of heart disease. Regular bars have from 28 to 32 g of carbohydrates each, depending on the flavor, and Smart-Carb bars have from 6 to 8 g net carbs each.

DHA

See chapter 7 Resources.

Flax

The Flax Council of Canada (204–982–2115; www.flaxcouncil.ca) endeavors to provide general flax facts of interest to consumers, as well as more specialized information for nutritionists, dietitians, food producers, manufacturers, and flax growers.

FiProFlax (ground flax), cold-milled by Health from the Sun from premium-quality flax with a high oil content, is available from Emerson Ecologics (800–654–4432 or 603–656–9778; www.emersonecologics.com).

Whole flax seed from Cathy's Country Store is organically grown golden flax. Available from Emerson Ecologics (800–654–4432 or 603–656–9778; www.emersonecologics.com).

Dakota Flax Gold. This is an organic flaxseed grown at Heintzman Farms (888–333–5813 or 605–447–5823; www.heintzmanfarms.com) in South Dakota. A "starter kit" is available that consists of three one-pound bags of flaxseed and an electric grinder.

SUGGESTED READING
Bennett, M. (1998). *The Flaxseed Revolution: Nature's Source of Omega-3's, Lignans, and Fiber.* Vista, CA: Optimal Healthspan Publications.

Traditional Chinese Medicine

Acupuncture, used alone or in conjunction with herbs, is very effective for relieving hot flashes, insomnia, night sweats, anxiety, restlessness, emotional instability, moodiness, menstrual cramps, and excessive bleeding. It's ideal to get a referral to an acupuncturist from your health care practitioner, but if you can't find one this way, contact the American Association of Oriental Medicine (866–455–7999 or 916–443–4770; www.aaom.org).

Chinese herbs. Your best option for obtaining Chinese herbs is to see a good practitioner of Chinese medicine, but if that's not an option where you live, you can purchase them from Quality Life Herbs (207–842–4929; www.qualitylifeherbs.com). Quality Life Herbs is run by my personal acupuncturist, Fern Tsao, and her daughter Maureen, both experts in the use of Chinese herbs. All the Chinese herbs mentioned in this book, as well as numerous others, are available through mail order from this company. Their products meet the highest standards possible for effectiveness and quality. I have been referring patients with a wide variety of conditions to Fern for many years, with excellent results.

> **Dong quai** (also known as dang gui, tang kuei, or angelica). Dong quai is the foundation of almost all menopausal formulations, including Joyful Change (see below), and can be taken indefinitely. Sometimes called angelica root, it can be found in many herb shops and health food stores. It is also processed into capsules, tablets, and tinctures, although I would avoid alcohol-based tinctures. The recommended dosages for most over-the-counter dong quai preparations are probably too low to

be helpful. Increasing the dosage to four or five of the tiny pills twice per day is unlikely to cause any problems, but it's always best to be under the supervision of a certified herbalist or Chinese medicine practitioner if you're going to do this. Dong quai is available from Enzymatic Therapy (800–783–2286 or 920–469–1313; www.enzy.com). (Enzymatic Therapy products are also widely available at health food stores.)

Joyful Change. I highly recommend this formula, which contains dong quai, because it addresses menopausal symptoms at their root and helps rebalance the body. Dosage is three tablets two times per day before meals. Available from Quality Life Herbs (207–842–4929; www.qualitylifeherbs.com).

Yun Nan Bai Yao (also known as Yunna Pai Yao). This formula stops or slows excessive bleeding but should not be used long-term. It also doesn't address the root cause of the problem. Still, it is very helpful for temporarily controlling the flooding, or heavy bleeding, so common in perimenopausal women. Recommended dosage: one or two capsules four times daily. Available from Quality Life Herbs (207–842–4929; www.qualitylifeherbs.com).

Xiao Yao Wan Plus (also known as Soothing Flow). This is a Chinese nutritional supplement that helps women with PMS, menstrual cramps, and perimenopausal symptoms. This supplement contains Paeonia, a well-known female tonic. Recommended dosage: four or five tablets four times per day, beginning two weeks before period is due and continuing through first day of bleeding. It may take up to three months to experience optimal results. Available from Quality Life Herbs (207–842–4929; www.qualitylifeherbs.com).

Chapter 7: The Menopause Food Plan

Dietary Supplements

COENZYME Q_{10}
Recommended dose: 10–100 mg/day. USANA's **CoQuinone 30** contains 30 mg coenzyme Q_{10} and 12.5 mg alpha-lipoic acid per capsule. Available through USANA (888–950–9595 or 905–264–9863; www.usana.com). I also recommend **Pure Coenzyme Q_{10}** by Verified Quality; available from Emerson Ecologics (800–654–4432 or 603–656–9778; www.emersonecologics.com).

DOCOSAHEXÆNOIC ACID (DHA/EPA)
Recommended dose: 100–400 mg per day. Made from algae, Neuromins is my first choice for taking this oil in supplement form. For more consumer

information on DHA, contact the DHA Information Center (888–652–7246 or 410–740–0081; www.dhadepot.com).

OptOmega. This blend of organic, cold-pressed flax, sunflower seed, pumpkin seed, and extra-virgin olive oils provides a high ratio of omega-3 to omega-6 fatty acids that supports cardiovascular health, improved immune function, mental acuity, and healthy skin. Available through USANA (888–950–9595 or 905–264–9863; www.usana.com).

Neuromins, manufactured by Nature's Way, are available from Emerson Ecologics (800–654–4432 or 603–656–9778; www.emersonecologics. com).

Martek Biosciences Neuromins Products
(888–OK–BRAIN or 410–740–0081; www.dhadepot.com)
Martek's DHA Depot website sells Neuromins gelcaps (both 100 mg and 200 mg, as well as a 100 mg product for children).

BiOmega-3 contains both DNA and EPA derived from cold water fish oil. Available through USANA (888–950–9595 or 905–264–9863; www.usana .com).

Multivitamins/Minerals
My top pick in multivitamins is the **USANA Health Pak 100** or **USANA Essentials,** manufactured by USANA Health Sciences, Inc. (888–950–9595 or 905–264–9863; www.usana.com).

I also like **Super Multi-Complex,** manufactured by Verified Quality, a comprehensive vitamin-mineral-trace element supplement containing twenty-eight essential nutritional ingredients, including copper and natural beta-carotene. Available from Emerson Ecologics (800–654–4432 or 603–656–9778; www.emersonecologics.com).

Proanthocyanidins
These powerful antioxidants are found in grape pips and pine bark. Recommendations: Start with 1 mg per pound of body weight per day, divided into three doses. After two weeks, cut back to 40–80 mg per day.

Proflavanol and Proflavanol 90 are available from USANA (888–950–9595 or 905–264–9863; www.usana.com).

OPC Pine Gold and OPC Grape Gold, manufactured by Primary Source, are available from Emerson Ecologics (800–654–4432 or 603–656–9778; www.emersonecologics.com).
Many excellent brands of OPCs are also available at pharmacies and natural food stores.

PROBIOTICS

Probiotic supplements provide gastrointestinal nutritional support by augmenting naturally occurring intestinal bacteria. The intestinal microecosystem typically carries up to four hundred strains of bacteria. From the point of view of intestinal health, a product that provides bacteria for multiple probiotic "niches" makes sense. These flora may become depleted in a number of ways, including antibiotic therapy, poor diet, and disease. Probiotics are useful for individuals bothered by intestinal gas and bloating, and may also be used when taking an antibiotic to prevent yeast infection. Be sure to take a probiotic whenever you're on antibiotics, but take them at different times of the day, so the antibiotic won't kill off the new friendly bacteria. Continue to take the probiotic for a week or so after you've finished your course of antibiotics. That way you'll be much less likely to get a yeast infection or GI upset from the antibiotic.

I recommend **PB 8 Probiotic,** manufactured by Nutrition Now. PB 8 does not contain sugar or FOS, and does not require refrigeration to maintain its potency, as most probiotics do. Take as directed on the bottle. PB 8 is available at health food stores. **Gastro Flora,** manufactured by Nutricology, is available from Emerson Ecologics (800–654–4432 or 603–656–9778; www.emersonecologics.com).

VITAMIN C

Vitamin C is vital to many body systems and processes, especially immune health, skin health, and cardiovascular function.

USANA's **Poly C** is comprised of several mineral ascorbates, bioflavonoids, rutin, and quercetin. Available through USANA (888–950–9595 or 905–264–9863; www.usana.com).

Pure Vitamin C Caps by Nutricology contain 1,000 mg vitamin C per capsule. Available from Emerson Ecologics (800–654–4432 or 603–656–9778; www.emersonecologics.com).

Digestive Aids

ENTERIC-COATED PEPPERMINT OIL

Most of the studies performed have utilized enteric-coated peppermint oil at a dosage of 0.2 ml twice daily between meals.

Pepogest, manufactured by Nature's Way, is available from Emerson Ecologics (800–654–4432 or 603–656–9778; www.emersonecologics.com).

Peppermint Plus, manufactured by Enzymatic Therapy (800–783–2286 or 920–469–1313; www.enzy.com). Enzymatic Therapy products are widely available at health food stores.

DEGLYCYRRHIZINATED LICORICE (*Glycyrrhiza Glabra*) (DGL)
Please note that the cortisol-like activity of this herb may cause a problem in people prone to hypertension. If you are taking licorice root, your blood pressure should be monitored to ensure that it stays stable.

Gaia Herbs Licorice Root A/F (also called **Licorice Root Glycerite**), an alcohol-free liquid product, is available from Emerson Ecologics (800–654–4432 or 603–656–9778; www.emersonecologics.com). **Wise Woman Herbals Licorice Root Solid Extract** is also available from Emerson Ecologics. Recommended dose for the solid extract is ¼ to ½ teaspoon, two to three times a day.

Licorice Root Capsules are manufactured by Nature's Way to provide 450 mg deglycyrrhizinated licorice with a guaranteed natural potency of not more than 6.5 percent glycyrrhizin. Recommended dose is one to two capsules three times daily with water at mealtimes. Available from Emerson Ecologics (800–654–4432 or 603–656–9778; www.emersonecologics.com).

ADDITIONAL DIGESTIVE SUPPORT

Seacure. Manufactured by Proper Nutrition, SeaCure is a concentrated fish protein that is gaining increasing recognition for its nutritional benefits in a wide range of disease conditions. Recommended for all digestive dysfunctions, e.g., Crohn's disease, irritable bowel syndrome, and ulcerative colitis. Also helpful after chemotherapy for nutritional support and immune system support. It is certified to be free of mercury and other heavy metals. Recommended dose is three capsules in the morning and three capsules in the afternoon. Available through Emerson Ecologics (800–654–4432 or 603–656–9778; www.emersonecologics.com).

Swedish Bitters. This tonic, which is excellent for stomach upset, is widely available in health food stores in liquid or capsule form. Swedish Bitters Elixir by Gaia Herbs is available from Emerson Ecologics (800–654–4432 or 603–656–9778; www.emersonecologics.com).

JOINT SUPPORT
Procosa II. This product from USANA (888–950–9595 or 905–264–9863; www.usana.com) contains a higher amount of glucosamine sulfate as well as tumeric (a natural form of COX-II inhibitor), a combination not found in any other joint health products.

Chapter 8: Creating Pelvic Health and Power

See chapter 5 Resources for information on progesterone.

Fibroids

EDUCATIONAL RESOURCES

Fibroid Network

(www.fibroidnetwork.com)

The mission of the United Kingdom–based Fibroid Network is to promote education, information, support services, and research on fibroids. They maintain an international database of current research on fibroids and recommended doctors, hospitals, and natural health practitioners providing treatment for fibroids. Information is provided (printed and online) in English, French, Spanish, Italian, Hungarian, Japanese, and Hindi.

Fibroid Treatment Collective

(866–362–6463 or 310–208–2442; www.fibroids.com)

A medical group of fibroid experts dedicated to curing fibroids with minimally invasive therapy, the Fibroid Treatment Collective in Los Angeles performed the very first uterine fibroid embolization in the U.S. The organization's website has a wealth of information about fibroids and their treatment.

Cleveland Clinic's Menstrual and Fibroid Treatment Center

(800–223–2273, ext. 46601, or 216–444–6601; www.clevelandclinic.org/obgyn)

This new arm of the famed Cleveland Clinic was designed to give women minimally invasive options to treat menstrual aberrations and alternatives to hysterectomy. The center also gives patients access to groundbreaking clinical trials, clinical research opportunities, and education programs.

Menstrual Pain

Bupleurum (Xiao Yao Wan, also known as Hsiao Yao Wan). Xiao Yao Wan Plus is a Chinese nutritional supplement that helps women with PMS, menstrual cramps, and perimenopausal symptoms. The **Soothing Flow** formulation from Quality Life Herbs (207–842–4929; www.qualitylifeherbs.com) also contains Paeonia (peony), a well-known female tonic.

Menastil. Menastil's active ingredient is calendula oil. The United States Food and Drug Administration and the Homeopathic Pharmacopoeia U.S. recognize this pure grade of calendula oil for the temporary relief of menstrual pain, as a nonprescription, over-the-counter, topically applied homeopathic product. Available from Claire Ellen Products (508–366–6311; www.menastil.com).

Castor Oil Packs

A castor oil pack consists of castor oil and wool flannel. Directions: Saturate a piece of flannel with castor oil and apply directly to area to be treated. On the side opposite the skin, lay a sheet of plastic, then apply a hot-water bottle. Use for thirty to sixty minutes five times weekly, or as directed by a practitioner. Area can be wiped clean with a dilute solution of warm water and baking soda.

Cold-Pressed Castor Oil and **Wool Flannel,** as well as **Disposable Castor Oil Packs,** by Baar Products, are available from Emerson Ecologics (800–654–4432 or 603–656–9778; www.emersonecologics.com).

Heavy Bleeding/Iron Deficiency

Iron 27+ is a time-released, chelated source of iron without gastrointestinal side effects. It is easily and readily absorbed, and is often the only source of iron that women tolerate easily. Available from Advanced Nutritional Research (ANR) (800–836–0644 or 716–699–2020).

Iron Drops. Manufactured by Levine Health Products, Iron Drops is a nonconstipating, impressively bioavailable form of iron. Recommended dose: 1.5 ml (cc) twice per day. Available from Emerson Ecologics (800–654–4432 or 603–656–9778; www.emersonecologics.com).

Yun Nan Bai Yao. This herbal combination is superb for stopping bleeding without causing clotting or disrupting circulation. Available from Quality Life Herbs (207–842–4929; www.qualitylifeherbs.com).

See chapter 5 Resources for information on formulary pharmacies.

Prepare for Surgery

Note: Avoid taking vitamin E for two weeks preoperatively and one week postoperatively. It may enhance bleeding.

Successful surgery. Guided-imagery audio program by Belleruth Naparstek. Available from Health Journeys (800–800–8661 or 330–633–3831; www.healthjourneys.com).

A two-tape set designed to help the listener imagine a successful surgery experience, surrounded by protection and support, with the body cooperating fully by slowing down blood flow and speeding up its mending capacity. Side B has affirmations. Tape 2 has continuous music to be taken into the operating room (the same music that underscores the imagery on Tape 1). This was the title that was studied so successfully at the Cleveland Clinic, Kaiser Permanente, and University of California at Davis Medical Center.

Prepare for Surgery, Heal Faster. Book and relaxation/healing audio program by Peggy Huddleston (800–726–4173 or 303–487–4440;

www.healfaster.com), available separately or as a combination. I found Peggy Huddleston's book very beneficial in my own recovery from surgery. Her work has helped thousands of others as well.

Urological Problems

Estriol vaginal cream is available by prescription from any formulary pharmacy that carries bioidentical hormones. If your doctor isn't familiar with one of these, have her or him call a formulary pharmacy where the pharmacists specialize in individualized hormone replacement. Usual strength is 0.5 mg/g.

Probiotics. To treat recurrent vaginal yeast infections, I recommend **PB 8 Probiotic** by Nutrition Now, as well as **Gastro Flora,** manufactured by Nutricology. (See chapter 7 Resources for more information.)

Uterine Prolapse
Inlet Medical, Inc. (800–969–0269 or 952–942–5034; www.inletmedical.org) can assist you in finding a physician who performs uterine repositioning/suspension.

Vaginal Weights/Pessaries
FemTone Weights and FPI (Feminine Personal Trainer) Vaginal Weight. Both available from As We Change (800–203–5585 or 619–213–2200; www.aswechange.com).

Educational Resources
National Association for Continence (formerly Help for Incontinent People) (800–252–3337 or 843–377–0900; www.nafc.org)

National Institute on Aging, NIA Information Center (800–222–2225 or 301–496–1752; www.nih.gov/nia)

National Kidney and Urologic Diseases Information Clearinghouse (800–891–5390; www.niddk.nih.gov)

Chapter 9: Sex and Menopause

Vaginal Lubricants

Crème de la Femme. This all-natural, nonhormonal vaginal lubricant is made entirely with pure botanicals. It contains no irritating alcohol dyes or glycerine (sugars), so it's even safe for diabetics. Available through www.drnorthrup.com.

See chapter 4 Resources for information on hormone testing laboratories.

Chapter 10: Nurturing Your Brain

See chapter 3 Resources for information on feng shui, and chapter 6 Resources for information on herbs.

Insomnia

Melatonin appears to regulate sleep/wake cycles, and supplements can thereby help the body adjust to different time zones. Usual dosage: 1–3 mg. I recommend **Time Release Melatonin** by Nutricology, available from Emerson Ecologics (800–654–4432 or 603–656–9778; www.emerson ecologics.com).

Valerian (*Valeriana officinalis*). Nature's Way Valerian Root is available from Emerson Ecologics (800–654–4432 or 603–656–9778; www.emersonecologics.com). Recommended dosage is 15–300 mg (standardized to 0.8 percent valerenic acid) at bedtime.

Babuna and amantilla tinctures from NutraMedix (800–730–3130 or 561–745–2917; www.nutramedix.net).

NutraMedix specializes in high-quality Peruvian botanicals. The specially designed extraction process the company uses results in highly bioavailable, whole-herb, broad-spectrum extracts that give excellent results.

Headaches and Menstrual Migraines

See chapter 6 Resources.

Seasonal Affective Disorder/Light Therapy

Women with SAD are often helped by light therapy. Full-spectrum lighting can also help PMS, perimenopausal symptoms, and ovulatory and other menstrual cycle disturbances. It can also increase serotonin levels.

Light for Health (800–468–1104 or 303–823–0274; www.lightforhealth.com)

Light for Health manufactures high-quality full-spectrum lighting in the form of UL-approved light boxes, fluorescent tubes, and compact fluorescents. The company's Indoor Sunshine lights are made with the highest quality mix of phosphors to produce a light that has the beneficial red, orange, yellow, green, blue, violet, and even trace ultraviolet A & B balanced to emit light like natural sunshine. Light for Health's BlueStar Lights work faster, allowing users to raise their serotonin levels in fifteen to twenty minutes.

Chromalux lightbulbs, though not truly full-spectrum, are color-corrected, so they are far superior to conventional lightbulbs. Chromalux bulbs are widely available in natural food stores and on the Internet.

Supplements for Brain Support

5-HTP is a precursor to serotonin, a neurohormone needed for melatonin production, appetite regulation, and mood regulation. 5-HTP is a natural product extracted from the seeds of *Griffonia simplicifolia,* unlike tryptophan supplements, which are produced synthetically or through bacterial fermentation. Recommended dose is 100–200 mg three times per day. Nature's Way Enteric-coated 5-HTP is available from Emerson Ecologics (800–654–4432 or 603–656–9778; www.emersonecologics.com). Also available from Enzymatic Therapy (as Calming Sleep) (800–783–2286 or 920–469–1313; www.enzy.com), Web Vitamins (800–919–9122 or 860–627–6627; www.webvitamins.com), or Solgar Vitamin & Herb Co. (877–765–4274 or 201–944–2311; www.solgar.com).

Chai Hu Long Gu Mu Li Wan. According to Traditional Chinese Medicine (TCM), most menopausal problems are due to liver and kidney *yin* deficiency, so strengthening energy in these organs will eliminate imbalances. This combination moves the liver *chi* and sedates the spirit. It is helpful for moodiness, emotional instability, outbursts of anger, and feelings of frustration. It is also beneficial for insomnia. It can be taken indefinitely and is commonly used by the general population in China, not just menopausal women. Available from Quality Life Herbs (207–842–4929; www.qualitylifeherbs.com).

DHA (docosahexænoic acid). See chapter 7 Resources for more information.

Ginkgo biloba is widely used to enhance memory and concentration, as well as to treat peripheral artery narrowing. I recommend **Ginkgo-PS** from USANA (888–950–9595 or 905–264–9863; www.usana.com) and Nature's Way Ginkgo biloba, available through natural food stores or Emerson Ecologics (800–654–4432 or 603–656–9778; www.emersonecologics.com). Recommended dosage is 40 mg three times per day.

Saint-John's-wort (0.3 percent hypericin). More than twenty double-blind clinical studies have shown that Saint-John's-wort is as effective as standard antidepressants at relieving symptoms of depression, but is much better tolerated and has fewer side effects. The herb's active ingredients are hypericin and hyperforin, which increase levels of brain neurotransmitters that maintain normal mood and emotional stability. **Hi Potency St.-John's-Wort** by Verified Quality is standardized to 3 percent hypericin and 3 percent hyperforin. Available from Emerson Ecologics (800–654–4432 or 603–656–9778; www.emersonecologics.com), and in health food stores. Take 300 mg three times per day, or as directed.

Inositol. Many studies indicate a therapeutic dose of 12 g per day. It's best to take it with food. I recommend **Inositol Powder,** manufactured by Verified Quality, a mildly sweet substance that dissolves instantly in water. Available from Emerson Ecologics (800–654–4432 or 603–656–9778; www.emer-sonecologics.com).

Pregnenolone is a precursor to DHEA and also to progesterone. Recommended starting dose is 10–50 mg per day, but it has been safely used in doses as high as 100–200 mg per day. Start low and gradually increase if needed. Douglas Laboratories' Pregnenolone (sublingual 5-mg tablets) is available from Emerson Ecologics (800–654–4432 or 603–656–9778; www.emersonecologics.com).

Proanthocyanidins. See chapter 7 Resources for more information.

SAM-e (S-adenosyl-L-methionine) is indicated for mood and emotional well-being, as well as joint health, mobility, and comfort. Also boosts antioxidant activity and supports immune function. The optimal dose for most people and conditions is 800–1,600 mg per day. Proper dosage is essential for optimal results. SAM-e by Nutricology is available from Emerson Ecologics (800–654–4432 or 603–656–9778; www.emersonecologics.com). Also widely available at natural food stores and in pharmacies.

Mercury-Free Fish Oil Supplements

BiOmega-3 contains both DNA and EPA derived from cold water fish oil. Available through USANA (888–950–9595 or 905–264–9863; www.usana.com).

Vital Choice Alaskan Sockeye Salmon Oil (800–608–4825 or 360–293–9525; www.vitalchoice.com). Wild salmon is preferable to farmed fish because it's much healthier and safer. Vital Choice is a particularly good source of wild salmon and wild salmon oil (in 1,000 mg softgels that provide 260 mg of total omega-3 fatty acids, including 150 mg of EPA and DHA).

Chapter 11: From Rosebud to Rose Hip

1. Skin Care

Sensé
USANA Health Sciences, Inc.
(888–950–9595 or 905–264–9863; www.usana.com)
This full skin-care line contains a wide range of highly effective antioxidants, including coenzyme Q_{10}, Proflavenol-T (a powerful cyanadin antioxidant), a lipid-soluble vitamin C known as Proteo-C (which helps build collagen), and vitamin A—along with a unique liposomal system to deliver those antioxidants to skin cells. The products have also been formulated so they don't cause irritation, even in those with sensitive skin. The Sensé line contains plant oils (calendula, orange peel, and ginseng) and fat-soluble

forms of oligomeric proanthocyanidins (OPCs) and proline, both of which have been shown to help thicken collagen. In addition, the Sensé products contain boron nitrate, which gives skin a healthy glow. Malic, lactic, and glycolic acids give the beauty serum exfoliating properties as well. All ingredients are present in sufficient concentrations to be effective. Clinical studies have shown that Sensé significantly increases the moisture content of skin and decreases wrinkles and fine lines. The Sensé products (all paraben-free) are also the only self-preserving skin care product line on the market. They contain *no* parabens or other preservatives. I've seen very impressive results with this line. To sample the products, order a Prelude pack.

Trienelle
Aspen Benefits Group
(800–539–5195 or 208–292–2400; www.trienelle.com)

Trienelle products are rich in the vitamin E complex, especially the tocotrienols, as well as a wide variety of other skin-specific antioxidants such as coenzyme Q_{10}, AHAs, procyanidins, and a clinically proven collagen-supporting ingredient known as microcollagen pentapeptides. In addition, Trienelle contains fruit acids and green apple extract. All the ingredients are present in the amounts that are clinically effective. Trienelle also contains a very high quality sunscreen and is nonirritating, making it ideal for daily use. I've personally been very impressed with this line, which includes **Daily Renewal Crème, Nightly Restoration Formula, Eye Reviving Gel,** and several other excellent products, including their **Acne Treatment Kit.**

Internal Hair and Skin Care

USANA Health Pak 100 or USANA Essentials
(888–950–9595 or 905–264–9863; www.usana.com)

Shou Wu Pian, a Chinese herbal supplement for hair growth, is available from Quality Life Herbs (207–842–4929; www.qualitylifeherbs.com). It works for both male and female hair loss.

Surgery

See chapter 8 Resources for information on preparing for surgery.

Chapter 12: Standing Tall for Life

Urine Bone Density Testing

Bone Resorption Assessment from Genova Diagnostics (800–522–4762 or 828–253–0621; www.gsdl.com) determines the rate at which you are excreting bone breakdown products and, hence, losing bone (available with a doctor's prescription).

Osteomark is marketed directly to doctors and is available through their offices.

Supplements for Bone Health

CALCIUM/MAGNESIUM SUPPLEMENTS
Calcium Complex, manufactured by Nature's Way, offers calcium and magnesium in a 1:1 ratio, and also contains boron and vitamin K. Recommended dose of Calcium Complex is three capsules, twice per day. Available from Emerson Ecologics (800–654–4432 or 603–656–9778; www.emersonecologics.com).
USANA's **Active Calcium** and **Active Calcium Chewables (Body Rox)** contain calcium as citrate and carbonate; magnesium as citrate, amino acid chelate, and oxide; vitamin D3, boron citrate, and silicon. Available through USANA (888–950–9595 or 905–264–9863; www.usana.com).

HERBAL INFUSIONS
Organically grown herbs are available from the following suppliers.

Avena Botanicals
(866–282–8362 or 207–594–0694; www.avenabotanicals.com)
    For dried organic herbs in 3-oz size.

Blessed Herbs
(800–489–4372; www.blessedherbs.com)
    For bulk herb sales.

VITAMIN D
Vitamin D supplementation can be important for women who spend little time outdoors, as well as those whose diets do not contain significant vitamin D.

Vitamin D from Verified Quality supplies 400 IU vitamin D3 per capsule. Available from Emerson Ecologics (800–654–4432 or 603–656–9778; www.emersonecologics.com).

Cod liver oil contains vitamins A and D, EPA (eicosaspentænoic acid), and DHA (docosahexænoic acid). Its cardiovascular benefits include lowering blood pressure, decreasing triglycerides, and reducing angina. **Norwegian Cod Liver Oil** provides 1,250 IU vitamin A, 130 IU vitamin D, 33–41 mg EPA, and 34–42 DHA per gelcap. Available from Emerson Ecologics (800–654–4432 or 603–656–9778; www.emersonecologics.com).

ADDITIONAL MUSCULOSKELETAL SUPPORT

Procosa II. This product from USANA (888–950–9595 or 905–264–9863; www.usana.com) contains 500 mg glucosamine sulfate and 125 mg turmeric extract per tablet, as well as vitamin C and manganese. Usual dose: two tablets daily.

Joint Synergy+, by Metabolic Response Modifiers, is a combination product containing 250 mg glucosamine per capsule, with chondroitin, collagen manganese, bromelain, MSM, ginseng, white willow, and turmeric, among other factors. Usual dose: four tablets daily. Available from Emerson Ecologics (800–654–4432 or 603–656–9778; www.emersonecologics.com). **Osteoking** is a 100 percent natural formula derived from Traditional Chinese Medicine (TCM) that is designed to optimize bone health. It comes in liquid form and includes a combination of six herbs. Available from Nature's Healing Solutions (800–550–9285; www.osteoking.com).

I also recommend **turmeric, ginger,** and **green tea** extracts by Nature's Way, available from Emerson Ecologics (800–654–4432 or 603–656–9778; www.emersonecologics.com).

Proanthocyanidins. See chapter 7 Resources for more information.

Strength Training

Strong Women Stay Young
Videotape program and books by Miriam Nelson, Ph.D. (800–203–5585 or 619–213–2200; www.strongwomen.com).

Pilates
For more information on finding a certified instructor or a training program in your area, or on obtaining Pilates method materials, visit the Pilates website at www.pilates-studio.com.

The Firm
(800–613–0414; www.firmdirect.com)
Videotape programs on aerobic workouts with weights. I personally used *The Firm* workouts with weights for nearly ten years. I consider these the most effective weight workouts available on video.

Chapter 13: Creating Breast Health

See chapter 8 Resources for more information on where to obtain supplies for castor oil packs.

Breast Cancer Information and Treatment

Voell, J., and Chatfield, C. (2005). *The Cancer Report: The Latest Research in Psychoneuroimmunology (How Thousands Are Achieving Permanent*

Recoveries). Naples, FL: Change Your World Press. (For more information on this research, visit www.cancer-report.com.)

National Cancer Institute Cancer Information Service
(1–800–4–CANCER; www.cancer.gov)
Call this number to request information about genetic counseling and testing services at cancer centers supported by the institute.

Sanoviv Medical Institute
(800–726–6848 or 801–954–7600; www.sanoviv.com)
This fully licensed medical facility along the Baja Coast of Mexico (about an hour from San Diego) combines both traditional and complementary medical practices to treat the whole person, addressing physical, mental, and spiritual health. It offers everything from surgery to spa facilities. Although Sanoviv helps cancer patients, it also treats those with autoimmune diseases, including lupus, multiple sclerosis, diabetes, chronic fatigue, and neurodegenerative diseases such as Parkinson's and Alzheimer's.

Dixie Mills, M.D. (www.drdixiemills.com). Breast health expert Dr. Mills maintains an excellent website that includes information on breast health, including *Honoring Our Breasts,* her guided self-exam on CD (with music).

Lymphedema

National Lymphedema Network
(800–541–3259 or 510–208–3200; www.lymphnet.org)
An internationally recognized, nonprofit information and networking organization to help those with lymphedema, either primary (the kind one is born with) or secondary (the kind one gets after an operation or injury, notably mastectomy and lymph node dissection). They provide referrals and educational courses for health care professionals and patients, publish a very helpful quarterly newsletter, host a biennial national conference on lymphedema, and maintain an extensive computer database.

Supplements for Breast Health

Coenzyme Q$_{10}$. See chapter 7 Resources for more information.

Flaxseed. See chapter 6 Resources for more information.

Revival Soy. See chapter 6 Resources for more information.

Chapter 14: Living with Heart, Passion, and Joy

Depression

See chapter 10 Resources for more information.

Forgiveness

See chapter 2 Resources for more information.

Transdermal Magnesium

Biogenics Magnesium Lotion
(888–242–6105 or 417–267–2900; www.normshealy.com)
The magnesium in this product, developed by holistic health pioneer Norm Shealy, M.D., Ph.D., is well absorbed through the skin. Dr. Shealy is the founder of The Shealy Institute, the first comprehensive pain and stress management facility in the U.S.

Supplements for Heart Health

Many of the sources for dietary supplements recommended for heart health are detailed in chapter 7 Resources.

Cod liver oil. See chapter 12 Resources for more information.

Garlic. Garlic EC from USANA (888–950–9595 or 905–264–9863; or www.usana.com) contains 650 mg garlic powder per tablet, standardized to yield 6,000 mcg allicin. **Garlicin,** manufactured by Nature's Way, contains at least 300 mg of high-potency dried garlic, providing release of at least 2,500 mcg of allicin per tablet. Garlicin is available from Emerson Ecologics (800–654–4432 or 603–656–9778; www.emersonecologics.com).

Hawthorn (*Crataegus* spp.). Widely available in health food stores as berries for tea infusions. Also available in pill form. If you prefer to take this in pill form, look for a standardized extract, a product that contains 10 percent procyanidins or 1.8 percent vitexin-4"-rhamnoside. Take 100–250 mg three times per day. Nature's Way and Enzymatic Therapy are reliable brands. **HeartCare,** manufactured by Nature's Way, is available from Emerson Ecologics (800–654–4432 or 603–656–9778; www.emersonecologics.com). To order hawthorn from Enzymatic Therapy, contact Enzymatic Therapy (800–783–2286 or 920–469–1313; www.enzy.com).

Proanthocyanidins. See chapter 7 Resources for more information.

Vitamin C. See chapter 7 Resources for more information.

Vitamin E consists of several fractions, including alpha, beta, delta, and gamma tocopherols, plus alpha, delta, and gamma tocotrienols. USANA's **E-Prime** (888–950–9595 or 905–264–9863; www.usana.com) provides a full spectrum of tocopherols and tocotrienols from natural sources. **Care Diem,** manufactured by Aspen Benefits Group, delivers 100 mg Nutriene, a 30 percent tocotrienol/tocopherol natural complex derived from rice bran oil. Care Diem is available from Emerson Ecologics (800–654–4432 or 603–656–9778; www.emersonecologics.com).

Notes

Chapter 1: Menopause Puts Your Life Under a Microscope

1. Sams, J., & Carson, D. (1988). *Medicine Cards* (p 150). Santa Fe: Bear & Co.

Chapter 2: The Brain Catches Fire at Menopause

1. Seymour, L. J. (ed.) (April 1999). News from Redbook. *Redbook, 16.*
2. Oren, D. A., et al. (April 2002). An open trial of morning light therapy for treatment of antepartum depression. *Am J of Psychiatry, 159* (4), 666–669.
3. Larsson, C., & Hallman, J. (1997). Is severity of premenstrual symptoms related to illness in the climacteric? *J Psychosomatic Obstetrics & Gynecology, 18,* 234–243; Novaes, C., & Almeida, O. P. (1999). Premenstrual syndrome and psychiatric morbidity at the menopause. *J Psychosomatic Obstetrics & Gynecology, 20,* 56–57; Arpels, J. C. (1996). The female brain hypoestrogenic continuum from PMS to menopause: A hypothesis and review of supporting data. *J Reproductive Medicine, 41* (9), 633–639.
4. Schmidt, P., et al. (1998). Differential behavioral effects of gonadal steroids in women with and in those without premenstrual syndrome. *NEJM, 338* (4), 209–216.
5. Larsson, C., & Hallman, J. (1997). Is severity of premenstrual symptoms related to illness in the climacteric? *J Psychosomatic Obstetrics & Gynecology, 18,* 234–243; Novaes, C., & Almeida, O. P. (1999). Premenstrual syndrome and psychiatric morbidity at the menopause. *J Psychosomatic Obstetrics & Gynecology, 20,* 56–57.

6. Benedek, T., & Rubenstein, B. (1939). Correlations between ovarian activity and psychodynamic processes: The ovulatory phase. *Psychosomatic Medicine, 1* (2), 245–270.

7. Weitoft, G. R., et al. (2000). Mortality among lone mothers in Sweden: A population study. *Lancet, 355,* 1215–1219.

8. Taylor, S. E., et al. (October 2002). Biobehavioral responses to stress in females: Tend-and-befriend, not fight-or-flight. *Psychol Rev, 109* (4), 745–50.

9. Herzog, A. (1997). Neuroendocrinology of epilepsy. In S. C. Schacter & O. Devinsky (eds.), *Behavioral Neurology and the Legacy of Norman Geschwind,* 235–236. Philadelphia: Lippincott, Williams & Wilkins; Moyer, K. E. (1976). *The Psychology of Aggression.* New York: Harper & Row; Albert, I., et al. (1987). Inter-male social aggression in rats: Suppression by medical hypothalamic lesions independently of enhanced defensiveness of decreased testicular testosterone. *Physiology & Behavior, 39,* 693–698; Post, R. M. (1992). Transduction of psychosocial stress into the neurobiology of recurrent affective disorder. *Am J Psychiatry, 149,* 999–1010.

10. Linehan, M. (1993). *Skills Training Manual for Treating Borderline Personality Disorder,* 143. New York: Guilford Press.

11. Herzog, A. G. (1989). Perimenopausal depression: Possible role of anomalous brain substrates. *Brain Dysfunction, 2,* 146–154.

12. Ledoux, J. E. (1986). Sensory systems and emotions: A model of affective processing. *Integrative Psychiatry, 4,* 237–243. For a complete scientific discussion of this area, see Schulz, M. L. (1998). *Awakening Intuition,* 113–135. New York: Harmony.

13. Musante, L., et al. (1989). Potential for hostility and dimensions of anger. *Health Psychology, 8,* 343; Mittleman, M. A., et al. (1995). Triggering of acute MI onset of episodes of anger. *Circulation, 92,* 1720–1725. For an exhaustive listing of the scientific studies documenting the emotional risk factors for heart attack, see Schulz, M. L., op. cit. (chapter 9, 216–250).

14. Porges, S., et al. (1996). Infant regulation of the vagal "brake" predicts child behavior problems: A psychobiological model of social behavior. *Developmental Psychobiology, 29* (8), 697–712; Porges, S. (1992). Vagal tone: A physiological market of stress vulnerability. *Pediatrics, 90,* 498–504; Donchin, Y., et al. (1992). Cardiac vagal tone predicts outcome in neurosurgical patients. *Critical Care Medicine, 20,* 941–949.

15. Heim, C., et al. (2000). Pituitary-adrenal and autonomic responses to stress in women after sexual and physical abuse in childhood, *JAMA, 284* (5), 592–596.

16. Lipton, B. (2005). *The Biology of Belief.* Santa Rosa, CA: Elite Books.

17. Schulz, M. L., M.D., Ph.D., behavioral neuroscientist and neuropsychiatrist (personal communication, March 20, 2000).

18. Van Der Kolk, B. A. (1996). The body keeps the score: Approaches to the psychobiology of posttraumatic stress disorder. In *Traumatic Stress: The Effects of Overwhelming Experience on Mind, Body, and Society.* New York: Guilford Press.

19. Clow, B. H. (1996). *The Liquid Light of Sex: Kundalini Rising at Mid-Life Crisis*. Berkeley, CA: Bear & Co. This book comes complete with charts that allow the reader to determine exactly when their key life passages will or have happened, thus allowing one to take full advantage of what might otherwise be considered a crisis without meaning.

Chapter 3: Coming Home to Yourself:
From Dependence to Healthy Autonomy

1. I originally learned to do this through a process called Proprioceptive Writing, taught by Linda Metcalf and Tobin Simon. (See Resources.)
2. Brody, E. M. (1989). *Family at Risk in Alzheimer's Disease*, 2–49. DHHS Publication no. 89–1569. Bethesda, MD: National Institute of Mental Health.
3. The research of Julie Brines, a sociologist at the University of Washington who studies so-called status-reversal couples, was covered in "Excuse Me, I'm the Breadwinner." *Money for Women Magazine* (May–June 2000), 16–17.

   Here is the data: Men whose wives earn all of the family cash spend four fewer hours a week on housework on average than do men who make just as much as their partners. When the husband works and his wife stays home, the husband spends three hours per week on housework versus his wife's twenty-five hours. When both husband and wife work and earn equal amounts, the husband does nine hours of housework per week and his wife does seventeen hours. But when the wife works and the husband stays home, the husband spends only five hours per week on housework, while his wife spends sixteen hours per week.

Chapter 4: This Can't Be Menopause, Can It?
The Physical Foundation of the Change

1. Randolph, J., & Sowers, M. F. (1999). Research on perimenopausal changes in 500 Michigan women, reported in *Midlife Women's Health Sourcebook*. Atlanta, GA: American Health Consultants.
2. McKinlay, S. M., et al. (1992). The normal menopause transition. *Maturitas, 14*, 103; Treloar, A. E., et al. (1981). Menstrual cyclicity and the perimenopause. *Maturitas, 3*, 249.
3. Munster, K., et al. (1992). Length and variation in the menstrual cycle—a cross-sectional study from a Danish county. *British J Obstetrics & Gynecology, 99* (5), 422; Collett, M. E., et al. (1954). The effect of age upon the pattern of the menstrual cycle. *Fertility & Sterility, 5*, 437.
4. Rannevik, G. (1995). A longitudinal study of the perimenopausal transition: Altered profiles of steroid and pituitary hormones, SHBG and bone mineral density. *Maturitas, 21*, 103.
5. Coulam, C. B., Adamson, S. C., & Annegers, J. F. (1986). Incidence of premature ovarian failure. *Am J Obstetrics & Gynecology, 67* (4), 604–606;

Miyake, T., et al. (1988). Acute oocyte loss in experimental autoimmune oophoritis as a possible model of premature ovarian failure. *Am J Obstetrics & Gynecology, 158* (1), 186–192; Coulam, C. B. (1982). Premature gonadal failure. *Fertility & Sterility, 38,* 645; Gloor, H. J. (1984). Autoimmune oophoritis. *Am J Clinical Pathology, 81,* 105–109; Leer, M., Patel, B., Innes, M., et al. (1980). Secondary amenorrhea due to autoimmune ovarian failure. *Australian, New Zealand J Obstetrics & Gynecology, 20,* 177–179; International Medical News Service (November 1985). Evidence of autoimmune etiology in some premature menopause. *OB-GYN News, 20* (21), 1, 30.

6. Sumiala, S., et al. (1996). Salivary progesterone concentrations after tubal sterilization. *Obstetrics & Gynecology, 88,* 792–796.

7. Aksel, S., et al. (1976). Vasomotor symptoms, serum estrogens and gonadotropin levels in surgical menopause. *Am J Obstetrics & Gynecology, 126,* 165–169. Judd, H. L., & Meldrum, D. R. (1981). Physiology and pathophysiology of menstruation and menopause. In S. L. Romney, M. J. Gray, & A. B. Little, et al. (eds.), *Gynecology and Obstetrics: The Health Care of Women.* (2nd ed., 885–907). New York: McGraw-Hill.

8. Saliva as a Diagnostic Fluid (September 20, 1993). Proceedings of the New York Academy of Sciences, *694,* 1–348; Lawrence, H. P. (March 2002). Salivary markers of systemic disease: noninvasive diagnosis of disease and monitoring of general health. *J Can Dent Assoc., 68* (3), 170–4; Vining, R. F., and McGinley, R. A. (1987). The measurement of hormones in saliva: Possibilities and pitfalls. *J Steroid Biochem, 27* (1–3), 81–94; Boothby, L. A., Doering, P. L., and Kipersztok, S. (May–June 2004). Bioidentical hormone therapy: A review. *Menopause, 11* (3), 356–67; Rakel, D. (ed.), (2003). *Integrative Medicine.* Philadelphia: Saunders.

9. Massoudi, M. S., et al. (1995). Prevalence of thyroid antibodies among healthy middle-aged women. Findings from the thyroid study in healthy women. *Annals of Epidemiology, 5* (3), 229–233.

10. Jefferies, W. McK. (1996). *The Safe Uses of Cortisone.* Springfield, IL: Charles C. Thomas.

11. Guthrie, J., et al. (1996). Hot flushes, menstrual status, and hormone levels in a population-based sample of midlife women. *Obstetrics & Gynecology, 88,* 437–442.

12. Leonetti, H., et al. (1999). Transdermal progesterone cream for vasomotor symptoms and postmenopausal bone loss. *Obstetrics & Gynecology, 94,* 227–228.

13. Freedman, R. R., & Woodward, S. (1992). Behavioral treatment of menopausal hot flashes: Evaluation by ambulatory monitoring. *Am J Obstetrics & Gynecology, 167,* 436–439; Stevenson, D. W., & Delprato, D. J. (1983). Multiple component self-control program for menopausal hot flashes. *J Behavioral Therapy & Experimental Psychology, 14* (2), 137–140; Domar, A. D., & Dreher, H. (1997). *Healing Mind, Healthy Woman,* 291–292. New York: Delta.

Chapter 5: Hormone Replacement: An Individual Choice

1. Writing Group for the Women's Health Initiative Investigators (2002). Risks and benefits of estrogen plus progestin in healthy postmenopausal women: Principal result from the Women's Health Initiative randomized controlled trial. *JAMA, 288,* 327–333.
2. Lacey, J. V., et al. (2002). Menopausal hormone replacement therapy and risk of ovarian cancer. *JAMA, 288,* 334–341.
3. Grodstein, F., Manson, J. E., Stampfer, M. J. (Jan./Feb. 2006). Hormone therapy and coronary heart disease: The role of time since menopause and age at hormone initiation. *J Womens Health (Larchmt), 15* (1), 35–44.
4. Shen, L., Qiu, S., Chen, Y., Zhang, F., van Breemen, R. B., Nikolic, D., & Bolton, J. L. (1998). Alkylation of 2'-deoxynucleosides and DNA by the Premarin metabolite 4-hydroxyequilenin semiquinone radical. *Chemical Research in Toxicology, 11,* 94–101; Bhavnani, B. (1998). Pharmacokinetics and pharmacodynamics of conjugated equine estrogens: Chemistry and metabolism. *Proceedings of the Society for Biological Medicine, 217* (1), 6–16; Zhang, F., et al. (1999). The major metabolite of equilin, 4-hydroxyequilin, autoxidizes to an σ-quinone which isomerizes to the potent cytotoxin 4-hydroxyequilenin-σ-quinone. *Chemical Research in Toxicology, 12,* 204–213.
5. Cole, W., et al. (June 26, 1995). The estrogen dilemma, *Time,* 46–53 (cover story).
6. Brody, J. (September 3, 2002). Sorting through the confusion about hormone replacemnt therapy. *New York Times.*
7. Shaak, C. (in press). Restoration of early luteal phase hormone levels in menopausal women by transdermal application of progesterone, estradiol, and testosterone. *Note:* Dr. Shaak's study used the following patented formulation of bioidentical hormones, known as TransproET: 150 mg progesterone, 0.5 mg estradiol, and 0.5 mg of testosterone per cc of cream. Patients were instructed to use some portion of a teaspoon of cream (⅛–¼ tsp), usually twice daily, depending upon their baseline endogenous hormone levels. For further information, write to Dr. Shaak at WomanWell, 405 Great Plain Avenue, Needham, MA 02492. Tel.: 781–453–0321; Hargrove, J., et al. (1998). Absorption of estradiol and progesterone delivered via Jergens lotion used as hormone replacement therapy. Poster session presented at the annual meeting of the North American Menopause Society, Philadelphia.
8. Hargrove, J. T., & Beckum, J. (September 1999). Utility of estradiol and progesterone suspended in propylene glycol and administered by the drop for more accurate individualization of HRT. Presented at the annual meeting of the North American Menopause Society, New York.
9. Follingstad, A. (1978). Estriol, the forgotten hormone. *JAMA, 239* (1), 29–39; Lemon, H. (1977). Clinical and experimental aspects of the anti-mammary carcinogenic activity of estriol. *Frontiers of Hormonal Research, 5* (1), 155–173; Lemon, H. (1975). Estriol prevention of mammary carci-

noma induced by 7, 12-dimethylbenzathracene and procarbazine. *Cancer Research, 35,* 1341–1353; Lemon, H. (1973). Oestriol and prevention of breast cancer. *Lancet, 1* (802), 546–547; Lemon, H. (1980). Pathophysiologic considerations in the treatment of menopausal patients with oestrogens: The role of oestriol in the prevention of mammary cancer. *Acta Endocrinologica, 233, suppl.,* 17–27; Lemon, H., Wotiz, H., Parsons, L., et al. (1966). Reduced estriol excretion in patients with breast cancer prior to endocrine therapy. *JAMA, 196,* 1128–1136.

10. Heimer, G. M., & Englund, D. E. (1992). Effects of vaginally administered oestriol on postmenopausal urogenital disorders: A cytohormonal study. *Maturitas, 3,* 171–179; Iosif, C. S. (1992). Effects of protracted administration of estriol on the lower urinary tract in postmenopausal women. *Archives of Gynecology and Obstetrics, 3* (251), 115–120; Kirkengen, A. L., Andersen, P., Gjersoe, E., et al. (June 1992). Oestriol in the prophylactic treatment of recurrent urinary tract infections in postmenopausal women. *Scandinavian Journal of Primary Health Care,* 139–142; Raz, K., & Stamm, W. (1993). A controlled trial of intravaginal estriol in postmenopausal women with recurrent urinary tract infections. *NEJM, 329,* 753–756.

11. The American College of Obstetricians and Gynecologists. (Oct 1, 2004). Cognition and dementia. *Obstetrics and Gynecology, 104* (suppl. 4), 25S–40S.

12. Speroff, L., et al. (1999). *Clinical Gynecologic Endocrinology and Infertility* (6th ed., 56–64). Philadelphia, PA: Lippincott, Williams & Wilkins.

13. Speroff, L. (September 1999). Commentary: Postmenopausal therapy reduces the risk of colorectal cancer. *OB/GYN Alert,* 35.

14. Love, R. R., Cameron, L., Connell, B. L. (1991). Symptoms associated with tamoxifen treatment in postmenopausal women. *Arch Intern Med 151,* 1842–1847.

15. Zimniski, S. J., et al. (1993). Induction of tamoxifen-dependent rat mammary tumors. *Cancer Res, 53,* 2937–2939; Powell-Jones, W., et al. (1975). Influence of anti-oestrogens on the specific binding in vitro of (3H)oestradiol by cytosol of rat mammary tumors and human breast carcinomata. *Biochem J, 150,* 71–75; Vancutsem, P. M., et al. (1994). Frequent and specific mutations of the rat p53 gene in eptocarcinomas induced by tamoxifen. *Cancer Res, 54,* 3864–3867; Shuibutani, S., et al. (1997). Mis-coding potential of tamoxifen-derived DNA adducts: Alpha-(N2-deoxyguanosinyl) tamoxifen. *Biochem, 36,* 13010–13017; Simon, R. (1995). Discovering the truth about tamoxifen: Problems of multiplicity in statistical evaluation of biomedical data. *J Natl Cancer Inst, 87,* 627–629.

16. Koenig, H., et al. (1995). Progesterone synthesis and myelin formation by Schwann cells. *Science, 268,* 1500–1503.

17. When I was a resident in OB/GYN at St. Margaret's Hospital in Boston in the mid-1970s, I routinely saw women in their late thirties and forties who had a number of children and continued to get pregnant year after year, until they welcomed a hysterectomy as a way to avoid further pregnancies. Their lives, beliefs, and biology stand in sharp contrast to today's thirty-six-year-old professional woman who started worrying that she wouldn't be

able to get pregnant as soon as she turned thirty-five. Our beliefs have subtle yet powerful effects on our biology—effects that are confirmed by research. Brant Secunda is an American-born shaman who was trained by the Huichol Indians, who live in a remote region of Mexico. Brant reports that Huichol women routinely get pregnant in their fifties and some even in their sixties. The work of Dr. Alice Domar, of the Beth Israel Deaconess Center for Mindbody Medicine, reports a 50 percent increase in pregnancy rates in previously infertile women, most of whom are professionals in their thirties and forties, when they participate in programs characterized by group support, deep relaxation, and attention to self-care. These pregnancies become possible because of the ability of the mind and beliefs to effect hormonal levels that better favor conception.

18. Hully, S., et al. (1998). Randomized trial of estrogen plus progestin for secondary prevention of coronary heart disease in postmenopausal women. *JAMA, 280,* 605–618; Sullivan, J. M., et al. (1995). Progestin enhances vasoconstrictor responses in postmenopausal women receiving estrogen replacement therapy. *Menopause, 4,* 193–197; Williame, J. K., et al. (1994). Effects of hormone replacement therapy on reactivity of atherosclerotic coronary arteries in cynomologous monkeys. *J Am Coll Cardiol, 24,* 1757–1761; Sarrel, P. (1999). The differential effects of oestrogens and progestins on vascular tone. *Human Reproduction Update, 5* (3), 205–209.

19. Tang, G. W. K. (1994). The climacteric of Chinese factory workers. *Maturitas, 19,* 177–182.

20. Hammond, C. B. (1994). Women's concerns with hormone replacement therapy—compliance issues. *Fertility & Sterility, 62* (suppl. 2), 157S–160S.

21. The Postmenopausal Estrogen/Progestin Intervention (PEPI) trial (1995). Effects of estrogen or estrogen/progestin regimens on heart disease risk factors in postmenopausal women. *JAMA, 273,* 199–206.

22. The American College of Obstetricians and Gynecologists (Oct 1, 2004). Coronary heart disease. *Obstetrics and Gynecology, 104* (suppl. 4), 415–485.

23. Yaffe, K., Lui, L.-Y., Grady, D., Cauley, J., Kramer, J., & Cummings, S. R. (2000). Cognitive decline in women in relation to non-protein-bound estradiol concentrations. *Lancet, 356* (9231), 708–712.

24. Grodstein, F., Newcomb, P. A., & Stampfer, M. J. (1999). Postmenopausal hormone therapy and the risk of colorectal cancer: A review and meta-analysis. *Am J Medicine, 106* (5), 574–582.

25. Kolata, G. (July 9, 2002). Citing risks, U.S. will halt study of drugs for hormones. *New York Times.*

Chapter 6: Foods and Supplements to Support the Change

1. Hudson, T. (1994). A pilot study using botanical medicine in the treatment of menopausal symptoms. Portland, Oregon, National College of Naturopathic Medicine and the Bastyr University of Natural Health Sciences.

2. Tyler, V. E. (1993). *The Honest Herbal: A Sensible Guide to the Use of Herbs and Related Remedies* (3rd ed.). Binghamton, NY: Haworth Press.

3. Elghamry, M. I., & Shihata, I. M. (1965). Biological activity of phytoestrogens. *Planta Medica, 13,* 352–357.
4. Knight, D., & Eden, J. (1996). A review of the clinical effects of phytoestrogens. Part 2. *Obstetrics & Gynecology, 87* (5), 897–904; Kaldas, R. S., & Hughes, C. L. (1989). Reproductive and general metabolic effects of phytoestrogens in mammals. *Reproductive Toxicology, 3,* 81–89.
5. Rose, D. P. (1992). Dietary fiber, phytoestrogens, and breast cancer. *Nutrition, 8,* 47–51.
6. Tamaya, T., et al. (1986). Inhibition by plant herb extracts of steroid bindings in uterus, liver, and serum of the rabbit. *Acta Obstetrica Gynecologica Scandinavia, 65,* 839–842.
7. Yoshiro, K. (1985). The physiological actions of tan-kwei and cnidium. *Bull. Oriental Healing Arts Institute USA, 10,* 269–278; Harada, M., Suzuki, M., & Ozaki, Y. (1984). Effects of Japanese *Angelica* root and peony root on uterine contraction in the rabbit *in situ. J Pharmacol Dynam, 7,* 304–311; Zhu, D. P. O. (1987). Dong quai. *Am J Chinese Medicine, 15,* 117–125.
8. Bohnert, K.-J. (Spring 1997). The use of *Vitex agnus-castus* for hyperprolactinemia. *Quarterly Review of Natural Medicine,* 19–20; American Botanical Council (1992). *Kommission E monograph: Agnus casti fructus (chaste tree fruits).* Fort Worth, TX.
9. Duker, E. M., et al. (1991). Effects of extracts from *Cimicifuga racemosa* on gonadotropin release in menopausal women and ovariectomized rats. *Planta Medica, 57,* 420–424, 1991.
10. Cassidy, A., Bingham, S., & Setchell, K. (1994). Biological effects of a diet of soy protein rich in isoflavones on the menstrual cycle of premenopausal women. *Am J Clin Nutr, 60,* 333–340; Anderson, J. W., et al. (1998). Effects of soy protein on renal function and proteinuria in patients with type 2 diabetes. *Am J Clin Nutr, 68* (suppl. 6), 1347S–1353S.
11. Wong, W. W., Heird, W. C., & Smith, E. O. (April 2000). Potential health benefits of soy in postmenopausal women. Data presented at the Experimental Biology Meeting, San Diego, CA.
12. Foth, D., & Cline, J. M. (1998). Effects of mammalian and plant estrogens on mammary glands and uteri of macaques. *Am J Clin Nutr, 68* (suppl.), 1413S–1471S.
13. Scheiber, M., & Setchell, K. (June 1999). Dietary soy isoflavones favorably influence lipids and bone turnover in healthy postmenopausal women. The Endocrine Society's 81st Annual Meeting Synopsis.
14. Zhuo, X. G., Melby, M. K., and Watanabe, S. (Sept. 2004). Soy isoflavone intake lowers serum LDL cholesterol: A meta-analysis of 8 randomized controlled trials in humans. *J Nutr, 134,* 2395–2400.
15. Anderson, J. W., Johnstone, B. M., and Cook-Newell, M. E. (Aug. 3, 1995). Meta-analysis of the effects of soy protein intake on serum lipids. *N Engl J Med, 333,* (5), 276–282.
16. Hall, W. L., et al. (Dec. 2005). Soy-isoflavone-enriched foods and inflammatory biomarkers of cardiovascular disease risk in postmenopausal women: Interactions with genotype and equol production. *Am J Clin Nutr, 82* (6), 1260–1268.

17. Desrochesm, S., et al. (March 2004). Soy protein favorably affects LDL size independently of isoflavones in hypercholesterolemic men and women. *J Nutr, 134* (3), 574–579; Nagata, C., et al. (March 2003). Soy product intake is inversely associated with serum homocysteine level in premenopausal Japanese women. *J Nutr, 133* (3), 797–800.

18. Food & Drug Administration, U.S. Department of Health and Human Services (1999). FDA talk paper: FDA approves new health claim for soy protein and coronary heart disease (T99–48).

19. William, K. (Nov. 1997). Interactive effects of soy protein and estradiol on arterial pathobiology. American Heart Association annual scientific sessions, Orlando, FL.

20. Alexandersen, P., et al. (2001). Ipriflavone in the treatment of postmenopausal osteoporosis: A randomized controlled trial. *JAMA, 285* (11), 1482–1488.

21. Roudsari, A. H., et al. (Oct. 29, 2005). Assessment of soy phytoestrogens' effects on bone turnover indicators in menopausal women with osteopenia in Iran: A before and after clinical trial. *Nutrition Journal, 4*, 30.

22. Bennink, M. R., Thiagarajan, L. D., et al. (Sept. 1999). Dietary soy is associated with decreased cell proliferation rate and zone in the colon mucosa of subjects at risk for colon cancer. Presented at the American Institute for Cancer Research Meeting, as reported on Reuters Health News Service.

23. Bruce, B., Spiller, G. A., & Holloway, L. (April 15–18, 2000). Soy isoflavones do not have an anti-thyroid effect in postmenopausal women over 64 years of age. Experimental Biology, San Diego, CA. Health Research and Studies Center, Los Altos, CA 94022; Palo Alto VA Health Care System, Palo Alto, CA 94034; Duncan, A. M., et al. (1999). Soy isoflavones exert modest hormonal effects in premenopausal women. *J Clinical Endocrinology & Metabolism, 84* (1), 192–197; Duncan, A. M., et al. (1999). Modest hormonal effects of soy isoflavones in postmenopausal women. *J Clinical Endocrinology & Metabolism, 84* (10), 3479–3484.

24. Albertazzi, P., et al. (1998). The effect of dietary soy supplementation on hot flashes. *Obstetrics & Gynecology, 91,* 6–11.

25. Ibid.

26. Dupree, K., et al. (June 4–7, 2005). Effects of soy on quality of life in postmenopausal women. The Endocrine Society Annual Meeting, San Diego, CA.

27. Handayani, R., et al. (Jan. 2006). Soy isoflavones alter expression of genes associated with cancer progression, including interleukin-8, in androgen-independent pc-3 human prostate cancer cells. *J Nutr, 136* (1), 75–82; Thelen, P., et al. (Oct. 20, 2005); Pharmacological potential of phytoestrogens in the treatment of prostate cancer. *Urologe A,* [Epub ahead of print] German; Sonn, G. A., Aronson, W., and Litwin, M. S. (2005). Impact of diet on prostate cancer: A review. *Prostate Cancer Prostatic Dis, 8* (4), 304–10.

28. Aldercreutz, H., et al. (1986). Determination of urinary lignans and phytoestrogen metabolites, potential antiestrogens and anticarcinogens in urine of women on various habitual diets. *J Steroid Biochemistry, 25* (5B), 791–797.

29. Aldercreutz, H. (1984). Does fiber-rich food containing animal lignan pre-

cursors protect against both colon and breast cancer? An extension of the "fiber hypothesis." *Gastroenterology, 86* (4), 761–764; Jenab, M., et al. (1996). The influence of flaxseed and lignans on colon carcinogenesis and beta-glucuronidase activity. *Carcinogenesis, 17* (6), 1343–1348; Johnstone, P. V. (1995). Flaxseed oil and cancer: Alpha-linolenic acid and carcinogenesis. In S. C. Cunnane & L. U. Thompson (eds.), *Flaxseed in Human Nutrition.* Champaign, IL: AOCS Press; Serraino, M., et al. (1991). The effect of flaxseed supplementation on early risk markers for mammary carcinogenesis. *Cancer Letter, 60,* 135–142; Serraino, M., et al. (1992). The effect of flaxseed supplementation on the initiation and promotional stages of mammary tumorigenesis. *Nutrition & Cancer, 17,* 153–159.

30. Lampe, J. W., et al. (1994). Urinary lignan and isoflavonoid excretion in premenopausal women consuming flaxseed powder. *Am J Clin Nutr, 60,* 122–128; Mousavi, Y., et al. (1992). Enterolactone and estradiol inhibit each other's proliferative effect on MCF and breast cancer cells in culture. *J Steroid Biochemistry & Molecular Biology, 41,* 615–619.

31. Bierenbaum, M. L., et al. (1993). Reducing atherogenic risk in hyperlipemic humans with flaxseed supplementation: A preliminary report. *J Am College Nutrition, 12* (5), 501–504.

32. Middleton, E., & Kandaswami, C. (Nov. 1994). Potential health-promoting properties of citrus bioflavonoids. *Food Technology,* 115–119.

33. I am indebted to Maureen Tsao, M.Ac., and her mother, Fern Tsao, for their assistance in preparing this section on Traditional Chinese Medicine and menopause.

34. Vernejoul, P., et al. (1985). Étude des meridiens d'acupuncture par les traceurs radioactifs [The study of acupuncture meridians using radioactive tracers]. *Bulletin Académie Nationale Médicine, 169* (7), 1071–1075.

Chapter 7: The Menopause Food Plan: A Program to Balance Your Hormones and Prevent Middle-Age Spread

1. Fine, J. T., Colditz, G. A., Coakley, E. H., Moseley, G., Manson, J. E., Willett, W. C., & Kawachi, I. (1999). A prospective study of weight change and health-related quality of life in women. *JAMA, 282,* 2136–2142.

2. *Dr. Atkins' New Diet Revolution* was the number-one best-selling diet book of the late 1990s. The research supporting the book is sound, though controversial.

3. A clinical study of the Atkins diet presented at the Southern Society of General Internal Medicine in New Orleans (1999) by lead researcher Dr. Eric Westman, assistant professor of medicine at North Carolina's Duke University, failed to show any adverse effects on kidney and liver function in the forty-one mildly obese study subjects who limited their carbohydrate intake to less than 20 g per day. They also took a multivitamin-mineral and fish oil supplement and exercised three times per week. The Durham study lasted for four months and test subjects dropped an average of twenty-one pounds each. Cholesterol levels dropped 6.1 percent and triglycerides dropped by 40 percent, while protective HDL cholesterol levels increased

by about 7 percent. Blood pressure and body composition also underwent favorable changes. The results of the Durham study were supported in a second, larger study of 319 overweight or obese patients conducted over a period of one year at the Atkins Center for Complementary Medicine in New York City. Results were similar, laying to rest any safety concerns. Under many perimenopausal conditions, however, even the Atkins diet may not be as effective as it is during other life stages, nor as it is for men.

4. Fukagawa, N. K., et al. (1990). Effect of age on body composition and resting metabolic rate. *Am J Physiology, 259,* E233; Ganesan, R. (1995). Aversive and hypophagic effects of estradiol. *Physiological Behavior, 55* (2), 279–285.

5. Groff, J. L., & Gropper, S. (2000). *Advanced Nutrition and Human Metabolism,* 147, 252, 447. Belmont, CA: Wadsworth.

6. Reaven, G. M. (2000). *Syndrome X: Overcoming the Silent Killer That Can Give You a Heart Attack.* New York: Simon & Schuster.

7. Eriksson, J., et al. (1989). Early metabolic defects in persons at increased risk for non-insulin-dependent diabetes mellitus. *NEJM, 321,* 337–343; Lillioja, S., et al. (1993). Insulin resistance and insulin secretory dysfunction as precursors of non-insulin-dependent diabetes mellitus: Prospective studies of the Pima Indians. *NEJM, 329,* 1988–1992.

8. Reaven, G. M. (1988). Role of insulin resistance in human disease. *Diabetes, 37,* 1595–1607; Zavaroni, I., et al. (1989). Risk factors for coronary artery disease in healthy persons with hyperinsulinemia and normal glucose tolerance. *NEJM, 320,* 702–706.

9. Fuh, M. M., et al. (1987). Abnormalities of carbohydrate and lipid metabolism in patients with hypertension. *Arch Intern Med, 147,* 1035–1038; Zavaroni, I., et al. (1987). Evidence that multiple risk factors for coronary artery disease exist in persons with abnormal glucose tolerance. *Am J Medicine, 83,* 609–612.

10. Nestler, J., et al. (1999). Ovulatory and metabolic effects of D-chiro-inositol in the polycystic ovary syndrome, *NEJM, 340,* 1314–1320.

11. Kazer, R. (1995). Insulin resistance, insulin-like growth factor 1 and breast cancer: A hypothesis. *International J Cancer, 62* (4), 403–406.

12. Bruning, P. F., Bonfrer, J. M., van Noord, P. A., Hart, A. A., de Jong-Bakker, M., & Nooijen, W. J. (1992). Insulin resistance and breast-cancer risk. *International J Cancer, 52* (4), 511–516; Seely, S. (1983). Diet and breast cancer: The possible connection with sugar consumption. *Medical Hypotheses, 11,* 319–327.

13. Bruning, P. F., et al. (1992). Ibid.

14. Kazer, R. (1995). Op. cit.

15. Huang, Z., Willett, W. C., Colditz, G. A., Hunter, D. J., Manson, J. E., Rosner, B., Speizer, F. E., & Hankinson, S. E. (1999). Waist circumference, waist:hip ratio, and risk of breast cancer in the Nurses' Health Study. *Am J Epidemiol, 150* (12), 1316–1324. Dr. Zhi-ping Huang from the Harvard School of Public Health, and his colleagues examined the association between waist circumference and waist-to-hip ratio with subsequent risk for breast cancer. Those with a waist circumference between 32 and 35.9

inches had a breast cancer risk 1.5 times greater than normal, while those with a waist circumference between 36 and 55 inches had a risk that was almost twice that of women whose waists were between 15 and 27.9 inches. Abdominal adiposity is associated with an excess of androgen and increased conversion of androgen to estrogen in fatty tissue. The research also concluded that "all postmenopausal hormone users were at increased risk of breast cancer regardless of central obesity."

16. Wild, R. D., et al. (1985). Lipoprotein lipid concentrations and cardiovascular risk in women with polycystic ovarian syndrome. *J Clinical Endocrinology & Metabolism, 61,* 946; Rexrode, K., et al. (1998). Abdominal adiposity and coronary heart disease in women. *JAMA, 280,* 1843–1848; Gillespie, L. (1999). *The Menopause Diet: Lose Weight and Boost Your Energy,* 18. Beverly Hills, CA: Healthy Life Publications.

17. Adams, K. F., et al. (2006). Overweight, obesity, and mortality in a large prospective cohort of persons age 50 to 71 years old. *NEJM, 355* (8), 763–778.

18. Huang, Z., et al. (1999). Op. cit.

19. Gillespie, L. (1999). *The Menopause Diet Mini Meal Cookbook,* 3. Beverly Hills, CA: Healthy Life Productions.

20. Michnobicz, J. (1987). Environmental modulation of estrogen metabolism in humans. *International Clinical Nutritional Review, 7,* 169–173; Anderson, K. E. (1984). The influence of dietary protein and carbohydrate on the principal oxidative biotranformations of estradiol in normal subjects. *J Clinical Endocrinology & Metabolism, 59* (1) 103–107.

21. Cutler, R. G. (1984). Carotenoids and retinol: Their possible importance in determining longevity of primate species. *Proceedings of the National Academy of Sciences, 81,* 7627–7631.

22. Murakoshi, M., et al. (1992). Potent preventive action of alpha-carotene against carcinogenesis. *Cancer Research, 52,* 6583–6587.

23. Franceschi, S., et al. (1994). Tomatoes and risk of digestive-tract cancers. *International J Cancer, 59,* 181–184.

24. Opara, E. C., et al. (1996). L-glutamine supplementation of a high fat diet reduces body weight and attenuates hyperglycemia and hyperinsulinemia in C57BL/6J mice. *J Nutrition, 126* (1), 273–279; Rogers, L. L., et al. (1955). Voluntary alcohol consumption by rats following administration of glutamine. *J Biological Chemistry, 214,* 503–507.

25. Hornstra, G. (2000). Essential fatty acids in mothers and their neonates. *Am J Clin Nutr, 71* (suppl.), 1262S–1269S.

26. I was introduced to this concept by Drs. Mary Dan Eades and Michael Eades, authors of *Protein Power* (New York: Bantam, 1996), and have found it to be true. Remember, however, that it is possible to produce too much insulin from overeating anything and also during times of stress—even when there aren't any carbohydrates around.

27. Strand, Ray. (2005). *Healthy for Life: Developing Healthy Lifestyles That Have a Side Effect of Permanent Fat Loss,* 228–229. Rapid City, SD: Real Life Press.

28. Ianoli, P., et al. (1998). Glucocorticoids upregulate intestinal nutrient transport in a time-dependent substrate-specific fashion. *Gastrointestinal Surgery, 2* (5), 449–457.

29. McGuigan, J. E. (1994). Peptic ulcer and gastritis. In K. Isselbacher, et al. (eds.), *Harrison's Principles of Internal Medicine, vol. 2* (13th ed., 1369). New York: McGraw-Hill.

30. Murray, M., & Pizzorno, J., (1998). *Encyclopedia of Natural Medicine,* 134–137. Rocklin, CA: Prima Publishing; van Marle, J., et. al. (1981). Deglycyrrhizinised licorice (DGL) and renewal of the rat stomach epithelium. *European J Pharmacology, 72,* 219–275.

Chapter 8: Creating Pelvic Health and Power

1. Helms, J. M. (1987). Acupuncture for the management of primary dysmenorrhea. *Obstetrics & Gynecology, 69* (1), 51–56.

2. Lepine, L. A., et al. (1997). Hysterectomy surveillance—United States, 1980–1993. *MMWR, 46,* 1–15.

3. Bradley, L., & Newman, J. (2000). Uterine artery embolization for treatment of fibroids: From scalpel to catheter. *The Female Patient, 25,* 71–78.

4. West, S. (1994). *The Hysterectomy Hoax.* New York: Doubleday.

5. Garcia, C.-R., & Cutler, W. B. (1984). Preservation of the ovary: A reevaluation. *Fertility & Sterility, 42* (4), 510–514.

6. Cutler, W. B. (1999). Human sex-attractant pheromones: discovery research, development, and application in sex therapy. *Psychiatric Annals, 29,* 54–9.

7. Hasson, H. (1993). Cervical removal at hysterectomy for benign disease: Risks and benefits. *J Reproductive Medicine, 58* (10), 781–789.

8. Carlson, K., Miller, B., & Fowler, F. (1994). The Maine Women's Health Study. I. Outcomes of hysterectomy. *Obstetrics & Gynecology, 83,* 556–565.

9. Rohner T. J., Jr., & Rohner. J. F. (1997). Urinary incontinence in America: The social significance. In P. D. O'Donnel (ed.), *Urinary Incontinence.* St. Louis, MO: Mosby-Yearbook, Inc.

10. Resnick, N. (1998). Improving treatment of urinary incontinence. *JAMA, 280* (23), 2034–2035.

11. Pandit, M., et al. (2000). Quantification of intramuscular nerves within the female striated urogenital sphincter muscles. *Obstetrics & Gynecology, 95,* 797–800.

12. Bhatia, N., Tchou, D. C. H., et al. (1988). Pelvic floor musculature exercises in treatment of anatomical urinary stress incontinence. *Physical Therapy, 68,* 652–655; Diokno, A. (1996). The benefits of conservative management in SUI. *Contemporary Urology, 8,* 36–48.

13. Singla, A. (2000). An update on the management of SUI. *Contemporary Ob/Gyn, 45* (1), 68–85.

14. Burgio, K., et al. (1998). Behavioral vs. drug treatment for urge incontinence in older women: A randomized trial. *JAMA, 280* (23), 1995–2000.

15. Galloway, N., et al. (June–July 1998). *Multicenter trial: Extracorporeal magnetic resonance therapy (EMRT) for the treatment of stress urinary incontinence.* First International Consultation on Incontinence, Monaco. (Abstract no. 31.)

16. Eckford, S. D., Jackson, S. R., Lewis, P. A., et al. (1996). The continence

control pad—a new external occlusion device in the management of stress incontinence. *British J Urology, 77,* 538–540.

17. Staskin D., et al. (1996). Effectiveness of a urinary control insert in the management of SUI: Early results of a multicenter study. *Urology, 47,* 629–636.

18. Lose G., & Versi, E. (1996). Pad-weighing tests in the diagnosis and quantification of incontinence. *International J Urogynecology, 3,* 324–328; Versi, E., et al. (1996). Evaluation of the home pad test in the investigation of female urinary incontinence. *British J Obstet Gynaecol, 103,* 162–167.

19. Davila, G. W., et al. (1994). The bladder neck support prosthesis: A nonsurgical approach to stress urinary incontinence in adult women. *Am J Obstetrics & Gynecology, 171,* 206–211.

20. Bergman, A., & Elia, G. (1995). Three surgical procedures for genuine stress incontinence. Five-year follow-up of a prospective randomized study. *Am J Obstetrics & Gynecology, 173,* 66–71.

21. Singla, A. Op. cit., 77.

22. Santarosa, R. P., & Blaivas, J. G. (1994). Periurethral injection of autologous fat for the treatment of sphincteric incontinence. *J Urology, 151,* 607–611; Bard, C. R. (1990). PMAA submission to U.S. Food & Drug Administration for IDE #G850010.

23. Burgio, K., et al. Op. cit.

Chapter 9: Sex and Menopause: Myths and Reality

1. Hartmann, U., et al. (2004). Low sexual desire in midlife and older women: Personality factors, psychosocial development, present sexuality. *Menopause, 11* (6, part 2), 726–40.

2. Basson, R. (Nov./Dec. 2004). Recent advances in women's sexual function and dysfunction. *Menopause, 11* (6, part 2), 714–25.

3. *NAMS Supplement—Update on Sexuality at Menopause and Beyond: Normative, Adaptive, Problematic, Dysfunctional,* North American Menopause Society, vol. 11, no. 6, (Nov. 2004), 708–86.

4. Bancroft, J., Loftus, J., & Long, J. S. (June 2003). Distress about sex: A national survey of women in heterosexual relationships. *Archives of Sexual Behavior, 32* (3), 193–208.

5. Sarrel, P. & Whitehead, M. I. (1985). Sex and menopause: Defining the issues. *Maturitas, 7,* 217–24.

6. van Lunsen, R. H., & Laan, E. (Nov.–Dec. 2004). Genital vascular responsiveness and sexual feelings in midlife women: Psychophysiologic, brain, and genital imaging studies. *Menopause, 11* (6, part 2), 741–8.

7. Avis, N., et al. (July/Aug. 2005). Correlates of sexual function among multiethnic middle-aged women: Results from the Study of Women's Health Across the Nation (SWAN). *Menopause, 12* (4), 385–98; Dennerstein, L., & Lehert, P. (Nov./Dec. 2004). Women's sexual functioning, lifestyle, mid-age, and menopause in 12 European countries. *Menopause, 11* (6, part 2), 778–85.

8. Bergmark, K., et al. (1999). Vaginal changes and sexuality in women with a history of cervical cancer. *NEJM, 340,* 1383–1389.

9. Savage, L. (1999). *Reclaiming Goddess Sexuality, 23.* Carlsbad, CA: Hay House.
10. Bodansky, S., & Bodansky, V. (2000). *Extended Massive Orgasm: How You Can Give and Receive Intense Sexual Pleasure.* Alameda, CA: Hunter House.
11. Love, P., & Robinson, J. (1994). *Hot Monogamy: Essential Steps to More Passionate, Intimate Lovemaking, 371.* New York: Dutton.
12. Hurlburth, D. F. (1991). The role of assertiveness in female sexuality: A comparative study between sexually assertive and sexually non-assertive women. *J Sex & Marital Ther, 12,* 183–190; Hoch, Z., et al. (1981). An evaluation of sexual performance comparison between sexually dysfunctional couples. *J Sex & Marital Ther, 17,* 90–102.
13. Zussman L., et al. (1981). Sexual responses after hysterectomy-oophorectomy: Recent studies and reconsideration of psychogenesis. *Am J Obstetrics & Gynecology, 40* (7), 725–729.
14. Bachman, G. A. (1985). Correlates of sexual desire in postmenopausal women. *Maturitas, 3,* 211.
15. Graziottin, A., & Basson, R. (Nov.–Dec. 2004). Sexual dysfunction in women with premature menopause. *Menopause, 11* (6, part 2), 766–77.
16. Alexander, J. L., et al. (Nov.–Dec. 2004). The effects of postmenopausal hormone therapies on female sexual functioning: A review of double-blind, randomized controlled trials. *Menopause, 11* (6, part 2), 749–65.
17. Sarrel, P. (1990). Sexuality and menopause. *Obstetrics & Gynecology, 75* (suppl. 4), 26S–35S; Sarrel, P. (1982). Sex problems after menopause: A study of 50 married couples treated in a sex counseling programme. *Maturitas, 4* (4), 231–239.
18. van Lunsen, R. H., & Laan, E. Op. cit.
19. Sarrel, P. (1990). Op. cit.
20. Sarrel, P., et al. (1998). Estrogen and estrogen-androgen replacement in postmenopausal women dissatisfied with estrogen-only therapy. *J Reproductive Medicine, 43* (10), 847–856; Sherwin, B., et al. (1985). Differential symptom response to parenteral estrogen and/or androgen administration in the surgical menopause. *Am J Obstetrics & Gynecology, 151,* 153–160.
21. Love, P., & Robinson, J. (1994). Op. cit. (73–76), commenting on the study of Schreiner-Engel, P. (1981). Sexual arousability and the menstrual cycle. *Psychosomatic Medicine, 43,* 1999–2212.
22. Collins, G. (2000). Safe sex: Important at any age. *The Female Patient, 20,* 4–8.
23. Love, P., & Robinson, J. (1994). Op. cit., 234–235.

Chapter 10: Nurturing Your Brain: Sleep, Depression, and Memory

1. Bliwise, D. L., et al. (1992). Prevalence of self-reported poor sleep in a healthy population age 50–65. *Social Science Medicine, 34* (49), 49.
2. Walsh, J. K., et al. (1992). Insomnia. In S. Chokroverty (ed.), *Sleep Disorders Medicine: A Comprehensive Textbook* (100). Stoneham, MA: Butterworth.

3. Rapkin, A., et al. (1997). Progesterone metabolite allopregnenolone in women with premenstrual syndrome. *Obstetrics/Gynecology, 90* (5), 709–714.

4. Cowden, W. L., Saenz, A., and Icaza, J. (Sept. 4–Oct. 21, 2005). The treatment of insomnia in patients of 4 hospitals in Guayaquil, Ecuador, using two novel herbal extracts: A double-blind, randomized, multiple crossover, placebo controlled, multicenter study. Unpublished study sponsored by Nutramedix LLC and Bionatus S. A. in Guayaquil, Ecuador; available online at www.bionatus.com/nutramedix/pages/moreinfo_babuna.html.

5. Leathwood, P. D., et al. (1985). Aqueous extract of valerian root (*Valeriana officinalis* L.) reduces latency to fall asleep in man. *Planta Medica, 54,* 144–148.

6. Murray, M. (1998). *5-HTP: The Natural Way to Overcome Depression, Obesity, and Insomnia.* New York: Bantam Books.

7. Holm, E., Staedt, U., Heep, J., Kortsik, C., Behne, F., Kaske, A., & Mennicke, I. (1991). *Untersuchungen zum Wirkungsprofil von D, L-Kavain: Zerebrale Angriffsorte und Schlaf-Wach-Rhythmus im Tierexperiment.* [The action profile of D, L-kavain: Cerebral sites and sleep-wakefulness rhythm in animals.] *Arzneimittelforschung, 41* (7), 673–683; ANPA Committee on Research (2000). The use of herbal alternative medicines in neuropsychiatry: A report of the ANPA Committee on Research. *J Neuropsychiatry & Clinical Neurosciences, 12,* 177–192.

8. McKinlay, J. B., et al. (1987). The relative contribution of endocrine changes and social circumstances to depression in mid-aged women. *J Health & Social Behavior, 28,* 345–363; Woods, N. F., & Mitchell, E. S. (1996). Patterns of depressed mood in midlife women: Observations from the Seattle Midlife Women's Health Study. *Research in Nursing & Health, 19* (2), 111–123; Martinsen, E. W. (1990). Benefits of exercise for the treatment of depression. *Sports Medicine, 9* (6), 380–389; Morgan, J., et al. (1970). Psychological effects of chronic physical activity. *Medical Science & Sports, 2* (4), 213–217; Kessler, R. C., et al. (1993). Sex and depression in the National Comorbidity Survey. I: Lifetime prevalence, chronicity and recurrence. *J Affective Disorders, 29,* 85.

9. Pratt, L. (1996). Depression, psychotropic medication and risk of myocardial infarction. *Circulation, 94* (12), 3123–3129; Michelson, D., et al. (1996). Bone mineral density in women with depression. *NEJM, 335,* 1176–1181; Denollet, J., et al. (1996). Personality as independent predictor of long-term mortality in patients with coronary heart disease. *Lancet, 347,* 417–421; Frasure-Smith, N., Lesperance, F., & Talajic, M. (1995). Depression and 18-month prognosis after myocardial infarction. *Circulation, 91* (4), 999–1005.

10. Sarno, J. (1991). *Healing Back Pain: The Mind-Body Connection,* 26–27. New York: Warner Books; Shealy, N. (1995). *Miracles Do Happen* (250). Rockport, MA: Element Books.

11. Woods, N. F., Mitchell, E. S., & Adams, C. (2000). Memory functioning among midlife women: Observations from the Seattle Midlife Women's Health Study. *Menopause, 7* (4), 257–265.

12. Aleem, F. A. (1985). Menopausal syndrome: Plasma levels of beta-endorphin in postmenopausal women measured by a specific radioimmunoassay. *Maturitas, 7,* 329–334; Genazzani, A. R., et al. (1988). Steroid replacement treatment increases beta-endorphin and beta-lipotropin plasma levels in postmenopausal women. *Gynecology & Obstetrical Investigation, 26,* 153–159.

13. Roca, C. A., et al. (1999). Gonadal steroids and affective illness. *Neuroscientist, 5* (4), 227–237; Halbreich, U. (1997). Role of estrogen in postmenopausal depression. *Neurology, 48* (5, suppl. 7), S16–S20.

14. Garcia-Segura, L. M., et al. (Nov. 1996). Effect of sex steroids on brain cells. In B. G. Wren (ed.), *Progress in the Management of the Menopause. The Proceedings of the 9th International Congress on the Menopause, Sydney, Australia,* 278–285. New York: Parthenon Publishing.

15. Young, R. J. (1979). Effect of regular exercise on cognitive functioning and personality. *British J Sports Medicine, 13* (3), 110–117; Gutin, B., (1966). Effect of increase in physical fitness on mental ability following physical and mental stress. *Research Quarterly, 37* (2), 211–220.

16. Doogan, D. P., & Caillard, V. (1992). Sertraline in the prevention of depression. *British J Psychiatry, 160,* 217–222; Eric, L. (1991). A prospective, double-blind, comparative, multicenter study of paroxitine and placebo preventing recurrent major depressive episodes. *Biological Psychiatry, 29* (suppl. 1), 254S–255S.

17. Pert, C. B. (Oct. 20, 1997). Letter to the editor. *Time, 150* (16).

18. Coppen, A. (1967). The biochemistry of affective disorders. *British J Psychiatry, 113,* 1237–1264; Stewart, J. W., et al. (1984). Low B6 levels in depressed outpatients. *Biol Psychiatry, 19* (4), 613–616; Hall, R. C. W., & Joffe, J. R. (1973). Hypomagnesemia: Physical and psychiatric symptoms. *JAMA, 224* (13), 1749–1751; Lieb, J., Karmali, R., & Horrobin, D. (1983). Elevated levels of prostaglandin E2 and thromboxane B2 in depression. *Prostaglandins Leukot Med, 10* (4), 361–367.

19. Fux, M., Levine, J., Aviv, A., & Belmaker, R. H. (1996). Inositol treatment of obsessive-compulsive disorder. *Am J Psychiatry, 153* (9), 1219–1221; Levine, J., et al. (1995). Double-blind, controlled trial of inositol treatment of depression. *Am J Psychiatry, 152,* 792–794.

20. DeVenna, M., & Rigamoni, R. (1992). Oral S-adenosyl-L-methionine in depression. *Curr Ther Res, 52,* 478–485; Di Benedetto, P., et al. (1993). Clinical evaluation of S-adenosyl-L-methionine versus transcutaneous electrical nerve stimulation in primary fibromyalgia. *Curr Ther Res, 53,* 222–229; Muskin, P. R., ed. (2000). *Complementary and Alternative Medicine and Psychiatry (Review of Psychiatry).* (Vol. 19, 8–18). Washington, D.C.: American Psychiatric Association Press; Shehin, V. O., et al. (1990). SAM-e in adult ADHD. *Psychopharmacology Bulletin, 25,* 249–253.

21. Evans, P. H. (1991). Cephaloconiosis: A free radical perspective on the proposed particulate-induced etiopathogenesis of Alzheimer's dementia and related disorders. *Medical Hypotheses, 34* (3), 209–219.

22. Freedman, M., et al. (1984). Computerized axial tomography in aging. In M. L. L. Albert (ed.), *Clinical Neurology of Aging.* New York: Oxford

University Press; Lehr, J., & Schmitz-Scherzer, R. (1976). Survivors and non-survivors: Two fundamental patterns of aging. In H. Thomae (ed.), *Patterns of Aging: Findings from the Bonn Longitudinal Study of Aging.* Basel: S. Karger; Benton, M. L., et al. (1981). Normative observations on neuropsychological test performance in old age. *J Clinical Neuropsychiatry, 3,* 33–42.

23. Jorm, A. F., et al. (1987). The prevalence of dementia: A quantitative integration of the literature. *Acta Psychiatrica Scandinavia, 76,* 465–479; Aronson, M. S., et al. (1990). Women, myocardial infarction, and dementia in the very old. *Neurology, 40,* 1102–1106.

24. Nash, J. M. (July 24, 2000). The new science of Alzheimer's. *Time, 156* (4), 51.

25. Snowdon, D., et al. (1996). Linguistic ability in early life and cognitive function and Alzheimer's disease in late life: Findings from the Nun Study. *JAMA, 275* (7), 528–532; Snowdon, D., et al. (1997). Brain infarction and the clinical expression of Alzheimer's disease: The Nun Study. *JAMA, 277* (10), 813–817.

26. Baldereschi, M., et al. (1998). Estrogen replacement therapy and Alzheimer's disease in the Italian Longitudinal Study on Aging. *Neurology, 50,* 996–1002; Kawas, C., et al. (1997). A prospective study of estrogen replacement therapy and the risk of developing Alzheimer's disease: The Baltimore Longitudinal Study of Aging. *Neurology, 48,* 1517–1521; Paganini-Hill, A., & Henderson, V. W. (1996). Estrogen replacement therapy and risk of Alzheimer's disease. *Arch Intern Med, 156* (19), 2213–2217; Tang, M. X., et al. (1996). Effect of œstrogen during menopause on risk and age at onset of Alzheimer's disease. *Lancet, 358,* 429–432; Ohkura, V., et al. (1994). Evaluation of estrogen treatment in female patients with dementia of Alzheimer's type. *Endocrinology J, 41,* 361–371; Henderson, V., et al. (1994). Estrogen replacement therapy in older women: Comparisons between Alzheimer's disease cases and nondemented control subjects. *Archives of Neurology, 51,* 896–900; Paganini-Hill, A., et al. (1994). Estrogen deficiency and risk of Alzheimer's disease in women. *Am J Epidemiol, 140,* 256–261; Brenner, D. E., et al. (1994). Postmenopausal estrogen replacement therapy on the risk of Alzheimer's disease: A population-based case control study. *Am J Epidemiol, 140,* 262–267; Honjo, H., et al. (1993). An effect of conjugated estrogen to cognitive impairment in women with senile dementia, Alzheimer's type: A placebo-controlled double-blind study. *J Japanese Menopause Society, 1,* 167–171; Kantor, H., et al. (1973). Estrogen for older women. *Am J Obstetrics & Gynecology, 116,* 115–118; Caldwell, B. M. (1954). An evaluation of psychological effects of sex hormone administration in aged women. *J Gerontology, 9,* 168–174.

27. McEwen, B. S., et al. (1999). Inhibition of dendritic spine induction on hippocampal ca-1 pyramidal neurons by nonsteroidal estrogen antagonists in female rats. *Endocrinology, 140,* 1044–1047.

28. Manly, J. J., et al. (2000). Endogenous estrogen levels and Alzheimer's disease among postmenopausal women. *Neurology, 54,* 833–837.

29. Baldereschi, M., et al. (1998). Op. cit.; Schneider, L. S., et al. (1996). Effects of estrogen replacement therapy on response to tacrine in patients with Alzheimer's disease. *Neurology, 46,* 1580–1584; Brinton, R. D., et al. (1997). 17-beta-estradiol increases the growth and survival of cultured cortical neurons. *Neurochemical Research, 22,* 1339–1351; Brinton, R. D., et al. (1997). Equilin, a principal component of the estrogen replacement therapy Premarin, increases the growth of cortical neurons via an NMDA receptor-dependent mechanism. *Experimental Neurology, 147,* 211–220; Matsumoto, A., et al. (1985). Estrogen stimulates neuronal plasticity in the deafferented hypothalamic arculate nucleus in aged female rats. *Neuroscience Research, 2,* 412–418; Okhura, T., et al. (1995). Estrogen increases cerebral and cerebellar blood flow in postmenopausal women. *Menopause, 2,* 13–18; Singh, M., et al. (1994). Ovarian steroid deprivation results in a reversible learning impairment and compromised cholinergic function in female Sprague-Dawley rats. *Brain Research, 644,* 305–312; Singh, M., et al. (1996). The effect of ovariectomy and estradiol replacement on brain derived neurotrophic factor messenger hippocampal brain expression in cortical and hippocampal brain regions of female Sprague-Dawley rats. *Endocrinology, 136,* 2320–2324.

30. Sherwin, B. (1997). Estrogen effects of cognition in menopausal women. *Neurology, 48* (suppl. 7), S21–S26.

31. McEwen, B. S., & Wooley, C. S. (1994). Estradiol and progesterone regulate neuronal structure and synaptic connectivity in adult as well as developing brain. *Experimental Gerontology, 29,* 431–436; Wooley, C. S., & McEwen, B. S. (1993). Roles of estradiol and progesterone in regulation of hippocampal dendritic spine density during the estrous cycle in the rat. *J Comparative Neurology, 336,* 293–306.

32. McLaughlin, I. J., et al. (1990). Zinc in depressive disorder. *Acta Psychiatr Scandinavia, 82,* 451–453.

33. Shaw, D. M., et al. (1988). Senile dementia and nutrition [letter]. *British Medical J, 288,* 792–793.

34. Gibson, Q. E., et al. (1988). Reduced activities of thiamine dependent enzymes in the brains and peripheral tissues of patients with Alzheimer's disease. *Archives of Neurology, 45,* 836–840.

35. Strachan, R. N., & Henderson, J. G. (1967). Dementia and folate deficiency. *Quarterly J Medicine, 36,* 189–204; Perkins. A. J., et al. (1999). Association of antioxidants and memory in multiethnic elderly sample using the Third National Health and Nutrition Examination Study. *Am J Epidemiol, 150,* 37–44.

36. Rovio, S., et al. (Nov. 2005). Leisure-time physical activity at midlife and the risk of dementia and Alzheimer's disease. *Lancet Neurol, 4* (11), 705–711.

37. Petrovitch, H., and White, L. (Nov. 2005). Exercise and cognitive function. *Lancet Neurol, 4* (11), 690–691.

38. Hoffman and Herbert (1990). Beware of cold remedies in the elderly. *Courtlandt Forum,* 28–41.

39. Lim, S. Y., and Suzuki, H. (June 2000). Intakes of dietary docosahexaenoic

acid ethyl ester and egg phosphatidylcholine improve maze-learning ability in young and old mice. *J Nutr, 130* (6), 1629–1632; Gamoh, S., et al. (1999). Chronic administration of docosahexaenoic acid improves reference memory-related learning ability in young rats. *Neuroscience, 93* (1), 237–241; Calon, F., et al. (Sept. 2, 2004). Docosahexaenoic acid protects from dendritic pathology in an Alzheimer's disease mouse model. *Neuron, 43* (5), 633–645.

40. Kalmijn, S., et al. (Jan. 27, 2004). Dietary intake of fatty acids and fish in relation to cognitive performance at middle age. *Neurology, 62* (2), 275–280.

41. Pan, Y., et al. (2000). Soy phytoestrogens improve radial arm maze performance in ovariectomized retired breeder rats and do not attenuate benefits of 17-beta-estradiol treatment. *Menopause, 7* (4), 230–235; Kim, H., et al. (2000). Attenuation of neurodegeneration-relevant modifications of brain proteins by dietary soy. *Biofactors, 12* (1–4), 243–250. Review.

42. Pan, Y., et al. (1999). Effect of estradiol and soy phytoestrogens on choline acetyltransferase and nerve growth factor mRNAs in the frontal cortex and hippocampus of female rats. *Proc Soc Exp Biol Med, 221* (2), 118–125.

43. Zeng, H., Chen, Q., & Zhao, B. (Jan. 15, 2004). Genistein ameliorates beta-amyloid peptide (25–35)-induced hippocampal neuronal apoptosis. *Free Radic Biol Med, 36* (2), 180–8; Sonee, M., Sum, T., Wang, C., & Mukherjee, S. K. (Sept. 2004). The soy isoflavone, genistein, protects human cortical neuronal cells from oxidative stress. *Neurotoxicology, 25* (5), 885–91.

44. File, S. E., et al. (Oct. 2001). Eating soya improves human memory. *Psychopharmacology (Berl), 157* (4), 430–6.

45. File, S. E., et al. (March 2005). Cognitive improvement after 6 weeks of soy supplements in postmenopausal women is limited to frontal lobe function. *Menopause, 12* (2), 193–201.

46. Kritz-Silverstein, D., Von Muhlen, D., Barrett-Connor, E., & Bressel, M. A. (May–June 2003). Isoflavones and cognitive function in older women: The Soy and Postmenopausal Health In Aging (SOPHIA) Study. *Menopause, 10* (3), 196–202.

47. Refat, S. L., et al. (1990). Effect of exposure of miners to aluminum powder. *Lancet, 336,* 1162–1165.

48. Council on Scientific Affairs (1985). Aspartame: Review on safety issues. *JAMA, 254* (3), 400–402; U. S. Department of Health and Human Services (1980). *Decision of the Public Board of Inquiry* (DHHS docket 75F–0335). Rockville, MD: Food & Drug Administration; Wurtman, R. J. (1983). Neurochemical changes following high-dose aspartame with dietary carbohydrates. *NEJM, 309,* 429–430; Yokogoshi, H., et al. (1984). Effects of aspartame and glucose administration on brain and plasma levels of large neutral amino acids and brain 5-hydroxyindoles. *Am J Clin Nutr, 40* (1), 1–7; Aspartame Consumer Safety Network, P.O. Box 780634, Dallas, TX 75378. Tel: 214–352–4268.

49. McEwen, B. S., et al. (1999). Op. cit.

50. Levy, B. R., Slade, M. D., Kunkel, S. R., & Kasl, S. V. (Aug. 2002).

Longevity increased by positive self-perceptions of aging. *J Pers Soc Psychol, 83* (2), 261–70.

51. Connor, J. R., Melone, J. H., & Yuen, A. R. (1981). Dendritic length in aged rats' occipital cortex: An environmentally induced response. *Experimental Neurology, 73* (3), 827–830; Connor, J. R., Diamond, M. C., & Johnson, R. E. (1980). Aging and environmental influences on two types of dendritic spines in the rat occipital cortex. *Experimental Neurology, 70* (2), 371–379.

52. Eriksson, P., et al. (1998). Neurogenesis in the adult human hippocampus. *Nature Medicine, 4* (11), 1313–1317.

53. Diamond, M., et al. (1985). Plasticity in the 904-day male rat cerebral cortex. *Experimental Neurology, 87,* 309–317.

54. Hausdorff, J., et al. (1999). The power of ageism on physical function of older persons: Reversibility of age-related gait changes. *J Am Geriatric Soc, 47,* 1346–1349.

55. Langer, E. (1989). *Mindfulness,* 113. Reading, MA: Addison-Wesley.

Chapter 11: From Rosebud to Rose Hip: Cultivating Midlife Beauty

1. Fisher, G. J., et al. (1997). Pathophysiology of premature skin aging induced by ultraviolet light. *NEJM, 337* (20), 1419–1428.

2. Van Scott, E. J., & Yu, R. J. (March 1989). Alpha hydroxy acids: Procedures for use in clinical practice. *Cutis, 43* (3), 222–228.

3. Van Scott, E. J., & Yu, R. J. (Nov. 1984). Hyperkeratinization, corneocyte cohesion, and alpha hydroxy acids. *J Am Acad Dermatol, 11* (5 pt. 1), 867–879; Stiller, M. J., et al. (June 1996). Topical 8% glycolic acid and 8% L-lactic acid creams for the treatment of photodamaged skin: A double-blind vehicle-controlled clinical trial. *Arch Dermatol, 132* (6), 631–636.

4. Steenvoorden, D. P., & van Henegouwen, G. M. (Nov. 1997). The use of endogenous antioxidants to improve photoprotection. *J Photochem Photobiol B, 41* (1–2), 1–10.

5. Fuchs, J., & Kern, H. (Dec. 1998). Modulation of UV-light-induced skin inflammation by D-alpha-tocopherol and L-ascorbic acid: a clinical study using solar simulated radiation. *Free Radic Biol Med, 25* (9), 1006–1012; Steenvoorden, D. P., and Beijersbergen van Henegouwen, G. (June 1999). Protection against UV-induced systemic immunosuppression in mice by a single topical application of the antioxidant vitamins C and E. *Int J Radiat Biol, 75* (6), 747–755.

6. Serbinova, E., et al. (1991). Free radical recycling and intermembrane mobility in the antioxidant properties of alpha-tocopherol and alphatocotrienol. *Free Radical Biology & Medicine, 10,* 263–275.

7. Traber, M. G., et al. (Jan. 1998). Penetration and distribution of alpha-tocopherol, alpha- or gamma-tocotrienols applied individually onto murine skin. *Lipids, 33* (1), 87–91.

8. Hoppe, U., et al. (1999). Coenzyme Q_{10}, a cutaneous antioxidant and energizer. *Biofactors, 9* (2–4), 371–378.

9. Sinatra, S. (1998). *The Coenzyme Q_{10} Phenomenon.* Chicago: Keats Publishing.

10. Bangha, E., Elsner, P., Kistler, G. S. (Aug. 1996). Suppression of UV-induced erythema by topical treatment with melatonin (N-acetyl-5-methoxytryptamine): A dose response study. *Arch Dermatol Res, 288* (9), 522–526.

11. Zhao, J., Wang, J., Chen, Y., & Agarwal, R. (Sept. 1999). Anti-tumor-promoting activity of a polyphenolic fraction isolated from grape seeds in the mouse skin two-stage initiation-promotion protocol and identification of procyanidin B5-3'-gallate as the most effective antioxidant constituent. *Carcinogenesis, 20* (9), 1737–1745; Kanda, T., et al. (July 1998). Inhibitory effects of apple polyphenol on induced histamine release from RBL-2H3 cells and rat mast cells. *Biosci Biotechnol Biochem, 62* (7), 1284–1289; Tomen, Inc. (1994–1999). Unpublished data.

12. Owen, D. R., et al. (Feb. 1999). Anti-aging technology for skincare '99. *Global Cosmetic Industry,* 38–43.

13. Katayama, K., et al. (May 15, 1993). A pentapeptide from type I procollagen promotes extracellular matrix production. *J Biol Chem, 268* (14), 9941–9944.

14. Ibid.

15. Sederma, Inc. Unpublished data.

16. Wilkinson, R. E. Photoaging: The role of UV radiation in premature skin aging and a review of effective defense strategies. Article published on the Trienelle website at www.trienelle.com/research-monograph.aspx.

17. Schmidt, J., et al. (1998). Treatment of skin aging with topical estrogens. *International J of Pharmaceutical Compounding, 2* (4), 270–274.

18. Draelos, Z. (Nov. 2005). The effect of Revival soy on the health and appearance of the skin, hair, and nails in postmenopausal women. Results of unpublished study available online at www.revivalsoy.com/home/newsletter/v08n01/art2.html?flash6=yes.

19. Kim, S. Y., et al. (April 2004). Protective effects of dietary soy isoflavones against UV-induced skin-aging in hairless mouse model. *J Am Coll Nutr, 23* (2), 157–162; Miyazaki, K., Hanamizu, T., Iizuka, R., and Chiba, K. (May–June 2002). Genistein and daidzein stimulate hyaluronic acid production in transformed human keratinocyte culture and hairless mouse skin. *Skin Pharmacol Appl Skin Physiol, 15* (3), 175–83; DiSilvestro, R. (Sept. 2003). A diversity of soy antioxidant effects. Presented at the fifth annual International Symposium on the Role of Soy in Preventing and Treating Chronic Disease, Orlando, FL; Djuric, Z., Chen, G., Doerge, D. R., Heilbrun, L. K., & Kucuk, O. (Oct. 22, 2001). Effect of soy isoflavone supplementation on markers of oxidative stress in men and women. *Cancer Lett, 172* (1), 1–6.

20. Saliou, C., et al. (1999). French *Pinus maritima* bark extract prevents ultraviolet-induced NF-KB–dependent gene expression in a human keratinocyte cell line. Abstract of a poster presentation at the Oxygen Club of California, 1999 World Congress.

21. Lopez-Torres, M., et al. (1998). Op. cit.; Eberlein-Konig, B., et al. (1998). Protective effect against sunburn of combined systemic ascorbic acid and vitamin E. *J Am Academy of Dermatology, 38,* 45–48.

22. Engels, W. D. (1982). Dermatological disorders: Psychosomatic illness

review (No. 4 in the series). *Psychosomatics, 23* (12), 1209–1219; Bick, E. (1968). Experience of the skin in early object relations. *International J of Psychoanalysis, 49,* 484–486.

23. Strauss, J. S., & Pochi, P. E. (1963). The human sebaceous gland: Its regulation by steroidal hormones, and its use as an end organ for assaying androgenicity *in vivo. Recent Progress in Hormonal Research, 19,* 385–444.
24. Peck, G. L., et al. (1979). Prolonged remissions of cystic and conglobate acne with 13-retinoic acid. *NEJM, 300,* 329–333.
25. Engels, W. D. (1982). Op. cit.; Bick, E. (1968). Op. cit.; Kaplan, H. I., & Sadock, B. J. (eds.) (1989). *Comprehensive Textbook of Psychiatry* (5th ed., 1221). Philadelphia, PA: Lippincott, Williams & Wilkins.
26. DeVille, R. L., et al. (1994). Androgenic alopecia in women: Treatment with 2% topical minoxidil solution. *Arch Dermatol, 130* (3), 303–307.
27. Lewenberg, A. (1996). Minoxidil-tretinoin combination for hair regrowth: Effects of frequency, dosage, and mode of application. *Advances in Therapy, 13* (5), 274–283.
28. Halsner, U. E., & Lucas, M. W. (1995). New aspects in hair transplantation for women. *Dermatol Surg, 21* (7), 605–610.
29. Hayden, T., et al. (August 9, 1999). Our quest to be perfect. *Newsweek,* 52–59.
30. Burkitt, D. P., et al. (1974). Dietary fiber and disease. *JAMA, 229* (8), 1068–1074; Braunwald, E. (ed.) (1987). *Harrison's Principles of Internal Medicine* (11th ed.). New York: McGraw-Hill.
31. Grismond, G. L. (1981). Treatment of pregnancy-induced phlebopathies. *Minerva Ginecol, 33,* 221–230.
32. Ries, W. (1976). Prevention of venous disease from nutritional-physio-logic aspect. *ZFA, 31* (4), 383–388; Braunwald, E. (ed.) (1987). Op. cit.
33. Ako, H., et al. (1981). Isolation of fibrinolysis enzyme activator from commercial bromelain. *Arch Int Pharmacodyn, 254,* 157–167.

Chapter 12: Standing Tall for Life: Building Healthy Bones

1. NIH Consensus Development Panel on Osteoporosis Prevention, Diagnosis, and Therapy. (Feb. 14, 2001). Osteoporosis prevention, diagnosis, and therapy. *JAMA, 285* (6), 785–95.
2. Cummings, S., et al. (1985). Epidemiology of osteoporosis and osteoporotic fractures. *Epidemiology Review, 7,* 178–208.
3. Lindsay, R. (1995). The burden of osteoporosis: Cost. *Am J Medicine, 98* (2A), 9S–11S.
4. Shipman, P., et al. (1985). *The Human Skeleton.* Cambridge, MA: Harvard University Press; Brown, J. (1990). *The Science of Human Nutrition.* New York: Harcourt Brace Jovanovich.
5. Lanyon, L. E. (1993). Skeletal responses to physical loading. In G. Mundy & J. T. Martin (eds.), *Physiology & Pharmacology of Bone, 107,* 485–505. Berlin: Springer-Verlag.
6. Travis, J. (2000). Boning up: Turning on cells that build bone and turning off ones that destroy it. *Science News, 157,* 41–42.

7. Manolagas, S. C. (1995). Sex steroids, cytokines, and the bone marrow: New concepts on the pathogenesis of osteoporosis. *Ciba Foundation Symposium, 191,* 187–202.

8. Riggs, B., et al. (1986). In women dietary calcium intake and rates of bone loss from midradius and lumbar spine are not related. *J Bone & Mineral Research, 1* (suppl.), 167; Genant, H. K., et al. (1985). Osteoporosis: Assessment by quantitative computed tomography. *Orthopedic Clinics of North America, 16* (3), 557–568.

9. Trotter, M., et al. (1974). Sequential changes in weight, density, and percentage weight of human skeletons from an early fetal period through old age. *Anatomical Record, 179,* 1–8.

10. Adams, P., et al. (1970). Osteoporosis and the effects of aging on bone mass in elderly men and women. *J Medical News Series, 39,* 601–615.

11. Harris, S., et al. (1992). Rates of change in bone mineral density of the spine, heel, femoral neck and radius in healthy postmenopausal women. *Bone Mineralization, 17* (1), 87–95; Riggs, B., et al. (1985). Rates of bone loss in the appendicular and axial skeletons of women: Evidence of substantial vertebral bone loss before menopause. *J Clinical Investigation, 77,* 1487–1491.

12. Fujita, T., et al. (1992). Comparison of osteoporosis and calcium intake between Japan and the United States. *Proc Soc Experimental Biology & Medicine, 200* (2), 149–152.

13. Frost, H. (1985). The pathomechanics of osteoporosis. *Clinical Orthopedics, 200,* 198–225.

14. Chappard, D., et al. (1988). Spatial distribution of trabeculae in iliac bones from 145 osteoporotic females. *Maturitas, 10,* 353–360; Biewener, A. A. (1993). Safety factors in bone strength. *Calcified Tissue International, 53* (suppl. 1), S68–S74.

15. Brown, S. (1996). *Better Bones, Better Body: Beyond Estrogen and Calcium.* Los Angeles: Keats Publishing.

16. Lees, B., et al. (1993). Differences in proximal femur bone density over two centuries. *Lancet, 341,* 673–675; Eaton, S., et al. (1991). Calcium in evolutionary perspective. *Am J Clinical Nutr, 54* (suppl.), 281S–287S.

17. Bauer, D. C., et al. (1993). Factors associated with appendicular bone mass in older women. *Ann Internal Medicine, 118* (9), 647–665.

18. Rigotti, N. A., et al. (1984). Osteoporosis in women with anorexia nervosa. *NEJM, 311* (25), 1601–1605.

19. Prior, J., et al. (1990). Spinal bone loss and ovulatory disturbances. *NEJM, 323* (18), 1221–1227; Cann, C., et al. (1984). Decreased spinal mineral content in amenorrheic women. *JAMA, 251* (5), 626–629.

20. Schuckit, M. (1994). Section 5: Alcohol and alcoholism. In K. Isselbacher, et al. (eds.), *Harrison's Principles of Internal Medicine, vol. 2* (13th ed., 2420). New York: McGraw-Hill.

21. Diamond, T., et al. (1989). Ethanol reduces bone formation and may cause osteoporosis. *Am J Medicine, 86,* 282–288; Bikler, D. D., et al. (1985). Bone disease in alcohol abuse. *Ann Internal Medicine, 103,* 42–48.

22. Gold, P. W., et al. (1986). Responses to corticotropin-releasing hormone in

the hypercortisolism of depression and Cushing's disease: Pathophysiology and diagnostic implications. *NEJM, 314,* 1329–1335; Michelson, D., et al. (1996). Bone mineral density in women with depression. *NEJM, 335* (16), 1176–1181.

23. Tatemi, S., et al. (1991). Effect of experimental human magnesium depletion on parathyroid hormone secretion and 1,25-dihyroxyvitamin D metabolism. *J Clin Endocrinol Metab, 73* (5), 1067–1072; Gaby, A., & Wright, J. (1988). *Nutrients and Bone Health.* Seattle, WA: Wright/Gaby Nutrition Institute.

24. Adinoff, A. D., & Hollister, J. R. (1983). Steroid-induced fracture and bone loss in patients with asthma. *NEJM, 309* (5), 265–268.

25. Hahn, T. J., et al. (1988). Altered mineral metabolism in glycocorticoidinduced osteopaenia: Effect of 25-hydroxyvitamin D administration. *J Clinical Investigation, 64,* 655–665.

26. Crilly, R. G., et al. (1981). Steroid hormones, ageing and bone. *Clinical Endocrinology & Metabolism, 10* (1), 115–139.

27. Johnell, O., et al. (1979). Bone morphology in epileptics. *Calcified Tissue International, 28* (2), 93–97.

28. Franklin, J. A., et al. (1992). Long-term thyroxine treatment and bone mineral density. *Lancet, 340,* 9–13; Paul, T. L., et al. (1988). Long-term L-thyroxine therapy is associated with decreased hip bone density in pre-menopausal women. *JAMA, 259,* 3137–3141; Coindre, J. M., et al. (1986). Bone loss in hypothyroidism with hormone replacement: A histomorphometric study. *Arch Intern Med, 146,* 48–53.

29. Brincat, M. P., et al. (1996). A screening model for osteoporosis using dermal skin thickness and bone densitometry. In B. G. Wren (ed.), *Progress in the Management of the Menopause: The Proceedings of the 8th International Congress on the Menopause,* 175–178. Sydney: Parthenon Publishing Group.

30. Robins, S. P. (1995). Collagen crosslinks in metabolic bone disease. *Acta Orthopedica Scandinavia, 66* (266, suppl.), S171–S175; Garnero, P., et al. (1994). Comparison of new biochemical markers of bone turnover in late postmenopausal osteoporotic women in response to alendronate treatment. *J Clin Endocrinol Metab, 79,* 1693–1700; Chesnut, C., et al. (1997). Hormone replacement therapy in postmenopausal women: Urinary N-telopeptide of type I collagen monitors therapeutic effect and predicts response of bone mineral density. *Am J Medicine, 102,* 29–37.

31. Cummings, S. R., et al. (in press). Regression to mean in clinical practice: Women who seem to lose bone density during treatment for osteoporosis usually gain if treatment is continued. *JAMA.* Cited in B. Ettinger (2000). Sequential osteoporosis treatment for women with postmenopausal osteoporosis. *Menopausal Medicine, Newsletter of the American Society for Reproductive Medicine, 8* (2), 3.

32. Munger, R. G. (1999). Prospective study of dietary protein intake and risk of hip fracture in postmenopausal women. *Am J Clin Nutr, 69* (1), 147–152.

33. Potter, S. M., Baum, J. A., Teng, H., Stillman, R. J., Shay, N. F., & Erdman,

J. W. (1998). Soy protein and isoflavones: Their effects on blood lipids and bone density in postmenopausal women. *Am J Clin Nutr, 68* (6, suppl.), 1375S–1379S.

34. Zhang, X., et al. (Sept. 12, 2005). Prospective cohort study of soy food consumption and risk of bone fracture among postmenopausal women. *Arch Intern Med, 165* (16), 1890–1895.

35. Lydeking-Olsen, E., et al. (Aug. 2004). Soymilk or progesterone for prevention of bone loss—a 2-year randomized, placebo-controlled trial. *Eur J Nutr, 43* (4), 246–57. Epub Apr 14, 2004.

36. Bonfield, T. (June 15, 1999). Research backs benefits of soy—postmenopausal women take note. *Cincinnati Enquirer.* This study, which was conducted by Dr. Michael Scheiber, of the Obstetrics and Gynecology Department at the University of Cincinnati, and Dr. Kenneth Setchell, director of mass spectrometry at Children's Hospital Medical Center, demonstrated that eating three servings of soy foods per day containing a total of about 70 mg of soy isoflavones had definite bone-building effects that may be as good as those of estrogen.

37. Hegarty, V., et al. (2000). Tea drinking and bone mineral density in older women. *Am J Clin Nutr, 71,* 1003–1007.

38. Watts, N. B., et al. (1995). Comparison of oral estrogens and estrogens plus androgen on bone mineral density, menopausal symptoms, and lipid-lipoprotein profiles in surgical menopause. *Obstetrics & Gynecology, 85,* 529–537.

39. Cummings, S., et al. (1998). Endogenous hormones and the risk of hip and vertebral fractures among older women. *NEJM, 339,* 733–738.

40. Riggs, B., & Melton, L. (1986). Involutional osteoporosis. *NEJM, 26,* 1676–1686. Buchanan, J. R., et al. (1988). Early vertebral trabecular bone loss in normal premenopausal women. *J Bone & Mineral Research, 3* (5), 583–587.

41. Carter, M. D., et al. (1991). Bone mineral content at three sites in normal perimenopausal women. *Clinical Orthopedics, 266,* 295–300; Harris, S., & Dawson-Hughes, B. (1992). Rates of change in bone mineral density of the spine, heel, femoral neck and radius in healthy postmenopausal women. *J Bone & Mineral Research, 17* (1), 87–95.

42. Heaney, R. P. (1990). Estrogen-calcium interactions in the post-menopause: A quantitative description. *J Bone & Mineral Research, 11* (1), 67–84.

43. Speroff, L. (Oct. 1999). Treatment options for the prevention of osteoporosis. *Ob/Gyn Clinical Alert, 46.*

44. Lee, J. (1991). Is natural progesterone the missing link in osteoporosis prevention and treatment? *Medical Hypotheses, 35,* 316–318; Prior, J. (1991). Progesterone and the prevention of osteoporosis. *Can J Ob-Gyn & Women's Healthcare, 3* (4), 178–183; Lee, J. (1990). Osteoporosis reversal: The role of progesterone. *Clinical Nutritional Review, 10,* 884–889; Prior, M. C., et al. (1994). Cyclic medroxyprogesterone increases bone density: A controlled trial in active women with menstrual cycle disturbances. *Am J Medicine, 96,* 521–530; Adachi, J. D., et al. (1997). A double-blind randomized controlled trial of the effects of medroxyprogesterone acetate on

bone density of women taking oestrogen replacement therapy. *British J Obstet Gynaecol, 104,* 64–70; Prior, J. C., et al. (1997). Premenopausal ovariectomy-related bone loss: A randomized, double-blind, one-year trial of conjugated estrogen or medroxyprogesterone acetate. *J Bone & Mineral Research, 12* (11), 1851–1863.

45. Rossouw, J. E., et al. (July 17, 2002). Risks and benefits of estrogen plus progestin in healthy postmenopausal women: Principal results from the Women's Health Initiative randomized controlled trial. *JAMA, 288* (3), 321–333.

46. Lindsay, R., Gallagher, J. C., Kleerekoper, M., & Pickar, J. H. (May 22–29, 2002). Effect of lower doses of conjugated equine estrogens with and without medroxyprogesterone acetate on bone in early postmenopausal women. *JAMA, 287* (20), 2668–2676.

47. Tremollieres, F. A., Strong, D. D., Baylink, D. J., & Mohan, S. (April 1992). Progesterone and promegestone stimulate human bone cell proliferation and insulin-like growth factor-2 production. *Acta Endocrinol (Copenh), 26* (4), 329–337.

48. Abraham, G. (1991). The importance of magnesium in the management of primary postmenopausal osteoporosis: A review. *J Nutritional Medicine, 2,* 165–178; Gaby, A., & Wright, J. (1990). Nutrients and osteoporosis: A review article. *J Nutritional Medicine, 1,* 63–72.

49. Buckley, L. M., et al. (1996). Calcium and vitamin D_3 supplementation prevents bone loss in the spine secondary to low-dose corticosteroids in patients with rheumatoid arthritis. A randomized, double-blind, placebo-controlled trial. *Ann Internal Medicine, 125* (12), 961–968.

50. Nielson, B. E., et al. (1987). Effects of dietary boron on mineral, estrogen, and testosterone metabolism in postmenopausal women. *FASEB, 1,* 394–397.

51. Dawson-Hughes, G., et al. (1990). A controlled trial of the effects of calcium supplementation on bone density in postmenopausal women. *NEJM, 323,* 878–883.

52. McGuigan, J. (1994). Peptic ulcer and gastritis. In K. Isselbacher, et al. (eds.), *Harrison's Principles of Internal Medicine, vol. 2* (13th ed., 1369). New York: McGraw-Hill.

53. Chu, J. Y., et al. (1975). Studies in calcium metabolism, II. Effects of low calcium and variable protein intake on human calcium metabolism. *Am J Clin Nutr, 28,* 1028–1035; Abelow, B., et al. (1992). Cross-cultural association between dietary animal protein and hip fracture: A hypothesis. *Calcified Tissue International, 50,* 14–18.

54. Gillespie, L. (1999). *The Menopause Diet: Lose Weight and Boost Your Energy,* 36. Beverly Hills, CA: Healthy Life Publications.

55. Aiello, L., & Wheeler, P. (1995). The expensive tissue hypothesis: The brain and the digestive system in human and primate evolution. *Current Anthropology, 36* (2), 199–221; Lorenz, K., & Lee, V. A. (1997). The nutritional and physiological impact of cereal products in human nutrition. *Critical Reviews in Food Science & Nutrition, 8,* 383–456; Cassiday, C. M. (1980). Nutrition and health in agriculturalists and hunter-gatherers: A

case study of two prehistoric populations. In R. F. Kandel, G. H. Pelto, & N. W. Jerome (eds.), *Nutritional Anthropology: Contemporary Approaches to Diet and Culture*, 117–145. Pleasantville, NY: Redgrave Publishing Company; Eaton, S. B., & Nelson, D. A. (1991). Calcium in evolutionary perspective. *Am J Clinical Nutrition*, *54* (suppl.), 281S–287S; Goodman, A. H., Dufour, D., & Pelto, G. H. (2000). *Nutritional Anthropology: Biocultural Perspectives on Food and Nutrition*. Mountain View, CA: Mayfield Publishing. See also *The Paleopathology Newsletter*, published by the Paleopathology Association. Contact: Ms. Eve Cockburn, 18655 Parkside, Detroit, MI 48221–2208.

56. Sources for this table are: U.S. Department of Agriculture, *Composition of Foods*, handbooks no. 8 and 456 (Washington, D.C.: U.S. Government Printing Office, 1963); J. A. Duke and A. A. Atchley, *Handbook of Proximate Analysis—Tables of Higher Plants* (Boca Raton: CRC Press, 1986); Leonard Jacobs, article in *East/West Journal*, (May 1985); John Lee, Osteoporosis reversal: The role of progesterone. *International Clinical Nutrition Review*, *vol. 10* (1990), 384–91; Judith Cooper Madlener, *The Sea Vegetable Book* (New York: Clarkson N. Potter, 1977); Nutrition Search, Inc., John Kirschmann, dir. comp., *Nutrition Almanac*, rev. ed. (New York: McGraw-Hill, 1979); U.S. Department of Agriculture, *Nutritive Value of Foods*, handbook no. 72 (Washington, D.C.: U.S. Government Printing Office, 1971); Mark Pedersen, *Nutritional Herbology* (Bountiful, UT: Pedersen, 1987); and Maine Coast Sea Vegetables Co., Shore Road, Franklin, ME 04634.

57. Caspit, A. (1994). Alendronate: An investigational agent for the prevention and treatment of osteoporosis. *Drug Therapy*, *24*, 41.

58. Guyatt, G. H., et al. (Sept. 2002). Summary of meta-analyses of therapies for postmenopausal osteoporosis and the relationship between bone density and fractures. *Endocrinol Metab Clin North Am*, *31* (3), 659–679, xii; Cranney, A., et al. (Aug. 2002). Meta-analyses of therapies for postmenopausal osteoporosis. IX: Summary of meta-analyses of therapies for postmenopausal osteoporosis. *Endocr Rev*, *23* (4), 570–578; Black, D. M., et al. (Dec. 7, 1996). Randomised trial of effect of alendronate on risk of fracture in women with existing vertebral fractures. Fracture Intervention Trial Research Group. *Lancet*, *348* (9041), 1535–1541; McClung, M. R., et al. (Feb. 1, 2001). Effect of risedronate on the risk of hip fracture in elderly women. Hip Intervention Program Study Group. *N Engl J Med*, *344* (5), 333–340; Harris, S. T., et al. (Oct. 13, 1999). Effects of risedronate treatment on vertebral and nonvertebral fractures in women with postmenopausal osteoporosis: a randomized controlled trial. Vertebral Efficacy with Risedronate Therapy (VERT) Study Group. *JAMA*, *282* (14), 1344–52.

59. DeGroen, P. C. (1996). Esophagitis associated with the use of alendronate. *NEJM*, *335*, 1016–1021.

60. Delmas, P., et al. (1997). Effects of raloxifene on bone mineral density, serum cholesterol concentrations, and uterine endometrium in postmenopausal women. *NEJM*, *337*, 1641–1647; Ettinger, B., et al. (Aug. 18,

1999). Reduction of vertebral fracture risk in postmenopausal women with osteoporosis treated with raloxifene: Results from a 3-year randomized clinical trial. Multiple Outcomes of Raloxifene Evaluation (MORE) Investigators. *JAMA, 282* (7), 637–45.

61. Silverman, S. L., and Azria, M. (Nov. 2002,). The analgesic role of calcitonin following osteoporotic fracture. *Osteoporos Int, 13* (11), 858–867.

62. Nelson, M., et al. (1994). Effects of high-intensity strength training on multiple risk factors for osteoporotic fractures: A randomized controlled trial. *JAMA, 272* (24), 1909–1914.

63. Nelson, M. (2000). *Strong Women Stay Young.* New York: Bantam.

64. Fiatarone, M., et al. (1994). Exercise training and nutritional supplementation for physical frailty in very elderly people. *NEJM, 330* (25), 1769–1775.

65. Rosen, C., et al. (1994). The effects of sunlight and diet on bone loss in elderly women from rural Maine. *Maine J Health Issues, 1* (2), 35–48. (Study done by Michael Holick in Bangor, Maine.)

66. Vieth, R. (1999). Vitamin D supplementation, 25-hydroxyvitamin D concentrations, and safety. *Am J Clin Nutr, 69,* 842–856. (Anyone who is serious about gathering more information on vitamin D and sunlight should read this impressive review article on the subject.)

67. Ibid.

68. Neer, R. M., et al. (1971). Stimulation by artificial lighting of calcium absorption in elderly human subjects. *Nature, 229,* 255.

69. Holick, M. F. (1995). Environmental factors that influence the cutaneous production of Vitamin D. *Am J Clin Nutr, 61* (suppl. 3), 638S–645S.

70. Dawson-Hughes, B., et al. (1991). Effect of vitamin D supplementation on wintertime and overall bone loss in healthy postmenopausal women. *Ann Internal Medicine, 115* (7), 505–511.

71. McNeil, T. (Spring 1998). The vitamin D guru: School of medicine professor sees the light and spreads the news. *Bostonia,* 34–35.

72. Veith, R. (1999). Op. cit.

73. Berger, J. (1998), 64–72. *Herbal Rituals.* New York: St. Martin's Press.

74. Weed, S. (1989). *Healing Wise: Wise Woman's Herbal* (262). Woodstock, NY: Ashtree Publications.

Chapter 13: Creating Breast Health

1. Toikkanene, S., et al. (1991). Factors predicting late mortality from breast cancer. *European J Cancer, 27* (5), 586–591.

2. Chen, C. C., et al. (1995). Adverse life events and breast cancer: Case-control study. *British Medical J, 311,* 1527–1530.

3. Dreher, Henry (personal communication, October 12, 2005).

4. Levy, S., et al. (1987). Correlation of stress factors with sustained depression of natural killer cell activity and predicted prognosis in patients with breast cancer. *J Clinical Oncology, 5,* 348–353.

5. Spiegel, D., et al. (1989). The effect of psychosocial treatment on survival of patients with metastatic breast cancer. *Lancet, 2* (8668), 888–891.

6. Prior, J. (1992). Critique of estrogen treatment for heart attack prevention: The Nurses' Health Study. *A Friend Indeed, 8* (8), 3–4; Schairer, C., et al. (2000). Menopausal estrogen and estrogen-progestin replacement therapy and breast cancer risk. *JAMA, 283* (4), 485–491.

7. Bulbrook, P. D., Swain, M. C., Wang, D. Y., et al. (1976). Breast cancer in Britain and Japan: Plasma oestradiol-17b, oestrone, and progesterone, and their urinary metabolites in normal British and Japanese women. *European J Cancer, 12,* 725–735.

8. Chlebowski, R. T., et al. (May 16, 2005). Dietary fat reduction in post-menopausal women with primary breast cancer: Phase III women's intervention nutrition study (WINS). Presented at the annual meeting of the American Society of Clinical Oncology (ASCO), Orlando.

9. Seely, S., et al. (1983). Diet and breast cancer: The possible connection with sugar consumption. *Medical Hypotheses, 11,* 319–327; Kazer, R. (1995). Insulin resistance, insulin-like growth factor I and breast cancer: A hypothesis. *International J Cancer, 62,* 403–406; Bruning, P., et al. (1992). Insulin resistance and breast-cancer risk. *International J Cancer, 52,* 511–516.

10. Tavani, A., et al. (Oct. 25, 2005). Consumption of sweet foods and breast cancer risk in Italy, *Annals of Oncology,* [Epub ahead of print].

11. Willett, W. C., et al. (1987). Moderate alcohol consumption and the risk of breast cancer. *NEJM, 316,* 1174–1180.

12. Ginsburg, E. (1996). Effects of alcohol ingestion on estrogens in post-menopausal women. *JAMA, 276* (21), 1747–1751.

13. Zhang, S., et al. (1989). A prospective study of folate intake and the risk of breast cancer. *JAMA, 281* (17), 1632–1637.

14. Ambrosone, C., et al. (1996). Cigarette smoking, N-acetyltransferase 2 genetic polymorphisms, and breast cancer risk. *JAMA, 276* (18), 1494–1501.

15. Bernstein, L., et al. (Nov. 16, 2005). Lifetime recreational exercise activity and breast cancer risk among black women and white women. *J Natl Cancer Inst., 97* (22), 1671–9.

16. Thune, I., et al. (1997). Physical activity and the risk of breast cancer. *NEJM, 336,* 1269–75.

17. Verkasalo, P. K., et al. (Oct. 15, 2005). Sleep duration and breast cancer: A prospective cohort study. *Cancer Res, 65* (20), 9595–9600.

18. Blask, D. E., et al. (Dec. 1, 2005). Melatonin-depleted blood from pre-menopausal women exposed to light at night stimulates growth of human breast cancer xenografts in nude rats. *Cancer Res, 65* (23), 11174–11184.

19. Schernhammer, E. S., & Hankinson, S. E. (July 20, 2005). Urinary melatonin levels and breast cancer risk. *J Natl Cancer Inst. 97* (14), 1084–1087.

20. Schernhammer, E. S., et al. (Oct. 17, 2001). Rotating night shifts and risk of breast cancer in women participating in the Nurses' Health Study. *J Natl Cancer Inst, 93* (20), 1563–1568.

21. Coleman, B. C. (March 10, 1999). Fatty diet and breast cancer: No link? *Portland Press Herald.*

22. Adlercreutz, H., et al. (1982). Excretion of the lignans enterolactone and enterodiol and of equol in omnivorous and vegetarian postmenopausal women and in women with breast cancer. *Lancet, 2* (8311), 1295–1299.

23. Goldin, B. R., Adlercreutz, H., et al. (1982). Estrogen excretion patterns and plasma levels in vegetarian and omnivorous women. *NEJM, 307,* 1542–1547.

24. Percival, M. (1997). Phytonutrients and detoxification. *Clinical Nutrition Insights,* (1–4). Published by the Foundation for the Advancement of Nutritional Education. Available from Metagenics North East, P.O. Box 848, Kingston, NH 03848.

25. Zava, D., & Duwe, G. (1997). Estrogenic and antiproliferative properties of genistein and other flavonoids in human breast cancer cells *in vitro. Nutrition & Cancer, 27* (1), 31–40.

26. Thomsen, A. R., et al., Influence of Prevastein, an isoflavone-rich soy product, on mammary gland development and tumorigenesis in Tg.NK (MMTV/c-neu) mice. (2005). *Nutr Cancer, 52* (2), 176–188; Allred, C. D., et al., Soy processing influences growth of estrogen-dependent breast cancer tumors. (2004). *Carcinogenesis, 25* (9), 1649–1657.

27. Allred, C. D., et al. (2004). Soy processing influences growth of estrogen-dependent breast cancer tumors. *Carcinogenesis, 25* (9), 1649–1657.

28. Nagata, C., et al. (1997). Decreased serum estradiol concentration associated with high dietary intake of soy products in premenopausal Japanese women. *Nutr Cancer, 29* (3), 228–233; Lu, L. J., et al. (2000). Increased urinary excretion of 2-hydroxyestrone but not 16alpha-hydroxyestrone in premenopausal women during a soya diet containing isoflavones. *Cancer Res, 60* (5), 1299–305; Cassidy, A., Bingham, S., and Setchell, K. D. (1994). Biological effects of a diet of soy protein rich in isoflavones on the menstrual cycle of premenopausal women. *Am J Clin Nutr, 60* (3), 333–40.

29. Xu, X., et al. (1998). Effects of soy isoflavones on estrogen and phytoestrogen metabolism in premenopausal women. *Cancer Epidemiol Biomarkers Prev, 7* (12), 1101–1108.

30. Wood, C. E., et al. (2004). Breast and uterine effects of soy isoflavones and conjugated equine estrogens in postmenopausal female monkeys. *J Clin Endocrinol Metab, 89* (7), 3462–3468.

31. Bagga, D., et al. (1997). Dietary modulation of omega-3/omega-6 polyunsaturated fatty acid ratios in patients with breast cancer. *J Nat Cancer Inst, 89* (15), 1123–1131.

32. Lockwood, K., et al. (1994). Partial and complete regression of breast cancer in patients in relation to dosage of coenzyme Q_{10}. *Biochemical & Biophysical Research Communications, 199* (3), 1504–1508.

33. Welch, H. G., & Black, W. C. (1997). Using autopsy series to estimate the disease "reservoir" for ductal carcinoma in situ of the breast: How much more breast cancer can we find? *Ann Internal Medicine, 127* (11), 1023–1028; Nielsen, M., et al. (1987). Breast cancer and atypia among young and middle-aged women: A study of 110 medicolegal autopsies. *British J Cancer, 56* (6), 814–819.

34. Welch, H. G., & Black, W. C. (1997). Op. cit., 1023.

35. Moody-Ayers, S., et al. (2000). "Benign" tumors and "early detection" in mammography-screened patients of a natural cohort with breast cancer. *Arch Intern Med, 160* (8), 1109–1115.

36. National Institutes of Health Consensus Development Panel. (1997). National Institutes of Health Consensus Development Conference Statement: Breast cancer screening for women ages 40–49. *J Natl Cancer Inst, 89* (14), 1015–26.

37. Prager, K. (1996). Outrage over mammogram screening unwarranted. *Medical Tribune.* Quoted by Gina Kolata in the *New York Times* (Jan. 28, 1997).

38. Harris, R. (July 20, 2005). Effectiveness: The next question for breast cancer screening. *Journal of the National Cancer Institute, 97* (14), 1021–3.

39. Berry, D. A., et al. (Oct. 27, 2005). Effect of screening and adjuvant therapy on mortality from breast cancer. *NEJM, 353* (17), 1784–92.

40. van Netten, J. P., et al. (April 16, 1994). Physical trauma and breast cancer. *Lancet, 343* (8903), 978–9.

41. Christiansen, C. L., et al. (2000). Predicting the cumulative risk of false-positive mammograms. *J Natl Cancer Inst, 92* (20) 1657–66.

42. Elmore, J. G., et al. (April 16, 1998). Ten-year risk of false positive screening mammograms and clinical breast exams. *NEJM, 338* (16), 1089–96.

43. Gotzsche, P. C., & Olsen, O. (2001). Is screening for breast cancer with mammography justifiable? *Lancet, 355,* 129–34; Gotzsche, P. C., & Olsen, O. (2001). Cochrane review on screening for breast cancer with mammography. *Lancet, 358,* 1340–2.

44. Miller, A. B., et al. (Sept. 20, 2000). Canadian National Breast Screening Study-2: 13-year results of a randomized trial in women aged 50–59 years. *Journal of the National Cancer Institute, 92,* 18, 1490–9.

45. Kerlikowske, K., et al. (Dec. 8, 1999). Continuing screening mammography in women aged 70 to 79 years: Impact on life expectancy and cost-effectiveness. *JAMA, 282,* 22, 2156–63.

46. Baines, C. (2005). Rethinking breast screening—again. *British Medical Journal, 331,* 1031.

47. Moore, F. (1978). Breast self-examination. *NEJM, 299* (6), 304–305.

48. Thomas, D. B., et al. (2002). Randomized trial of breast self-examination in Shanghai: Final results. *J Natl Cancer Inst, 94,* 1445–1457.

49. Personal communication from Dana Wyrick. Dana Wyrick is a registered massage therapist who developed this self-massage routine for breast health after studying with lymphedema therapy specialists in Europe and Australia, where the technique is far more common.

50. Kerlikowske, K., et al. (1993). Positive predictive value of screening mammography by age and family history of breast cancer. *JAMA, 270* (2), 444.

51. National Council on Aging (1997). *Myths and Perceptions About Aging and Women's Health.* Washington, D.C. (1997). Assessing the odds. *Lancet, 350* (9091), 1563.

52. Love, S. (2005). *Dr. Susan Love's Breast Book* (145). Cambridge, MA: Da Capo Lifelong Books.

53. Ries, L. A. G., Eisner, M. P., Kosary, C. L., Hankey, B. F., Miller, B. A., Kleg, L., & Edwards, B. K. (eds.) (2000). *SEER Cancer Statistics Review, 1973–1993.* Bethesda, MD: National Cancer Institute; Black, W. C., et al.

(1995). Perceptions of breast cancer risk and screening effectiveness in women younger than 50 years old. *J Nat Cancer Inst, 87,* 720–731.

54. Phillips, K. A. (1999). Putting the risk of breast cancer in perspective. *NEJM, 340* (2), 141–144.

55. Hirshaut, Y., & Pressman, P. (2000). *Breast Cancer: The Complete Guide* (256). New York: Bantam.

56. American College of Obstetrics & Gynecology, Committee on Genetics (Oct. 1996). *Breast–Ovarian Cancer Screening* (Committee Opinion no. 176). Washington, D.C.

57. Collins, F. S. (1986). BRCA1—lots of mutations, lots of dilemmas. *NEJM, 334* (3), 186–188.

58. Weisberg, T. (Oct. 1996). Genetic testing for breast cancer. *Maine Cancer Perspectives, 2* (4), 3.

59. Kesaniemi, Y. A. (unpublished data). Cited in A. Viitanen (1996), A new estrogen gel: Clinical benefits. In B. G. Wren (ed.), *Progress in the Management of the Menopause: The Proceedings of the 8th International Congress on the Menopause* (168). Sydney, Australia: Parthenon.

60. LaVecchia, C., Negri, E., Franceschi, S., et al. (1995). Hormone replacement therapy and breast cancer risk: A cooperative Italian study. *British J Cancer, 72,* 244–248.

61. Campagnoli, C., et al. (1999). HRT and breast cancer risk: A clue for interpreting the available data. *Maturitas, 33,* 185–190; Collaborative Group on Hormonal Factors in Breast Cancer (1997). Breast cancer and hormone replacement therapy: Collaborative reanalysis of data from 51 epidemiological studies of 52,705 women with breast cancer and 108,411 without breast cancer. *Lancet, 350,* 1047–1059.

62. Bhavani, B. R., et al. (1994). Pharmacokinetics of 17-B-dihydroequilin sulfate and 17-B-dihydroequilin in normal postmenopausal women. *J Clin Endocrinol & Metab, 78,* 197–204.

63. Hargrove, J., & Eisenberg, E. (1995). Menopause. *Med Clin North Am, 79* (6), 1337–1363.

64. Campagnoli, C. (1999). Op. cit.; Collaborative Group on Hormonal Factors in Breast Cancer (1997). Op. cit.

65. Beral V., Million Women Study Collaborators (2003). Breast cancer and hormone-replacement therapy in the Million Women Study. *Lancet, 362* (9382), 419–27.

66. Coombs, N. J., et al. (2005). Hormone replacement therapy and breast cancer: Estimate of risk. *BMJ, 331* (7512) 347–9.

67. Coombs, N. J., et al. (Nov.–Dec. 2005). Hormone replacement therapy and breast cancer risk in California. *Breast J, 11* (6), 410–5.

68. Campagnoli, C. (1999). Op. cit. Given the results of the WHI study on Prempro and the financial losses suffered by Wyeth Ayerst as a result, it's doubtful that we'll ever have the data needed to prove this!

69. Huang, Z., Willett, W. C., Colditz, G. A., Hunter, D. J., Manson, J. E., Rosner, B., Speizer, F. E., & Hankinson, S. E. (1999). Waist circumference, waist:hip ratio, and risk of breast cancer in the Nurses' Health Study. *Am J Epidemiol, 150* (12) 1316–1324. "Furthermore," they write, "it has been

proposed that abdominal adiposity is associated with an excess of androgen and increased conversion of androgen to estrogen in adipose tissue." They also point out that hormone use by postmenopausal women likely raises hormone levels in all those women. "[A]s a result, all postmenopausal hormone users were at increased risk of breast cancer regardless of central obesity," they reason.

70. Melamed, M., et al. (Nov. 1997). Molecular and kinetic basis for the mixed agonist/antagonist activity of estriol. *Molecular Endocrinology, 11*, 12, 1868–78.

71. Rajkumar, L., et al. (2004). Prevention of mammary carcinogenesis by short-term estrogen and progestin treatments. *Breast Cancer Research, 6*, 1, R31–7.

72. Henrich, J. B. (1992). The postmenopausal estrogen/breast cancer controversy. *JAMA, 268*, 1900–1902; Wotiz, H. H., Beebe, D. R., & Muller, E. (1984). Effect of estrogen on DMBA-induced breast tumors. *J Steroid Biochem, 20*, 1067–1075.

73. Drife, J. O. (1986). Breast development in puberty. *Ann NY Acad Sci, 464*, 58–65; Dulbecco, R., et al. (1982). Cell types and morphogenesis in the mammary gland. *Proc Natl Acad Sci USA, 79*, 7346–7350; Long-acre, T., & Bartow, S. (1986). A correlative morphologic study of human breast and endometrium in the menstrual cycle. *Am J Surgical Path, 10* (6), 382–393; Weinberg, R. A. (Sept. 1996). How cancer arises. *Scientific American*, 62–70.

74. Lemon, H. (1973). Oestriol and prevention of breast cancer. *Lancet, 1* (802), 546; Lemon, H. (1975). Estriol prevention of mammary carcinoma induced by 7,12-dimethyl-benzanthracene and procarbazine. *Cancer Res, 35*, 1341–1353; Lemon, H. (1980). Pathophysiologic considerations in the treatment of menopausal patients with oestrogens: The role of oestriol in the prevention of mammary cancer. *Acta Endocrinol, 1*, 17–27; Lemon, H., Wotiz, H., Parsons, L., et al. (1966). Reduced estriol excretion in patients with breast cancer prior to endocrine therapy. *JAMA, 196*, 1128–1136.

75. Bu, S. Z., et al. (1997). Progesterone induces apoptosis and upregulation of p53 expression in human ovarian carcinoma cell lines. *Cancer, J American Cancer Society, 79* (10), 1944–1950.

76. Zava, D. T., & Duwe, G. (1997). Estrogen and antiproliferative properties of genistein and other flavonoids in human breast cancer cells *in vivo*. *Nutr & Cancer, 27* (1), 31–40.

77. Cowan, A. D., et al. (1961). Breast cancer incidence in women with a history of progesterone deficiency. *Am J Epidemiol, 114* (2), 209.

78. Chang, K. J., et al. (1995). Influences of percutaneous administration of estradiol and progesterone on human breast epithelial cell cycle *in vivo*. *Fertil & Steril, 63*, 785–791.

79. Badwe, R. A., et al. (1991). Timing of surgery during menstrual cycle and survival of premenopausal women with operable breast cancer. *Lancet, 337*, 1261–1264.

80. Hrushesky, W. (1996). Breast cancer, timing of surgery, and the menstrual cycle: Call for prospective trial. *J Women's Health, 5* (6), 555–566.

81. Wren, B., & Eden, J. A. (1996). Do progestogens reduce the risk of breast

cancer? A review of the evidence. *Menopause: The J of the N Am Menopause Soc, 3,* (1), 4–12.

82. Wren, B., & Eden, J. A. (1996). Do progestogens reduce the risk of breast cancer? A review of the evidence. *Menopause: The J of the N Am Menopause Soc, 3,* (1), 4–12.

83. McEwen, B. S., et al. (1999). Inhibition of dendritic spine induction on hippocampal ca-1 pyramidal neurons by nonsteroidal estrogen antagonist in female rats. *Endocrinology, 140,* 1044–1047; McEwen, B. S., & Wooley, C. S. (1994). Estradiol and progesterone regulate neuronal structure and synaptic connectivity in adult as well as developing brain. *Experimental Gerontology, 29,* 431–436; Wooley, C. S., & McEwen, B. S. (1993). Roles of estradiol and progesterone in regulation of hippocampal dendritic spine density during the estrous cycle in the rat. *J Comparative Neurology, 336,* 293–306.

84. Timmerman, D., et al. (1998). A randomized trial on the use of ultrasonography or office hysteroscopy for endometrial assessment in postmenopausal patients with breast cancer who were treated with tamoxifen. *Am J Obstetrics & Gynecology, 179,* 62–70; Franchi, M., et al. (1999). Endometrial thickness in tamoxifen-treated patients: An independent predictor of endometrial disease. *Obstetrics & Gynecology, 93,* 1004–1008; Ramonetta, L. M., et al. (1999). Endometrial cancer in polyps associated with tamoxifen use. *Am J Obstetrics & Gynecology, 180,* 340–341.

85. Osborne, C. K. (1999). Questions and answers about tamoxifen. In *Tamoxifen for the Treatment and Prevention of Breast Cancer.* V. Craig, ed. Melville, NY. (1995). NSABP halts B-14 trial: No benefit seen beyond 5 years of tamoxifen use. *J Nat Cancer Inst, 87,* 1829.

86. Fisher, B. (1998). Tamoxifen for prevention of breast cancer: Report of the National Surgical Adjuvant Breast and Bowel Project P-1 Study. *J Nat Cancer Inst, 90* (18), 1371–1388.

87. Gail, M. H., et al. (1989). Projecting individualized probabilities of developing breast cancer for white females who are being examined annually. *J Nat Cancer Inst, 81* (24), 1879–1886.

88. Melnikow, J., et al. (2006). Chemoprevention: Drug pricing and mortality: The case of tamoxifen. *Cancer,* published online July 24, 2006, in advance of print.

89. Gandey, A. (2006). Tamoxifen fails to reduce breast cancer risk in most women. *Medscape Medical News,* July 26, 2006; http://www.medscape.com/viewarticle/54157.

Chapter 14: Living with Heart, Passion, and Joy: How to Listen to and Love Your Midlife Heart

1. Svendsen, N. A. (Oct. 1999). Personal letter, excerpted in *Health Wisdom for Women, 6* (10), 8. Used here with permission from the author.

2. Tremollieres, F. A., et al. (1999). Coronary heart disease risk factors and menopause: A study in 1,684 French women. *Atherosclerosis, 142* (2), 415–423.

3. Clow, B. H. (1996). *Liquid Light of Sex: Kundalini Rising at Mid-Life Crisis* (103–104). Santa Fe, NM: Bear & Co.

4. National Center for Health Statistics (1996). *Vital Statistics of the United States, 1992, Vol. 11: Morality, Part A* (DHHS Publication 96–1101). Hyattsville, MD: U.S. Dept. of Health and Human Services, Public Health Service.

5. American Heart Association (1997). *Heart and Stroke Statistical Update.* Dallas, TX; Centers for Disease Control and Prevention, National Center for Health Statistics (1996). *Health, United States, 1995* (PHS Publication 96–1232). Hyattsville, MD: U.S. Dept. of Health and Human Services, Public Health Service; Leiman, J. M., Meyer, J. E., Rothschild, N., & Simon, L. J. (March 1997). *Selected Facts on U.S. Women's Health: A Chart Book.* New York: The Commonwealth Fund; Maynard, C., et al. (1992). Gender differences in the treatment and outcome of acute myocardial infarction. Results from the Myocardial Infarction Triage and Intervention Registry. *Arch Intern Med, 152* (5), 972–976.

6. *Selected Facts on U.S. Health,* Op. cit.

7. Childre, D., & Martin, H. (1999). *The HeartMath Solution* (foreword). San Francisco: HarperSanFrancisco.

8. Skinner, J. (1993). Neurocardiology: Brain mechanisms underlying fatal cardiac arrhythmias. *Neurologic Clinics, 11* (2), 325–351.

9. Kudenchuk, P. J., et al. (1996). Comparison of presentation, treatment and outcome of acute myocardial infarction in men vs. women (The Myocardial Infarction Triage and Intervention Registry). *Am J Cardiology, 78* (1), 9–14.

10. Cooper, G. S. (1999). Menstrual and reproductive risk factors for ischemic heart disease. *Epidemiology, 10* (3), 255–259; Hazeltine, F. P., & Jacobson, B. (1997). *Women's Health Research: A Medical and Policy Primer* (173). Washington, D.C.: APA Press.

11. Iribarren, C., et al. (2000). Association of hostility with coronary artery calcification in young adults: The CARDIA Study. *JAMA, 283* (19), 2546–2551.

12. Friedman, M., & Rosenman, R. (1974). *Type A Behavior and Your Heart.* New York: Alfred A. Knopf.

13. Webber, L. S., et al. (1979). Occurrence in children of multiple risk factors for coronary artery disease: The Bogalusa Heart Study. *Preventive Medicine, 8,* 407–418; Khoury, P., et al. (1980). Clustering and interrelationships of coronary heart disease risk factors in schoolchildren, ages 6–19. *Am J Epidemiol, 112,* 524–538.

14. Stampfer, M., et al. (2000). Primary prevention of coronary heart disease in women through diet and lifestyle. *NEJM, 343,* 16–22.

15. Mo-Suwan, L., & Lebel, L. (1996). Risk factors for cardiovascular disease in obese and normal school age children: Association of insulin with other cardiovascular risk factors. *Biomed Environ Sci, 9* (2–3), 269–275; Wing, R. R., & Jeffery, R. W. (1995). Effect of modest weight loss on changes in cardiovascular risk factors: Are there differences between men and women between weight loss and maintenance? *Int J Obes Relat Metab Disord, 19* (1), 67–73.

16. Manson, J. E., et al. (1992). The primary prevention of myocardial infarction. *NEJM, 326* (21), 1406–1416; Mosca, L., et al. (1999). Guide to preventive cardiology for women. AHA/ACC Scientific Statement Consensus panel statement. *Circulation, 99* (18), 2480–2484.

17. Grundy, S. M., et al. (July 13, 2004). Implications of recent clinical trials for the National Cholesterol Education Program Adult Treatment Panel III guidelines. *Circulation, 110* (2), 227–239.

18. ALLHAT Officers and Coordinators for the ALLHAT Collaborative Research Group (Dec. 18, 2002). Major outcomes in moderately hypercholesterolemic, hypertensive patients randomized to pravastatin vs usual care: The Antihypertensive and Lipid-Lowering Treatment to Prevent Heart Attack Trial (ALLHAT-LLT). *JAMA, 288* (23), 2998–3007.

19. Heart Protection Study Collaborative Group (July 6, 2002), MRC/BHF Heart Protection Study of cholesterol lowering with simvastatin in 20,536 high-risk individuals: A randomised placebo-controlled trial. *Lancet, 360* (9326), 7–22.

20. Matsuzaki, M., et al. (Dec. 2002). Large-scale cohort study of the relationship between serum cholesterol concentration and coronary events with low-dose simvastatin therapy in Japanese patients with hypercholesterolemia. *Circ J, 66* (12), 1087–1095.

21. Newman, C. B., et al. (Sept. 15, 2003). Safety of atorvastatin derived from analysis of 44 completed trials in 9,416 patients. *Am J Cardio, 92* (6), 670–676.

22. Sever, P. S., et al. (April 5, 2003). Prevention of coronary and stroke events with atorvastatin in hypertensive patients who have average or lower-than-average cholesterol concentrations, in the Anglo-Scandinavian Cardiac Outcomes Trial—Lipid Lowering Arm (ASCOT-LLA): A multicentre randomised controlled trial. *Lancet, 361* (9364), 1149–1158.

23. Jenkins, A. J. (Oct. 18, 2003). Might money spent on statins be better spent? *BMJ, 327* (7420), 933.

24. Laise, E. (Nov. 2003). The Lipitor dilemma. *Smart Money: The Wall Street Journal Magazine of Personal Business, 12* (11), 90–96.

25. Langsjoen, P. H., and Langsjoen, A. M. (2003). The clinical use of HMG CoA-reductase inhibitors and the associated depletion of coenzyme Q_{10}. A review of animal and human publications. *Biofactors, 18* (1–4), 101–111.

26. Gaist, D., et al. (May 14, 2002). Statins and risk of polyneuropathy: A case-control study. *Neurology, 58* (9), 1333–1337.

27. Schwartz, G. G., et al. (April 4, 2001). Effects of atorvastatin on early recurrent ischemic events in acute coronary syndromes: The MIRACL study: A randomized controlled trial. *JAMA, 285* (13), 1711–1718.

28. Suarez, E. C. (May–June 1999). Relations of trait depression and anxiety to low lipid and lipoprotein concentrations in healthy young adult women. *Psychosom Med, 61* (3), 273–279.

29. Newman, T. B., & Hulley, S. B. (Jan. 3, 1996). Carcinogenicity of lipid-lowering drugs. *JAMA, 275* (1), 55–60.

30. Folkers, K., et al. (May 19, 1997). Activities of vitamin Q_{10} in animal models and a serious deficiency in patients with cancer. *Biochem Biophys Res*

Commun, 234 (2), 296–299; Lockwood, K., et al. (July 6, 1995). Progress on therapy of breast cancer with vitamin Q_{10} and the regression of metastases. *Biochem Biophys Res Commun, 212* (1), 172–177.

31. Sinatra, S. (2000). *Heart Sense for Women,* 108. Washington, D.C.: Lifeline.

32. Sacks, F. M., et al. (Oct. 3, 1996). The effect of pravastatin on coronary events after myocardial infarction in patients with average cholesterol levels. Cholesterol and Recurrent Events Trial investigators. *N Engl J Med, 335* (14), 1001–1009.

33. Boudreau, D. M., et al. (June 1, 2004). The association between 3-hydroxy-3-methylglutaryl coenzyme A inhibitor use and breast carcinoma risk among postmenopausal women: A case-control study. *Cancer, 100* (11), 2308–2316.

34. Manson, J. E., et al. (1990). A prospective study of obesity and risk of coronary heart disease in women. *NEJM, 332* (13), 882–889.

35. Kelly, P., et al. (June 1997). Unmetabolized folic acid in serum: Acute studies in subjects consuming fortified food and supplements. *Am J Clin Nutr, 65* (6), 1790–1795; Morita, H., et al. (April 15, 1997). Genetic polymorphism of 5,10-methylenetetrahydrofolate reductase (MTHFR) as a risk factor of coronary artery disease. *Circulation, 95* (8), 2032–2036.

36. Wu, T., et al. (2000). Periodontal disease and risk of cerebrovascular disease: The first national health and nutrition examination survey and its follow-up study. *Arch Intern Med, 160* (18), 2749–2755; Hujoel, P. P., et al. (2000). Periodontal disease and coronary heart disease risk. *JAMA, 284* (11), 1406–1410.

37. American Cancer Society (1997). *Cancer Facts and Figures,* 5008. Atlanta.

38. Hollenbach, K. A., et al. (1993). Cigarette smoking and bone mineral density in older men and women. *Am J Public Health, 83,* 1265–1270.

39. Berenson, G. S., et al. (1998). Association between multiple cardiovascular risk factors and atherosclerosis in children and young adults. *NEJM, 338,* 1650–1656.

40. Mann, D. (May 2, 1996). Job stress can cause fatal MI. *Medical Tribune, Primary Care Edition,* 21; Suadicani, P., Hein, H. O., & Gyntelberg, F. (1993). Are social inequalities as associated with the risk of ischaemic heart disease a result of psychosocial working conditions? *Atherosclerosis, 101* (2), 165–175; Legault, S. E., et al. (1995). Pathophysiology and time course of silent myocardial ischemia during mental stress: Clinical, anatomical, and physiological correlates. *British Heart J, 73,* 242–249; Kaplan, G. A., & Keil, J. E. (1993). Socioeconomic factors and cardiovascular disease: A review of the literature. *Circulation, 88,* 1973–1998.

41. Castelli, W. P. (1988). Cardiovascular disease in women. *Am J Obstetrics & Gynecology, 158* (6), 1553–1560, 1566–1567; Lacroix, A. Z. (1994). Psychosocial factors in risk of coronary heart disease in women: An epidemiologic perspective. *Fertility-Sterility, 62* (suppl. 2), 133S–139S; Mahoney, L. T., et al. (1996). Coronary risk factors measured in childhood and young adult life are associated with coronary artery calcification in young adults: The Muscatine Study. *J Am Coll Cardiol, 27* (2), 277–284; Schaefer, E. J., et al. (1994). Factors associated with low and

elevated plasma HDL cholesterol and apolipoprotein A-I levels in the Framingham Offspring Study. *J Lipid Research, 35* (5), 871–872; Garrison, R. J., et al. (1993). Educational attainment and coronary heart disease risk: The Framingham Offspring Study. *Prevention Medicine, 22* (1), 54–64.

42. Mann, S. J. (1999). *Healing Hypertension: A Revolutionary New Approach* (2). New York: John Wiley.

43. Ferketich, A. K., et al. (2000). Depression as an antecedent to heart disease among women and men in the NHANES I Study. *Arch Intern Med, 160,* 1261–1268.

44. Jeppesen, J. (1997). Effects of low-fat high-carbohydrate diets on risk for ischemic heart disease in postmenopausal women. *Am J Clin Nutr, 65* (4), 1027–1033.

45. Kearney, M. T., et al. (1997). William Heberden revisited: Postprandial angina—interval between food and exercise and meal composition are important determinants of time to onset of ischemia and maximal exercise tolerance. *J Am College of Cardiology, 29* (2), 302–307.

46. Crapo, P. A., et al. (1976). Plasma glucose and insulin responses to orally administered simple and complex carbohydrates. *Diabetes, 25* (9), 741–747; Crapo, P. A. (1977). Postprandial plasma-glucose and -insulin responses to different complex carbohydrates. *Diabetes, 26* (12), 1178–1183.

47. Modan, M., et al. (1985). Hyperinsulinemia: A link between hypertension, obesity and glucose intolerance. *J Clin Invest, 75,* 809–817.

48. Ridker, P. M., et al. (2000). C-reactive protein and other markers of inflammation in the prediction of cardiovascular disease in women. *NEJM, 342* (12), 836–843; Black, H. R. (1990). Coronary artery disease paradox: The role of hyperinsulinemia and insulin resistance and its implications for therapy. *J Cardiovascular Pharmacology, 15* (suppl. 5), 26S–38S; Brindley, D. M., & Rolland, Y. (1989). Possible connections between stress, diabetes, obesity, hypertension, and altered lipoprotein metabolism that may result in arteriosclerosis. *Clinical Science, 77* (5), 453–461; DeFronzo, R., & Ferrannini, E. (1991). Insulin resistance: A multifaceted syndrome responsible for NIDDM, obesity, hypertension, dyslipidemia, and atherosclerotic cardiovascular disease. *Diabetes Care, 14* (3), 173–194; Eades, M., & Eades, M. D. (1996). *Protein Power.* New York: Bantam; Kazer, R. (1995). Insulin resistance, insulin-like growth factor I and breast cancer: A hypothesis. *International J Cancer, 62,* 403–406; Lehninger, A. L. (1993). *Principles of Biochemistry.* New York: Worth; Jeppesen, J. (1997). Op. cit.

49. Tribble, D. L. (1999). AHA science advisory. Antioxidant consumption and risk of coronary heart disease: Emphasis on vitamin C, vitamin E, and beta-carotene: A statement for health care professionals from the American Heart Association. *Circulation, 99* (4), 591–595.

50. Anderson, J. W., et al. (1995). Meta-analysis of the effects of soy protein intake on serum lipids. *NEJM, 333* (5), 276–282.

51. Nelson, G. J., & Chamberlain, J. G. (1995). The effects of dietary alpha-linolenic acid on blood lipids and lipoproteins in humans. In Cunnane,

S. C., & Thompson, L. U. (eds.). *Flaxseed in Human Nutrition*. Champaign, IL: AOCS Press; Nestel, P. J., Pomeroy, S. E., Sasahard, T., et al. (1997). Arterial compliance in obese subjects is improved with dietary plant n-3 fatty acid from flaxseed oil despite increased LDL oxidizability. *Arterioscler Throm Vasc Biol, 17,* 1163–1170.

52. Witteman, J. C., et al. (1994). Reduction of blood pressure with oral magnesium supplementation in women with mild to moderate hypertension. *Am J Clin Nutrition, 60* (1), 129–135.

53. Eisenberg, M. J. (1992). Magnesium deficiency and sudden death. *American Heart Journal, 124,* 2, 544–9; Turlapaty, P. D., & Altura, B. M. Magnesium deficiency produces spasms in coronary arteries: Relationship to etiology of sudden death ischemic heart disease. *Science, 208,* 4440 (April 11, 1980), 198–200; Altura, B. M. (Aug. 1979). Sudden death ischemic heart disease and dietary magnesium intake: Is the target site coronary vascular smooth muscle? *Medical Hypotheses, 5,* 8, 843–8.

54. Altura, B. M., et al. (1991). Cardiovascular risk factors and magensium: Relationships to atherosclerosis, ischemic heart disease, and hypertension. *Magnes Trace Elem, 10,* 182–192; Bostick, R. M. (1999). Relation of Ca+, vitamin D, and dairy food intake to ischemic heart disease mortality among postmenopausal women. *Am J Epidemiol, 149* (2), 151–161; Morrison, H., et al. (1996). Serum folate and risk of fatal coronary heart disease. *JAMA, 275* (24), 1893–1896; Stampfer, M. J., et al. (1993). Vitamin E consumption and the risk of coronary disease in women. *NEJM, 328,* 1444–1449; Yochum, L., et al. (1999). Dietary flavonoid intake and risk of cardiovascular disease in postmenopausal women. *Am J Epidemiol, 149* (10), 943–949; Kushi, L. H., et al. (1996). Dietary antioxidant vitamins and death from coronary heart disease in postmenopausal women. *NEJM, 334,* 1156–1162.

55. Digiesi, V., et al. (1990). Effect of coenzyme Q_{10} on essential hypertension. *Current Therapy Research, 47,* 841–845.

56. Ghirlanda, G., et al. (1993). Evidence of plasma CoQ_{10}-lowering effects by HMG-CoA reductase inhibitors: A double-blind, placebo-controlled study. *J Clinical Pharmacology, 33,* 226–229.

57. Singh, R. B., et al. (1999). Effect of hydrosoluble coenzyme Q_{10} on blood pressures and insulin resistance in hypertensive patients with coronary artery disease. *J Human Hypertension, 13* (3), 203–208.

58. Yamagami, T., et al. (1977). Study of coenzyme Q_{10} in essential hypertension. In K. Folkers & Y. Yamamura (eds.), *Biochemical and Clinical Aspects of Coenzyme Q_{10}, vol. 1* (231–242). Amsterdam: Elsevier.

59. Singh, R. B., et al. (April 2003). Effect of coenzyme Q_{10} on risk of atherosclerosis in patients with recent myocardial infarction. *Mol Cell Biochem, 246* (1–2), 75–82.

60. Sinatra, S. (1998). *The Coenzyme Q_{10} Phenomenon*. Los Angeles: Keats Publishing.

61. Howard, A. N., et al. (1996). Do hydroxycarotenoids prevent coronary heart disease? A comparison between Belfast and Toulouse. *International J Vitamin & Nutritional Research, 66,* 113–118.

62. Stampfer, M. J., et al. (May 20, 1993). Vitamin E consumption and the risk of coronary disease in women. *NEJM, 328* (20), 1444–1449.
63. Stephens, N. G., et al. (1996). Randomized controlled trial of vitamin E in patients with coronary disease. Cambridge Heart Antioxidant Study (CHAOS). *Lancet, 347,* 781–786.
64. Miller, E. R. (Jan. 4, 2005). Meta-analysis: High-dosage vitamin E supplementation may increase all-cause mortality. *Annals of Internal Medicine, 142* (1), 37–46.
65. Bostick, R. M., et al. (Sept. 15, 1993). Reduced risk of colon cancer with high intakes of vitamin E: The Iowa women's health study. *Cancer Research, 53* (18), 4230–4237.
66. Zandi, P. P. (Jan. 2004). Reduced risk of Alzheimer disease in users of antioxidant vitamin supplements: The Cache county study. *Archives of Neurology, 61* (1), 82–88.
67. Lu, M. (May 15, 2005). Prospective study of dietary fat and risk of cataract extraction among US women. *American Journal of Epidemiology, 161* (10), 948–959.
68. Newaz, M. A., & Nawal, N. N. (Nov. 1999). Effect of gamma-tocotrienol on blood pressure, lipid peroxidation and total antioxidant status in spontaneously hypertensive rats (SHR). *Clin Exp Hyperens, 21* (8), 1297–1313; Qureshi, A. A., & Peterson, D. M. (May 2001). The combined effects of novel tocotrienols and lovastatin on lipid metabolism in chickens. *Atherosclerosis, 156* (1), 39–47; Sen, C. K., Khanna, S., Roy, S., and Packer, L. (April 28, 2000). Molecular basis of vitamin E action. Tocotrienol potently inhibits glutamate-induced pp60(c-Src) kinase activation and death of HT4 neuronal cells. *J Biol Chem, 275* (17), 13049–13055; Theriault, A., et al. (July 1999). Tocotrienol: a review of its therapeutic potential. *Clin Biochem, 32* (5), 309–319.
69. Janson, M. (1997). Drug free management of hypertension. *Am J Natural Medicine, 4* (8), 14–17.
70. Gaziano, J. M. (1994). Antioxidant vitamins and coronary artery disease risk. *Am J Medicine, 97* (suppl.), 3S–18S, 3S–21S; Nenseter, M. S., Volden, V., Berg, T., et al. (1995). No effect of beta-carotene supplementation on the susceptibility of low-density lipoprotein to *in vitro* oxidation among hypercholesterolaemic postmenopausal women. *Scan J Clin Lab Invest, 55,* 477–485; Riemersma, R. A., et al. (1991). Risk of angina pectoris and plasma concentrations of vitamin A, E, C, and carotene. *Lancet, 337* (8732), 1–5; Stampfer, M. J., Hennekens, C. H., Manson, J. E., et al. (1993). Vitamin E consumption and the risk of coronary disease in women. *NEJM, 328* (20), 1444–1449; Steinberg, E., et al. (1992). Antioxidants in the prevention of human atherosclerosis. *Circulation, 85* (6), 2238–2343; Street, D. A., Comstock, G. W., Salkeld, R. M., Schuep, W., & Klag, M. J. (1994). Serum antioxidants and myocardial infarction. Are low levels of carotenoids and alpha-tocopherol risk factors for myocardial infarction? *Circulation, 90* (3), 1154–1161.
71. Rimm, E. B. (1998). Folate and vitamin B_6 from diet and supplements in relation to risk of coronary heart disease among women. *JAMA, 279,* 359–364.

72. Leaf, A., et al. (1988). Cardiovascular effect of n-3 fatty acids. *NEJM, 318* (9), 549–557; von Schaky, C., et al. (1999). The effect of dietary omega-3 fatty acids in coronary atherosclerosis: A randomized, double-blind, placebo-controlled trial. *Ann Internal Medicine, 130* (7), 554–562.

73. Hertog, M. G., et al. (1997). Antioxidant flavonols and coronary heart disease. *Lancet, 349* (9053), 699.

74. Jain, A. K., et al. (1993). Can garlic reduce levels of serum lipids? A controlled clinical study. *Am J Medicine, 94,* 632–635; Kleijnen, J., et al. (1989). Garlic, onions, and cardiovascular risk factors: A review of the evidence from human experiments with emphasis on commercially available preparations. *Br J Clin Pharmacol, 28,* 535–544; Mader, F. H. (1990). Treatment of hyperlipidemia with garlic powder tablets. *Arzneim-Forsch, 40,* 1111–1116; McMahon, F. G., & Vargas, R. (1993). Can garlic lower blood pressure? A pilot study. *Pharmacotherapy, 13* (4), 406–407.

75. Berger, J. (1998). *Herbal Rituals* (132–138). New York: St. Martin's Press.

76. Anderson, J. W., Johnstone, B. M., and Cook-Newell, M. E. (Aug. 3, 1995). Meta-analysis of the effects of soy protein intake on serum lipids. *N Engl J Med, 333* (5), 276–282; Zhuo, X. G., Melby, M. K., and Watanabe, S. (Sept. 2004). Soy isoflavone intake lowers serum LDL cholesterol: A meta-analysis of 8 randomized controlled trials in humans. *J Nutr, 134* (9), 2395–2400.

77. Hall, W. L., et al. (Dec. 2005). Soy-isoflavone–enriched foods and inflammatory biomarkers of cardiovascular disease risk in postmenopausal women: Interactions with genotype and equol production. *Am J of Clin Nutr, 82* (6), 1260–1268.

78. Desroches, S., et al. (March 2004). Soy protein favorably affects LDL size independently of isoflavones in hypercholesterolemic men and women. *J Nutr, 134* (3), 574–579; Nagata, C., et al. (March 2003). Soy product intake is inversely associated with serum homocysteine level in premenopausal Japanese women. *J Nutr, 133* (3), 797–800.

79. Anderson, J. J., et. al. (Dec. 1999). Health potential of soy isoflavones for menopausal women. *Public Health Nutr, 2* (4), 489–504.

80. Jenkins, D. J., et. al. (Aug. 2002). Effects of high- and low-isoflavone soyfoods on blood lipids, oxidized LDL, homocysteine, and blood pressure in hyperlipidemic men and women. *Am J Clin Nutr, 76* (2), 365–372.

81. Food & Drug Administration, U.S. Department of Health and Human Services (1999). FDA talk paper: FDA approves new health claim for soy protein and coronary heart disease (T99–48).

82. Anderson, J. W., and Hoie, L. H. (June 2005). Weight loss and lipid changes with low-energy diets: Comparator study of milk-based versus soy-based liquid meal replacement interventions. *J Am Coll Nutr, 24* (3), 210–216.

83. Skrabal, F. (1981). Low sodium/high potassium diet for the prevention of hypertension: Probable mechanisms of action. *Lancet, 2* (8252), 895–900.

84. Alpers, G. W., et al. (1999). Antiplatelet therapy: New foundations for optimal treatment decisions. *Neurology, 53* (7, suppl. 4), 25S–31S; Antiplatelet Trialists' Collaboration (1994). Collaborative overview of randomised trials of antiplatelet therapy—1: Prevention of death, myocardial

infarction, and stroke by prolonged antiplatelet therapy in various categories of patients. *British Medicine J, 308,* 81–106; DeAbago, F. J., et al. (1999). Association between SSRIs and upper GI bleeding. *British Medicine J, 319,* 1106–1109; Easton, J. D., et al. (1999). Antiplatelet therapy: Views from the experts. *Neurology, 53* (7, suppl. 4), 32S–37S; Rong, Y., et al. (1994). Pycnogenol protects vascular endothelial cells from induced oxidant injury. *Biotechnol Therapy, 5* (3–4), 117–126.

85. Ridker, P. M., et al. (March 31, 2005). A randomized trial of low-dose aspirin in the primary prevention of cardiovascular disease in women. *N Engl J Med, 352* (13), 1293–1304.

86. Joshipura, K. J., et al. (Oct. 6, 1999). Fruit and vegetable intake in relation to risk of ischemic stroke. *JAMA, 282* (13), 1233–1239.

87. Osganian, S. K., et al. (June 2003). Dietary carotenoids and risk of coronary artery disease in women. *Am J Clin Nutr, 77* (6), 1390–1399.

88. Duffy, S. J., et al. (July 10, 2001). Short- and long-term black tea consumption reverses endothelial dysfunction in patients with coronary artery disease. *Circulation, 104* (2), 151–156.

89. Keli, S. O., et al. (March 25, 1996). Dietary flavonoids, antioxidant vitamins, and incidence of stroke: The Zutphen study. *Arch Intern Med, 156* (6), 637–642.

90. Quereshi, A. A., & Quereshi, N. (1993). Tocotrienols: Novel hypocholesterolemic agents with antioxidant properties. In Packer, L., and Fuchs, J. (eds.), *Vitamin E in Health and Disease.* New York: Marcel Dekker.

91. Oh, R. (Jan.–Feb. 2005). Practical applications of fish oil (omega-3 fatty acids) in primary care. *J Am Board Fam Pract, 18* (1), 28–36; Mozaffarian, D., et al. (Jan. 24, 2005). Fish consumption and stroke risk in elderly individuals: the cardiovascular health study. *Arch Intern Med, 165* (2), 200–206; Iso, H., et al. (Jan. 17, 2001). Intake of fish and omega-3 fatty acids and risk of stroke in women. *JAMA, 285* (3), 304–312.

92. Hambrecht, R., et al. (2000). Effect of exercise on coronary endothelial function in patients with coronary artery disease. *NEJM, 342,* 454–460; Goldman, E., (Nov. 1, 1999). Exercise equals estrogen for lowering heart risk. *Internal Medicine News, 16.*

93. Belardinelli, R., et al. (1998). Effects of moderate exercise training on thallium uptake and contractile response to low-dose dobutamine of dysfunctional myocardium in patients with ischemic cardiomyopathy. *Circulation, 97,* 553–561.

94. Lemole, J. (Feb. 1999). Personal interview for *Health Wisdom for Women.*

95. Herrington, D., et al. (2000). Effects of estrogen replacement on the progression of coronary artery atherosclerosis. *NEJM, 343,* 522–529; Hulley, S., et al., for the Heart and Estrogen/Progestin Replacement Study (HERS) Research Group (1998). Randomized trial of estrogen plus progestin for secondary prevention of coronary heart disease in postmenopausal women. *JAMA, 280,* 605–613; No authors listed (March 13, 2000). Estrogen replacement and atherosclerosis (ERA). Presented at the 49th annual meeting of the American College of Cardiology, Anaheim, CA.

96. Grodstein, F., Manson, J. E., & Stampfer, M. J. (Jan./Feb. 2006). Hormone

therapy and coronary heart disease: the role of time since menopause and age at hormone initiation. *J Womens Health (Larchmt), 15* (1), 35–44.

97. Koh, K. K., Mincemoyer, R., Bui, M. N., et al. (1997). Effects of hormone replacement therapy on fibrinolysis in postmenopausal women. *NEJM, 336,* 683–690; Nasr, A., & Breckwoldt, M. (1998). Estrogen replacement therapy and cardiovascular protection: Lipid mechanisms are the tip of an iceberg. *Gynecol Endocrinol, 12,* 43–59; Oparil, S. (1999). Arthur C. Corcoran Memorial Lecture: Hormones and vasoprotection. *Hypertension, 33,* 170–176; Pines, A., Mijatovic, V., van der Mooren, M. J., et al. (1997). Hormone replacement therapy and cardioprotection: Basic concepts and clinical considerations. *Eur J Gynecol Reprod Biol, 71,* 193–197; van der Mooren, M. J., Mijatovic, V., & van Baal, W. M. (1998). Hormone replacement therapy in postmenopausal women with specific risk factors for coronary artery disease. *Maturitas, 30,* 27–36; Rosano, G. (1996). 17-ß-estradiol therapy lessens angina in postmenopausal women with syndrome X. *J Am Coll Cardiol, 28,* 1500–1505.

98. Clarkson, T. B., & Anthony, M. S. (1997). Effects on the cardiovascular system: Basic aspects. In Lindsay, R., Dempster, D. W., & Jordan, V. C. (eds.). *Estrogens and Antiestrogens* (89–118). Philadelphia: Lippincott-Raven; Gerhard, M., & Ganz, P. (1995). How do we explain the clinical benefits of estrogen? From bedside to bench. *Circulation, 92,* 5–8; Reis, S. E., Gloth, S. T., Blumenthal, R. S., et al. (1994). Ethinyl estradiol acutely attenuates abnormal coronary vasomotor responses to acetylcholine in postmenopausal women. *Circulation, 89* (1), 52–60; Sullivan, J. M. (1996). Hormone replacement therapy in cardiovascular disease: The human model. *British J Obstet Gynaecol, 103* (suppl. 13), 50S–67S.

99. Darling, G. M., Johns, J. A., McCloud, P. L., et al. (1997). Estrogen and progestin compared with simvastatin for hypercholesterolemia in postmenopausal women. *NEJM, 337,* 595–601; Davidson, M. H., Testolin, L. M., Maki, K. C., et al. (1997). A comparison of estrogen replacement, pravastatin, and combined treatment for the management of hypercholesterolemia in postmenopausal women. *Arch Intern Med, 157,* 1186–1192; Koh, K. K., Cardillo, C., Bui, M. N., et al. (1997). Vascular effects of estrogen and cholesterol-lowering therapies in hypercholesterolemic postmenopausal women. *Circulation, 99,* 354–360.

100. Fitzgerald, F. T. (1986). The therapeutic value of pets. *Western J Medicine, 144,* 103–105.

101. Ibid.

102. Friedmann, E., Katcher, A., Lunch, J. J., & Thomas, S. A. (1980). Animal companions and the one-year survival of patients after discharge from a coronary care unit. *Public Health Reports, 95,* 307–312.

103. Beck, A., & Katcher, A. (1983). *Between Pets and People: The Importance of Animal Companionship.* New York: Putnam; Katcher, A., & Beck, A. (1983). *New Perspectives on Our Lives with Companion Animals.* Philadelphia: University of Pennsylvania Press.

Index

About the Author

Christiane Northrup, M.D., trained at Dartmouth Medical School and Tufts New England Medical Center. She is a board-certified obstetrician/gynecologist with more than twenty years of clinical and medical teaching experience. As past president of the American Holistic Medical Association, and past Clinical Assistant Professor of Obstetrics and Gynecology through the University of Vermont College of Medicine's program at Maine Medical Center, she appreciates the need for a partnership between the best of conventional and complementary medicine. Dr. Northrup is the author of the *New York Times* best-selling book *Women's Bodies, Women's Wisdom* and *Mother-Daughter Wisdom*—a Quill Award nominee in 2005. She is the editor of the monthly e-letter *Women's Health Wisdom* and the *Dr. Christiane Northrup* bimonthly newsletter. She has hosted five successful public television specials and her work has been featured on *The Oprah Winfrey Show, The Today Show, Nightly News with Tom Brokaw, The View,* and *Good Morning America*. She lives in Maine.